T0217951

Lecture Notes
in Business Information Processing   **468**

Series Editors

Wil van der Aalst⬭, *RWTH Aachen University, Aachen, Germany*
Sudha Ram⬭, *University of Arizona, Tucson, AZ, USA*
Michael Rosemann⬭, *Queensland University of Technology, Brisbane, QLD, Australia*
Clemens Szyperski, *Microsoft Research, Redmond, WA, USA*
Giancarlo Guizzardi⬭, *University of Twente, Enschede, The Netherlands*

LNBIP reports state-of-the-art results in areas related to business information systems and industrial application software development – timely, at a high level, and in both printed and electronic form.

The type of material published includes

- Proceedings (published in time for the respective event)
- Postproceedings (consisting of thoroughly revised and/or extended final papers)
- Other edited monographs (such as, for example, project reports or invited volumes)
- Tutorials (coherently integrated collections of lectures given at advanced courses, seminars, schools, etc.)
- Award-winning or exceptional theses

LNBIP is abstracted/indexed in DBLP, EI and Scopus. LNBIP volumes are also submitted for the inclusion in ISI Proceedings.

Marco Montali · Arik Senderovich ·
Matthias Weidlich
Editors

Process Mining Workshops

ICPM 2022 International Workshops
Bozen-Bolzano, Italy, October 23–28, 2022
Revised Selected Papers

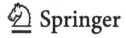 Springer

Editors
Marco Montali
Free University of Bozen-Bolzano
Bozen-Bolzano, Italy

Arik Senderovich
York University
Toronto, ON, Canada

Matthias Weidlich
Humboldt-Universität zu Berlin
Berlin, Germany

ISSN 1865-1348   ISSN 1865-1356 (electronic)
Lecture Notes in Business Information Processing
ISBN 978-3-031-27814-3   ISBN 978-3-031-27815-0 (eBook)
https://doi.org/10.1007/978-3-031-27815-0

This Springer imprint is published by the registered company Springer Nature Switzerland AG
The registered company address is: Gewerbestrasse 11, 6330 Cham, Switzerland

Preface

The International Conference on Process Mining (ICPM) was established three years ago as the conference where people from academia and industry could meet and discuss the latest developments in the area of process mining research and practice, including theory, algorithmic challenges, and applications. Although the ICPM conference series is very young, it has attracted innovative research of high quality from top scholars and industrial researchers.

This year the conference took place in Bolzano, Italy and included co-located workshops that were held on October 24, 2022. The workshops presented a wide range of outstanding research ideas and excellent paper presentations. In addition, the resulting workshop programs were complemented with keynotes, round-table panels, and poster sessions, providing a lively discussion forum for the entire community. ICPM 2022 featured eight workshops, each focusing on particular aspects of process mining, either a particular technical aspect or a particular application domain:

- 3rd International Workshop on Event Data and Behavioral Analytics (EDBA)
- 3rd International Workshop on Leveraging Machine Learning in Process Mining (ML4PM)
- 3rd International Workshop on Responsible Process Mining (RPM) (previously known as Trust, Privacy and Security Aspects in Process Analytics)
- 5th International Workshop on Process-Oriented Data Science for Healthcare (PODS4H)
- 3rd International Workshop on Streaming Analytics for Process Mining (SA4PM)
- 7th International Workshop on Process Querying, Manipulation, and Intelligence (PQMI)
- 1st International Workshop on Education Meets Process Mining (EduPM)
- 1st International Workshop on Data Quality and Transformation in Process Mining (DQT-PM)

The proceedings present and summarize the work that was discussed during the workshops. In total, the ICPM 2022 workshops received 89 submissions, of which 42 papers were accepted for publication, leading to a total acceptance rate of about 47%. Supported by ICPM, each workshop also conferred a best workshop paper award. Finally, it is worth mentioning that to promote open-research, ICPM proudly offered to publish the proceedings as open-access.

We would like to thank all the people from the ICPM community, who helped to make the ICPM 2022 workshops a success. We particularly thank the entire organization committee for delivering such an outstanding conference. We are also grateful to the workshop organizers, the numerous reviewers, and, of course, the authors for their contributions to the ICPM 2022 workshops.

November 2022

Marco Montali
Arik Senderovich
Matthias Weidlich

Contents

5th International Workshop on Process-Oriented Data Science for Healthcare (PODS4H'22)

1st International Workshop on Education Meets Process Mining (EduPM'22)

3rd International Workshop on Event Data and Behavioral Analytics (EdbA'22)

Third International Workshop on Event Data and Behavioral Analytics (EdbA'22)

In recent decades, capturing, storing, and analyzing event data has gained attention in various domains such as process mining, clickstream analytics, IoT analytics, e-commerce, and retail analytics, online gaming analytics, security analytics, website traffic analytics, and preventive maintenance, to name a few. The interest in event data lies in its analytical potential as it captures the dynamic behavior of people, objects, and systems at a fine-grained level.

Behavior often involves multiple entities, objects, and actors to which events can be correlated in various ways. In these situations, a unique, straightforward process notion does not exist, is unclear or different processes or dynamics could be recorded in the same data set.

The objective of the Event Data & Behavioral Analytics (EdbA) workshop series is to provide a forum to practitioners and researchers for studying a quintessential, minimal notion of events as the common denominator for records of discrete behavior in all its forms. The workshop aims to stimulate the development of new techniques, algorithms, and data structures for recording, storing, managing, processing, analyzing, and visualizing event data in various forms. To this end, different types of submissions are welcome such as original research papers, case study reports, position papers, idea papers, challenge papers, and work in progress papers on event data and behavioral analytics.

The third edition of the EdbA workshop attracted 15 submissions. After careful multiple reviews by the workshop's program committee members, seven were accepted for a full-paper presentation at the workshop. All full-paper papers have been included in the proceedings. This year's papers again cover a broad spectrum of topics, which can be organized into three main themes: human behavior and IoT, detecting anomalies and deviations, and event data beyond control-flow.

In the final plenary discussion session, the workshop's participants had a very fruitful discussion about several topics including (i) the possibility to build general approaches to event abstraction instead of domain-dependent ones, (ii) the goals of event abstraction, (iii) the usefulness of offline process mining, (iv) data awareness and decision points in human processes, and (v) guidelines for object-centric logs.

The organizers wish to thank all the people who submitted papers to the EdbA'22 workshop, the many participants creating fruitful discussion and sharing insights and the EdbA'22 Program Committee members for their valuable work in reviewing the submissions. A final word of thanks goes out to the organizers of ICPM 2022 for making this workshop possible.

November 2022

Benoît Depaire
Dirk Fahland
Francesco Leotta
Xixi Lu

Organization

Workshop Chairs

Benoît Depaire	Hasselt University, Belgium
Dirk Fahland	Eindhoven University of Technology, The Netherlands
Francesco Leotta	Sapienza University of Rome, Italy
Xixi Lu	University of Utrecht, The Netherlands

Program Committee

Massimiliano de Leoni	University of Padua, Italy
Jochen De Weerdt	Katholieke Universiteit Leuven, Belgium
Claudio Di Ciccio	Sapienza University of Rome, Italy
Chiara Di Francescomarino	University of Trento, Italy
Bettina Fazzinga	University of Calabria, Italy
Marwan Hassani	Eindhoven University of Technology, The Netherlands
Gert Janssenswillen	Hasselt University, Belgium
Felix Mannhardt	Eindhoven University of Technology, The Netherlands
Niels Martin	Hasselt University, Belgium
Jan Mendling	Humboldt-Universität zu Berlin, Germany
Marco Montali	Free University of Bozen-Bolzano, Italy
Marco Pegoraro	RWTH Aachen University, Germany
Stef van den Elzen	Eindhoven University of Technology, The Netherlands
Greg Van Houdt	Hasselt University, Belgium

Do You Behave Always the Same?
A Process Mining Approach

Gemma Di Federico[✉] and Andrea Burattin

Technical University of Denmark, Kgs. Lyngby, Denmark
`gdfe@dtu.dk`

Abstract. Human behavior could be represented in the form of a process. Existing process modeling notations, however, are not able to faithfully represent these very flexible and unstructured processes. Additional non-process aware perspectives should be considered in the representation. Control-flow and data dimensions should be combined to build a robust model which can be used for analysis purposes. The work in this paper proposes a new hybrid model in which these dimensions are combined. An enriched conformance checking approach is described, based on the alignment of imperative and declarative process models, which also supports data dimensions from a statistical viewpoint.

1 Introduction

A process is a series of activities that are executed with the aim of achieving a specific goal. The notion of process can be used to describe most of the behaviors we adopt in our daily life. Whenever we deal with an ordered series of activities, that are performed repetitively, we can leverage the notion of *process* [10]. A process model is a formalization of a process, it abstracts activities and dependencies in a conceptual model. A process modeling language offers the set of rules and structural components to represent a process in form of a model. An example of a process is the procedure to get medications from a prescription, as well as the process that a person follows in order to get ready for work in the morning. In the former example, the procedure is strict and follows a well-defined and ordered set of activities; in the latter example, the process is flexible and can vary based on daily preferences, meaning that the process does not necessarily enforce a static structure. To some extent, existing process modeling languages are able to represent processes related to human behavior, however, several important aspects cannot be expressed by those languages. Dealing with human processes is challenging [8] since human beings are not forced to follow a strict procedure while executing activities, which results in high variability of the process, and the model. What is more, human behavior can be influenced by external factors, such as the environment. Modeling languages have structural limitations which restrict the expressiveness of the models they can represent. Among these is the fact that a process model primarily focuses on the control flow perspective. Consider a process executed in an environment with a temperature of 18°,

© The Author(s) 2023
M. Montali et al. (Eds.): ICPM 2022, LNBIP 468, pp. 5–17, 2023.
https://doi.org/10.1007/978-3-031-27815-0_1

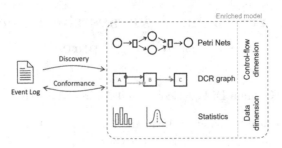

Fig. 1. Approach overview

in which a person is drinking 5 glasses of water per day. If the ambient temperature rises, the frequency of the activity "drinking" is expected to increase as well. Let's now consider a new instance of the same process, in which a person is drinking 5 glasses of water but the temperature is 32°. Just considering a control-flow perspective, the two instances are perfectly compliant. However, combining the drinking activity with both its frequency and the environment temperature, leads to a more detailed representation of the behavior. Additionally, most of the imperative languages only allow the design of uncountable loops, while this aspect could be relevant when representing human behavior. Declarative languages only specify the workflow through the use of constraints, i.e., only the essential characteristics are described. Hence, the model over-generalizes the process, often allowing too many different behaviors. As process models are conceptual models, they actually are abstractions of reality, focusing only on the aspects that are deemed relevant. The reality can be captured by observing the actual process, resulting in a set of events collected in an event log. When trying to workshops establish a relation between a process model and the reality, in which both refer to the same process execution, it can be easily noted how far from each other they can be. Even if numerous process modeling languages exist, the control-flow and the constraints discovery (both referring to imperative and declarative processes) are not always sufficient to capture all the characteristics of some kind of process. Other dimensions must be considered and included in the analysis. Among the tasks investigated in Process Mining [6], *conformance checking* [4] assumes process models to be *prescriptive* (a.k.a. *normative*) and thus it tries to establish the extent to which executions are compliant with the reference model. Therefore, if conformance checking tasks are needed, the model should be as robust and realistic as possible.

The work presented in this paper aims at improving conformance checking techniques by extending them in such a way that the control-flow is used alongside other dimensions. As depicted in Fig. 1, we suggest a hybrid approach in which process and data dimensions are combined, and we implement an enriched conformance checking approach based on the alignment of imperative and declarative process models, which also supports data dimensions form a statistical viewpoint.

The paper is structured as follows. Section 2 presents related work and motivate the paper. In Sect. 3 the solution is presented. Evaluated and discussion is in Sect. 4. Section 5 concludes the paper and presents future work.

2   Background

2.1   State of the Art

The difference between a business process and a human-related process lies in the rigidity of the structure: human processes can be extremely flexible, involving additional perspectives [8] on top of the control-flow.

Although it is possible to define the set of activities that compose human behavior, we cannot define (or restrict) with certainty their order of execution. The reason is that activities are typically combined based on the specific cases, i.e. they are heavily case-dependent [18], and the behavior changes according to known or unknown factors, in a conscious or unconscious way [13]. Even though they share many characteristics with knowledge intensive processes [7], they have a lower degree of uncertainty. Traditional process modeling languages manifest significant limitations when applied to such unstructured processes, usually resulting in describing all possible variants [9] in form of complex and chaotic process models. A process model representing human behavior must abstract the underlying process, allowing for variability, but without over-generalizing.

In order to combine rigid and flexible parts of the models, and thus take advantage of both imperative and declarative process modeling languages [16], hybrid approaches have emerged. Hybrid models combine several process dimensions to improve the understandability of a process model and to provide a clearer semantic of the model itself. According to Andaloussi et al. [2] three process artifacts are usually combined in hybrid approaches, and are static, dynamic or interactive artifacts. Schunselaar et al. [17] propose a hybrid language which combines imperative and declarative constructs. The approach firstly derives an imperative process model (a process tree) and then the less structured parts are replaced with declarative models to improve the overall model precision. López et al., in [12], combine texts with the Dynamic Condition Response (DCR) language. The declarative model is discovered directly from text, and then a dynamic mapping between model components and text is provided. The approach aims to improve the understandability of declarative models. An interactive artifact is proposed in [14] where authors combine the static representation of a process model (DCR graph) and its execution through a simulation. The work presents a tool in which the user can interact directly with the process model. Hybrid approaches focus on the combination of a graphical representation of the process model, together with either another static component (e.g. a process model in a different notation, alongside or hierarchically integrated) or a dynamic or interactive artifact such as a simulation. Although they improve the representation of a process model, the control-flow only is not expressive enough.

Felli et al. [11] recognized the importance of enriching a process model with other perspectives, by proposing a framework to compute conformance metrics and data-aware alignments using Data Petri Nets. However, they consider, in a combined way, the control-flow and the data that the process manipulates, without considering non-process aware perspectives. In the work presented in this paper, the data dimension refers to all those attributes of the activities that are not directly captured by process discovery algorithms, hence not represented in a process model. Without considering these additional perspectives, a process model would be too general, always leading to a successful alignment between the model and new process instances. As a result, if a new process instance varies in activities frequency or duration, it will always fit the model. In this respect, conformance checking fails in its principle.

2.2   Problem Description

Behaviour modelling is a demanding task [8]. In view of the fact that human beings have their own minds and their own interests, their behavior cannot be entirely defined *ex-ante*. There are logical reasons behind the execution of an ordered series of activities, but the way in which these activities are coordinated is not necessarily a single and unique pattern. This makes the control-flow of behaviors highly *variable*. Additionally, a considerable part of human behavior is composed of *repeatable activities*. Human beings perform a *semi-defined* set of activities every day, but part of it is repeated several times throughout the day [3]. Whenever an activity is executed, it may be part of a different set of circumstances, a.k.a. *context*.

Moreover, the *duration* of the activities is also a key factor that allows us to distinguish situations. An activity, based on its duration, can have different meanings. E.g. the *sleeping* activity executed for 8 h can be interpreted differently from the same activity executed only for 2 h. Both scenarios are represented by the

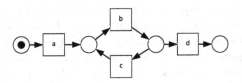

Fig. 2. WF-net derived from $L = [\langle a, b, c, b, d \rangle^2, \langle a, b, c, b, c, b, d \rangle^{10}]$

same process model, but the duration is not directly captured and encoded in the model. As a consequence, the two situations cannot be distinguished. This case can be observed in Fig. 2, in which a simple WF-Net is derived from the traces in L. From the model we cannot distinguish whether activity a was performed for one minute or for one hour. The last aspect we focus on is the *frequency* of activities. As for the duration, the frequency of occurrence of an activity can affect the meaning of the process. Although process modeling languages are capable of representing the repetitions of activities (such as loops), information on the recurrence of the frequency is not included. Loops and repetitions are therefore uncountable. For instance, from the model in Fig. 2 we can't differentiate if the loop between the activities b and c is executed one time or ten times. A trace $t = \langle a, b, c, b, c, b, c, b, c, b, d \rangle$ can perfectly be executed in the model, even though previous examples from the log show only fewer repetitions.

To tackle the above-mentioned issues, we implemented an enriched conformance checking approach, in which we provide information on the process based on different points of view, i.e. control-flow dimensions (both declarative and imperative) along with data dimensions. The work presented in this paper aims to answer the following research question:

RQ: *Does a hybrid process model help in describing human behavior, with the goal of understanding whether such behavior has changed or whether it is consistent with previous observations?*

3   Approach

A process model by itself is not always capable to faithfully capture human behavior. As introduced in the above section, several types of hybrid approaches have been developed, but they all focus only on the process dimension. Especially when dealing with human behavior, typical process representations are not enough. We therefore analyzed human behavior processes and investigated whenever the process representation does not relate to the real process. The conformance checking approach presented in this paper consists of an integrated solution that combines discovery and conformance of both a process and a data dimension. As introduced in Fig. 1, our discovery produces process models as well as a list of statistics for the activities in the event log. The models represent the control-flow perspective, while the statistics the data perspective. In this first version of the approach, the statistics focuses on three data aspects which allow to capture other dimensions of the process, and are the duration of activities, their frequency and the absolute time. The conformance checking produces an enriched fitness value that is based on the verification between each trace in the event log and the enriched discovered model. The enriched fitness value is the composition of the six fitness measures, and it is calculated according to the procedure described in the next subsections. It is important to highlight the importance of the enriched fitness value obtained by the application of the approach presented in this paper. In fact, the value does not refer only to a control-flow perspective, but takes into consideration other dimensions that are not strictly process related.

3.1   Control-Flow and Data Discovery

Control-Flow Representation and Discovery. The main challenge in behavioral modeling is to observe the process from different points of view. The first viewpoint is the control-flow perspective, which can be represented using imperative or declarative languages. Although a declarative language allows to abstract from the problem of variability, as it represents the process in form of constraints, an imperative language has a clearer and more structured representation. The two language categories have different characteristics and, based on the usage, the most appropriate one can be chosen. However, to allow the discovery and the conformance, only languages with a clear execution semantic are considered in the presented approach. The main purpose beyond this paper is that a process model representing human behavior is visually clear and representative of the process. As argued before, imperative and declarative languages have pros and cons in this task. Therefore, to avoid to restrict the final user through a specific representational direction, we decided to include both language families in the proposed approach. In particular, the process discovery includes the *Heuristic* [19] and *Inductive Miner* [15], which produce Petri Nets, and the *DisCoveR* [15] algorithm which produces a DCR Graph.

Data Representation and Discovery. The data dimension focuses on the derivation of relevant statistics under the frequency of activities, their duration, and their occurrence time point of view. As introduced in Sect. 2.2, the *frequency* of activities is a relevant feature to discover repetitions of activities inside the process. To compute the frequency, the occurrence of each unique activity identifier is counted in each trace of the event log. Then, the frequencies are aggregated to the entire event log, and basic statistics are calculated for each activity. The statistics are the mean, the standard deviation, the median, the minimum frequency and the maximum frequency. The values computed enrich the discovered process from a frequency perspective, allowing to have information on the occurrence of each activity identifier.

The second element modelling the data perspective is the *duration*, used to investigate the duration of each activity over time. A different duration in the execution of an activity can completely change the meaning with respect to the process. The duration of the activities is calculated based on the mean duration of each unique activity identifier in each trace. Given an activity identifier, mean, median, min and max duration are calculated for each trace. The values are then aggregated to obtain more accurate results which describe the entire event log.

Always remaining in the time dimension, the *absolute time* when activities happen is another relevant factor in behavioral modeling. Even if conceptually activities are not executed at the same precise time, the absolute time is a powerful tool for identifying delays in the execution of activities. This dimension is treated by considering the histogram of how often each activity has been observed within a certain time interval (e.g., hours of the day).

3.2   Control-Flow and Data Conformance

Once the enriched model is derived, conformance checking algorithms can be used to relate the process model with instance of the process collected in an event log. The conformance checking tries to align both the control-flow and the data perspectives, producing an enriched fitness value as output.

Conformance of the Control-Flow Dimension. The enriched model is represented both in form of Petri Nets and a DCR Graph. According to these languages, the conformance checking algorithms included are the alignment [1] for the Petri Nets, and a rule checker [5] for the DCR Graph. An alignment algorithm establishes a link between a trace in the event log and a valid execution sequence of the process model. For each trace in the event log, a fitness value is obtained. The rule checker verifies if a trace violates the constraints of the graph. For each trace, a fitness value is obtained.

Conformance of the Data. While for the control-flow perspective there are conformance checking techniques available, for the data part it was necessary to investigate the most suitable ways to compare the reference data with the actual instance. For each component of the data dimension, we implement a comparison function. To verify if the frequency statistics in the enriched model conform to the event log, we will assume that activities are normally distributed. The normal distribution is used to show that values close to the mean are more frequent in occurrence than values far from the mean. Assuming that the mean value is our reference value for the frequency, by means of the computed probability density function we can interpret the likelihood that the mean frequency value (for each activity identifier) in the trace, is close to the reference. Then, we consider the likelihood as the fitness value for the frequency dimension. What is more, the frequency value under analysis has to be in the range from the minimum number of occurrences up to the maximum number of occurrences (defined in the model), otherwise a zero fitness value is returned.

The same approach explained for frequencies is used for the duration of activities. Activity durations are assumed to be normally distributed and hence the same strategy is used.

Concerning the absolute time, the approach used in the previous two cases cannot be used, primarily because the absolute time is not cumulative. E.g., we may have the same activity repeated multiple time within the same trace and therefore it might not be possible to aggregate the time of those activities. We decided to use the histogram of the frequencies of each activity over time intervals. To compute the conformance we normalize the frequencies in the interval 0–1 (where 1 indicates the most frequent time interval and 0 the least frequent time interval) and the conformance of new absolute time is then computed as the normalized frequency for the time interval the new absolute time belongs to.

The final fitness value is an aggregation of six values, that are the results of the application of conformance checking algorithms together with the results of the conformance of the statistics. Let's call $\bigoplus$ the aggregation function for the individual measures, the overall conformance becomes:

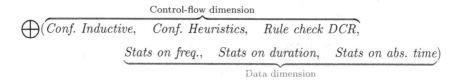

Examples of possible aggregations functions (i.e., $\bigoplus$) could be the (weighted) average, the maximum, and the minimum. The (weighted) average would be useful when all dimensions should be considered, the minimum would be a bit more restrictive as it'd require all measures to be high in order to return a high value itself. The fitness value shows how the discovered hybrid model reflects the behavior in the event log, both under a control-flow and a data dimension. By means of the enriched conformance checking approach presented in this paper, we have a powerful tool to explain and identify variations and discrepancies even under a non-process aware dimension.

4   Evaluation

The approach presented in this work aims to demonstrate that behavioral modeling cannot be represented solely by the control-flow: additional perspectives not referring to the control-flow must be considered. The evaluation conducted is based on trying different scenarios and verifying how the control-flow and the data perspectives respond to the identification of the variations. We identified three different scenarios, and we built (via simulation) a total of 8 synthetic event logs[1], with 1000 traces each. Each scenario contains a "normal" situation (the reference event log) and "anomalous situations" (the event logs used for verifying the conformance). Each scenario aims at identifying the advantages and limitations of both process and data perspectives.

4.1   Scenarios and Logs Description

Scenario 1 (S1) *Description* - The first scenario describes the night routine of a person. The idea is that a person sleeps all night but wakes up between zero and two times to go to the bathroom. *Variations* - The first variation describes a situation in which a person goes to the bathroom very frequently during the night, from four to ten times. In the second variation the person goes to the toilet a normal number of times but stays in the bathroom for a long period of time. *Objective* - The main objective of S1 is to highlight the importance of the data perspective. In fact, the variation is in the frequency and the duration, perspectives that are usually not represented on top of process models.

Scenario 2 (S2) *Description* - The second hypothetical scenario focuses on repetitive activities. The log synthesizes a day where a person eats lunch, leaves the apartment and then comes back for eating dinner, and relaxes on the couch until sleeping time. In a normal scenario, the person has lunch between 11:30 and 13:00, and dinner between 18:00 and 20:00. Both having lunch and having dinner are referred to as the activity of *eating*. *Variations* - Eating lunch or dinner outside the predefined ranges is considered an anomalous behavior. In the first variation, the person has lunch around 14:00 and dinner on time, or has lunch on time and delayed dinner between 21:30 and 23:00. The second variation skips one or both of the meals. *Objective* - The objective of S2 is to verify the behavior of the modeling languages with repetitive activities, both in terms of execution time and actual occurrence. We should be able to identify if a person is skipping meals, or if they are having delayed meals.

Scenario 3 (S3) *Description* - The last scenario describes a hypothetical morning routine: the person wakes up and has breakfast. Right after they go to the bathroom and then get dressed, ready to go out. *Variations* - In the variation the person does not follow the normal control-flow of the activities but mixes the execution of them. The process always starts with waking up but then the get dressed activity can be skipped and executed later. After that, the breakfast, bathroom, and get dressed activities can be executed in any order.

---

[1] All the event logs can be found at https://doi.org/10.5281/zenodo.6632042.

Table 1. Fitness values for control-flow perspective

Scenario		CCHeu	CCInd	CCDCR	Avg
S1 Norm vs	S1 Freq	1.00	1.00	1.00	1.00
	S1 Duration	1.00	1.00	1.00	1.00
S2 Norm vs	S2 Absence	0.75	0.75	0.00	0.50
	S2 Delay	1.00	1.00	1.00	1.00
S3 Norm vs	S3 Shuffle	0.76	0.76	0.00	0.50

Table 2. Fitness values for data perspective

Scenario		CCFreq	CCDur	CCTime	Avg
S1 Norm vs	S1 Freq	0.33	0.52	0.73	0.53
	S1 Duration	0.76	0.46	0.90	0.71
S2 Norm vs	S2 Absence	0.75	0.67	0.90	0.77
	S2 Delay	1.00	0.70	0.48	0.72
S3 Norm vs	S3 Shuffle	1.00	0.67	0.82	0.83

In the end, the person goes out. *Objective* - The purpose of S3 is to focus solely on the control-flow. In this scenario we introduce variability in the execution of activities, starting from a structured and linear situation.

4.2   Log Evaluation

The approach presented in this paper is implemented as Java and Python applications[2]. We constructed a Python script to orchestrate the execution of all algorithms and return a final conformance value. For each scenario, the base event log is used to derive the reference model. Conformance checking is then applied on the reference model together with each variation log. The results are stored in a CSV file. The created logs aim at demonstrating that there are cases in which the control-flow cannot explain the process by itself and cases in which the statistics alone do not give a clear overview of the problem. In particular, scenario S1 focuses entirely on the data perspective, showing how frequency and duration affect the analysis. S3 highlights the importance of the control-flow perspective, while S2 combines both of them with missing activities on one hand and the delay on the other hand.

4.3   Results and Discussion

The results of the application of the approach are presented below. The values obtained are referred as: CCHeu for the alignment between the log and the Petri

---

[2] The implementation can be found at https://doi.org/10.5281/zenodo.6631366.

Table 3. Fitness values for control-flow and data perspective

Scenario		$\oplus$ = min	$\oplus$ = avg
S1 Norm vs	S1 Freq	0.33	0.76
	S1 Duration	0.46	0.85
S2 Norm vs	S2 Absence	0.00	0.64
	S2 Delay	0.48	0.86
S3 Norm vs	S3 Shuffle	0.00	0.67

Net obtained by the Heuristic Miner, CCInd for the Inductive, and CCDCR for the rule checker of DCR. Similarly for the other measures: conformance on the frequency is CCFreq, on duration is CCDur, and on absolute time is CCTime.

To highlight the importance of the two dimensions, the results are firstly presented separately. Table 1 shows the fitness values obtained in each conformance evaluation under a control-flow perspective. Only in two cases the conformance is not perfect, that is the case of S2 Absence and S3 Shuffle. In the first one, since one activity can be skipped, the fitness value for both the Petri Nets is lowered. The fitness of the conformance with the DCR graph is zero because the constraints between *eating* and *leave* activities, and between *eating* and *relax* activities are violated when the execution of the *eating* activity is missing. In the second case instead, the order of the activities is violated. To sum up, perfect fitness values can be observed in 3 cases, while 0.5 is the average for the remaining two cases. The conclusion that can be drawn from this table is that by analyzing the processes only from the control-flow perspective, no anomaly is identified in the form of variation of frequency, duration or absolute time.

Table 2 shows all the fitness values obtained in each conformance evaluation under a data perspective. The conformance between the model from S1 and the log with frequency variation returns a fitness value of 0.33, as expected. Discrepancies also emerge in the same scenario, but in the duration variation, under the duration statistic. A significant divergence between the reference model and the actual data is observed in Scenario S2, in the delay variation, under a time perspective. In fact, the conformance of the absolute time statistic returns a low fitness value, while all the other values are optimal. By computing the average fitness for each scenario/variation, highlights the discrepancies between the data perspective and the control-flow perspective. The average values in Table 2 are much lower then the average values in Table 1.

To obtain more consistent results, all the individual values of conformance must be combined. Table 3 compares the two perspectives together, returning aggregated values in form of average and minimum for each scenario/variation. The table reveals the gap between the fitness of the control-flow dimension and the fitness of the data dimension. In almost all the scenarios, the minimum fitness value obtained (over all the perspectives) is close to zero. The total average in the table is the arithmetic mean. According to the situation at hand, other aggregation functions might also be used (e.g. by using a weighted mean, thus providing different weights for different aspects). In the case of this experiment, none of the logs evaluated returned a perfect fitness value as instead observed in Table 1, where the focus was only on the control-flow.

Based on the results shown in Table 3 we can conclude that, while individual dimensions might show perfect fitness by themselves, even when the logs should not be explainable by the model (cf. both Table 1 and Table 2); a hybrid approach is instead always able to discriminate non-compliant behavior (observable by having no entries with value 1 in Table 3), even when different aggregation functions are used. Therefore, the research question stated in Sect. 2 can be positively answered.

4.4   Limitations

Although the evaluation pointed out promising results, there are several limitations. The first aspect to consider regards the statistics: the statistics on the duration assume a normal probability distribution. Remaining on the perspective of the accuracy of time, the histogram used in the absolute time statistics is calculated by aggregating the executions per hour. Hence, if an activity is delayed but still within the same hour (with respect to the reference model), the fitness is not affected. Finally, choosing a proper aggregation function might not be trivial. In fact, the enriched conformance checking proposed should include a tuning function capable of balancing all the dimensions.

5   Conclusions and Future Work

In order to deal with human behavioral, and in particular, in order to understand whether the behavior is compliant with a normative model, new conformance checking techniques are needed. The control-flow is not enough and it does not provide all information needed for the application of conformance checking techniques when dealing with human behavior. The process must be analyzed from different point of view: the control-flow perspective and the data perspective. The method proposed in this paper produces an enriched fitness value that balances control-flow alignment and data statistics. The control-flow alignments investigates whether the order of the activities is compliant with expectations, whereas the statistics focus on the activity frequency, activity duration, and absolute time. By creating synthetic event logs, we have demonstrated that the application of this methodology allows the identification of variations and discrepancies between a reference model and an event log where the typical conformance techniques were failing. In a previous work (see [8]), we identified all the requirements that a process modeling language must fulfill in order to represent human behavior. These requirements have been used to identify the two perspectives to include in the hybrid model. To reply the research question introduced in Sect. 2.2, taking advantage from the evaluation conducted in this paper, especially from the results in Table 3, it emerged that to properly verify the conformance of a process representing human behavior, a hybrid process model is needed. The first step as a future work, is to refine the statistics, such as the duration, and evaluate other perspectives to be included. After that, we would like to combine the two dimensions together from a semantic point of view.

Acknowledgements. We would like to thank Anton Freyr Arnarsson and Yinggang Mi who helped with the formulation of some of the ideas of this paper.

References

1. van der Aalst, W., Adriansyah, A., van Dongen, B.: Replaying history on process models for conformance checking and performance analysis. Wiley Interdiscip. Rev.: Data Min. Knowl. Discov. **2**(2), 182–192 (2012)
2. Andaloussi, A.A., Burattin, A., Slaats, T., Kindler, E., Weber, B.: On the declarative paradigm in hybrid business process representations: a conceptual framework and a systematic literature study. Inf. Syst. **91**, 101505 (2020)
3. Banovic, N., Buzali, T., Chevalier, F., Mankoff, J., Dey, A.K.: Modeling and understanding human routine behavior. In: Proceedings of the CHI Conference, pp. 248–260 (2016)
4. Carmona, J., van Dongen, B., Solti, A., Weidlich, M.: Conformance Checking. Springer, Cham (2018)
5. Debois, S., Hildebrandt, T.T., Laursen, P.H., Ulrik, K.R.: Declarative process mining for DCR graphs. In: Proceedings of SAC, pp. 759–764 (2017)
6. van Der Aalst, W.: Process Mining: Data Science in Action, 2nd edn. Springer, Heidelberg (2016). https://doi.org/10.1007/978-3-662-49851-4
7. Di Ciccio, C., Marrella, A., Russo, A.: Knowledge-intensive processes: characteristics, requirements and analysis of contemporary approaches. J. Data Semant. **4**(1), 29–57 (2015)
8. Di Federico, G., Burattin, A., Montali, M.: Human behavior as a process model: which language to use? In: Italian Forum on BPM, pp. 18–25. CEUR-WS (2021)
9. Diamantini, C., Genga, L., Potena, D.: Behavioral process mining for unstructured processes. J. Intell. Inf. Syst. **47**(1), 5–32 (2016). https://doi.org/10.1007/s10844-016-0394-7
10. Dumas, M., La Rosa, M., Mendling, J., Reijers, H.A.: Introduction to business process management. In: Fundamentals of Business Process Management, pp. 1–33. Springer, Heidelberg (2018). https://doi.org/10.1007/978-3-662-56509-4_1
11. Felli, P., Gianola, A., Montali, M., Rivkin, A., Winkler, S.: CoCoMoT: conformance checking of multi-perspective processes via SMT. In: Polyvyanyy, A., Wynn, M.T., Van Looy, A., Reichert, M. (eds.) BPM 2021. LNCS, vol. 12875, pp. 217–234. Springer, Cham (2021). https://doi.org/10.1007/978-3-030-85469-0_15
12. López, H.A., Debois, S., Hildebrandt, T.T., Marquard, M.: The process highlighter: from texts to declarative processes and back. In: BPM (Dissertation/Demos/Industry) vol. 2196, pp. 66–70 (2018)
13. Lull, J.J., Bayo, J.L., Shirali, M., Ghassemian, M., Fernandez-Llatas, C.: Interactive process mining in IoT and human behaviour modelling. In: Fernandez-Llatas, C. (ed.) Interactive Process Mining in Healthcare. HI, pp. 217–231. Springer, Cham (2021). https://doi.org/10.1007/978-3-030-53993-1_13
14. Marquard, M., Shahzad, M., Slaats, T.: Web-based modelling and collaborative simulation of declarative processes. In: Motahari-Nezhad, H.R., Recker, J., Weidlich, M. (eds.) BPM 2015. LNCS, vol. 9253, pp. 209–225. Springer, Cham (2015). https://doi.org/10.1007/978-3-319-23063-4_15

15. Nekrasaite, V., Parli, A.T., Back, C.O., Slaats, T.: Discovering responsibilities with dynamic condition response graphs. In: Giorgini, P., Weber, B. (eds.) CAiSE 2019. LNCS, vol. 11483, pp. 595–610. Springer, Cham (2019). https://doi.org/10.1007/978-3-030-21290-2_37

16. Pichler, P., Weber, B., Zugal, S., Pinggera, J., Mendling, J., Reijers, H.A.: Imperative versus declarative process modeling languages: an empirical investigation. In: Daniel, F., Barkaoui, K., Dustdar, S. (eds.) BPM 2011. LNBIP, vol. 99, pp. 383–394. Springer, Heidelberg (2012). https://doi.org/10.1007/978-3-642-28108-2_37

17. Schunselaar, D.M.M., Slaats, T., Maggi, F.M., Reijers, H.A., van der Aalst, W.M.P.: Mining hybrid business process models: a quest for better precision. In: Abramowicz, W., Paschke, A. (eds.) BIS 2018. LNBIP, vol. 320, pp. 190–205. Springer, Cham (2018). https://doi.org/10.1007/978-3-319-93931-5_14

18. Stefanini, A., Aloini, D., Benevento, E., Dulmin, R., Mininno, V.: A process mining methodology for modeling unstructured processes. Knowl. Process. Manag. **27**(4), 294–310 (2020)

19. Weijters, A., van Der Aalst, W.M., De Medeiros, A.A.: Process mining with the heuristics miner-algorithm. TU/e, Technical report WP 166 (2017), 1–34 (2006)

Enhancing Data-Awareness of Object-Centric Event Logs

Alexandre Goossens[1]([⊠])(iD), Johannes De Smedt[1](iD), Jan Vanthienen[1](iD), and Wil M. P. van der Aalst[2](iD)

[1] Leuven Institute for Research on Information Systems (LIRIS), KU Leuven, Leuven, Belgium
{alexandre.goossens,johannes.smedt,jan.vanthienen}@kuleuven.be
[2] Process and Data Science (PADS) Chair, RWTH Aachen University, Aachen, Germany
wvdaalst@pads.rwth-aachen.de

Abstract. When multiple objects are involved in a process, there is an opportunity for processes to be discovered from different angles with new information that previously might not have been analyzed from a single object point of view. This does require that all the information of event/object attributes and their values are stored within logs including attributes that have a list of values or attributes with values that change over time. It also requires that attributes can unambiguously be linked to an object, an event or both. As such, object-centric event logs are an interesting development in process mining as they support the presence of multiple types of objects. First, this paper shows that the current object-centric event log formats do not support the aforementioned aspects to their full potential since the possibility to support dynamic object attributes (attributes with changing values) is not supported by existing formats. Next, this paper introduces a novel enriched object-centric event log format tackling the aforementioned issues alongside an algorithm that automatically translates XES logs to this Data-aware OCEL (DOCEL) format.

Keywords: Object-centric event logs · Process mining · Decision mining

1 Introduction

In the last few years, object-centric event logs have been proposed as the next step forward in event log representation. The drive behind this is the fact that the eXtensible Event Stream (XES) standard [15] with a single case notion does not allow capturing reality adequately [14]. A more realistic assumption instead is to view a process as a sequence of events that interact with several objects. Several

This work was supported by the Fund for Scientific Research Flanders (project G079519N) and KU Leuven Internal Funds (project C14/19/082).

M. Montali et al. (Eds.): ICPM 2022 Workshops, LNBIP 468, pp. 18–30, 2023.
https://doi.org/10.1007/978-3-031-27815-0_2

object-centric event log representations have been proposed such as eXtensible Object-Centric (XOC) event logs [18], Object-Centric Behavioral Constraint model (OCBC) [4], and most recently Object-Centric Event Logs (OCEL) [14]. The first two event log representations face scalability issues related to the storage of an object model with each event or to the duplication of attributes [14]. However, there is a difficult trade-off to be made between expressiveness and simplicity, leaving the recent OCEL proposal as the most suitable for object-centric process mining as it strikes a good balance between storing objects, attributes and their relationships and yet keeping everything simple.

OCEL offers interesting new research opportunities not only for process mining with, e.g., object-centric Petri nets [1] or object-centric predictive analysis [11], but also for decision mining [16]. OCEL is already well on its way to become an established standard with a visualization tool [12], log sampling and filtering techniques [5], its own fitness and precision notions [2], its own clustering technique [13], an approach to define cases and variants in object-centric event logs [3] and a method to extract OCEL logs from relational databases [23]. In this paper, attributes are considered to be logged together with events and objects in an event log and should relate clearly to their respective concepts, i.e., events, objects or both. As such, OCEL could provide more analysis opportunities by supporting attributes having several values simultaneously, allowing attributes to change values over time and to unambiguously link attributes to objects, all of which is currently not fully supported but common in object-centric models such as structural conceptual models like the Unified Modeling Language (UML) [20].

For this purpose, this paper proposes an extension to OCEL called, Data-aware OCEL or DOCEL, which allows for such dynamic object attributes. The findings are illustrated through a widely-used running example for object-centric processes indicating how this standard can also support the further development of object-centric decision/process mining and other domains such as Internet of Things (IoT) related business processes. This paper also presents an algorithm to convert XES logs to DOCEL logs. Since many event logs are available in a "flat" XES format for every object involved in the process, not all information can be found in one event log. As such, providing an algorithm that merges these XES files into one DOCEL log would centralize all the information in one event log without compromising on the data flow aspects that make XES such an interesting event log format.

The structure of this paper is as follows: Sect. 2 explains the problem together with a running example applied on the standard OCEL form. Section 3 introduces the proposed DOCEL format together with an algorithm to automatically convert XES log files into this novel DOCEL format. Next, the limitations and future work of this work are discussed in Sect. 4. Finally, Sect. 5 concludes this paper.

2 Motivation

The IEEE Task Force conducted a survey during the 2.0 XES workshop[1] concluding that complex data structures, especially one-to-many or many-to-many object relationships, form a challenge for practitioners when pre-processing event logs. By including multiple objects with their own attributes, object-centric event logs have the opportunity to address these challenges. This does entail that the correct attributes must be unambiguously linked to the correct object and/or activity to correctly discover the process of each object type as well as the relevant decision points [1]. The next subsection discusses the importance object attribute analysis had on single case notion event logs.

2.1 Importance of Object Attributes in Single Case Notion Event Logs

Various single case notion process mining algorithms make use of both event and case attributes, e.g., in [7], a framework is proposed to correlate, predict and cluster dynamic behavior using data-flow attributes. Both types of attributes are used to discover decision points and decision rules within a process in [17]. For predictive process monitoring, the authors of [9] develop a so-called clustering-based predictive process monitoring technique using both event and case data. Case attributes are also used to provide explanations of why a certain case prediction is made within the context of predictive process monitoring [10].

The same challenges apply to decision mining which aims to discover the reasoning and structure of decisions that drive the process based on event logs [22]. In [8], both event and case attributes are used to find attribute value shifts to discover a decision structure conforming to a control flow and in [19], these are used to discover overlapping decision rules in a business process. Lastly, within an IoT context, it has been pointed out that contextualization is not always understood in a similar fashion as process mining does [6]. As such object-centric event logs offer an opportunity for these different views of contextualization to be better captured.

The previous paragraphs show (without aiming to provide an exhaustive overview) that various contributions made use of attributes that could be stored and used in a flexible manner. Unfortunately, as will be illustrated in the next subsections, the aforementioned aspects related to attribute analysis are currently not fully supported in object-centric event logs.

2.2 Running Example

Consider the following adapted example inspired from [8] of a simple order-to-delivery process with three object types: Order, Product, Customer. Figure 1[2] visualizes the process.

---

[1] https://icpmconference.org/2021/events/category/xes-workshop/list/?tribe-bar-date=2021-11-02.

[2] All figures are available in higher resolution using the following <u>link</u>.

A customer places an order with the desired quantity for Product 1,2 or 3.
Next, the order is received and the order is confirmed. This creates the value
attribute of order. Afterwards, the ordered products are collected from the ware-
house. If a product is a fragile product, it is first wrapped with cushioning material
before being added to the package. The process continues and then the shipping
method needs to be determined. This is dependent on the value of the order, on
whether there is a fragile product and on whether the customer has asked for a
refund. If no refund is asked, this finalizes the process. The refund can only be
asked once the customer has received the order and requests a refund. If that is
the case, the order needs to be reshipped back and this finalizes the process.

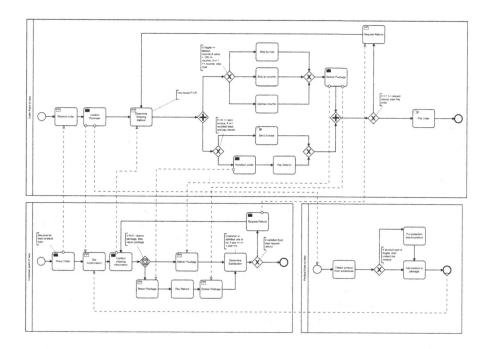

Fig. 1. BPMN model of running example

2.3   OCEL Applied to the Running Example

In this subsection, the standard OCEL representation visualizes a snippet of this
process. Table 1 is an informal OCEL representation of events and Table 2 is an
informal OCEL representation of objects. Figure 2 visualizes the meta-model
of the original OCEL standard. Several **observations** can be made about the
standard OCEL representation:

**A: Attributes that are stored in the events table can not unambigu-
ously be linked to an object.** The OCEL standard makes the assumption

Table 1. Informal representation of the events in an OCEL format

ID	Activity	Timestamp	Customer	Order	Product Type	Q1	Q2	Q3	Refund	Order Value	Resource	Shipping Method
e1	Place Order	09:00	{c1}	{o1}	{p1,p2}	5	2	0	0			
e2	Receive Order	10:00		{o1}							Jan	
e3	Confirm Purchase	11:00		{o1}						95	Jan	
e4	Collect product from warehouse	12:00		{o1}	{p2}						Johannes	
e5	Collect product from warehouse	12:00		{o1}	{p1}						Johannes	
e6	Put protection around the product	12:15		{o1}	{p1}						Johannes	
e7	Add product to package	12:30		{o1}	{p1}						Johannes	
e8	Add product to package	12:30		{o1}	{p2}						Johannes	

Table 2. Informal representation of the objects in an OCEL format

ID	Type	Name	Bank account	Value	Fragile
c1	Customer	Elien	BE24 5248 54879 2659		
o1	Order				
p1	Product			15	1
p2	Product			10	0
p3	Product			20	1

that attributes that are stored in the events table can only be linked to an event. This assumption was taken for its clear choice of simplicity and it holds in this running example, which has straightforward attributes relationships and no changing product values over time. Even though the given example is very obvious regarding how the attributes relate to the objects given the attribute names, this is not always the case. If the value of a product could change over time, the product value attributes would have to be added to the events table but then there would be 4 attributes storing values, i.e., order value, product 1 value, product 2 value and product 3 value. Knowing which attribute is linked to which object would then require domain knowledge as it is not explicitly made clear in the events table. As such, this can be an issue in the future for generic OCEL process discovery or process conformance algorithms since prior to running such an algorithm, the user would have to specify how attributes and objects are related to one another.

B: Based on the OCEL metamodel (Fig. 2), it is unclear whether attributes can only be linked to an event or an object individually or whether an attribute can be linked to both an event and an object simultaneously. Since the OCEL standard did not intend for attribute values to be shared between events and objects by design to keep things compact and clear and since the OCEL UML model (Fig. 2) can not enforce the latter, Object-Constraint Language (OCL) constraints would have made things clearer. Therefore, it might be beneficial to support the possibility *to track an attribute change*, e.g., the *refund* attribute of object *Order* can change from 0 to 1 and back to 0 across the process.

C: Attributes can only contain exactly one value at a time according to the OCEL metamodel (see Fig. 2). This observation entails two aspects. First, it is unclear, based on the metamodel of Fig. 2, whether an attribute can contain a list of values. It is not difficult to imagine situations with a list of values, e.g., customers with multiple bank accounts or emails, products can have more than one color. Currently, OCEL supports multiple values by creating a separate column for each value in the object or event table. This means that each value is treated as a distinct attribute , e.g., in the running example, a customer orders a quantity of product 1, 2 and 3. This can be considered as 1 attribute with 3 values. However, in Table 1, the columns Q1, Q2 and Q3 are considered to be separate attributes even though they could be considered as being from the same overarching attribute Quantity. Secondly, even if an attribute only has 1 value at a time, its value could change over time as well. Such an attribute can be considered to have multiple values at different points in time. If a value were to change, currently, one would have to create a new object for each attribute change. Unfortunately, this only works to some degree since there are no object-to-object references (only through events) in the standard OCEL format. Another possibility would require to unambiguously track the value of an attribute of an object to a certain event that created it. This is also valid within an IoT context with sensors having multiple measurements of the same attributes over time. As such, the first three observations clearly go hand in hand.

D: Both the event and object tables seem to contain a lot of columns that are not always required for each event or object. When looking at the events table, attribute *Order Value* is only filled once with event 'confirm purchase' when it is set for order 1. One could either duplicate this value for all the next events dealing with order 1 or one could simply keep it empty. Therefore, in a big event log with multiple traces one could expect a lot of zero padding or duplication of values across events. Even though this issue is not necessarily present in a storage format, it still shows that ambiguity about attribute relationships might lead to wrongly stored attributes without domain knowledge.

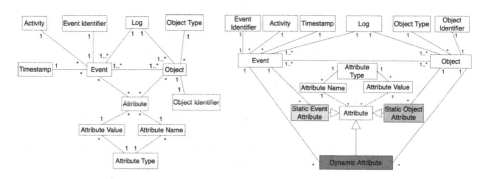

Fig. 2. OCEL UML model from [14]   **Fig. 3.** DOCEL UML model

3   Data-Aware OCEL (DOCEL)

Subsection 3.1 introduces the DOCEL UML metamodel. Next, Subsect. 3.2 applies DOCEL to the running example. Finally, Subsect. 3.3 introduces an algorithm to convert a set of XES files into this DOCEL format.

3.1   DOCEL UML Metamodel

To formally introduce the DOCEL standard, a UML class diagram is modeled (Figure 3). UML diagrams clearly formalize how all concepts relate to one another in OCEL or DOCEL. Based on the observations from Sect. 2.3, the key differences with the UML class diagram of OCEL (Fig. 2) are indicated in color in Fig. 3 to enrich OCEL even further:

> **1: Attribute values can be changed and these changes can be tracked.** By allowing ambiguities, domain knowledge becomes indispensable to make sensible and logical conclusions. In the DOCEL UML model, attributes are considered to be an assignment of a value to an attribute name in a particular context event and/or object. A distinction is made between static and dynamic attributes. Static event attributes and static object attributes are assumed to be linked to an event or an object respectively and only contain fixed value(s). Static attributes are stored in a similar fashion as with the standard OCEL format, namely in the event or the object table, except that now each object type has an individual table to avoid having null values for irrelevant columns. On the other hand, dynamic attributes are assumed to have changing values over time. Dynamic attributes are linked to both an object and an event so that a value change of an attribute can easily be tracked. Another design choice would be to store a timestamp with the attribute value instead of linking it to the event, however, this might lead to ambiguity in case two events happened at the exact same moment. As such, this proposal tackles observation **A**.
>
> **2: Event attributes can unambiguously be linked to an object.** This issue goes hand in hand with the previous proposal and is solved at the same time. By distinguishing between dynamic and static attributes all relations between attributes, events and objects are made clear and ambiguities have been reduced. A static attribute is either linked to an object or an event and its value(s) can not change over time. A dynamic attribute is clearly linked to the relevant object and to the event that updated its value. The DOCEL UML model (Fig. 3) can enforce that a static attribute must be linked with at least 1 event or at least 1 object since a distinction is made between static event attributes and static object attributes. For dynamic attributes, this issue does not apply since it needs to both connected to both an object and an event anyhow. This proposal solves both observations **A & B**.
>
> **3: Attributes can contain a list of values.** Even though not all attributes have a list of values, supporting this certainly reflects the reality that multiple values do occur in organizations. In the DOCEL UML model (Fig. 3) the 1

cardinality for Attribute Value allows both dynamic and static attributes to have complex values, e.g., lists, sets and records containing multiple values. In practice, these values are stored in the relevant attribute tables with a list of values. This proposal solves observation **C**.

3.2 DOCEL Applied to the Running Example

Table 3 is the events table containing all the events together with their **static event attributes** (in green) in this case *Resource*. Complying with the DOCEL UML model, only static event attributes are found in this table which are solely linked to events. The main changes from the OCEL to the DOCEL tables have been highlighted using the same color scheme as in the DOCEL UML model to show where the columns have been moved to in the DOCEL tables.

Table 3. Informal representation of events with static attributes in a DOCEL format

EID	Activity	Timestamp	Customer	Order	Product Type	Resource
e1	Place Order	1/01/22 09:00	{c1}	{o1}	{p1,p2}	
e2	Receive Order	1/01/22 10:00	{c1}	{o1}	{p1,p2}	Jan
e3	Confirm Purchase	1/01/22 11:00		{o1}	{p1,p2}	Jan
e4	Collect product from warehouse	1/01/22 12:00		{o1}	{p2}	Johannes
e5	Collect product from warehouse	1/01/22 12:00		{o1}	{p1}	Johannes
e6	Put protection around the product	1/01/22 12:15		{o1}	{p1}	Johannes
e7	Add product to package	1/01/22 12:30		{o1}	{p1}	Johannes
e8	Add product to package	1/01/22 12:30		{o1}	{p2}	Johannes

Tables 4, 5 and 6 represent object type tables where the objects are stored. Each object is given an object ID. In this data-aware format, aligned with the UML model, a distinction is made between static attributes and dynamic attributes. Static attributes are assumed to be immutable and, therefore, the **static object attributes** (in blue) are stored together with the objects themselves, e.g., *customer name, product value, fragile* and *bank account*. Notice how here, once again, the attributes can be clearly linked to an object. Table 5 only contains primary keys because its attributes are dynamic attributes in this example.

Table 4. Product Type table

Products		
PID	**Value**	**Fragile**
p1	15	1

Table 5. Order table

Orders
OrderID
o1

Table 6. Customer table

Customer		
CID	**Name**	**Bank account**
c1	Elien	BE24 5248 5487 2659

The red Tables 7, 8, 9 and 10 are **dynamic attribute** tables. Dynamic attributes are assumed to be mutable and its values can change over time. Using two foreign keys (event ID and object ID), the attribute and its value can be traced back to the relevant object as well as the event that created it. Each attribute value is given an attribute value ID with the value(s) being stated in the following column. This complies with the proposed UML model in Fig. 3 where dynamic attributes are clearly linked to the relevant event and relevant object.

Table 7. Quantity table

Quantity			
QID	**Quantity**	**EID**	**OID**
q1	{5,2,0}	*e1*	*o1*

Table 8. Order Value table

Order Value			
VID	**Value**	**EID**	**OID**
v1	95	*e3*	*o1*

Table 9. Refund table

Refund			
RID	**Refund Value**	**EID**	**OID**
r1	0	*e1*	*o1*
r2	1	*e15*	*o1*
r3	0	*e24*	*o1*

Table 10. Shipping method table

Shipping method			
SID	**Method**	**EID**	**OID**
s1	courrier	*e11*	*o1*
s2	express courrier	*e18*	*o1*

From the DOCEL log, the following things are observed:

Attributes can unambiguously be linked to an object, to an event or to both an event and an object with the use of foreign keys.

Attributes can have different values over time, with value changes directly tracked in the dynamic attributes tables. This means one knows when the attribute was created and for how long it was valid, e.g., refund was initialized to 0 by event 1, then event 15 set it to 1 and finally event 24 sets it back to 0.

Static and dynamic attributes can contain a list of values in the relevant attributes table, e.g., attribute Quantity.

The amount of information stored has only increased with foreign keys. Previously, the dynamic attributes would have been stored anyhow in the events table with the unfortunate side-effect of not being explicitly linked to the relevant object and with more columns in the events table. This essentially is a normalization of an OCEL data format. Even though it starts resembling a relational database structure, it was decided for this DOCEL format to not include relations between objects. Deciding on whether to include object models within event logs is essentially a difficult trade-off between complexity/scalability and available information within the event log. From this perspective, the design choice of XOC and OCBC was mostly focused on reducing complexity [14], where we aim for an event log format that offers more information in exchange of a slightly increased complexity. As such, the DOCEL standard has decreased the amount of columns per table and thus observation **D** is solved as well.

3.3   Automatically Converting XES Logs to DOCEL Logs

Currently, research is focused on automatically converting XES logs to OCEL logs with a first proposal introduced in [21]. Automatically transforming XES logs or an OCEL log to the proposed DOCEL log would mainly require domain knowledge to correctly link all attributes to the right object, but this is also required for a normal process analysis of an OCEL log. Our algorithm can be found in Algorithm 1. This algorithm takes as input a set of XES files describing the same process and assumes that each XES file describes the process from the point of view of one object type. The main ideas of the algorithm are as follows:

- Line 3 starts the algorithm by looping over all XES-logs.
- Lines 4–8 create the object type tables with all their objects and static object attributes. In line 7, it is assumed that the trace attributes are not changing and solely linked to one object. Since the assumption is made that an XES file only contains one object type, these trace attributes can be considered as static object attributes belonging to that object.
- Lines 10–12 require the user to identify the static event attributes and the other event attributes that can be linked to an object. Next, a new EventID is made to know from which log an event comes from.
- In line 15, the dynamic attributes tables are constructed under the assumption that attributes that have not yet been identified as static object attributes or static event attributes are dynamic attributes.
- Lines 17–18 create the new chronologically ordered events Table E.
- Line 20 matches the events with the relevant objects based on the dynamic attributes tables using the new EventID. It should definitely also include the object related to the original traceID related to that event.
- Finally, lines 21–22 will create the final DOCEL eventIDs and update the eventID across all dynamic attribute tables.

Algorithm 1. Algorithm to go from XES logs to DOCEL logs

```
 1: L ← l                                                          ▷ List of XES logs (l)
 2: OT ← ot                                              ▷ List of present object types
 3: for l ∈ L do
 4:     for ot ∈ (OT ∈ l) do
 5:         Create empty object type table
 6:         for o ∈ ot do                                 ▷ Find all objects of an object type
 7:             Create row with objectID and trace attributes    ▷ Trace attributes = static object attributes
 8:     for e ∈ L do
 9:         Match event attributes to the event or to an object
10:         Create newEventID with log identifier            ▷ To distinguish similar events of different logs
11:     Create event table e_l with static event attributes.
12:     Create dynamic attributes table with valueID, value(s) and two foreign keys {newEventID, objectID}
13: Create empty event table E with a column for every object type.
14: Merge all e_l tables chronologically in E.
15: for e ∈ E do
16:     Find and insert all objects related to e in the relevant object type column
17:     Create unique DOCELeventID
18:     Update all foreign keys of linked dynamic attributes with new DOCELeventID
```

4   Limitations and Future Work

To better store information about attributes, DOCEL comes with a variable number of tables. However, the tables should be smaller as there are fewer columns compared to the standard OCEL format. It is still possible to only use certain attributes or attribute values for analysis by extracting the relevant attributes/values. Instead of selecting a subset of columns with OCEL, the user selects a subset of tables in DOCEL which offer more information. Next, neither OCEL or DOCEL include the specific roles of objects of the same object type in an event, in case of a *Send Message* event from person 1 to person 2, making it currently impossible to distinguish between the sender and the receiver.

To further validate the DOCEL format, the authors are planning to develop a first artificial event log together with a complete formalization of the DOCEL UML with OCL constraints. Furthermore, directly extracting DOCEL logs from SAP is also planned. Regarding the algorithm to automatically convert XES logs to DOCEL logs, the authors are planning to extend the algorithm with a solution to automatically discover which attributes are linked to objects or events. Secondly, an extension to create a DOCEL log based on a single XES file with multiple objects is also planned. DOCEL however offers many other research opportunities such as novel algorithms for object-centric process discovery, conformance checking or enhancements which would further validate or improve the DOCEL format. Also other domains such as IoT-related process mining can be interesting fields to apply DOCEL on.

5   Conclusion

This paper illustrates that the OCEL standard has certain limitations regarding attribute analysis, such as unambiguously linking attributes to both an event and an object or not being able to track attribute value changes. To deal with these challenges, an enhanced Data-aware OCEL (DOCEL) is proposed together with an algorithm to adapt XES logs into the DOCEL log format. With DOCEL, the authors hope that new contributions will also take into account this data-flow perspective not only for object-centric process and decision mining algorithms but also for other domains such as IoT-oriented process analysis.

References

1. van der Aalst, W., Berti, A.: Discovering object-centric Petri nets. Fundam. Inform. **175**(1–4), 1–40 (2020)
2. Adams, J.N., van der Aalst, W.: Precision and fitness in object-centric process mining. In: 2021 3rd International Conference on Process Mining (ICPM), pp. 128–135. IEEE (2021)
3. Adams, J.N., Schuster, D., Schmitz, S., Schuh, G., van der Aalst, W.M.: Defining cases and variants for object-centric event data. arXiv preprint arXiv:2208.03235 (2022)
4. Artale, A., Kovtunova, A., Montali, M., van der Aalst, W.M.P.: Modeling and reasoning over declarative data-aware processes with object-centric behavioral constraints. In: Hildebrandt, T., van Dongen, B.F., Röglinger, M., Mendling, J. (eds.) BPM 2019. LNCS, vol. 11675, pp. 139–156. Springer, Cham (2019). https://doi.org/10.1007/978-3-030-26619-6_11
5. Berti, A.: Filtering and sampling object-centric event logs. arXiv preprint arXiv:2205.01428 (2022)
6. Bertrand, Y., De Weerdt, J., Serral, E.: A bridging model for process mining and IoT. In: Munoz-Gama, J., Lu, X. (eds.) ICPM 2021. LNBIP, vol. 433, pp. 98–110. Springer, Cham (2022). https://doi.org/10.1007/978-3-030-98581-3_8
7. De Leoni, M., van der Aalst, W.M.P., Dees, M.: A general process mining framework for correlating, predicting and clustering dynamic behavior based on event logs. Inf. Syst. **56**, 235–257 (2016)
8. De Smedt, J., Hasić, F., van den Broucke, S.K., Vanthienen, J.: Holistic discovery of decision models from process execution data. Knowl.-Based Syst. **183**, 104866 (2019)
9. Di Francescomarino, C., Dumas, M., Maggi, F.M., Teinemaa, I.: Clustering-based predictive process monitoring. IEEE Trans. Serv. Comput. **12**(6), 896–909 (2016)
10. Galanti, R., Coma-Puig, B., de Leoni, M., Carmona, J., Navarin, N.: Explainable predictive process monitoring. In: 2020 2nd International Conference on Process Mining (ICPM), pp. 1–8. IEEE (2020)
11. Galanti, R., de Leoni, M., Navarin, N., Marazzi, A.: Object-centric process predictive analytics. arXiv preprint arXiv:2203.02801 (2022)
12. Ghahfarokhi, A.F., van der Aalst, W.: A python tool for object-centric process mining comparison. arXiv preprint arXiv:2202.05709 (2022)
13. Ghahfarokhi, A.F., Akoochekian, F., Zandkarimi, F., van der Aalst, W.M.: Clustering object-centric event logs. arXiv preprint arXiv:2207.12764 (2022)
14. Ghahfarokhi, A.F., Park, G., Berti, A., van der Aalst, W.: OCEL standard. Process and Data Science Group, RWTH Aachen University, Technical report 1 (2020)
15. Günther, C.W., Verbeek, H.M.W.: XES standard definition. IEEE Std (2014)
16. Hasić, F., Devadder, L., Dochez, M., Hanot, J., De Smedt, J., Vanthienen, J.: Challenges in refactoring processes to include decision modelling. In: Teniente, E., Weidlich, M. (eds.) BPM 2017. LNBIP, vol. 308, pp. 529–541. Springer, Cham (2018). https://doi.org/10.1007/978-3-319-74030-0_42
17. de Leoni, M., van der Aalst, W.M.P.: Data-aware process mining: discovering decisions in processes using alignments. In: Proceedings of the 28th Annual ACM Symposium on Applied Computing, pp. 1454–1461. ACM (2013)

18. Li, G., de Murillas, E.G.L., de Carvalho, R.M., van der Aalst, W.M.P.: Extracting object-centric event logs to support process mining on databases. In: Mendling, J., Mouratidis, H. (eds.) CAiSE 2018. LNBIP, vol. 317, pp. 182–199. Springer, Cham (2018). https://doi.org/10.1007/978-3-319-92901-9_16
19. Mannhardt, F., de Leoni, M., Reijers, H.A., van der Aalst, W.M.P.: Decision mining revisited - discovering overlapping rules. In: Nurcan, S., Soffer, P., Bajec, M., Eder, J. (eds.) CAiSE 2016. LNCS, vol. 9694, pp. 377–392. Springer, Cham (2016). https://doi.org/10.1007/978-3-319-39696-5_23
20. OMG: Uml: Unified Modeling Language 2.5.1 (2017). https://www.omg.org/spec/UML/2.5.1/About-UML/. Accessed 23 June 2022
21. Rebmann, A., Rehse, J.R., van der Aa, H.: Uncovering object-centric data in classical event logs for the automated transformation from XES to OCEL. In: Business Process Management-20th International Conference, BPM, pp. 11–16 (2022)
22. Vanthienen, J.: Decisions, advice and explanation: an overview and research agenda. In: A Research Agenda for Knowledge Management and Analytics, pp. 149–169. Edward Elgar Publishing (2021)
23. Xiong, J., Xiao, G., Kalayci, T.E., Montali, M., Gu, Z., Calvanese, D.: Extraction of object-centric event logs through virtual knowledge graphs (2022). http://www.inf.unibz.it/~calvanese/papers/xiong-etal-DL-2022.pdf

Multi-perspective Identification of Event Groups for Event Abstraction

Adrian Rebmann[1]([✉]), Peter Pfeiffer[2,3], Peter Fettke[2,3], and Han van der Aa[1]

[1] Data and Web Science Group, University of Mannheim, Mannheim, Germany
{rebmann,han.van.der.aa}@uni-mannheim.de
[2] German Research Center for Artificial Intelligence, Saarbrücken, Germany
{peter.pfeiffer,peter.fettke}@dfki.de
[3] Saarland University, Saarbrücken, Germany

Abstract. In process mining settings, events are often recorded on a low level and cannot be used for meaningful analysis directly. Moreover, the resulting variability in the recorded event sequences leads to complex process models that provide limited insights. To overcome these issues, event abstraction techniques pre-process the event sequences by grouping the recorded low-level events into higher-level activities. However, existing abstraction techniques require elaborate input about high-level activities upfront to achieve acceptable abstraction results. This input is often not available or needs to be constructed, which requires considerable manual effort and domain knowledge. We overcome this by proposing an approach that suggests groups of low-level events for event abstraction. It does not require the user to provide elaborate input upfront, but still allows them to inspect and select groups of events that are related based on their common multi-perspective contexts. To achieve this, our approach learns representations of events that capture their context and automatically identifies and suggests interesting groups of related events. The user can inspect group descriptions and select meaningful groups to abstract the low-level event log.

Keywords: Process mining · Event abstraction · Multi-perspective analysis

1 Introduction

Process mining comprises methods to analyze event data that is recorded during the execution of organizational processes. Specifically, by automatically discovering process models from event logs, process discovery yields insights into how a process is truly executed [1]. Events recorded by information systems are often too fine-granular for meaningful analysis, though, and the resulting variability in the recorded event sequences leads to overly complex models. To overcome this issue, *event abstraction* techniques aim to lift the low-level events recorded in a log to a more abstract representation, by grouping them into high-level activities [17].

Existing techniques for event abstraction (cf., [4,17]) are either *unsupervised* or *supervised*. Unsupervised techniques do not require any input about targeted high-level activities. Instead, they rely on control-flow similarities between low-level event types.

© The Author(s) 2023
M. Montali et al. (Eds.): ICPM 2022 Workshops, LNBIP 468, pp. 31–43, 2023.
https://doi.org/10.1007/978-3-031-27815-0_3

Yet, they do not consider any other dependencies between events, such as the amount of time between their execution. Since the user of such techniques has no control over the abstraction result, there is no guarantee that they yield meaningful high-level activities, making it hard to ensure that an abstraction is appropriate for a specific analysis goal. For instance, if the goal is to understand interactions between employees in a process, grouping events based on control-flow similarity might lead to high-level activities that encompass different employees. This makes it difficult—if not impossible—to analyze interactions in the process. Supervised event abstraction techniques aim to overcome such issues by requiring input about high-level activities upfront, e.g., high-level process models [2] or predefined event patterns [10]. In this manner, such techniques give the user control over high-level activities. However, in practice the required information is often not available beforehand. For instance, when applying event abstraction as a preprocessing step to process discovery, high-level process models are typically not available [17]. Even if knowledge on the desired high-level activities is available, it may require a lot of manual effort to translate it into the necessary input, e.g., by defining how these high-level activities manifest themselves in low-level event patterns [10].

These two extremes, between not giving the user any control over high-level activities and requiring too much input, call for a common middle ground, i.e., a convenient means to support users in their abstraction tasks. In particular, users should be enabled to control the characteristics of high-level activities, while reducing the upfront knowledge they need about the data. This is particularly challenging in situations where the events' labels do not reveal the purpose of the high-level activities they relate to. An *Update record* event, for instance, could relate to any activity that modifies a business object. In such situations it is inevitable to look at the context of events and identify high-level activities in a more indirect manner.

To enable this, we propose an approach that allows the user to inspect groups of events based on their common context, thus, guiding them towards identifying meaningful high-level activities that can be used for abstraction without requiring upfront input about these activities. Our approach learns representations that capture complex contextual dependencies between low-level events, e.g., that events are executed within a short period of time and are performed by the same resource. Based on these representations, it automatically identifies and suggests groups of events. The user can select meaningful groups that can in turn be used to abstract the low-level log.

We motivate the need for the multi-perspective identification of event groups for abstraction in Sect. 2, before introducing preliminaries in Sect. 3. We present our approach in Sect. 4. Then, Sect. 5 describes a proof of concept demonstrating the potential of our approach. Section 6 summarizes related work; Finally, Sect. 7 discusses limitations of our work, gives an outlook on next steps, and concludes.

2   Problem Illustration

Our work deals with situations in which there are complex $n{:}m$ relations between low-level event classes and high-level activities, which means that events with the same label can relate to different activities, which themselves can relate to any number of events. Such low-level recording is a common issue, e.g., when dealing with UI logs, logs from messaging and document management systems, and logs of sensor data. In

Table 1. A single case of a request handling process recorded on a low level.

CaseID	EventID	Class	Timestamp	Role	Column
C1	e1	Receive email	05-23 07:45	Assistant	
C1	e2	Create record	05-23 09:07	Assistant	
C1	e3	Open document	05-23 10:40	Assistant	
C1	e4	Close document	05-23 10:51	Assistant	
C1	e5	Update record	05-23 10:52	Assistant	isComplete
C1	e6	Open document	05-25 15:03	Manager	
C1	e7	Update record	05-25 15:20	Manager	isAccepted
C1	e8	Close document	05-25 15:23	Manager	
C1	e9	Send email	05-26 10:03	Assistant	

such settings, individual events are often not informative and cause a high degree of variability in event logs resulting in the discovery of spaghetti models [17].

For illustration purposes, consider a request-handling process, which is supported by an information system logging events on a low level, i.e., on the level of database and document operations, such as *Open document, Update record*, and *Send email*. A single case of the low-level event log of this process is depicted in Table 1. On the activity level, blue events (*e1–e2*) record that a new request has been received, purple events (*e3–e5*) refer to checking required documents for completeness, whereas brown events (*e6–e8*) refer to a decision about a request. Finally, the gray event (*e9*) represents the notification about the outcome of the request.

Looking at the sequence of events in case *C1*, however, does not reveal these activities, because their purpose is not explicitly indicated in the available data. For instance, from an *Open document* event like *e3*, it is unclear if it refers to a check for completeness or a decision. Therefore, we have to discover meaningful activities in a more indirect manner, i.e., by looking for events that occur in a commonly recurring context. This may include the temporal context, e.g., that events occur within a short period of time, the organizational context, e.g., that events are executed by the same resource, and the data context associated with individual events. For instance, the purple events (*e3–e5*) happen within a short period of time (12 min), are executed by an assistant, while *e5* changes the value of the *isComplete* column. In contrast, the brown events (*e6–e8*) happen within 20 min, are executed by a manager, while *e7* changes the value of the *isAccepted* column. The events within these two groups share a common context from both the time and resource perspectives, whereas the different columns they update indicate a clear difference between the groups in *C1*, i.e., they hint at the purpose of an underlying business activity.

Therefore, our goal is to group events that have similar contexts, in order to make the purpose of activities that the low-level events represent more apparent. However, commonly recurring contexts of events, like the ones illustrated above, often cannot be identified from individual cases, because these represent single process instances in which contexts may not recur. Therefore, we have to consider the entire event log for this task, i.e., all events, across cases. The identification of these recurring contexts is highly complex from the low-level event log, though, which may have dozens of event classes and attributes and thousands of cases. Hence, this requires an automated identification of groups of events, yet, we also want to make sure that identified groups are actually meaningful for a user and their specific analysis purpose.

We tackle this through two main parts:

Multi-perspective Event Groups. We identify groups of events based on their multi-perspective context. In particular, we assign similar events that share commonly recurring contexts across process perspectives to the same group and distinct events that do not share such contexts to different groups. An example is shown in Fig. 1, where, e.g., an *Open document* is grouped with an *Update record* event, as both are executed by an assistant and happen within 20 min. In contrast, the *Update record* event executed by a manager changing the value of the *isAccepted* column is assigned to a different group. While these events belong to the same case *C1*, it is important to stress that we aim for groups of events that span individual cases. If, for instance, a hypothetical *Update record* event of a case *C2* is also executed by an assistant and changes the *isComplete* column, we aim to assign it to the same group as *e3* and *e5*, because they share contexts across cases.

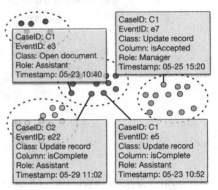

Fig. 1. Multi-perspective event groups.

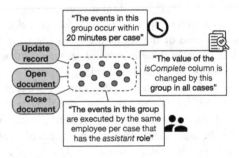

Fig. 2. Suggestion of a group of events.

Effective Group Suggestions. To ensure that identified groups are indeed meaningful, we support the user with understandable suggestions, allowing them to assess and select groups of related events based on their context. For instance, in our running example we identified that a group of events is executed within a short period of time by the same role, which changes the status of the request as shown in Fig. 2. Given that the events in this group occur in a similar context and there is a clear property that differentiates this from other groups, i.e., the change of the *isComplete* value, we aim to suggest it to the user. They might associate this group with a check for completeness in the request-handling process, select it for abstraction, and later assign it a suitable label.

3   Preliminaries

Events. We consider events recorded during the execution of a process and write $\mathcal{E}$ for the universe of all events. Events have unique identifiers and carry a payload containing their Class and optional contextual information, such as a timestamp, resource information, or relevant data values. We capture this payload by a set of attributes $\mathcal{D} = \{D_1, \ldots, D_p\}$, with $dom(D_i)$ as the domain of attribute D_i, $1 \leq i \leq p$. We write $e.D$ for the value of attribute D of an event e. For instance, for event $e1$ in Table 1, we write $e1.\texttt{Class} = \textit{Receive email}$ and $e1.\texttt{Role} = \textit{Assistant}$.

Event Log. An event log is a set of *traces* L, with each trace a sequence of events $\sigma \in \mathcal{E}^*$, representing a single execution of a process, i.e., a case. An event belongs to exactly one trace. We write E_L for the set of all events of the traces in L.

Event Groups. An event group is a set of events $g \subseteq E_L$. A grouping of events $G = \{g_1, \ldots, g_k\}$ is a set of event groups, such that G's members are disjoint and cover all events in E_L, i.e., $\bigcup_i^k g_i = E_L \wedge \bigcap_i^k g_i = \emptyset$.

4 Approach

As visualized in Fig. 3, our approach takes as input an event log and consists of four steps to create event group suggestions for event abstraction. Step 1 learns contextual dependencies between events and establishes multi-perspective representations. Step 2 groups the events based on these representations, which yields event groups as visualized in Fig. 1. Step 3 then computes key properties per group, which Step 4 uses to create suggestions by selecting groups with interesting properties and generating descriptions of the common contexts in which a groups' events occur. The output is a set of group suggestions and textual descriptions per group, such as shown in Fig. 2. The user can inspect these suggestions and select meaningful groups that serve their analysis purpose. The selected groups can then be used to abstract the low-level event log.

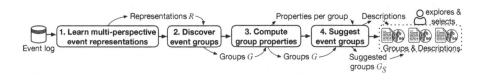

Fig. 3. The main steps of our approach.

4.1 Step 1: Learn Multi-perspective Event Representations

In the first step, we establish event representations that capture the multi-perspective context of low-level events, i.e., we aim to derive a representation r for each low-level event e, which contains contextual information available in e's attributes as well as its context in terms of surrounding events in its trace. As illustrated in Sect. 2, it is essential to consider this multi-perspective context of events to obtain meaningful event groups. The challenge here lies in generating representations that contain the relevant context required to create such groups. To this end, we leverage the ability of the Multi-Perspective Process Network (MPPN) [11]. The approach processes traces with various perspectives of different types, i.e., categorical, numerical, and temporal event attributes, as well as the trace-based context.

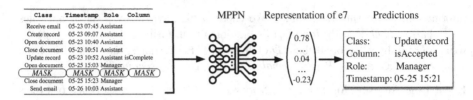

Fig. 4. Masked event prediction to learn multi-perspective representations.

For a trace σ, MPPN transforms the sequence of each available attribute's values into distinct 2D "images". Each image is processed by a pre-trained convolutional neural network (CNN) and results in one feature vector per attribute. Then, in order to obtain multi-perspective representations, the individual per-attribute vectors are pooled and processed by a fully-connected neural network resulting in one representation of adjustable size per trace, which contains features of all perspectives. Through the transformation of sequences of attribute values into images and the use of CNNs, the approach can focus on detecting similar patterns across traces in L, rather than focusing on the specific order in which events occur in individual traces. This flexibility in terms of how traces are processed makes MPPN a good choice for the task at hand, since, especially in event abstraction settings, we need to account for the considerable degree of variability present in low-level event sequences. Moreover, the learned representations include all process perspectives and thus, can be used for multi-perspective clustering tasks.

Originally, MPPN was developed to learn representations per trace $\sigma \in L$. Therefore, we have to adapt its learning strategy during training to be able to obtain one representation r per event $e \in E_L$, which captures e's multi-perspective context. To this end, we randomly mask all attribute values of events and train MPPN to predict these masked values given all other information in σ. For instance, as shown in Fig. 4, we replace the values of $e7$.Class, $e7$.Timestamp, $e7$.Role, and $e7$.Column with *MASK*. The task of MPPN is to predict all masked attribute values of $e7$ using the information from the trace's other events. If MPPN is able to accurately predict the attribute values of the masked events, this indicates that the learned representations capture their events' contexts well. Since MPPN has access to all events and their attributes before and after $e7$, rich contextual information can be incorporated into r.

After being trained in this manner on the whole event log, we obtain a set R of representations: for each event e, we mask all attribute values of e, process σ with MPPN, and add the generated representation r to R.

4.2 Step 2: Discover Event Groups

Step 2 discovers groups of events with commonly recurring multi-perspective contexts, which may represent high-level activities. To establish a set G of event groups, we cluster events with similar learned representations since they are likely to share a similar context, for instance, because they are executed by the same resources and occur within a short period of time. For performance reasons, we reduce the complexity of the representations using *Principal Component Analysis* (PCA). Then, we apply the well-known

Table 2. Exemplary group properties used by our approach.

Level	Perspective	Property	Example description based on template sentences
Group	Control-flow	# of event classes	*This group has "Open document" and "Close document" events*
	Resource	# of resources	*All events of this group are executed by 20 different resources.*
	Resource	# of roles	*All events of this group are executed by the "Assistant" role.*
	Time	Day of occurrence	*90% of events in this group happened on a Wednesday.*
	Time	Time of occurrence	*All events in this group happened before noon.*
	Data (cat.)	Distinct values	*All events have the value "Loan takeover" for the* Goal *attribute.*
	Data (num.)	Value range	*The* Cost *attribute ranges between 1,000 and 1,500 in this group.*
Case	Control-flow	# of event classes	*For this group, there are on average 3 events per case.*
	Control-flow	Range of positions	*The events of this group occur in a range of 2 to 3 events.*
	Resource	# of resources	*All events in this group are executed by the same resource per case.*
	Resource	# of roles	*All events in this group are executed by the "Manager" role.*
	Time	Duration	*This group of events takes 45 min on average per case.*
	Data (cat.)	Distinct values	*The value of the* isAccepted *attribute changes once on average.*
	Data (num.)	Value range	Cost *attribute has a range of 50 on average for this group per case*

k-means algorithm to obtain clusters. Instead of setting a specific number of clusters k, we use the *elbow method* [15] to select an appropriate k from a range of values (from 2 up to twice the number of event classes).

This clustering yields a grouping G as illustrated in Fig. 1. By assigning labels to each group $g \in G$, we could build a mapping between low-level events and high-level activities at this point already, which can be used to abstract a low-level event log. However, the remaining steps further process the groups to suggest only interesting ones to the user to make sure that they can assess how meaningful groups are for abstraction.

4.3 Step 3: Compute Group Properties

Next, based on the available event attributes, we compute a set of properties for each group $g \in G$, which jointly describe the multi-perspective common context of the events in g. These are later used to (1) assess how interesting a group is and (2) create textual descriptions of the group as exemplified in Fig. 2. An overview of considered properties is provided in Table 2. These do not necessarily consider all aspects of a particular input event log, yet, our approach can be easily extended with additional ones. As the table shows, properties either refer to all events in g or to the events in g per case. Moreover, each property refers to one attribute and, as such, to one main process perspective, i.e., the control-flow, resource, time, or data perspective. For instance, a group-based, resource-related property would be *the number of distinct roles that execute events within a group*, whereas a case-based one would be *the average number of distinct roles in a group per case*.

We compute group-level properties by aggregating the attribute values of events in a group, i.e., we collect distinct categorical and sum, average, and compute the range of numerical attribute values. For case-level properties, we first aggregate per trace and then take the average, minimum, and maximum. For instance, for a case-level property that explains the maximum number of distinct resources per trace, we count distinct resources that executed a group's events for each trace and take the maximum.

Handling Noise. There may be events with attribute values that occur infrequently in the established groups, which may pollute otherwise clear, representative group properties. To deal with such noise, we introduce a noise-filtering threshold τ, which can take values between 0 and 1 with a default value of 0.2 (the commonly used noise filtering threshold to separate frequent from infrequent behavior). We remove an event from a group g if the value's relative frequency in g is less than τ times the values' relative frequency in the log and recompute the property.

4.4   Step 4: Suggest Event Groups

In the final step, we select those groups that have properties that are actually interesting, i.e., we establish a set $G_s \subseteq G$ of groups to be suggested to the user. For these, we then create textual descriptions providing the most interesting properties per group, such as visualized in Fig. 2 of our running example.

Selecting Groups to Suggest. Using the properties that have been derived for a group g, we make a selection of groups to present to the user based on the interestingness of their properties. We argue that there are primarily two aspects that determine if a property is interesting for multi-perspective event abstraction: *distinctness* and *uniqueness*.

Distinctness. The distinctness of a property assumes that the more a property of a group differs from that of others, the more interesting it is. For instance, if a group of events is the only one that contains the *Manager* role, this makes it interesting. We compute the *earth mover's distance* [13] using the property's value sets for categorical properties and the property's averages per case for numerical ones for each group versus all other groups. The sum of the distances is the distinctness score of a property. The larger this score, the more distinct this group is from others for the respective property.

Uniqueness. The uniqueness of a property reflects how similar events in a group are with respect to a specific property. For instance, a group that contains events that all refer to the *Assistant* role makes this group more interesting than a group, whose events refer to five different roles. The uniqueness of a categorical property is the number of distinct values that occur for it in this group, whereas for numerical ones, we calculate the variance of the values within a group. On the case level, the uniqueness can be quantified using the mean number of distinct values per case for categorical properties, respectively the mean value range (difference between minimum and maximum) for numerical ones. The smaller this score, the more unique a group is for the property.

Inclusion Criterion. We rank the groups per property and include a group g in G_s if it ranks highest for at least one property for either uniqueness or distinctness.

Generating Textual Group Descriptions. Next, we provide understandable explanations for the groups in G_s. To this end, we create natural language descriptions of the properties of a group g, such as exemplified in Fig. 2. For each property, we fill slots of pre-defined template sentences. Examples of already filled template sentences are provided in the rightmost column of Table 2.

4.5   Output

Our approach outputs the set G_s of event group suggestions for event abstraction along with their corresponding textual descriptions. A user can inspect the generated descriptions and select meaningful groups. In this manner, we introduce a means to ensure that the groups that are ultimately used for abstraction are actually useful for the user with respect to their downstream analysis goal. While these textual descriptions are a means to explain the generated suggestions in an intuitive manner, the set of suggested groups in G_s are the important output for the actual event abstraction. They can be used to build a mapping from low-level events to higher-level activities, once each selected group is assigned a label. The concrete abstraction of the low-level event log can then be instantiated in various manners. For instance, we can replace each low-level event's class with the label associated with its group, i.e., high-level activity, and only retain the last event with the same label per trace. An important aspect is to consider multiple instances of the same high-level activity within a trace [8], which we will address when further developing our approach.

5   Proof of Concept

We implemented our approach as a Python prototype and simulated an event log that mirrors the scenario outlined in the problem illustration (Sect. 2)[1]. We aim to show that our approach can find groups of low-level events that correspond to meaningful high-level activities and that these can be used for event abstraction.

Data. There are no public logs available that record data as considered in our work and for which a ground truth is known. Therefore, we modeled a high-level and corresponding low-level Petri net. We simulated the low-level net introducing multi-perspective contextual dependencies and n:m relationships between the event classes and high-level activities. For instance, the execution of the *Decide on acceptance* activity (cf. Fig. 5) yields *Open document*, *Close document*, and *Update record* events, is performed by one manager per case, and takes at most 20 min.

Settings. We trained MPPN on the event log (cf. Sect. 4.1) generating vectors r of size 128. It reached almost 100% accuracy on all attributes except `Resource` with 73%. For PCA, we chose an explained variance of 0.99 to minimize information loss.

Results. Table 3 shows the groups suggested by our approach, including the multi-perspective context found in their event attributes. How these groups relate to the original high-level activities is indicated in Fig. 5.

We found that our approach identified three groups of events that exactly resemble high-level activities. Group 2 corresponds to the *Examine thoroughly* activity, Group 3 to *Decide on acceptance*, and Group 4 to *Communicate decision*. Notably, *Decide on acceptance* consist of the same set of low-level event classes as *Examine thoroughly*. However, Group 1 represents the whole initial phase of the process, which actually consists of four high-level activities, i.e., our approach could not discriminate the intended

---

[1] The source code, high-level as well as low-level process models, simulation, and a detailed scenario description are all available at https://github.com/a-rebmann/exploratory-abstraction.

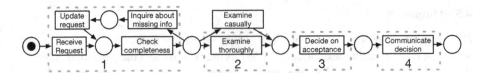

Fig. 5. High-level process model with groups suggested by our approach.

Table 3. Group suggestions found by our approach.

Group	1	2	3	4
Event classes	Open email, Open document, Create record, Update record, Close document, Send email	Open document, Query record, Update record, Close document	Open document, Update record, Close document	Generate document, Query record, Send email
Context	Roles: Assistant Resource: avg. 2.5 per case Duration: 3 h 30 m per case Status: complete, incomplete	Roles: Expert Resource: 1 per case Duration: 20 m per case Status: complete	Roles: Manager Resource: 1 per case Duration: 15 m per case Status: accept, reject	Roles: Assistant Resource: 1 per case Duration: 8 m per case Status: accept, reject

high-level activities. This could be due to ambiguous contextual information, e.g., because the events all happen at the beginning of their case and are executed by the same role. However, depending on the specific analysis purpose, this event group may still be meaningful. If, for instance, a user is interested in how requests are examined and how decisions are made, they do want to abstract from the details of this initial phase.

To highlight the usefulness of the suggested groups for abstraction, we applied them to the low-level event log, omitting events from groups not included in G_s. In particular, we map the low-level events of each group $g \in G_s$, to high-level activities. The DFG of the low-level event log and the DFG obtained after abstracting the log are visualized in Fig. 6. In the low-level DFG, the nodes refer to the distinct event classes in the log. Because one event class can be part of multiple high-level activities and one high-level activity can consist of multiple low-level event classes, limited insights can be obtained about the underlying process. From Fig. 6a it is, therefore, impossible to derive the actual relations to activities in Fig. 5. For instance, since *Send email* events relate to both inquiring about missing information (at the start of the process) and communicating a decision (at the end), there is a loop in the low-level DFG from the last to the first node, which obscures the distinct activities. However, our approach was able to group events in a way, such that a meaningful structure becomes visible (Fig. 6b), e.g., by assigning *Send email* events with different contexts (start vs. end of the process) to different groups. The initial process phase has been abstracted into a single activity, i.e., *Initial check* (the values of the *Status* attribute, i.e., *complete* and *incomplete*, hint at a checking activity). Moreover, clear behavioral patterns that were "hidden" in the low-level DFG are revealed for the later phase of the process: there is a choice between doing a thorough examination or not and there is a sequence between first examining the request, deciding on it, and finally communicating the decision. Note that we manually assigned meaningful labels to the new activities, since this is not yet supported by the approach. However, the descriptions of the multi-perspective event contexts our approach creates already provide the user with hints on how to label the groups.

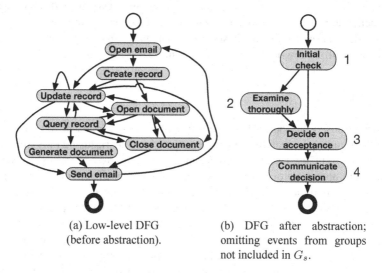

(a) Low-level DFG (before abstraction).

(b) DFG after abstraction; omitting events from groups not included in G_s.

Fig. 6. Abstraction impact achieved with the suggested groups.

These results indicate the potential of the approach to identify meaningful groups of events for event abstraction without any knowledge of true high-level activities. Also, the necessity to involve the user becomes clear, who can inspect group descriptions and make the final decision if a group is meaningful and which activity it resembles.

6   Related Work

A broad range of event abstraction techniques has been proposed in the context of process mining [4, 17]. To conduct meaningful abstraction, techniques require explicit input about high-level activities, which has to be provided by the user beforehand. For instance, some techniques assume a data attribute to indicate higher abstraction levels [7, 9], whereas others assume high-level process models as input [2]. While a recent technique explains the relations between low-level events and activities, the high-level activities and a mapping to low-level event classes are still required [6]. Other techniques do not require users to explicitly provide information about higher-level activities themselves, but criteria about when events are considered to be part of the same high-level activity, e.g., using temporal information [3] or requirements about the specific characteristics high-level activities should have [12]. In contrast to these techniques, our approach does not require the user to provide input about high-level activities upfront, but supports them in finding suitable groups of events based on their properties, which can then be used to abstract the event log in a meaningful manner.

Beyond the context of event abstraction, a recent study [18] examined exploratory analysis practices in process mining finding that few techniques support the user in the exploration of event data. A notable example is the work by Seeliger et al. [14] who introduced a system for trace clustering, which recommends clusters to analyze based on process performance indicators and thus, suggests groups of cases rather than events. Tsoury et al. [16] strive to augment logs with information derived from database records and transaction logs to allow for deeper insights when exploring event data. While these works provide the user with valuable support when analyzing complex event logs, they do not consider lifting low-level event data to a more meaningful level of abstraction.

7   Conclusion

This paper proposed an approach to identify and suggest groups of low-level events based on their multi-perspective recurring contexts that it learns using only information available in the event log. Users can inspect and select suggested groups, which supports the meaningful abstraction of event logs without the need to provide elaborate input about high-level activities upfront. In an initial proof of concept, we showed that the approach can indeed identify groups that correspond to high-level activities.

The research presented in this workshop paper is work in progress. We aim to expand the current work in several directions. First, we aim to extend the scope of our approach by adding a phase in which users can explore groups and interactively refine meaningful but too coarse-grained ones (such as Group 1 in Sect. 5), e.g., by triggering a clustering of a single group. Also, we aim to provide the user with various options for abstracting events by clustering the same representations but with different settings. Furthermore, if a group is discarded by the user because it does not make sense to them, e.g., because events with *complete* as the value for a Status attribute were assigned to the same group as events with *incomplete*, we want to incorporate their decision. In such cases, a re-clustering could be applied that takes this feedback into account and suggest groups that adhere to it. Second, motivated by the shift towards conducting data-driven process analysis in an object-centric and view-based manner [5], we aim to overcome the assumption that low-level events belong to exactly one case. Finally, to assess the usefulness of our (extended) approach, we aim to go beyond an evaluation using synthetic logs, by applying it in real-word settings and involving participants in a user study to assess the value of the suggestions our approach provides.

References

1. van der Aalst, W.M.P.: Process Mining: Data Science in Action. Springer, Cham (2016)
2. Baier, T., Mendling, J., Weske, M.: Bridging abstraction layers in process mining. Inf. Syst. **46**, 123–139 (2014)
3. De Leoni, M., Dündar, S.: Event-log abstraction using batch session identification and clustering. In: Proceedings of the ACM Symposium on Applied Computing, pp. 36–44 (2020)
4. Diba, K., Batoulis, K., Weidlich, M., Weske, M.: Extraction, correlation, and abstraction of event data for process mining. Wiley Interdisc. Rev. **10**(3), 1–31 (2020)
5. Fahland, D.: Process mining over multiple behavioral dimensions with event knowledge graphs. In: van der Aalst, W.M.P., Carmona, J. (eds.) Process Mining Handbook. Lecture Notes in Business Information Processing, vol. 448, pp. 274–319. Springer, Cham (2022). https://doi.org/10.1007/978-3-031-08848-3_9

6. Fazzinga, B., Flesca, S., Furfaro, F., Pontieri, L.: Process mining meets argumentation: explainable interpretations of low-level event logs via abstract argumentation. Inf. Syst. **107**, 101987 (2022)
7. Leemans, S.J., Goel, K., van Zelst, S.J.: Using multi-level information in hierarchical process mining: balancing behavioural quality and model complexity. In: ICPM, pp. 137–144 (2020)
8. Li, C.Y., van Zelst, S.J., van der Aalst, W.M.: An activity instance based hierarchical framework for event abstraction. In: ICPM, pp. 160–167. IEEE (2021)
9. Lu, X., Gal, A., Reijers, H.A.: Discovering hierarchical processes using flexible activity trees for event abstraction. In: ICPM, pp. 145–152. IEEE (2020)
10. Mannhardt, F., de Leoni, M., Reijers, H.A., van der Aalst, W.M., Toussaint, P.J.: Guided process discovery - a pattern-based approach. Inf. Syst. **76**, 1–18 (2018)
11. Pfeiffer, P., Lahann, J., Fettke, P.: Multivariate business process representation learning utilizing gramian angular fields and convolutional neural networks. In: Polyvyanyy, A., Wynn, M.T., Van Looy, A., Reichert, M. (eds.) BPM 2021. LNCS, vol. 12875, pp. 327–344. Springer, Cham (2021). https://doi.org/10.1007/978-3-030-85469-0_21
12. Rebmann, A., Weidlich, M., van der Aa, H.: GECCO: constraint-driven abstraction of low-level event logs. In: ICDE 2022, pp. 150–163. IEEE (2022)
13. Rubner, Y., Tomasi, C., Guibas, L.J.: A metric for distributions with applications to image databases. In: Sixth International Conference on Computer Vision, pp. 59–66. IEEE (1998)
14. Seeliger, A., Sánchez Guinea, A., Nolle, T., Mühlhäuser, M.: ProcessExplorer: intelligent process mining guidance. In: Hildebrandt, T., van Dongen, B.F., Röglinger, M., Mendling, J. (eds.) BPM 2019. LNCS, vol. 11675, pp. 216–231. Springer, Cham (2019). https://doi.org/10.1007/978-3-030-26619-6_15
15. Tibshirani, R., Walther, G., Hastie, T.: Estimating the number of clusters in a data set via the gap statistic. J. Roy. Stat. Soc. **63**(2), 411–423 (2001)
16. Tsoury, A., Soffer, P., Reinhartz-Berger, I.: A conceptual framework for supporting deep exploration of business process behavior. In: Trujillo, J.C., et al. (eds.) ER 2018. LNCS, vol. 11157, pp. 58–71. Springer, Cham (2018). https://doi.org/10.1007/978-3-030-00847-5_6
17. van Zelst, S.J., Mannhardt, F., de Leoni, M., Koschmider, A.: Event abstraction in process mining: literature review and taxonomy. Granular Comput. 2 (2020)
18. Zerbato, F., Soffer, P., Weber, B.: Initial insights into exploratory process mining practices. In: Polyvyanyy, A., Wynn, M.T., Van Looy, A., Reichert, M. (eds.) BPM 2021. LNBIP, vol. 427, pp. 145–161. Springer, Cham (2021). https://doi.org/10.1007/978-3-030-85440-9_9

Detecting Complex Anomalous Behaviors in Business Processes: A Multi-perspective Conformance Checking Approach

Azadeh Sadat Mozafari Mehr$^{(\boxtimes)}$ ⓘ, Renata M. de Carvalho ⓘ,
and Boudewijn van Dongen ⓘ

Department of Mathematics and Computer Science, Eindhoven University of Technology,
Eindhoven, The Netherlands
{a.s.mozafari.mehr,r.carvalho,b.f.v.dongen}@tue.nl

Abstract. In recent years, organizations are putting an increasing emphasis on anomaly detection. Anomalies in business processes can be an indicator of system faults, inefficiencies, or even fraudulent activities. In this paper we introduce an approach for anomaly detection. Our approach considers different perspectives of a business process such as control flow, data and privacy aspects simultaneously. Therefore, it is able to detect complex anomalies in business processes like spurious data processing and misusage of authorizations. The approach has been implemented in the open source ProM framework and its applicability was evaluated through a real-life dataset from a financial organization. The experiment implies that in addition to detecting anomalies of each aspect, our approach can detect more complex anomalies which relate to multiple perspectives of a business process.

Keywords: Outlier behavior detection · Anomalous behavior · Data privacy · Conformance checking · Multi-perspective analysis

1 Introduction

Today, anomaly detection is essential for businesses. This concept refers to the problem of finding patterns in data that do not conform to regular behavior. Outliers and anomalies are two terms commonly used in regards to anomaly detection. The importance of outlier or anomaly detection lies in the fact that anomalies in data can be translated into valuable, and often critical and actionable information in a variety of applications such as fraud detection, intrusion detection for cyber-security, and fault detection in systems [4]. In the business process management domain, anomaly detection can be applied for detecting anomalous behaviors during business processes executions. Often, organizations look for anomalies in their business processes, as these can be indicators for inefficiencies, insufficiently trained employees, or even fraudulent activities. Mostly, companies rely on process-aware information systems to manage their daily processes. The event logs of these information systems are a great source of information capturing executed behavior of different elements involved in the business processes such as

© The Author(s) 2023
M. Montali et al. (Eds.): ICPM 2022 Workshops, LNBIP 468, pp. 44–56, 2023.
https://doi.org/10.1007/978-3-031-27815-0_4

employees and systems. They can be used to extract valuable information about the executions of a process (process instances) as they reflect executed behaviors. In the context of business processes, an anomaly is defined as a deviation from a defined behavior, i.e., the business process model [11].

Nowadays, business processes have a high level of complexity. On top of a daily process, many standards and regulations are implemented as business rules which should be considered in anomaly analysis. For compliance checking, business analysts should investigate the processes from multiple perspectives. This is a very challenging task since different aspects of processes should be considered in both isolating and combining views in order to detect hidden deviations and anomalous behaviors. For instance, generally employees are authorized to access sensitive data only in the context of working and for a defined purpose. Privacy violations may happen when employees misuse this authority for secondary purposes like personal or financial benefits. In this regards, one of the articles in the GDPR regulation is about purpose limitation emphasizing "Who can access data for which purpose?". Such data privacy rule is closely related to three different perspectives: i) the control flow, or the tasks being executed; ii) the data, or the flow and processing of information; and iii) the privacy, or the legitimate role allocation. This example clearly shows that the approaches which focus only on control flow or data flow aspects are not sufficient to detect deviations and anomalies in complex problems. The potential of multi-perspective process mining has been emphasized by several contributions [2,6,8]. Although these techniques consider data objects and/or the resources, in all of them control flow is a priority since they assume data objects or resources as attributes of activity instances in the process execution.

Previously, we presented a balanced multi-perspective approach for conformance checking and anomaly detection which considered control-flow, data and privacy perspectives all together and simultaneously without giving priority to one perspective [9]. In this paper, we extend our previous approach by considering the type of data operations (mandatory or optional) and their execution constraints in the calculation of alignments. To the best of our knowledge, no other approach takes data layer restrictions of data operation type and frequency into account. Furthermore, in our new approach, we made the concept of context (purpose) of data processing more clear. As another improvement, to avoid reporting false positive deviations in the control flow perspective, we consider partial order of activity executions. Similarly, Lu *et al.* [7] used partial order in event data to improve the quality of conformance checking results. However their approach checks only control flow alignment in contrast to our approach which is a multi-perspective conformance checking method.

The remainder of this paper is structured as follows. Section 2 introduces our multi-perspective conformance checking approach to detect complex anomalous behaviors in business processes. Section 3 presents the applicability of our approach through a real-life case study, discussing the experimental design and results. At last, the conclusion of this paper is presented in Sect. 4.

2   Methodology

Current conformance checking methods use alignments (in detail explained in [3]) to relate the recorded execution of a process with its model. Commonly, these techniques have a fundamental property, so-called synchronous product model. A synchronous product model links observed behavior and modeled behavior in a Petri net format. By using an A* based search strategy [1, 12], the conformance checking techniques can compute alignments for individual cases in an event log.

While traditional conformance checking approaches only consider control flow aspect of a process, we consider data and privacy aspects together with control flow perspective all at once. In the rest of this section, we explain the structure of the synchronous product model in our new approach for multi-perspective conformance checking and show the types of anomalies that our method is able to detect by employing A* algorithm on the designed synchronous product model.

2.1   Construction of Synchronous Product Model

To clarify the steps of constructing the synchronous product in our approach, let us consider the inputs shown in Fig. 1. Figure 1(a) shows a workflow-net as the process model. This process model starts with activity A by role R1 and continues with activities B, C, and D by role $R2$. According to the data model depicted in Fig. 1(b), for the completion of activity A, mandatory data operation $Read(x)$ should be executed and the actor is allowed to repeat this data operation. $Update(y)$ is another data operation in the context of activity A that is optional and the actor is allowed to execute this operation only once while performing A. Each of activities B, C, and D are expected to execute one mandatory data operation in order to fulfilment. Figure 1(c) shows the organisational model in our example. There are two roles in the organisational model. Actor (resource) $u1$ has the role $R1$ and the actor $u2$ has the role $R2$.

Figure 1(d) shows one trace of the process log. This trace contains eight process events that correspond to a single case. The start and complete events with the same activity name and id indicate the occurrence of an instance of a specific activity. For example, e_3 and e_4 both with id equal to 2 indicate the execution of one instance of activity B. The events are sorted by their occurrence time.

Figure 1(e) presents a data trace with three data operations $op1$, $op2$, and $op3$, which were executed on the data fields x, z, and m during the execution of case 100.

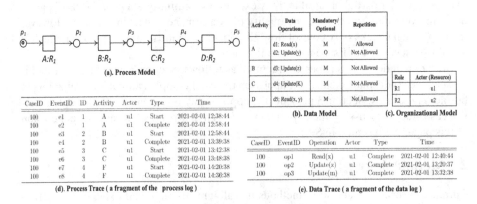

(a). Process Model

(b). Data Model

(c). Organizational Model

(d). Process Trace (a fragment of the process log)

(e). Data Trace (a fragment of the data log)

Fig. 1. The inputs of the proposed approach in the running example

Figure 1(d) together with Fig. 1(e) shape the observed behavior for case 100. A close inspection of the event logs already shows that there are some conformance issues. First, from the control flow perspective, activity D appears to be missing while activity F is an unexpected activity according to the process model. Second, from data perspective, two mandatory data operations $d4$ and $d5$ are missing and $op3$ implies the execution of a spurious data operation by user $u1$. Third, from privacy (resource) perspective, activities B and C are expected to be performed by a user playing role $R2$, but it appears that these activities and data operations were performed by user $u1$ who plays the role $R1$. From combined perspectives, although activity B was performed in correct order and expected by the process model and its executed data operation ($op2$) conforms with the data model, there is a deviation in the privacy aspect. Data operation $op2$ is only supposed to be executed within the context of activity B by an actor playing the role $R2$ however this data operation was accessed by a user who plays the role $R1$.

A traditional conformance checking technique, which focuses only on the control flow, would ignore the resource and data parts of the modeled behavior. To address this issue, now we present our approach which considers control flow, data and privacy aspects of a business process simultaneously for anomaly detection analysis and can automatically distinguish all kind of anomalies which were described earlier.

As a pre-processing step, to combine process, data and privacy (resource) aspects into a single prescribed behavior, we first shape the operation net of each activity in the process model considering corresponding data operations in the data model. For instance, the operation net of activity A is depicted in Fig. 2 surrounded by a red line. It represents how we model mandatory and optional data operations and their execution constraint in a Petri net format. In the operation net of an activity X, there are two corresponding transitions labelled with "Xs" (X+Start) and "Xc" (X+complete) (i.e. transition As and Ac in Fig. 2). For each expected data operation of the activity, one transition labeled with the name of data operation and two places are created: one is the input place and the other is the output place of the expected data operation. The input place of the expected data operation is an output place for the activity transition with the start type, while the output place of the expected data operation is an input place for the activity transition with the complete type. An invisible transition is created and connected to input and output places of each optional data operations (i.e. transition below $d2$ in Fig. 2). An invisible transition is created and connected to input and output places of each data operation that is allowed to be executed frequently. In this case, the input place of the invisible transition is an output place for that data operation while the output place of the invisible transition is an input place for that data operation (i.e. transition above $d1$ in Fig. 2).

The first foundation of the synchronous product in our approach is *Model net*. The model net (N_M) is constructed by replacing each activity in the original process model (i.e. Fig. 1(a)) with corresponding operation net. Figure 2 shows the model net for our running example. In this model, we enriched the process model (Fig. 1(a)) with the expected data operations shown in Fig. 1(b).

The second foundation of the synchronous product in our approach is *Process net*. The process net (N_P) represents a process trace. It shows a sequence of the transitions labelled with activities and their life cycle as they appeared in the process trace.

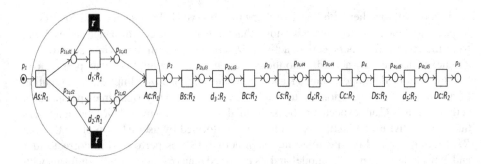

Fig. 2. Model net of the running example. The operation net of activity A is surrounded by the red line. (Color figure online)

The yellow part in the middle of Fig. 3 shows the process net constructed based on the process trace example in Fig. 1. Two concurrent transitions Ac And Bs in this model show the partial order of the completion of activity A (reflected in e_2) and the start of activity B (reflected in e_3) which have the same timestamp. To match start and complete events related to one instance of an activity, we consider a matching place labelled as C and the name of executed activity (we call these type of places as context places). The input and output of matching places are start and complete events related to one instance of an activity. It should be noted that context places are created if and only if the start and complete events related to one activity have the same "id" attribute.

The third foundation of the synchronous product in our approach is *Data net*. The data net (N_D) represents a data trace. It shows a sequence of the transitions labelled with executed data operations as they appeared in the data trace. The red part in the bottom of Fig. 3 shows the data net constructed based on the data trace example in Fig. 1.

Using the model net, process net and data net, we present the synchronous product model as the combination of these three nets with two additional sets of synchronous transitions. Figure 3 shows the synchronous product for our running example. For the sake of less complexity, in this model, we relabeled the transitions of model net as t_{mi}, transitions of process net as t_{pi}, and transitions in data net as t_{di}. We also chose new identifiers for the places in model net, process net and data net as p_{mi}, p_{pi} and p_{di}, respectively.

As shown in Fig. 3, other than transitions of the model, process and data nets, there are two sets of synchronous transitions called synchronous transitions and data synchronous transitions. *Synchronous transitions* only exist when an expected activity appears in the process net. *Data synchronous transitions* only exists when an expected data operation appears in the data net. Additionally, each data operation is associated to a so called matched activity. The matched activity is the activity instance that was executed by the same resource as the data operation and the timestamp of the data event should be between the start and completion time of the matched activity in the process net. These conditions are reflected in the model by input/output to the context place of matched activity. Input places of synchronous data operations contain: the input place

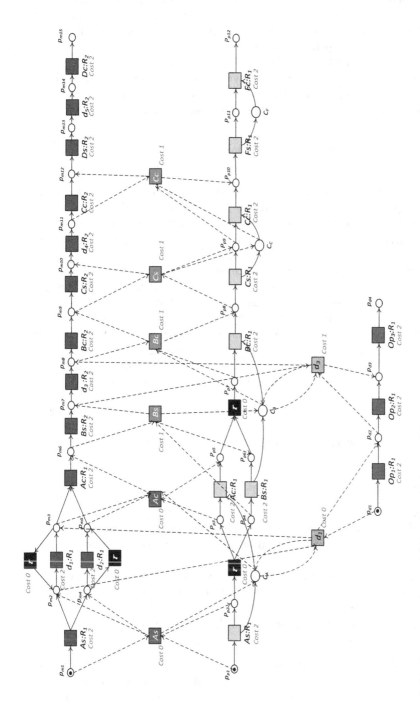

Fig. 3. Synchronous product model based on the inputs of the running example. The model net is depicted in the top part in purple color, the process net is depicted in the middle part in yellow color and the data net is depicted in the bottom part in red color. Synchronous moves and data synchronous moves are shown in blue and green colors, respectively. Synchronous moves and data synchronous moves with illegitimate roles are shown in light blue and orange colors, respectively (Color figure online).

of the corresponding executed data operation in the data net; the input place of the expected data operation in the model net; and the context place of matched activity in the process net. Output places of the synchronous data operations contain: the output places of the executed data operation; the output place of the expected data operation; and the context place of matched activity.

For including the privacy aspect in the synchronous transitions, we consider a penalty cost in case of expected activity and/or data operation done by an unexpected role. This will be discussed in the next section under the cost function definition.

2.2   Multi-layer Alignment and Cost Function

An alignment is a firing sequence of transitions from initial marking to the final marking in the synchronous product model. In our approach, initial marking m_i is the set of starting places of each model, process and data nets. Final marking m_f is the set of last places of each model, process and data nets. For instance, in Fig. 3, $m_i = \{p_{m1}, p_{p1}, p_{d1}\}$ is the initial marking and $m_f = \{p_{m15}, p_{p12}, p_{d4}\}$ is the final marking.

We need to relate "moves" in the logs to "moves" in the model in order to establish an alignment between the model, process trace and data trace. However, it might happen that some of the moves in the logs cannot be mimicked by the model and vice-versa. We explicitly denote such "no moves" by "≫". Formally, we represent a move as (t_m, t_p, t_d), where we set t_m to be a transition in the model net, t_p to be a transition of the events in the process net (process trace), and t_d to be a transition of the events in data net (data trace). Our approach separates moves into two categories: synchronous moves and deviations. Synchronous moves represent expected behavior:

- A *synchronous move* happens when an expected activity was performed by a legitimate role.
- A *data synchronous move* happens when an expected data operation was executed by a legitimate role.

We further distinguish six kinds of deviations:

- A *move on model* happens when there are unobserved activity instances.
- A *move on model* happens when there are unobserved data operations.
- A *move on process log* happens when an unexpected activity instance was performed.
- A *move on data log* happens when an unexpected data operation was executed.
- A *synchronous move with illegitimate role* happens when an expected activity was performed by an illegitimate role.
- A *data synchronous move with illegitimate role* happens when an expected data operation was performed by an illegitimate role.

The computation of an optimal alignment relies on the definition of a proper cost function for the possible kinds of moves. We extend the standard cost function to include data and privacy costs. We define our default multi-layer alignment cost function as follows:

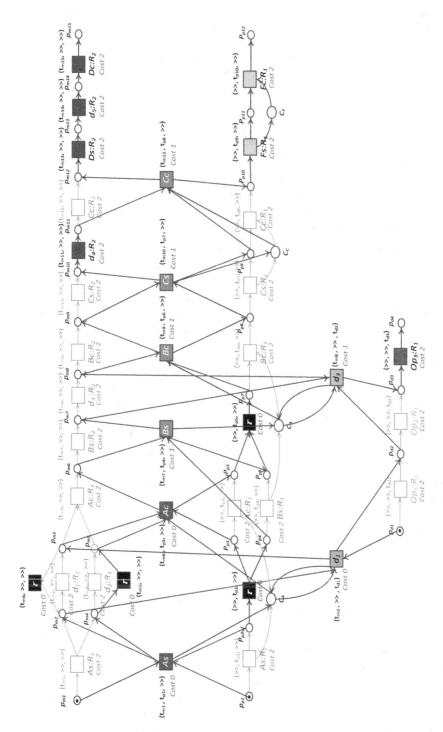

Fig. 4. Full run of the synchronous product corresponding to an optimal alignment, assuming a multi-layer cost function for the running example

Definition 1 (Multi-Layer Alignment Cost function). *Let* (t_m, t_p, t_d) *be a move in alignment between a model, process trace and a data trace. The cost* $K(t_m, t_p, t_d)$ *is:*

$$K(t_m, t_p, t_d) = \begin{cases} 2, & \textit{if } (t_m, t_p, t_d) \textit{ is a move on process log} \\ & \textit{or move on data log, or move on model} \\ 0, & \textit{if } (t_m, t_p, t_d) \textit{ is Process/Data sync. move} \\ & \textit{with legitimate role} \\ 1, & \textit{if } (t_m, t_p, t_d) \textit{ is process/Data sync. move} \\ & \textit{with illegitimate role} \end{cases}$$

Note that, to include the cost for deviations related to the privacy layer, we considered a penalty cost equal to 1 in our cost function. If the actor of observed behavior was not allowed to perform activity and/or data operation we add the penalty cost.

The alignment with the lowest cost is called an optimal alignment. We define Optimal Multi-Layer Alignment as follows:

Definition 2 (Optimal Multi-Layer Alignment). *Let* N *be a WFR-net,* σ_c *and* β_c *be a process trace and data trace, respectively. Assuming* A_N *as the set of all legal alignment moves, a cost function* K *assigns a non-negative cost to each legal move:* $A_N \rightarrow \mathbb{R}_0^+$. *The cost of an alignment* γ *between* σ_c, β_c *and* N *is computed as the sum of the cost of all constituent moves* $K(\gamma) = \sum_{(t_m, t_p, t_d) \in \gamma} K(t_m, t_p, t_d)$. *Alignment* γ *is an optimal alignment if for any alignment* γ' *of* σ_c, β_c *and* N, $K(\gamma) \leq K(\gamma')$.

For finding the optimal alignments we employed A* algorithm. Figure 4 illustrates an optimal alignment for running example, depicted on top of the synchronous product shown in Fig. 3. It shows that there are six kinds of deviations between observed behavior and modeled behavior, namely synchronous moves with illegitimate roles on transitions *Bs*, *Bc*, *Cs*, and *Cc* in light blue color, data synchronous move with illegitimate role showing spurious data operation on transitions *d3* in orange color, model moves showing missing data operations on transitions *d4* and *d5* and model moves showing skipped activities on transitions *Ds* and *Dc* in purple color, process log moves indicating unexpected activities on transitions *Fs* and *Fc* in yellow color, and a data log move showing unexpected data operations on transition *op3* in red color.

3 Evaluation

To evaluate the applicability of our approach to real-life scenarios, we used the event log recording the loan management process of a Dutch Financial Institute provided by BPI challenge 2017 [5]. After splitting the provided event log, the resulting process log and data log contain 301,709 workflow events and 256,767 data operations, respectively. These logs were recorded from managing 26,053 loan applications. The activities and data operations were performed by 146 resources (employees or system).

Figure 5 shows the loan management process in Petri net notation. In this process, there are four main milestones: receiving applications, negotiating offers, validating documents, and detecting potential fraud. The execution of activities may require performing certain mandatory or optional data operations. The data model of this process which presents the relationship between activities and data operations is shown in

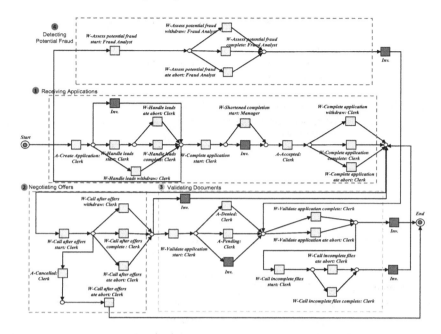

Fig. 5. Loan management process model [10]

Table 1. Such data model is created according to domain knowledge and also indicates whether the user is allowed to repeat the execution of the data operations. As shown in the process model (Fig. 5), three roles are supposed to conduct the activities. Most of the activities are supposed to be done by the role *clerk*. Activities related to fraud detection are supposed to be done by a *fraud analyst*. The activity "W Shortened completion"

Table 1. Data model of the loan management process. Type: Mandatory (M), Optional (O). Repetition: is allowed (True), is not allowed (False). A: Application, O: Offer, W: Workflow [10].

Activity	Data operation	Type	Repetition
A-Create Application	Create: (applicationID)	M	False
W-Shortened Completion start	Read: (applicationID, email)	M	False
A-Accepted	Create: (offerID)	M	False
	Read: (offerID)	M	False
	Read: (address, email)	M	False
	Read: (address)	O	False
A-Cancelled	Update: (OCancelledFlag)	M	True
W-Call after offer start	Update: (ACompletedFlag)	M	False
W-Call after offer complete	Update: (OAcceptedFlag)	M	False
W-Call after offer withdraw	Update: (OReturnedFlag)	M	False
W-Call after offer ate abort	Update: (OCancelledFlag)	M	False
W-Validate application start	Update: (AValidatedFlag)	M	False
A-Pending	Update: (OAcceptedFlag)	M	False
A-Denied	Update: (ORefusedFlag)	M	True
W-Validate application ate abort	Update: (OCancelledFlag)	M	True
W-Call incomplete files start	Update: (AInCompleteFlag)	M	False

Table 2. The result of experiment with real-life data

Category	Anomaly	Occurence
1	Ignored mandatory data operation "Update(OCancelledFlag)"	40,869
2	Unexpected data operation "Update (OReturnedFlag)"	18,291
3	Unexpected data operation "Read (offID)"	11,874
4	Unexpected data operation "Create (offID)"	11,874
5	Unexpected data operation "Read (address- email)"	9,640
6	Ignored mandatory data operation "Create(appID)"	9,354
7	Unexpected data operation "Update (OCancelledFlag)"	5,624
8	Unexpected activity "W Call incomplete files complete"	2,565
9	Skipped activity "W Call incomplete files ate abort"	1,919
10	Unexpected data operation "Read (email)"	1,874

can only be executed by a *manager*. Managers also have the authority to perform all the activities related to a clerk.

We implemented our approach as a package in the ProM framework called Multi Layer Alignment in the "MultiLayerAlignmentWithContext" plugin. Using this tool, we applied our approach on the described business process. A summary of our results that shows ten most frequent anomalies is reported in Table 2. In addition to detecting multi-layer deviations, the experiment remarks that the approach is capable to reconstruct and provide the link between performed activities in the process layer and executed data operations in the data layer to present the contexts of data processing. For example, Table 2 shows mandatory data operation *"Update(OCancelledFlag)"* was ignored 40,869 times. We have also developed a view that provides detailed information, described in [10], which finds that this anomaly happened 16,735 times in the context of activity *"W-Validate application ate abort"*, 16,184 times in the context of activity *"W-Call after offers ate abort"*, and 7,950 times in the context of activity *"A-Cancelled"*. Furthermore, it could detect who (in terms of roles and users) had the anomalous or suspicious behaviors during process executions.

4   Conclusion

In this work, we presented an approach for detecting complex anomalous behaviors in business processes. Through an example, we showed the structure of our multi-layer synchronous product model which is the foundation of conformance checking and applying alignment algorithms.

In existing multi-perspective conformance checking approaches, control flow perspective is a priority thus many deviations stay hidden and uncovered. In contrast, in our approach, different perspectives of a business process such as control flow, data and privacy aspects are considered simultaneously to detect complex anomalies which relates to multiple perspectives of a business process.

We showed the applicability of our approach using real-life event logs of a loan management process from a financial institute. The experiment demonstrated the approach's capability to return anomalies such as ignored data operations, suspicious activities and data operations, spurious and unexpected data operations. Additionally, our method could reconstruct the link between process layer and data layer from executed behavior and present the contexts of data processing. Thus, it can discover data accesses without clear context and purposes.

As future step, we plan a qualitative analysis of how useful the results of our approach are to the business analysts to detect anomalous and suspicious behaviors in business processes.

Reproducibility. The inputs required to reproduce the experiments can be found at https://github.com/AzadehMozafariMehr/Multi-PerspectiveConformanceChecking

Acknowledgement. The author has received funding within the BPR4GDPR project from the European Union's Horizon 2020 research and innovation programme under grant agreement No 787149.

References

1. Van der Aalst, W., Adriansyah, A., van Dongen, B.: Replaying history on process models for conformance checking and performance analysis. Wiley Interdisc. Rev. Data Min. Knowl. Discov. **2**(2), 182–192 (2012)
2. Alizadeh, M., Lu, X., Fahland, D., Zannone, N., van der Aalst, W.: Linking data and process perspectives for conformance analysis. Comput. Secur. **73**, 172–193 (2018)
3. Carmona, J., van Dongen, B., Solti, A., Weidlich, M.: Conformance Checking Relating Processes and Models. Springer, Cham (2018)
4. Chandola, V., Banerjee, A., Kumar, V.: Anomaly Detection. In: Sammut, C., Webb, G. (eds.) Encyclopedia of Machine Learning and Data Mining, pp. 1–15. Springer, Boston (2016). https://doi.org/10.1007/978-1-4899-7502-7_912-1
5. van Dongen, B.: BPI Challenge 2017 (2017). https://doi.org/10.4121/uuid:5f3067df-f10b-45da-b98b-86ae4c7a310b
6. de Leoni, M., van der Aalst, W.M.P.: Aligning event logs and process models for multi-perspective conformance checking: An approach based on integer linear programming. In: Daniel, F., Wang, J., Weber, B. (eds.) Business Process Management. LNCS, pp. 113–129. Springer, Heidelberg (2013). https://doi.org/10.1007/978-3-642-40176-3_10
7. Lu, X., Fahland, D., van der Aalst, W.M.P.: Conformance checking based on partially ordered event data. In: Fournier, F., Mendling, J. (eds.) BPM 2014. LNBIP, pp. 75–88. Springer, Cham (2015). https://doi.org/10.1007/978-3-319-15895-2_7
8. Mannhardt, F., Leoni, de, M., Reijers, H., Aalst, van der, W.: Balanced multi-perspective checking of process conformance. Computing **98**, 407–437 (2014)
9. Mozafari Mehr, A.S., de Carvalho, R.M., van Dongen, B.: Detecting privacy, data and control-flow deviations in business processes. In: Nurcan, S., Korthaus, A. (eds.) CAiSE 2021. LNBIP, pp. 82–91. Springer International Publishing, Cham (2021). https://doi.org/10.1007/978-3-030-79108-7_10
10. Mozafari Mehr, A.S., de Carvalho, R.M., van Dongen, B.: An association rule mining-based framework for the discovery of anomalous behavioral patterns. In: Chen, W., Yao, L., Cai, T., Pan, S., Shen, T., Li, X. (eds.) ADMA 2022. LNCS, vol. 13725, pp. 397–412. Springer, Cham (2022). https://doi.org/10.1007/978-3-031-22064-7_29

11. Nolle, T., Seeliger, A., Mühlhäuser, M.: BINet: multivariate business process anomaly detection using deep learning. In: Weske, M., Montali, M., Weber, I., vom Brocke, J. (eds.) BPM 2018. LNCS, vol. 11080, pp. 271–287. Springer, Cham (2018). https://doi.org/10.1007/978-3-319-98648-7_16

12. Dongen, B.F.: Efficiently computing alignments. In: Weske, M., Montali, M., Weber, I., vom Brocke, J. (eds.) BPM 2018. LNCS, vol. 11080, pp. 197–214. Springer, Cham (2018). https://doi.org/10.1007/978-3-319-98648-7_12

A Survey on the Application of Process Mining to Smart Spaces Data

Yannis Bertrand[1]([✉])[iD], Bram Van den Abbeele[1], Silvestro Veneruso[2][iD], Francesco Leotta[2][iD], Massimo Mecella[2][iD], and Estefanía Serral[1][iD]

[1] Research Centre for Information Systems Engineering (LIRIS), KU Leuven, Warmoesberg 26, 1000 Brussels, Belgium
{yannis.bertrand,estefania.serralasensio}@kuleuven.be,
bram.vandenabbeele@student.kuleuven.be
[2] Sapienza Università di Roma, Rome, Italy
{veneruso,leotta,mecella}@diag.uniroma1.it

Abstract. During the last years, a number of studies have experimented with applying process mining (PM) techniques to smart spaces data. The general goal has been to automatically model human routines as if they were business processes. However, applying process-oriented techniques to smart spaces data comes with its own set of challenges. This paper surveys existing approaches that apply PM to smart spaces and analyses how they deal with the following challenges identified in the literature: choosing a modelling formalism for human behaviour; bridging the abstraction gap between sensor and event logs; and segmenting logs in traces. The added value of this article lies in providing the research community with a common ground for some important challenges that exist in this field and their respective solutions, and to assist further research efforts by outlining opportunities for future work.

Keywords: Process mining · Smart spaces · Sensor logs

1 Introduction

Over the last few years, facilitated by the development of smart spaces, researchers and manufacturers have shown interest in analysing human behaviour via data collected by Internet of Things (IoT) devices. This information is then used to get insights about the behaviour of the user (e.g., sleep tracking), or to perform automated actions for the user (e.g., automatically opening the blinds).

While both PM and smart spaces have been evolving quickly as separate fields of study during the last years, researchers have recently explored combining both disciplines and obtained interesting results. Applying PM techniques to smart

The work of Yannis Bertrand and Estefanía Serral was partially supported by the Flemish Fund for Scientific Research (FWO) with grant number G0B6922N. The work of Silvestro Veneruso and Francesco Leotta was partially funded by the Sapienza project with grant number RM120172B3B5EC34.

M. Montali et al. (Eds.): ICPM 2022 Workshops, LNBIP 468, pp. 57–70, 2023.
https://doi.org/10.1007/978-3-031-27815-0_5

spaces data, enables modelling and visualising human habits as processes [19]. However, even though process models could be extracted from smart spaces data, multiple problems arose when applying techniques designed for BPs to human habits [19].

This paper studies how current approaches deal with well-known challenges in applying PM to smart spaces data and human behaviour [19]: modelling formalism for representing human behaviour, abstraction gap between sensor and event logs, and logs segmentation in traces. The main contribution of this article to the research community is therefore threefold: (1) providing an overview and comparison of PM techniques applied to smart spaces, (2) analysing how these techniques currently deal with the three challenges identified, and (3) providing an outline for future work.

The remainder of this paper is structured as follows: Sect. 2 introduces some background concepts and commonly used terminology in the fields of smart spaces and PM. Section 3 describes the related work. The methodology followed to perform the survey is defined in Sect. 4. Results are reported in Sect. 5. Section 6 discusses the results and provides an outline for future work. Lastly, Sect. 7 concludes the paper with an overview of the key findings.

2   Background

2.1   Smart Spaces

Smart spaces are cyber-physical environments where an information system takes as input raw sensor measurements, analyses them in order to obtain a higher level understanding of what is happening in the environment, i.e., the current context, and eventually uses this information to trigger automated actions through a set of actuators, following final user preferences. A smart space produces at runtime a sequence of sensor measurements called *sensor log* in the form shown in Table 1.

The following terminology is usually employed [21]:

- *Activities*, i.e., groups of human atomic interactions with the environment (actions) that are performed with a final goal (e.g., cleaning the house).
- *Habits, routines, or behaviour patterns*, i.e., an activity, or a group of actions or activities that happen in specific contextual conditions (e.g., what the user usually does in the morning between 08:00 and 10:00).

Human Activity Recognition (HAR) is a common task in smart spaces that aims at recognizing various human activities (e.g., walking, sleeping, watching tv) using machine learning techniques based on data gathered from IoT environments [16]. [24] argues that HAR is part of a bigger picture with the ultimate aim to provide assistance, assessment, prediction and intervention related to the identified activities.

2.2   Process Mining in Smart Spaces

The main goal of applying PM in a smart space is to automatically discover models of the behaviour of the user(s) of the smart space based on a log of the sensors present in the environment. Models can represent activities (or habits) that users perform in the smart space, e.g., eating, working, sleeping. It is important to highlight the following differences between PM and smart spaces:

- Whereas smart spaces techniques usually take as input sensor logs, process mining techniques use *event logs*. Events in event logs are execution of business activities, while sensor logs contain fine grained sensor measurements.
- The term *business process* in PM may correspond to the terms *activity, habit, routine, or behaviour pattern* in the smart space community.
- While event logs are typically split in traces (process executions), sensor logs are not segmented and may contain information related to different activities or habits.

Smart spaces usually produce and analyse data in the form of sensor logs. According to [27], in order to apply techniques from the PM area, the sensor log must be converted into an event log. The entries of an event log must contain at least three elements: *(i)* the case id, which identifies a specific process instance, *(ii)* the label of the activity performed and *(iii)* the timestamp. The conversion from a sensor log to an event log usually consists of two steps, respectively *(i)* bridging the granularity gap between sensor measurements and events and *(ii)* segmenting the event log into traces, i.e., to assign a case ID to each event.

Table 1. Example of a sensor log used in smart spaces

Timestamp	Sensor	Value
...	...	...
2022-05-31 12:34:52	M3	ON
2022-05-31 12:34:58	M5	OFF
2022-05-31 12:35:04	M3	OFF
2022-05-31 12:35:22	T2	22
2022-05-31 12:38:17	M29	OFF
...	...	...

3   Related Work

This section provides a short summary of the surveys and reviews that have previously been performed on the application of PM on human behaviour discovery.

[21] surveyed the modelling and mining techniques used to model human behaviour. They studied the model lifecycle of each approach and identified important challenges that typically came up when performing HAR. However, they reviewed all sorts of techniques used in HAR, not focusing on PM techniques.

[24] performed a literature review and created a taxonomy on the application of HAR and process discovery techniques in industrial environments. While focusing on PM for HAR, this study is restricted to one application domain.

[13] analysed how classic PM tasks (i.e., process discovery, conformance checking, enhancement) have taken advantage of artificial intelligence (AI) capabilities. The survey specifically focused on two different strategies: (1) using explicit domain knowledge and (2) the exploitation of auxiliary AI tasks. While [13] briefly covers the application of PM to smart spaces, this section is rather short as their focus lies on PM in general.

No recent survey has identified which existing PM approaches were applied to smart spaces and how these approaches deal with the challenges identified in [19].

4   Methodology

To perform the survey, a systematic literature review protocol was followed to maximise the reproducibility, reliability and transparency of the results [17]. The protocol consists of six phases: (1) specify research questions, (2) define search criteria, (3) identify studies, (4) screening, (5) data extraction and (6) results. Figure 1 shows the number of studies reviewed and excluded in each phase and the reasoning behind the exclusion.

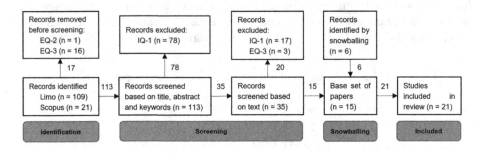

Fig. 1. Search methodology: included and excluded papers.

4.1   Research Questions

In this article, we will study the following research questions (RQs), focusing on the challenges identified in [19]:

- RQ-1: how do primary studies represent human behaviour? One of the challenges when applying PM to smart spaces data is to choose an appropriate formalism that can model human behaviour.
- RQ-2: how do PM techniques address the gap between sensor events and process events? The low-level sensor logs from smart spaces have to be translated to higher-level event logs [32,35].
- RQ-3: how do PM techniques tackle logs that are not split in traces? PM requires the log to be segmented into traces, which is typically not the case of sensor logs.

4.2   Search Criteria and Studies Identification

Since this paper is about using PM to model human behaviour from smart spaces data, three groups were identified: group 1 represents PM, group 2 represents human behaviour modelling and group 3 represents the smart space environment. Frequently used synonyms were added to ensure full coverage of the relevant literature on each topic, yielding the following search query:

("process mining" OR "process discovery") AND ("behaviour pattern" OR "behavior pattern" OR "habit" OR "routine" OR "activity of daily living" OR "activities of daily living" OR "daily life activities" OR "daily-life activities" OR "daily behaviour" OR "daily behavior") AND ("smart space" OR "smart home" OR "smart environment" OR "smart building")

The base set of papers was identified by searching the title, abstract and keywords using the Scopus and Limo online search engines, providing access to articles published by Springer, IEEE, Elsevier, Sage, ACM, MDPI, CEUR-WS, and IOS Press. The final set of articles was retrieved on 05/04/2022.

4.3   Screening

The papers identified by the search string must pass a quality and relevance assessment in order to be included in the survey. The assessment consists of exclusion and inclusion criteria.

The exclusion criteria EQ-x are defined as follows:

- EQ-1: the study is not written in English.
- EQ-2: the item is not fully accessible through the university's online libraries.
- EQ-3: the paper is a duplicate of an item already included in the review.
- EQ-4: the study is a survey or literature review primarily summarising previous work where no new contribution related to the research topic is provided.

The inclusion criterion IQ-x is defined as follows:

- IQ-1: the study is about discovering and modelling human behaviour using PM techniques using smart spaces data and answers at least one research question.

The first set of primary studies was formed by all articles that remain after the inclusion and exclusion criteria screening. Once these studies were selected, forward and backward snowballing was performed. Articles identified through snowballing were screened using the same criteria.

4.4   Data Extraction

First, generic information was extracted such as title, authors, year of publication, and the environment in which the included study is situated. Afterwards, the research questions were answered based on the content of each article.

Table 2. Overview of included primary studies

ID	Ref	Title	Year	Environment	Dataset	Type(s) of sensors	Labelled	Segmentation
S1	[11]	Process Mining for Individualized Behavior Modeling Using Wireless Tracking in Nursing Homes	2013	Healthcare	Own	Proximity	/	T
S2	[4]	Learning and Recognizing Routines and Activities in SOFiA	2014	Office	Own	Motion, Brightness, Light, Temperature, Pressure, Touch and Magnetic	Yes	A
S3	[5]	Incremental Learning of Daily Routines as Workflows in a Smart Home Environment	2015	Home	[6]	Motion, Temperature and Magnetic	Yes	A > A
S4	[7]	Process-Based Habit Mining: Experiments and Techniques	2016	Home	[6]	Motion	Partially	T
S5	[34]	Heuristic approaches for generating Local Process Models through log projections	2016	Home	[38]	Motion, Magnetic and Power	Yes	T
S6	[23]	Revealing daily human activity pattern using PM approach	2017	Home	[25]	Motion, Magnetic and Float	Yes	T
S7	[3]	Discovering Process Models of Activities of Daily Living from Sensors	2018	Home	[6]	Motion, Temperature and Magnetic	Yes	A > A
S8	[36]	Event Abstraction for Process Mining Using Supervised Learning Techniques	2018	Home	[38]	Motion, Magnetic and Power	Partially	T
S9	[29]	Addressing multi-users open challenge in habit mining for a PM-based approach	2018	Home	Own	Proximity	/	T
S10	[33]	Generating time-based label refinements to discover more precise process models	2019	Home	[38]	Motion, Magnetic and Power	No	T > T
S11	[9]	Analyzing of Gender Behaviors from Paths Using Process Mining: A Shopping Mall Application	2019	Commerce	Own	Proximity	No	T > T
S12	[2]	Extraction of User Daily Behavior From Home Sensors Through Process Discovery	2020	Home	[6]	Motion, Temperature and Magnetic	Yes	A > A
S13	[20]	Visual process maps: a visualization tool for discovering habits in smart homes	2020	Home	[6]	Motion	Yes	A
S14	[37]	Process Mining for Activities of Daily Living in Smart Homecare	2020	Healthcare	[30]	Not Specified	Yes	A
S15	[8]	Discovering Customer Paths from Location Data with Process Mining	2020	Commerce	Own	Proximity	No	T > T
S16	[26]	A Multi-case Perspective Analytical Framework for Discovering Human Daily Behavior from Sensors using Process Mining	2021	Home	[31]	Proximity	Yes	A
S17	[15]	Process Model Discovery from Sensor Event Data	2020	Home	[6]	Motion	Partially	T
S18	[10]	Unsupervised Segmentation of Smart Home Logs for Human Habit Discovery	2022	Home	[6]	Motion, Temperature and Magnetic	No	T > T
S19	[22]	Interactive Process Mining in IoT and Human Behaviour Modelling	2021	Home	Own	Motion	No	T
S20	[28]	Supporting Users in the Continuous Evolution of Automated Routines in their Smart Spaces	2021	Home	Simulated	Motion	Yes	T
S21	[18]	The Benefits of Sensor-Measurement Aggregation in Discovering IoT Process Models: A Smart-House Case Study	2021	Home	Simulated	Motion	Yes	T > T

5   Results

Table 2 gives an overview of the studies included in the survey, and provides general information about each study. Figure 2a shows the publication trend over the years.

5.1   Modelling Formalisms

An overview of the modelling formalisms used by the papers surveyed is shown on Fig. 2b (note that some papers used more than one modelling language). Petri Nets are by far the most used formalism, consistent with the fact that it is a very popular process modelling formalism and the output to several state-of-the-art discovery algorithms.

Petri Nets is followed by weighted directed graphs, mostly as the output of the fuzzy miner algorithm [14], which allows to mine flexible models.

A third noteworthy modelling language is timed parallel automata, a formalism introduced in [12] that is designed to be particularly expressive. Other formalisms are less spread, only used by at most two studies. In addition, only S20 uses a modelling formalism that incorporates the process execution context. Also note that S9 only derived an event log from the sensor log and did not mine a model, hence no formalism is used.

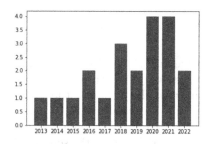

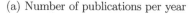

(a) Number of publications per year

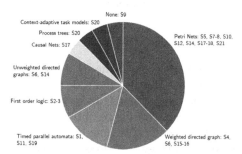

(b) Breakdown of the use of formalisms in the studies

Fig. 2. Statistics about the studies.

5.2   Abstraction Gap Between Sensor Events and Process Events

This section gives an overview of the techniques that the primary studies use to convert sensor events into process events. Among them, S14, S15, S20 and S21 do not require any conversion step because they already work with event logs instead of sensor logs. In particular, S20 and S21 make use of synthetic event logs produced by a simulator. All the other studies have validated their approaches with real-life datasets, as shown in Table 2. Six studies (S1, S2, S9, S11, S15,

S19) have performed the validation step on datasets they generated themselves, all the other ones have applied their methodologies on state-of-the-art datasets, namely [6,25,30,31,38].

Two general approaches to make groups of sensor measurements that correspond to higher-level events can be identified from the literature: (i) classical window-based, time-based or event-based segmentation, and (ii) more complex time-series analysis.

In order to translate raw sensor measurements into proper event labels, the most common method is to derive information from the sensor's location, as in S1, S5, S11, S12, S15, and S19. E.g., if the triggered sensor is above the bed then the activity "sleeping" is derived. However, this method has its drawbacks, acknowledged in S4: the information provided by motion sensors is not always detailed enough to derive activities accurately. These ambiguities could be addressed by introducing other types of sensor in the environment (e.g., cameras), but making the approach more intrusive.

In S13, authors perform the conversion task by adapting an already existing algorithm to automatically segment and assign human actions' labels (i.e., MOVEMENT, AREA or STAY), combined with their relative *location* inside the smart environment (e.g., STAY Kitchen_table).

Using a labelled dataset facilitates this conversion task. Studies S8, S10 and S16 have used such labelling to manually deduce event names. However, this approach can be very time consuming and error prone, and labels often corresponds to activities at a higher level of abstraction with respect to atomic events.

5.3   Log Segmentation into Traces

PM techniques typically need a log to be segmented in traces with a case ID [27], a requirement that is often not met by sensor logs (only the sensor log in S10 meets this requirement). To account for this, most of the included studies use a form of segmentation to obtain an event log made of distinct cases, as shown in Table 2, where T is time-based and A is activity-based. We assume that all studies, even those that do not state it explicitly, at least segment the sensor log in one trace per day to meet the requirement posed by PM techniques.

There are two types of segmentations applied in the studies: manual vs automatic. The following studies perform a manual activity-based segmentation:

- S7 performs activity-based segmentation to segment a log by creating one trace per day. Their approach uses the 'sleeping' activity to determine when two consecutive days should be split.
- S12 uses activity-based segmentation to segment a day into activities. Based on the annotations added by the user, artificial trace start and end events are added to the sensor log (e.g., when a user indicates that he or she is starting the 'cooking' activity, a start event is added to the sensor log).

Alternatively, some approaches try to automatically segment the log. This solution appears more feasible in real scenarios than manual labelling, which is time-consuming and error-prone. In the analysed works, automatic segmentation is performed according to the time dimension following different strategies:

- Using the time-based technique to split days using midnight as cut-off point; such as in S4 and S5.
- Segmenting each day into activities or visits by measuring the gap between two sensor events. When the gap is larger than a predefined threshold, the log is split in two traces; such as S11 or S21.

In addition, if the sensor log contains different human routines a clustering step is usually implemented, such as in S21.

6   Discussion

This section discusses the invistagated challenges and identifies future lines of research.

6.1   Modelling Formalisms

As discussed in Sect. 5.1, papers applying PM to smart spaces data must explicitly or implicitly choose a formalism to represent human processes.

Interestingly, while it is suggested in [19] that human routines are volatile and unpredictable, the most used formalism in the reviewed studies is Petri Nets, an imperative modelling language. This may simply be because Petri Nets are one of the most widely used languages in PM, which allow, a.o., process checking, simulation and enactment.

A certain number of studies opted for more flexible formalisms, e.g., weighted directed graphs. This enables the discovery of clearer and potentially better fitting models, though less precise and actionable. A solution to make those more actionable is to implement prediction techniques, as in S8. It is also remarkable that none of the studies mined declarative models, a widespread flexible paradigm that could be able to cope with the volatility of human behaviour. This may be explained by the fact that declarative models are usually harder to understand than imperative models, making it more complex for the users to interact with the smart space system.

Finally, another important aspect in smart spaces is context-awareness: the process model should be context-aware to adapt to the changes in the environment [1]. This is surprisingly still neglected in current research about PM applied to smart spaces. Only S20 supports the modelling of context adaptive routines by using context-adaptive task models and process trees.

6.2   Abstraction Gap Between Sensor Events and Process Events

The abstraction gap has been recognized as one of the main challenges in BP applied to IoT data [40].

The main challenge here is that the solutions proposed in the literature are dataset- and/or sensor-specific. In most cases only PIR sensor data are available, witnessing the human performing actions in specific areas of the house. This also makes the techniques proposed very sensitive to the distribution of sensors across the environment. In addition, the scarce availability of datasets makes it difficult to evaluate the proposed approaches across multiple scenarios. In most cases, datasets from the CASAS project[1] are used. This does not provide a sufficient heterogeneity to ensure a reliable evaluation.

Finally, input from the broader PM literature could help address this issue. More specifically, generic event abstraction techniques used in PM could also be used to abstract sensor events into process events (see [39]). In addition to this, IoT PM methodologies also propose techniques to extract an event log from sensor data such as, e.g., in S17; a deeper dive in this literature could identify relevant abstraction techniques for smart spaces.

6.3   Log Segmented into Traces

The proposed approaches for segmentation are usually naive (e.g., automatic daily based segmentation) or relying on extensive output from the user (i.e., in manual activity-based segmentation). From this point of view, the open research challenge is to perform segmentation by using the process semantics and the context. An initial proposal has been given in [10] where process model quality measures are used to iteratively segment the log.

In addition to this, segmentation is only a part of the problem, as traces must be clustered in order to produce event logs that are homogeneous from the point of view of instances, which is a prerequisite for PM. This is analogous to the general issue of case ID definition in PM, i.e., pinpointing what an instance of the process is.

6.4   Future Work

First of all, the study of the best modelling formalism for human behaviour is to be continued, as many different languages are used and some languages showing potentially useful characteristics have not been used yet (e.g., declarative models). The choice on the formalism may need to be adapted to the specific application, and transformations between formalisms may also be a viable option to meet diverse needs (understandability, actionability, expressiveness, flexibility, etc.). In addition, the use of contextual information to create more meaningful models remains for a large part unexplored.

Another issue that stands out is the frequent usage of the same datasets by the included studies. A large portion of the included studies use one of the most common datasets from smart homes to perform their research (see Table 2). The scarce availability of these datasets may explain the trend of studies focusing on the home environment (see Table 2). While the use of a common dataset makes

---

[1] See http://casas.wsu.edu/datasets/.

it easier to compare the different methods, it might make some of the techniques less generalisable to other data and other environments.

Another suggestion for future work is to source datasets from more varying environments. Diversifying the application scenario could benefit the research community as this might lead to new insights or techniques. Additionally, simulators could also be developed to generate labelled datasets that can be used to develop and validate PM techniques for different kinds of smart spaces and types of sensors.

7   Conclusions

In this paper, we surveyed the application of PM to smart spaces data. A total of 21 studies were included in the survey and classified according to how they handle three main identified challenges PM techniques need to deal with when analysing smart spaces' data [19]: 1) use of a suitable formalism to represent human behaviour; 2) abstraction gap between sensor events and process events; 3) log segmentation into traces.

The results showed that there are already some suitable solutions for these challenges, achieving the mining from sensor measurements to activities, and sometimes going a step further by identifying habits. However, some important issues still need to be addressed in future work, such as the selection of an appropriate modelling formalism for human behaviour mining, the exploitation of context information, the generalisability of the developed techniques or the challenge of multi-user environments.

References

1. Aztiria, A., Izaguirre, A., Basagoiti, R., Augusto, J.C., Cook, D.J.: Automatic modeling of frequent user behaviours in intelligent environments. In: 2010 IE, pp. 7–12 (2010)
2. Cameranesi, M., Diamantini, C., Mircoli, A., Potena, D., Storti, E.: Extraction of user daily behavior from home sensors through process discovery. IEEE IoT J. 7(9), 8440–8450 (2020)
3. Cameranesi, M., Diamantini, C., Potena, D.: Discovering process models of activities of daily living from sensors. In: Teniente, E., Weidlich, M. (eds.) BPM 2017. LNBIP, vol. 308, pp. 285–297. Springer, Cham (2018). https://doi.org/10.1007/978-3-319-74030-0_21
4. Carolis, B.D., Ferilli, S., Mallardi, G.: Learning and recognizing routines and activities in SOFiA. In: Aarts, E., et al. (eds.) AmI 2014. LNCS, vol. 8850, pp. 191–204. Springer, Cham (2014). https://doi.org/10.1007/978-3-319-14112-1_16
5. Carolis, B.D., Ferilli, S., Redavid, D.: Incremental learning of daily routines as workflows in a smart home environment. ACM TiiS 4(4), 1–23 (2015)
6. Cook, D.J., Crandall, A.S., Thomas, B.L., Krishnan, N.C.: CASAS: a smart home in a box. Computer 46(7), 62–69 (2012)
7. Dimaggio, M., Leotta, F., Mecella, M., Sora, D.: Process-based habit mining: experiments and techniques. In: 2016 Intl IEEE Conferences UIC, pp. 145–152 (2016)

8. Dogan, O.: Discovering customer paths from location data with process mining. EJEST **3**(1), 139–145 (2020)

9. Dogan, O., Bayo-Monton, J.L., Fernandez-Llatas, C., Oztaysi, B.: Analyzing of gender behaviors from paths using process mining: a shopping mall application. Sensors **19**(3), 557 (2019)

10. Esposito, L., Leotta, F., Mecella, M., Veneruso, S.: Unsupervised segmentation of smart home logs for human habit discovery. In: 2022 18th International Conference on Intelligent Environments (IE), pp. 1–8. IEEE (2022)

11. Fernández-Llatas, C., Benedi, J.M., García-Gómez, J.M., Traver, V.: Process mining for individualized behavior modeling using wireless tracking in nursing homes. Sensors **13**(11), 15434–15451 (2013)

12. Fernandez-Llatas, C., Pileggi, S.F., Traver, V., Benedi, J.M.: Timed parallel automaton: a mathematical tool for defining highly expressive formal workflows. In: Fifth Asia Modelling Symposium, pp. 56–61 (2011)

13. Folino, F., Pontieri, L.: Ai-empowered process mining for complex application scenarios: survey and discussion. JoDS **10**(1), 77–106 (2021)

14. Günther, C.W., van der Aalst, W.M.P.: Fuzzy mining – adaptive process simplification based on multi-perspective metrics. In: Alonso, G., Dadam, P., Rosemann, M. (eds.) BPM 2007. LNCS, vol. 4714, pp. 328–343. Springer, Heidelberg (2007). https://doi.org/10.1007/978-3-540-75183-0_24

15. Janssen, D., Mannhardt, F., Koschmider, A., van Zelst, S.J.: Process model discovery from sensor event data. In: Leemans, S., Leopold, H. (eds.) ICPM 2020. LNBIP, vol. 406, pp. 69–81. Springer, Cham (2021). https://doi.org/10.1007/978-3-030-72693-5_6

16. Jobanputra, C., Bavishi, J., Doshi, N.: Human activity recognition: a survey. Proc. Comput. Sci. **155**, 698–703 (2019)

17. Kitchenham, B.: Procedures for performing systematic reviews. Keele UK Keele Univ. **33**(2004), 1–26 (2004)

18. de Leoni, M., Pellattiero, L.: The benefits of sensor-measurement aggregation in discovering IoT process models: a smart-house case study. In: Marrella, A., Weber, B. (eds.) BPM 2021. LNBIP, vol. 436, pp. 403–415. Springer, Cham (2022). https://doi.org/10.1007/978-3-030-94343-1_31

19. Leotta, F., Mecella, M., Mendling, J.: Applying process mining to smart spaces: perspectives and research challenges. In: Persson, A., Stirna, J. (eds.) CAiSE 2015. LNBIP, vol. 215, pp. 298–304. Springer, Cham (2015). https://doi.org/10.1007/978-3-319-19243-7_28

20. Leotta, F., Mecella, M., Sora, D.: Visual process maps: a visualization tool for discovering habits in smart homes. JAIHC **11**(5), 1997–2025 (2020)

21. Leotta, F., Mecella, M., Sora, D., Catarci, T.: Surveying human habit modeling and mining techniques in smart spaces. Future Internet **11**(1), 23 (2019)

22. Lull, J.J., Bayo, J.L., Shirali, M., Ghassemian, M., Fernandez-Llatas, C.: Interactive process mining in IoT and human behaviour modelling. In: Fernandez-Llatas, C. (ed.) Interactive Process Mining in Healthcare. HI, pp. 217–231. Springer, Cham (2021). https://doi.org/10.1007/978-3-030-53993-1_13

23. Ma'arif, M.R.: Revealing daily human activity pattern using process mining approach. In: EECSI 2017, pp. 1–5 (2017)

24. Mannhardt, F., Bovo, R., Oliveira, M.F., Julier, S.: A taxonomy for combining activity recognition and process discovery in industrial environments. In: Yin, H., Camacho, D., Novais, P., Tallón-Ballesteros, A.J. (eds.) IDEAL 2018. LNCS, vol. 11315, pp. 84–93. Springer, Cham (2018). https://doi.org/10.1007/978-3-030-03496-2_10

25. Ordóñez, F.J., De Toledo, P., Sanchis, A.: Activity recognition using hybrid generative/discriminative models on home environments using binary sensors. Sensors **13**(5), 5460–5477 (2013)
26. Prathama, F., Yahya, B.N., Lee, S.L.: A multi-case perspective analytical framework for discovering human daily behavior from sensors using process mining. In: COMPSAC 2021, pp. 638–644 (2021)
27. Reinkemeyer, L.: Process mining in a nutshell. In: Reinkemeyer, L. (ed.) Process Mining in Action, pp. 3–10. Springer, Cham (2020). https://doi.org/10.1007/978-3-030-40172-6_1
28. Serral, E., Schuster, D., Bertrand, Y.: Supporting Users in the continuous evolution of automated routines in their smart spaces. In: Marrella, A., Weber, B. (eds.) BPM 2021. LNBIP, vol. 436, pp. 391–402. Springer, Cham (2022). https://doi.org/10.1007/978-3-030-94343-1_30
29. Sora, D., Leotta, F., Mecella, M.: Addressing multi-users open challenge in habit mining for a process mining-based approach. In: Integrating Research Agendas and Devising Joint Challenges, pp. 266–273 (2018)
30. Sztyler, T., Carmona, J.J.: Activities of daily living of several individuals (2015)
31. Tapia, E., Intille, S., Larson, K.: Activity recognisation in home using simple state changing sensors. Pervasive Comput. **3001**, 158–175 (2004)
32. Tax, N., Alasgarov, E., Sidorova, N., Haakma, R.: On generation of time-based label refinements. arXiv preprint arXiv:1609.03333 (2016)
33. Tax, N., Alasgarov, E., Sidorova, N., Haakma, R., van der Aalst, W.M.: Generating time-based label refinements to discover more precise process models. JAISE **11**(2), 165–182 (2019)
34. Tax, N., Sidorova, N., van der Aalst, W.M., Haakma, R.: Heuristic approaches for generating local process models through log projections. In: 2016 IEEE SSCI, pp. 1–8 (2016)
35. Tax, N., Sidorova, N., Haakma, R., van der Aalst, W.: Mining process model descriptions of daily life through event abstraction. In: Bi, Y., Kapoor, S., Bhatia, R. (eds.) IntelliSys 2016. SCI, vol. 751, pp. 83–104. Springer, Cham (2018). https://doi.org/10.1007/978-3-319-69266-1_5
36. Tax, N., Sidorova, N., Haakma, R., van der Aalst, W.M.P.: Event abstraction for process mining using supervised learning techniques. In: Bi, Y., Kapoor, S., Bhatia, R. (eds.) IntelliSys 2016. LNNS, vol. 15, pp. 251–269. Springer, Cham (2018). https://doi.org/10.1007/978-3-319-56994-9_18
37. Theodoropoulou, G., Bousdekis, A., Miaoulis, G., Voulodimos, A.: Process mining for activities of daily living in smart homecare. In: PCI 2020, pp. 197–201 (2020)
38. Van Kasteren, T., Noulas, A., Englebienne, G., Kröse, B.: Accurate activity recognition in a home setting. In: Proceedings of UbiComp 2008, pp. 1–9 (2008)
39. van Zelst, S.J., Mannhardt, F., de Leoni, M., Koschmider, A.: Event abstraction in process mining: literature review and taxonomy. Granular Comput. **6**(3), 719–736 (2021)
40. Zerbato, F., Seiger, R., Di Federico, G., Burattin, A., Weber, B.: Granularity in process mining: Can we fix it? In: CEUR Workshop Proceedings, vol. 2938, pp. 40–44 (2021)

Building User Journey Games
from Multi-party Event Logs

Paul Kobialka[1]([✉])[iD], Felix Mannhardt[2][iD], Silvia Lizeth Tapia Tarifa[1][iD],
and Einar Broch Johnsen[1][iD]

[1] University of Oslo, Oslo, Norway
{paulkob,sltarifa,einarj}@ifi.uio.no
[2] Eindhoven University of Technology, Eindhoven, The Netherlands
f.mannhardt@tue.nl

Abstract. To improve the user experience, service providers may systematically record and analyse user interactions with a service using event logs. User journeys model these interactions from the user's perspective. They can be understood as event logs created by two independent parties, the user and the service provider, both controlling their share of actions. We propose *multi-party event logs* as an extension of event logs with information on the parties, allowing user journeys to be analysed as weighted games between two players. To reduce the size of games for complex user journeys, we identify *decision boundaries* at which the outcome of the game is determined. Decision boundaries identify subgames that are equivalent to the full game with respect to the final outcome of user journeys. The decision boundary analysis from multi-party event logs has been implemented and evaluated on the BPI Challenge 2017 event log with promising results, and can be connected to existing process mining pipelines.

Keywords: User journeys · Event logs · Weighted games · Decision boundaries

1 Introduction

In a competitive market, a good user experience is crucial for the survival of service providers [1]. User journeys model the interaction of a user (or customer) with a company's services (service provider) from the user's perspective. One of the earliest works to map user journeys was proposed by Bitner *et al.* in the form of service blueprinting [2]. Current tools can model and analyse individual journeys with the aim to improve services from the customers' point of view [3,4].

User journey analysis methods based on event data exploit events recording the user interactions with a service and its underlying information systems. Due to the sequential nature of user-service interactions, process mining techniques

This work is part of the *Smart Journey Mining* project, funded by the Research Council of Norway (grant no. 312198).

© The Author(s) 2023
M. Montali et al. (Eds.): ICPM 2022 Workshops, LNBIP 468, pp. 71–83, 2023.
https://doi.org/10.1007/978-3-031-27815-0_6

that assume grouped sequences of events as input, have been used to analyse user journeys [5–8]. For example, Bernard *et al.* explore and discover journeys from events [7] and Terragni and Hassani use event logs of user journeys to give recommendations [5]. Input events are treated in the same way as for the analysis of business processes: each journey is an instance of a process (case) recorded in a sequence of events (trace) where each event represents an activity occurrence.

In contrast to a business process, which may include numerous actors and systems, a user journey is a sequence of very specific interactions between two parties: the user, and one or more service providers. This invites a specific view on the source event log, where some events are controlled by the user and others by service providers. At the end of the journey, some events represent desirable outcomes for the service provider (positive events) whereas others represent undesirable outcomes (negative events). Such partition of the event log into desired and undesired cases or process outcomes has been explored before. *Deviance mining* classifies cases to investigate deviations from expected behaviour [9]. A binary partition of the event log into positive and negative cases was used in, e.g., logic-based process mining [10,11] and error detection [12]. Outcome prediction aims to predict the outcome of a process case based on a partial trace [13,14]. However, these works do not consider the interactions between user and service providers in user journeys as interactions between independent parties. Results of game theory have previously been used by Saraeian and Shirazi for anomaly detection on mined process models [16] and by Galanti *et al.* for explanations in predictive process mining [17]; in contrast to our work, these works do not use game theory to account for multiple independent parties in the process model.

In this paper, we propose a *multi-party* view for user journeys event logs and present a model reduction based on game theory. We have recently shown how to model and analyse a user journey as a two-player weighted game, in a small event log (33 sequences) from a real scenario that could be manually analysed [15]. However, in scenarios with a large number of complex user journeys, the resulting game can be challenging for manual analysis. This paper introduces a k-sequence transition system extension on the directly follows graph of the multi-party game approach presented in [15], and proposes a novel method to automatically detect *decision boundaries* for user journeys. The method can be useful for the analysis of the journeys since it identifies the parts from where the game becomes deterministic with respect to the outcome of the journey, i.e., the service provider has no further influence on the outcome afterwards. We apply our method to the BPIC'17 dataset [18] as an example of complex user-service interactions, which is available in a public dataset. BPIC'17 does not include information on which activities are controlled by the user (a customer is applying for a loan) and which are controlled by the service provider (a bank). We add this information based on domain knowledge and define *multi-party event logs* as an extension of event logs with party information for user journeys. The application on BPIC'17 demonstrates the feasibility and usefulness of our approach. Our results show that we can automatically detect the most critical parts of the game that guarantees successful and, respectively, unsuccessful, user journeys.

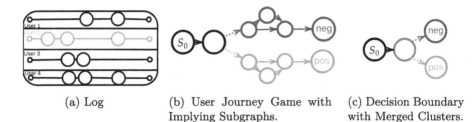

(a) Log

(b) User Journey Game with Implying Subgraphs.

(c) Decision Boundary with Merged Clusters.

Fig. 1. Construction of the decision boundary reduction.

This analysis could be extended with automated methods targeting predictive and prescriptive analysis, e.g., recommendations for process improvement.

The outline of our paper is illustrated in Fig. 1. Section 2 introduces necessary definitions and summarizes *user journey games*. These are extended with a novel game theoretical reduction method in Sects. 3 and 4. Section 5 illustrates our reduction method and the results on BPIC'17 and Sect. 6 concludes the paper.

2   User Journey Games

This section provides background on our previous work on user journey games [15]. The input to the user journey analysis is an *event log* [19] storing records of observations of interactions between a user and one or more service providers. An *event log* L is a multiset of observed *traces* over a set of actions [19]. Given a universe $\mathscr{A}$ of actions, traces $\tau \in L$ are finite, ordered sequences $\langle a_0, \ldots, a_n \rangle$ with $a_i \in \mathscr{A}$, i.e., $L \in \mathcal{B}(\mathscr{A}^*)$. Given an event log L, we introduce the concept of a *multi-party event log* $\mathcal{L} = \langle L, P, I \rangle$ in which each event belongs to a *party*, where P is the set of parties and the function I extends the traces $\tau \in L$ with information for each event about the initiating party from P.

Transition systems $S = \langle \Gamma, A, E, s_0, T \rangle$ have a set Γ of states, a set A of actions (or labels), a transition relation $E \subseteq \Gamma \times A \times \Gamma$, an initial state $s_0 \in \Gamma$ and a set $T \subseteq \Gamma$ of final states. A *weighted transition system* S extends a transition system S, with a weight function w indicating the impact of every event [20]. *Weighted games* partition the events and consider them as actions in a weighted transition system, *controllable* actions A_c and *uncontrollable* actions A_u [21]. Only actions in A_c can be controlled. Actions in A_u are decided by an adversarial environment. When analysing games, we look for a *strategy* that guarantees a desired property, i.e. winning the game by reaching a certain state. A strategy is a partial function $\Gamma \to A_c \cup \{\lambda\}$ deciding the actions of the controller in a given state (here, λ denotes the "wait" action, letting the adversary move).

User journeys capture how a user moves through a service by engaging in so-called *touchpoints*, which are either actions performed by the user or a communication event between the user and a service provider [3]. User journeys are inherently goal-oriented. Users engage in a service to reach a goal, e.g. receiving a loan or visiting a doctor. If they reach the goal, the journey is *successful*, otherwise *unsuccessful*. This can be modelled by a transition system with final states T, and successful goal states from a subset $T_s \subseteq T$: every journey ending in $t \in T_s$ is successful. A journey's success does not only depend on the actions of the service provider—the journey can be seen as a game between service provider and user, where both parties are self-interested and control their share of actions. We define *user journey games* as weighted transition systems with goals and self-interested parties [15]:

Definition 1 (User journey games). *A* user journey game *is a weighted game* $G = \langle \Gamma, A_c, A_u, E, s_0, T, T_s, w \rangle$, *where*

- Γ *are states that represent the touchpoints of the user journey,*
- A_c *and* A_u *are disjoint sets of actions respectively initiated by the service provider and the user,*
- $E \subseteq \Gamma \times A_c \cup A_u \times \Gamma$ *are the possible transitions between touchpoints,*
- $s_0 \in \Gamma$ *is an initial state,*
- $T \subseteq \Gamma$ *are the final states of the game,*
- $T_s \subseteq T$ *are the final states in which the game is successful, and*
- $w : E \to \mathbb{R}$ *specifies the weight associated with the different transitions.*

The analysis of services with a large number of users requires a notion of user feedback [3]: Questionnaires provide a viable solution for services with a limited number of users, but not for complex services with many users. In a user journey game, the weight function w denotes the impact that an interaction has on the journey. A user journey game construction is described in [15]. When building user journey games from event logs, we used Shannon entropy [22] together with majority voting to estimate user feedback without human intervention. The more certain the outcome of a journey becomes after an interaction, the higher the weight of the corresponding edge. *Gas* extends weights to (partial) journeys so they can be compared. Given an event log L and its corresponding weighted transition system S, the gas G of a journey $\tau \in L$ accumulates the weights when replaying τ along the transitions in S, $G(\tau) := \sum_{a_i \in \tau} w(a_i)$.

Formal statements about user journey games can be analysed using a model checker such as UPPAAL STRATEGO [23]. UPPAAL STRATEGO extends the UPPAAL system [24] by games and stochastic model checking, allowing properties to be verified up to a confidence level by simulations (avoiding the full state space exploration). If a statement holds, an enforcing strategy is computed. To strengthen the user-focused analysis of user journeys, we assume that an adversarial environment exposes the worst-case behaviour of the service provider by letting the service provider's actions be controllable and the user's actions uncontrollable. For example, let us define a strategy pos for always reaching a successful final state. Define two state properties positive for a successful and negative for an unsuccessful final state. The keyword control indicates a game with an adversarial environment and A<> searches for a strategy where the flag positive eventually holds at some state in all possible paths of the game:

Algorithm 1. Decision Boundary Detection

Input: User journey game $G = \langle \Gamma, A_c, A_u, E, s_0, T, T_s, w \rangle$, unrolling constant n
Output: Decision Boundary $M \subset \Gamma$
1: Assert Termination of Model Checker
2: Initialize mapping $R : \Gamma \rightarrow \{\mathbf{True}, \mathbf{False}\}$
3: **for** State $s \in \Gamma$ **do**
4:     Game $G' \leftarrow \text{DESCENDANTS}(s)$
5:     Game $G'' \leftarrow \text{ACYCLIC}(G', n)$
6:     Update $R(s) \leftarrow \text{QUERY}(G'')$
7: Set $\Gamma_P \leftarrow \{s \in \Gamma \mid \bigwedge R(s') \quad \forall s' \in \text{DESCENDANTS}(s)\}$
8: Set $\Gamma_N \leftarrow \{s \in \Gamma \mid \bigwedge \neg R(s') \quad \forall s' \in \text{DESCENDANTS}(s)\}$
9: Add State s_{pos} and s_{neg} to G ▷ States implying outcome
10: **for** State $s \in \Gamma$ **do**
11:     **if** $s \in \Gamma_P$ **then** $\text{MERGE}(G, s_{pos}, s)$
12:     **else if** $s \in \Gamma_N$ **then** $\text{MERGE}(G, s_{neg}, s)$
13: $M \leftarrow \emptyset$
14: **for** State $s \in \Gamma$ **do**   ▷ Build decision boundary
15:     **if** $\{s_{pos}, s_{neg}\} = \{t \mid t \in (s, t) \in E\}$ **then** $M \leftarrow M \cup \{s\}$
16: **return** M

```
strategy pos = control: A<> positive .
```

If the strategy pos exists, it can be further analysed and refined to, e.g., minimize
the number of steps or gas to reach a final state within an upper bound time T:

```
strategy min = minE(steps) [t<= T] : <> positive under pos .
```

Strategies can be stochastically evaluated using a number of runs X, e.g., evaluate
the minimal gas of the refined strategy within an upper bound time T:

```
E[t<=T; X] (min: gas) under min.
```

3   Decision Boundaries

A decision boundary abstracts a game to focus on crucial parts from where the
future outcome is decided. Finding the decision boundary in a complex game can
be useful; e.g., there might be no guarantee to find a successful game strategy
pos (see Sect. 2). Such a strategy can only be found for certain states in the
game, which may be scattered around and therefore hard to analyse when using
non-automatic methods. Moreover, detecting the decision boundary that lead
to outcomes in the game from where there is no possibility of recovery can be
used to propose further recommendations for service improvement. Figure 1b
and 1c illustrate the game abstraction using decision boundaries. The red and
green marked parts of the game in Fig. 1b display guaranteeing areas. Once the
journey reached a state within those areas, the outcome becomes deterministic.

Since all reachable states from a red or green state share the same outcome, they can be abstracted away (Fig. 1c).

Algorithm 1 computes the decision boundary for a game G. The mapping R, from states s to Boolean, stores whether there exists a successful strategy pos that starts from each state $s \in \Gamma$ (Lines 2–6). The algorithm computes a reachable sub-game G' for every state s using the function DESCENDANTS(s), which computes the parts of G which are reachable from s by path exploration. Function ACYCLIC(G', n) unrolls n times all loops in G', e.g. by a breadth-first search strategy. An example of loop-unrolling in games is displayed in Fig. 2. The resulting acyclic game G'' is then model checked with QUERY(G'') to look for a successful strategy pos. The result is stored in $R(s)$.

Furthermore, some states are segregated into two sets, Γ_P and Γ_N, based on the results from the previous computation (Lines 7–8). States from which it is only possible to reach positive, respectively negative, results are assigned to Γ_P, respectively Γ_N. States in these sets guarantee the outcome of the game. The game is simplified by abstracting all states in Γ_P, respectively Γ_N, into one state s_{pos}, respectively s_{neg}, using the function MERGE (Lines 9–12). Once one of these states is reached, the journey becomes deterministic; the service provider has no further influence on the final outcome. *The states which point to s_{pos} and s_{neg} form the decision boundary* (Lines 13–15).

4   Mining Decision Boundaries

Event logs obtained from user journeys record actions performed by several parties. A user can send messages to a service offered by a service provider and a service provider can send messages to a user currently using the service. It is common practice that artefacts of these actions are recorded in the service provider's event logs, particularly the order of actions. However, knowledge about which party has triggered which action is commonly ignored while collecting such logs.

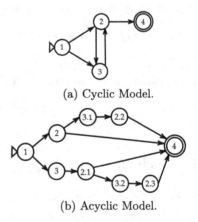

(a) Cyclic Model.

(b) Acyclic Model.

Fig. 2. Unrolling example.

In this paper, we approximate multi-party event logs $\mathcal{L}$ by pre-defining a party function I mapping actions a in event log L to a party in $P = \{C, U\}$, where C denotes the service provider and U the user. For simplicity, we assume that different service provider parties are captured by the same party C.

We can now build a user journey game from a multi-party event log following [15] (see Fig. 1 for an overview). We then extend the obtained directly follows graph to a k-sequence transition system $S_L^k = \langle \Gamma, A, E, s_0, T \rangle$ [25], which considers states that record the last k actions happening in the traces of L and stores them in a single state; e.g., the 2-action states of trace $\langle a, b, c \rangle$

are $\{\langle a \rangle, \langle a, b \rangle, \langle b, c \rangle\}$. This abstraction captures more information in the game, improving the precision of the game and the alignment between game and log.

We insert an initial state s_0 at the beginning of each trace $\tau \in L$, and a final state $t \in T$ at the end of each trace $\tau \in L$. Let H denote the set of states corresponding to the k-sequence abstraction for all traces in L, then the states are defined by $\Gamma \subseteq \{s_0\} \cup T \cup H$. The transition relation E is constructed over adjacent actions in all traces $\tau \in L$. An edge (s_i, a_{i+1}, s_{i+1}) is in E if there is a trace $\tau \in L$ where the last action in state s_i is followed by the last action a_{i+1} in s_{i+1}. A transition with action a_{i+1} in S_L^k, means that the corresponding action has also been performed in τ.

The constructed transition system S_L^k is transformed into a user journey game by computing the weights on the transitions (see Sect. 2), and applying function I to compute the set $A_c = \{a \mid I(a) = C\}$ of actions controlled by the service provider and the set $A_u = \{a \mid I(a) = U\}$ of actions controlled by the user. The user journey game is used to compute its decision boundary (Sect. 3). States behind the decision boundary are merged into *successful* and *unsuccessful* states (Fig. 1c). The result is a strongly reduced game preserving all information on the decision structure.

5   Evaluation on BPIC'17

The BPI Challenge 2017 (BPIC'17) [18] provides an event log recording actions in loan applications from a Dutch financial institute. Since this event log has records of interactions between users and a service provider, including calls, it is a suitable event log for user journey analysis. However, we needed to make assumptions to complete the missing information for our scenario, e.g., which journeys are successful or unsuccessful and infer the party function I with knowledge about which actions are triggered by which party.

The event log contains activities from the following groups: Application (A), Offer (O) and Workflow (W) [26]. Recorded journeys in the log can end with three different states: (1) an offer is accepted, (2) the application is declined, or (3) the application is cancelled. We define a party function I, based on domain knowledge and official information given in the BPIC'17 forum.[1] We assume that only users can *cancel*, *submit* or *complete* an application, and that users decide whether *calls* take place. We further assume that accepted offers are successful journeys, cancellations are unsuccessful journeys: both parties would prefer a different outcome since the user spent time in the service and the bank invested resources, and declined applications are neither successful nor unsuccessful journeys: users followed the whole process without achieving their goal (the bank has to decline certain offers to protect the users, e.g., from unsustainable debt). We exclude declined application journeys from the analysis, given their ambiguity.

BPIC'17 is known to include a substantial change in the service provider's process, called a *concept drift* [27], in July 2016. To investigate how this change impacts the user journey game, we split the log at this month and investigate

---

[1] https://www.win.tue.nl/promforum/categories/-bpi-challenge-2017.

both parts separately. The first part contains traces until 30.06.2016, while the second part contains traces after 01.08.2016.

5.1 User Journey Game Generation

We now report on the generation of the user journey game for the BPIC'17 event log, with focus on the preprocessing of the data. The full implementation is given in the accompanying artefact.[2] We pre-processed BPIC'17 by discretising the call durations according to their length, tagging different offers inside one trace, and ignoring incomplete journeys. This was necessary since records of call durations vary between seconds to hours and several call interactions in one journey consist of repeated adjacent occurrences of events associated to one call. To discretise the duration, we first aggregate repeated and adjacent calls. After the aggregation, we consider calls with duration under 10 min as "short"; between 10 min and 4 h as "long"; and above 4 h as "super long". Single calls with a speaking time below 60 s are omitted in the aggregation. Records of multiple offers can be present in the same journey. One of these offers can be accepted while the remaining are cancelled. To simplify journeys, every event associated to an offer or cancellation is ignored after one of the offers is accepted. Offers are automatically cancelled if there is no response after 20 days. We differentiate between actively cancelled offers and cancellations due to time-out, and ignore incomplete journeys and journeys with declined applications.

We further simplify the event log by removing events that do not influence the journey; e.g., *W_Call after offers* is always followed by *A_Complete*, therefore one of them can be removed systematically. We removed outliers and only kept journeys whose variance is present in the corresponding log more than once. Journeys resulting in a cancellation are considered unsuccessful, thus S_{neg} is attached to them; S_{pos} is attached to the successful ones. After preprocessing, we generated the user journey game, following the method of Sect. 4. We first generated the transition system S_L^3, with sequence history 3. The party function I and weight w transformed S_L^3 into a user journey game.

5.2 Simulation

Stochastic simulations can help a service provider to evaluate strategies, to guide their users along their services, before implementing them. We evaluated different strategies on the user journey game for BPIC'17 until July, using UPPAAL STRATEGO to learn and compare the outcomes. In the experiments reported in this section, we consider three strategies. In the strategy max, the service

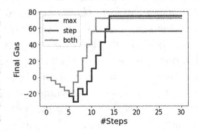

Fig. 3. Simulations under different strategies.

[2] https://github.com/smartjourneymining/bpi_games/releases/tag/EdbA22.

provider can guide the user through the service by maximizing the final gas, while in the strategy step the service provider is minimising the expected number of steps. We also consider a strategy with the combination of both, both. Furthermore, we treat the user as controllable to allow a comparative analysis between the strategies, so that all the strategies reach a positive final state.

The simulations in Fig. 3 show the developments of the gas value under different strategies. The simulations reveal that users have to endure a dip in their gas at the beginning of their journey to reach the positive final state. From the customer's perspective, it is not optimal to have negative experiences (negative gas) to complete the service successfully. The strategy max achieves the highest amount of gas, 33% above step, but it also causes the largest minimum, 50% more than step, within the dip. The strategy step reduces the number of taken steps by 30%, and improves the gas minimum by 33%, but it also reduces the final gas by 25%. The combined strategy both maximizes the final gas while minimising the expected number of steps, and yields a comparable high maximum as max, while reducing the number of steps by 22% and holding steps's improved minimum.

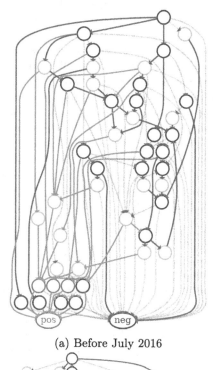

(a) Before July 2016

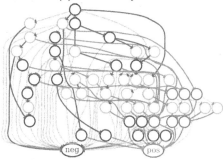

(b) From August 2016

Fig. 4. Decision boundaries (Blue) for both BPIC'17 Event Logs. (Color figure online)

5.3 Decision Boundary

An exhaustive search over all states revealed the decision boundaries for both BPIC'17 event logs, using the algorithm in Algorithm 1. Figure 4a shows the decision boundary for the first part, i.e. until July, and Fig. 4b for the second part. The states *positive* and *negative* incorporate all states with a certain outcome. Blue states mark the decision boundary. Time-out cancellation edges are violet, edges with a positive weight are green and edges with a negative weight are red.

We first report on the outcomes of the analysis for the first event log and then for the second one. Our analysis revealed the existence of few paths to successful final states, and that several journeys time-out very far into the application process.

Analysing the decision boundary reveals that most states are negatively biased and have a direct connection to *negative*. With uncontrollable user actions, the service provider has no means to guide the user to a successful outcome, except for a small positive cluster around *positive*. Most positive states require long journeys. A detailed analysis reveals that four out of five states in the decision boundary are related to calls. The action *"W_Call incomplete files"* leads to the decision boundary from two states and *"O_Sent (online only)"* (only sending the offer online) from two other states.

The figure reveals many time-out cancellations from various states during the journey, even for paths that are very far into the application process. Such cancellations are unsatisfactory for both the service provider and user, since both parties invested time and resources into the journey and preferred a different outcome. The service provider can draw two action recommendations: reaching the positive outcome should be simplified, thus the decision boundary could be extended, and well-progressed journeys should be increasingly prevented from time-outs, thus reducing the number of time-outs of progressed journeys.

Figure 4b shows the process model for the later data set. The figure shows that the process model changed significantly after the concept drift in Juli 2016. The new decision boundary inherits all states except one and contains one new state. The positioning of the new boundary has improved. The decision boundary improved in two parts: it reaches further into the negative part of the game and increased in size. While the previous decision boundary contained only five states, the updated decision boundary contains seven states. The updated decision boundary includes four out of five states of the previous decision boundary and the fifth state lies now before the decision boundary. Additionally, it contains three new states: one was previously in the positive cluster, one was prior to the decision boundary and one new state.

Besides the total number of nodes also the reachability of the decision boundary improved. The number of nodes reaching the decision boundary increased by $\frac{1}{3}$. The amount of timeouts within advanced journeys is reduced. Customers that continue far into the journey are more prone to finish successfully or to cancel by themselves. The average number of actions from start to time-out reduced from 5.4375 to 5, thus the user journey improved generally.

The service provider can now start to investigate the actions related to states in the decision boundary.

6   Conclusion

This paper proposes a novel view on user journey event logs by introducing multi-party event logs that differentiate between the actors of actions leading to events. To promote a user-centric view, the service provider is modelled as controllable and the user as uncontrollable. Based on such a multi-party event log, we show how to use user journey games to model the interaction between user and service provider, and use model checking to find strategies with guaranteed outcomes.

We introduce an analysis to identify *decision boundaries*; these constitute a crucial part of a game at which the outcome of the user journey is determined. Decision boundaries are useful since strategies that guarantee a positive outcome for all paths are unlikely in complex user journeys. The decision boundary additionally serves to reduce the size of the game. This enables us to apply the user journey game approach to the BPIC'17 dataset, which is a real-life event log of a complex user journey that can be transformed to a multi-party event log. The decision boundary gives clear insights into determining factors for the BPIC'17 user journey before and after a concept drift. Our analysis reveals the changes done in the workflow and demonstrates the support and applicability for further analysis through our method, assuming a transformation of the BPIC'17 event log into a multi-party event log, and assuming that users actually have an influence on their journey through their active decisions.

User journey games and decision boundary analysis open many interesting directions for future work. We plan to combine user journey games with well-established process mining tools to discover process models for behaviour leading to determining states. Furthermore, we would like to automate recommendations for improvement, based on the decision boundary. While the decision boundary is helpful for analysing the interaction between a user and service providers, the analysis is still hand-made. We also plan to generalise the approach to cyclic models to make it agnostic to the current unrolling bound n in each cycle. Furthermore, we would like to investigate probabilistic games to capture ambiguities within user actions. Finally, we would like to implement a multi-party event log in cooperation with companies to study real interactions between user and service provider.

References

1. Fornell, C., Mithas, S., Morgeson, F.V., Krishnan, M.: Customer satisfaction and stock prices: high returns, low risk. J. Mark. **70**(1), 3–14 (2006)
2. Bitner, M.J., Ostrom, A.L., Morgan, F.N.: Service blueprinting: a practical technique for service innovation. Calif. Manage. Rev. **50**(3), 66–94 (2008)
3. Rosenbaum, M.S., Otalora, M.L., Ramírez, G.C.: How to create a realistic customer journey map. Bus. Horiz. **60**(1), 143–150 (2017)
4. Halvorsrud, R., Kvale, K., Følstad, A.: Improving service quality through customer journey analysis. J. Serv. Theory Pract. **26**(6), 840–867 (2016)
5. Terragni, A., Hassani, M.: Optimizing customer journey using process mining and sequence-aware recommendation. In: Proceedings of the 34th Symposium on Applied Computing (SAC 2019), pp. 57–65. ACM Press (2019)
6. Bernard, G., Andritsos, P.: Contextual and behavioral customer journey discovery using a genetic approach. In: Welzer, T., Eder, J., Podgorelec, V., Kamišalić Latifić, A. (eds.) ADBIS 2019. LNCS, vol. 11695, pp. 251–266. Springer, Cham (2019). https://doi.org/10.1007/978-3-030-28730-6_16

7. Bernard, G., Andritsos, P.: A process mining based model for customer journey mapping. In: Proceedings of the Forum and Doctoral Consortium Papers at the 29th International Conference on Advanced Information Systems Engineering (CAiSE 2017). CEUR Workshop Proceedings, vol. 1848, pp. 49–56. CEUR-WS.org (2017)

8. Hassani, M., Habets, S.: Predicting next touch point in a customer journey: a use case in telecommunication. In: European Conference on Modeling and Simulation (2021)

9. Nguyen, H., Dumas, M., La Rosa, M., Maggi, F.M., Suriadi, S.: Mining business process deviance: a quest for accuracy. In: Meersman, R., et al. (eds.) OTM 2014. LNCS, vol. 8841, pp. 436–445. Springer, Heidelberg (2014). https://doi.org/10.1007/978-3-662-45563-0_25

10. Lamma, E., Mello, P., Riguzzi, F., Storari, S.: Applying inductive logic programming to process mining. In: Blockeel, H., Ramon, J., Shavlik, J., Tadepalli, P. (eds.) ILP 2007. LNCS (LNAI), vol. 4894, pp. 132–146. Springer, Heidelberg (2008). https://doi.org/10.1007/978-3-540-78469-2_16

11. Bellodi, E., Riguzzi, F., Lamma, E.: Probabilistic declarative process mining. In: Bi, Y., Williams, M.-A. (eds.) KSEM 2010. LNCS (LNAI), vol. 6291, pp. 292–303. Springer, Heidelberg (2010). https://doi.org/10.1007/978-3-642-15280-1_28

12. Rubin, V.A., Mitsyuk, A.A., Lomazova, I.A., van der Aalst, W.M.: Process mining can be applied to software too! In: Proceedings of the 8th ACM/IEEE International Symposium on Empirical Software Engineering and Measurement, pp. 1–8 (2014)

13. Teinemaa, I., Dumas, M., Rosa, M.L., Maggi, F.M.: Outcome-oriented predictive process monitoring: Review and benchmark. ACM Trans. Knowl. Discov. Data **13**(2), 17:1–17:57 (2019)

14. Kratsch, W., Manderscheid, J., Röglinger, M., Seyfried, J.: Machine learning in business process monitoring: a comparison of deep learning and classical approaches used for outcome prediction. Bus. Inf. Syst. Eng. **63**(3), 261–276 (2021)

15. Kobialka, P., Tapia Tarifa, S.L., Bergersen, G.R., Johnsen, E.B.: Weighted games for user journeys. In: Schlingloff, B.H., Chai, M. (eds.) SEFM 2022. LNCS, vol. 13550, pp. 253–270. Springer, Cham (2022). https://doi.org/10.1007/978-3-031-17108-6_16

16. Saraeian, S., Shirazi, B.: Process mining-based anomaly detection of additive manufacturing process activities using a game theory modeling approach. Comput. Industr. Eng. **146**, 106584 (2020)

17. Galanti, R., Coma-Puig, B., de Leoni, M., Carmona, J., Navarin, N.: Explainable predictive process monitoring. In: Proceedings of the ICPM, pp. 1–8. IEEE (2020)

18. van Dongen, B.: BPI Challenge 2017 (2017). https://doi.org/10.4121/uuid:3926db30-f712-4394-aebc-75976070e91f

19. van der Aalst, W.M.P.: Process Mining - Data Science in Action. Springer, Heidelberg (2016). https://doi.org/10.1007/978-3-662-49851-4

20. Thrane, C., Fahrenberg, U., Larsen, K.G.: Quantitative analysis of weighted transition systems. J. Log. Algebraic Program. **79**(7), 689–703 (2010)

21. Bouyer, P., Cassez, F., Fleury, E., Larsen, K.G.: Optimal strategies in priced timed game automata. In: Lodaya, K., Mahajan, M. (eds.) FSTTCS 2004. LNCS, vol. 3328, pp. 148–160. Springer, Heidelberg (2004). https://doi.org/10.1007/978-3-540-30538-5_13

22. Shannon, C.E.: A mathematical theory of communication. Bell Syst. Tech. J. **27**(3), 379–423 (1948)

23. David, A., Jensen, P.G., Larsen, K.G., Mikučionis, M., Taankvist, J.H.: UPPAAL STRATEGO. In: Baier, C., Tinelli, C. (eds.) TACAS 2015. LNCS, vol. 9035, pp. 206–211. Springer, Heidelberg (2015). https://doi.org/10.1007/978-3-662-46681-0_16

24. Larsen, K.G., Pettersson, P., Yi, W.: UPPAAL in a nutshell. Intl. J. Softw. Tools Technol. Transf. **1**(1–2), 134–152 (1997)

25. van der Aalst, W.M.P., Rubin, V., Verbeek, H.M.W., van Dongen, B.F., Kindler, E., Günther, C.W.: Process mining: a two-step approach to balance between under-fitting and overfitting. Softw. Syst. Model. **9**(1), 87–111 (2010)

26. Rodrigues, A.M.B., et al.: Stairway to value: mining a loan application process. https://www.win.tue.nl/bpi/lib/exe/fetch.php?media=2017:bpi2017_winner_academic.pdf

27. Adams, J.N., van Zelst, S.J., Quack, L., Hausmann, K., van der Aalst, W.M.P., Rose, T.: A framework for explainable concept drift detection in process mining. In: Polyvyanyy, A., Wynn, M.T., Van Looy, A., Reichert, M. (eds.) BPM 2021. LNCS, vol. 12875, pp. 400–416. Springer, Cham (2021). https://doi.org/10.1007/978-3-030-85469-0_25

Leveraging Event Data for Measuring Process Complexity

Maxim Vidgof[1][(✉)] [iD] and Jan Mendling[1,2] [iD]

[1] Wirtschaftsuniversität Wien, Welthandelsplatz 1, 1020 Vienna, Austria
`maxim.vidgof@wu.ac.at`
[2] Humboldt-Universität zu Berlin, Unter den Linden 6, 10099 Berlin, Germany
`jan.mendling@hu-berlin.de`

Abstract. Complexity is an important aspect of business processes. Numerous metrics have been introduced to measure process complexity, however, existing metrics view processes merely as sequences of activities, disregarding the corresponding data. This is a major omission since much of the complexity of business processes stems from the variation of data that is associated with it. In this paper, we refer to recent research on how behavioral complexity of business processes can be defined. More specifically, we extend entropy-based complexity metrics such that they are capable of capturing the variation of event data. We provide some first insights into the implications of applying these newly proposed metrics.

Keywords: Process complexity · Event data · Graph entropy

1 Introduction

The central objectives of Business Process Management (BPM) is the improvement of process performance [5]. One of the factors hampering process performance is complexity. For this reason, it is key prerequisite for process improvement to be able to, first, measure process complexity in an appropriate way and, then, define measures to address it.

Prior research has contributed to our understanding of how process complexity can be measured based on event logs [1]. However, it is an important omission that these event-log measures are defined purely based on the behaviour aspects of event sequences. This neglects observations from work on process standardization that identified eleven theoretical dimensions that are tied to process standardization [13]. Notably, two of them relate to inputs & outputs and to data. Also other fields like Machine Learning acknowledge the importance of data complexity and its impact on results of, e.g., prediction models. So far, there is no process complexity measure that reflects the complexity of data.

In this paper, we address this research problem and discuss how the complexity of process-related data can be integrated with process complexity measures. To this end, we extend an existing entropy-based process complexity metric with

© The Author(s) 2023
M. Montali et al. (Eds.): ICPM 2022 Workshops, LNBIP 468, pp. 84–95, 2023.
https://doi.org/10.1007/978-3-031-27815-0_7

aspects of process-related event data. We provide a preliminary evaluation on an artificial as well as a real-life event logs and discuss directions for future work.

The remainder of this paper is organized as follows. Section 2 introduces existing complexity metrics and their limitations. Section 3 presents our approach. Section 4 shows the preliminary evaluation, its discussion and limitations of this paper. Section 5 concludes the paper.

2   Background

This section discusses the background of our research. We first reflect upon prior contributions to measuring process complexity based on event logs. Then we turn to approaches from neighboring fields on how to measure data complexity.

2.1   Process Complexity Metrics

Over the years, several process complexity metrics have been introduced. They have focused on one of the following aspects: size, variability and distance. Size-based metrics count properties of an event log, such as the number of events, traces, average trace length, etc. Metrics related to variability show the variation in the event log, they often build transition matrices based on directly-follows relations observed in the event log [1] or use the number of unique sequences in the log [12]. Distance-based metrics measure the difference between traces in the event log, e.g. affinity of two event sequences, i.e. the extent to which the directly-follow relations of the sequences overlap [6].

Recently, complexity metrics based on graph entropy have been introduced: *variant entropy, normalized variant entropy, sequence entropy* and *normalized sequence entropy* [1]. The latter one has been proven to capture all the three aspects of process complexity and also correlate with the complexity of the discovered process models. A major drawback of all these metrics is, however, that they are sill solely focused on the behavior and ignore event data.

2.2   Data Complexity Metrics

Machine Learning domain has a long history of measuring data complexity. This is not surprising as the complexity of the input data is expected to influence the performance of the predictions. Researchers in the Machine Learning domain generally used three kinds of complexity metrics proposed in [7] and [8]:

1. Measure of overlap: Fisher's discriminant ratio (F1), volume of overlap region (F2), feature efficiency (F3).
2. Measure of class separability: The minimized sum of the error distance of a linear classifier (L1), training error of linear classifier (L2), the ratio of average intra/inter class nearest neighbor distance (N2), leave one out error rate of the 1-NN classifier (N3).

3. Measure of geometry, topology and density of manifolds: Nonlinearity of linear classifier by Linear programming (L3), nonlinearity of 1-NN classifier (N4), space covering by ϵ-neighborhoods (T1), average number of points per dimension (T2), density (D1).

These metrics have been widely used for different tasks, e.g. [9] uses them for the selection of suitable normalization technique for a particular classification problem, [10] uses some of the data complexity measures to estimate the significant intervals for oversampling.

However, such complexity metrics have limited applicability in the process mining domain. First, these metrics measure assume the data has class labels and, moreover, implicitly assume that these labels are fixed. They then measure complexity with respect to this classes, e.g. overlap between classes or class separability. While such metrics seem useful for some applications, e.g. categorical outcome prediction in Predictive Process Monitoring, they would provide little help when the data is not split into classes at all or these classes are not relevant for the problem at hand, e.g. remaining time prediction. Furthermore, even if useful, such metrics would give different results for the same data depending on the problem, e.g. if the same dataset is used for categorical outcome and next activity prediction, the classes for two problems would be different and thus the complexity measurements. Second, a study has shown that while some of the data complexity metrics provide useful information, e.g. are connected with classifier performance, they cannot be used to compare different datasets wihh different characteristics [2]. Finally, these metrics ultimately treat the data as a sample of independent observations, ignoring the process notion and the corresponding relations between the data points, i.e. events. This might be a critical drawbacks for process mining applications.

While the former drawbacks could theoretically be fixed by taking a step back and using entropy or Gini index of the entire dataset as a metric of complexity, the latter problem of losing the process notion would still persist. Thus, our goal in this paper is to extend an existing process complexity metric with the capability of considering data complexity as well.

3   Approach

In order to incorporate data complexity into a process complexity metric, we extend the existing complexity metrics based on graph entropy [1]. First, we introduce Enriched Extended Prefix Automata that include event data. Second, we introduce cumulative complexity metrics that allow to study in more detail how the complexity changes as new events are observed.

Extended Prefix Automata (EPA), introduced in [1], are a representation of business processes without abstraction. However, in its basic form, an EPA only contains information about the behavior. It means, the transitions between states are only labeled with activity labels, and the events in the EPA only contain activity label, case ID timestamp and a link to the predecessor event.

Enriched EPAs, or EEPAs for short, are EPAs enriched with other event data. In essence, it is achieved in the following way. First, an event in the EEPA does not only contain its basic attributes (case ID, activity label, timestamp and predecessor) but also an Attribute Container, where all trace and event attributes are stored. The distinction between trace and event attributes is made in order to prevent name collisions, otherwise these attributes are treated equally, and each event in the trace contains all trace attributes of its trace. The EEPA containing such events is then a state automaton with guards. Thus, the transitions of an EEPA are labeled not only with activity labels but also with corresponding attribute values. In order to follow a transition on EEPA, the event thus should have not only a matching activity label but also matching attributes. In case there is no matching transition, a new partition with new state and a corresponding new transition is added to an EEPA, in the same way as a new partition is added to an EPA on a previously unobserved prefix. One can then apply the same complexity metrics to an EEPA as to an EPA – *variant entropy, normalized variant entropy, sequence entropy* and *normalized sequence entropy* – but they will now take data into account as well because the underlying EEPA is partitioned based on behavior and the data.

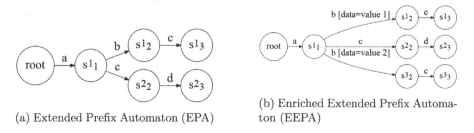

(a) Extended Prefix Automaton (EPA)   (b) Enriched Extended Prefix Automaton (EEPA)

Fig. 1. Difference between an extended prefix automaton and an enriched extended prefix automaton built from the same event log.

Figure 1 shows the difference between an EPA and an EEPA built from the same event log $L = [\langle a, b, c \rangle^2, \langle a, c, d \rangle]$ where in of the $\langle a, b, c \rangle$ traces the activity b carries event data *value*1 and in the second one *value*2. While the EPA only has 2 partitions and both $\langle a, b, c \rangle$ traces belong to partition 1, the corresponding EEPA makes difference between these two traces based on the event data and thus puts these traces in 2 different partitions and has 3 partitions in total. This necessarily means an EEPA would have more states and partitions than an EPA built from the same log, leading to higher variant entropy. An EEPA is also expected to have higher sequence entropy and normalized sequence entropy as it has more partitions with the same number of events. This is, however, not necessarily the case for normalized variant entropy exactly because an EEPA has more partitions but at the same time more states than a corresponding EPA.

It is important to note though that attribute selection plays a crucial role in building an EEPA. If an event log is rich in attributes, including them all might lead to an EEPA where every trace is represented with a separate partition, which is not too insightful. First, it is recommended to use only categorical variables, since numeric ones have a much lower probability to coincide on different events. Thus, existing numerical attributes should either be disregarded or transformed into categorical bins, where the size of the bins also has significant impact and thus should be chosen with caution. Second, for the same reason it might be meaningful to also perform similar binning even on categorical attributes in case they have a large number of values. Finally, one should consider based on the value ranges as well as the attribute description whether the attribute is relevant at all and possibly reduce the pool of attributes used.

Our claim is that data adds an additional layer of complexity on top of behavior. Thus, it is interesting to observe how complexity of a process increases over time by adding new data values while the behavior stays exactly the same. In order to do so, we also introduce the concept of cumulative complexity. That is, we want to not only measure the total complexity of the entire log but also want to see how it evolved, i.e. how new behavior and/or data influenced the complexity. To this end, we introduce the concept of an *active event* which is an event in the (E)EPA that happened (arbitrarily far in the past) before some threshold timestamp, i.e. an event having a timestamp smaller than some given threshold. Similarly, an *active state* is a state in an (E)EPA that includes at least one active event. Then we only consider active events/states for measuring sequence and variant entropy, respectively.

By gradually increasing the threshold, we can add more and more events to the (E)EPA as if we were building it in real time and get the complexity metrics at each point in time, e.g. at the end of each week, month, year, etc. It is equivalent to measuring complexity after each period and then continuing to build the (E)EPA, however, can be repeated indefinitely with different time granularity over the same automaton. In addition, it enables to use two kinds of normalization.

Normally, the variant and sequence entropy are calculated using all states/events in an EPA. Then, the normalization is done by dividing the metric by $|X|log(|X|)$, where $|X|$ is the total number of states/events in the EPA. When normalizing cumulative metrics, however, there are two possibilities. While variant and sequence entropy are obviously measured over active states/events, when it comes to normalization these metrics can be divided by either the number of active states/events or by the total number of the states/events in the full (E)EPA (containing the full event log). The former option would be indeed equivalent to measuring normalized metrics at the end of each time period, and the latter one allows to observe cumulative growth of the normalized metrics over time. These 6 cumulative complexity metrics – *variant entropy, variant entropy normalized over active states, variant entropy normalized over all states, sequence entropy, sequence entropy normalized over active events, sequence entropy nor-*

malized over all events – equip us with the means of observing how new events (carrying new behavior and/or data) influence the complexity.

4 Evaluation

In this section, we present the preliminary evaluation of our approach. First, with an artificial event log and then with real-life event logs. Next, we discuss our results and report current limitations. The implementation is publicly available on GitHub[1].

4.1 Artificial Event Log

We use an example loan process application from [5] shown in Fig. 2. We manually created an event log with 10 traces. All events have a user associated with it. The event *Loan application received* is always associated with a user *System*, which is not considered further. The events associated with the activity *Assess loan risk* have a categorical variable *Risk* and the events associated with the activity *Appraise property* have a numerical variable *Price*. In the first month, there are 4 traces following 2 variants with 1 user and 2 risk levels. In the second month, additional 2 variants are introduced. In the third month, additional user is added who follows the same variants. Finally, in the fourth month additional risk level is added, while the users and variants are kept the same. The prices vary over the entire event log.

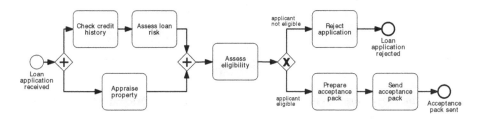

Fig. 2. Loan process, reused from [5].

We then computed the four complexity metrics – variant entropy, normalized variant entropy, sequence entropy and normalized sequence entropy – for this log but varied the data that we took into consideration. Table 1 shows the results. The first row corresponds to an EPA that only considers the behavior and uses no data. The second row corresponds to an EEPA that only uses the *User* variable of the events, and so on. We also split the numeric price into 3 bins to show how numeric data can also be incorporated.

As we can see, the complexity of the EEPAs using additional data on top of behavior is considerably higher than the complexity of an EPA. We also see

---

[1] https://github.com/MaxVidgof/process-complexity.

Table 1. Complexity of the artificial event log using different amount of event data.

Data	Variant entropy	Normalized variant entropy	Sequence entropy	Normalized sequence entropy
None	16.25	0.4	47.16	0.17
User	42.58	0.53	95.64	0.35
User & Risk	80.0	0.56	118.52	0.44
User & Risk & Price (binned)	109.12	0.59	135.94	0.50
User & Risk & Price (numeric)	109.12	0.59	135.94	0.50

that all metrics continue to grow as we consider more variables since it leads to higher partition counts in the EEPA.

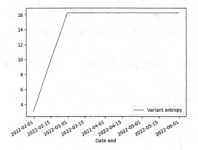
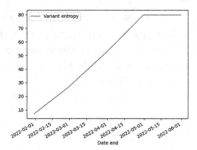

(a) Cumulative variant entropy of simple EPA

(b) Cumulative variant entropy of EEPA with *User* and *Risk*

Fig. 3. Cumulative variant entropy for simple EPA and an enriched EPA with *User* and *Risk* event data.

Cumulative complexity metrics also enable us to observe how the complexity changes as new events are observed. For instance, Fig. 3 shows the development of variant entropy. When only behavior is considered (Fig. 3a), the complexity stops growing as soon as all variants are observed. When the event data is also taken into account (Fig. 3b), however, variant entropy continues to grow even when all variants are observed because of the new data: new user introduced in March and new risk level added in April.

4.2   Real-Life Event Logs

We also conducted a preliminary evaluation of our technique on the Business Process Intelligence Challenge logs from years 2012 [4], 2013 [11] and 2015 [3].

For each event log, we did the following. First, we filtered the event logs such that they contain only categorical attributes, i.e. we removed all attributes having numeric values or representing dates. Second, we generated an Extended Prefix Automaton from each log. We will further refer to these automata as simple EPAs. We calculated variant entropy, normalized variant entropy, sequence entropy and normalized sequence entropy for each of these simple EPAs. Furthermore, we calculated cumulative metrics – variant entropy, variant entropy normalized over active states, variant entropy normalized over all states, sequence entropy, sequence entropy normalized over active events, sequence entropy normalized over all events – for each month from the month of the rirst event in the respective log to the month of the last event. Then, we generated Enriched Extended Prefix Automata (enriched EPAs or EEPAs) from the same logs repeated the same procedures, i.e. calculated the 4 total complexity metrics as well as 6 cumulative complexity metrics over time. As a result, for each log we had 4 complexity metrics for the corresponding simple EPA, 4 complexity metrics of the corresponding EEPA, 6 time series of cumulative complexity metrics for the EPA and 6 time series of cumulative complexity metrics for the EEPA.

First, we wanted to evaluate whether the new metrics adequately depict the additional complexity introduced by event data. Two-sided t-test reported significant difference between normalized sequence entropy of the enriched and the simple EPA. In all cases, except the normalized variant entropy, the metric for the enriched EPA was greater than of its simple counterpart. Thus, we also performed one-sided t-tests. While the p-values were considerably smaller in all cases, normalized sequence entropy still remained the only one with significant difference (p-value 0.01). Interestingly, difference in variant entropy was also close to significant (p-value 0.09). More observations might render it significant as well.

For each of the logs we also compared the time series of the 6 cumulative complexity metrics measured with the simple and enriched EPAs. Here, we not only performed two-sided t-tests that would say whether the difference in means of the two samples is significant but also performed two-sided Kolmogorov-Smirnov tests that would assess whether two samples come from the same continuous distribution. It is important to note that some event logs carry events from before the observation period, e.g. BPIC 2012 includes some events from late 2011. This introduces periods having only 1 event and thus entropy metrics equalling 0, which might influence the value distribution. Thus, in such cases we also filter the metrics for the corresponding event log, keeping only non-zero observations. Periods with non-zero observations are naturally the same for the metrics computed with EPA and EEPA.

The results of these tests can be seen in Table 2. The columns in the table represent the metric, the rows are different time series pairs (for a simple and enriched EPA) and cells indicate whether there was a significant difference between two time series. T means t-test reported significant difference and K means Kolmogorov-Smirnov test reported significant difference. We say the difference is significant when the p-value is below 0.05.

Table 2. Differences in cumulative complexity metrics of enriched extended prefix automata and extended prefix automata for real-life event logs. T stands for significant difference reported by t-test, K stands for significant difference reported by Kolmogorov-Smirnov test.

Data	Variant entropy	Normalized variant entropy (active)	Normalized variant entropy (all)	Sequence entropy	Normalized sequence entropy (active)	Normalized sequence entropy (all)
BPIC12	TK				TK	
BPIC13					K	
BPIC13 filtered					TK	
BPIC15_1	TK	K			TK	
BPIC15_2					K	
BPIC15_2 filtered					TK	
BPIC15_3	TK	K			TK	
BPIC15_3 filtered	TK	K			TK	
BPIC15_4		K			K	K
BPIC15_4 filtered	T	K			TK	
BPIC15_5	T				K	
BPIC15_5 filtered	T	K			TK	

As we can see, sequence entropy normalized over active events significantly differs for all event logs with Kolmogorov-Smirnov test and for almost all event logs with t-test. Variant entropy shows significant difference with Kolmogorov-Smirnov test in 4 logs and with t-test in 7 logs. Variant entropy normalized over active states shows significant difference in Kolmogorov-Smirnov test in 6 logs. Finally, sequence entropy normalized over all events shows significant difference with Kolmogorov-Smirnov test in 1 log.

4.3 Discussion

The evaluation on the artificial log shows that the new metrics are capable of highlighting the complexity introduced by new event data. While some of this increased complexity could be uncovered by using existing process complexity metric in conjunction with auxiliary metrics, e.g. the added user could be also spotted with Social Network Analysis and multimple risk levels could be extracted from internal documentation or a BPMS, this would not necessarily work with all data, especially if this data comes from external sources. It is also important to note that while binning indeed allows taking numerical data into consideration, the efficiency of such method largely depends on the granularity, since if set too high it might bring no additional value compared to directly using numerical data.

Evaluation on the real-life logs further confirms these results. Normalized sequence entropy seems to highlight the increase in complexity due to data in the most effective way. This is not surprising as normalized sequence entropy also the only one that significantly correlates with, e.g. model complexity [1] and may just be a better metric.

When it comes to the cumulative metrics, sequence entropy normalized over active events shows best significance, also confirming the above stated ideas. As expected, also the differences in variant entropy are significant. The underlying idea that with the same behavior more distinct data would lead to more branching and more partitions in the EEPA than in the EPA of the corresponding log, which would also logically lead to higher variant entropy, seems to have found its confirmation. The fact that such effect is observed not in all event logs may be attributed to lower difference in data in the other logs. However, it needs further and more detailed investigation.

4.4   Limitations

This paper is a work in progress and thus suffers from a range of limitations. First, there are limitations in terms of the implementation. While it is capable of handling smaller event logs, it does not scale well, thus restricting evaluation and, more importantly, real-life application of the metrics. Second, the attribute selection in the real-life log evaluation was superficial. It considered all of the categorical attributes and none of the numeric ones. More thorough selection of categorical attributes as well as meaningful binning of the numeric ones is expected to give more adequate results. Third, only basic statistical methods were used for the analysis, especially when it comes to cumulative metrics. While they are definitely time series, no analysis techniques specific to this kind of data has been applied yet.

5   Conclusion and Future Work

Complexity is important aspect of business processes that requires thorough studying. While existing process complexity metrics are successful in measuring behavioral complexity of the processes, they completely ignore the data associated with the events and thus miss the next layer of complexity that is added by this data. On the other hand, there exist data complexity metrics, however, they do not have the notion of process and also have other implicit assumptions that limit their usability in process mining.

In this paper, we proposed a set of new process complexity metrics that take into account event data in addition to behavior. These metrics are based on existing complexity metrics for Extended Prefix Automata but use an updated version of such automata – Enriched EPAs. We conducted preliminary evaluation on a small artificial example as well as on a set of real-life event logs.

The initial results show that our new metrics capture the data complexity in addition to behavior complexity. We plan to extend our evaluation on more real-life logs, improve the implementation and analyse the results in more detail.

References

1. Augusto, A., Mendling, J., Vidgof, M., Wurm, B.: The connection between process complexity of event sequences and models discovered by process mining. Inf. Sci. **598**, 196–215 (2022). https://doi.org/10.1016/j.ins.2022.03.072

2. Cano, J.R.: Analysis of data complexity measures for classification. Expert Syst. Appl. **40**(12), 4820–4831 (2013). https://doi.org/10.1016/j.eswa.2013.02.025, https://www.sciencedirect.com/science/article/pii/S0957417413001413

3. van Dongen, B.B.: BPI challenge 2015, May 2015. https://doi.org/10.4121/uuid: 31a308ef-c844-48da-948c-305d167a0ec1, https://data.4tu.nl/collections/BPI_Challenge_2015/5065424/1

4. van Dongen, B.: BPI Challenge 2012, April 2012. https://doi.org/10.4121/uuid: 3926db30-f712-4394-aebc-75976070e91f, https://data.4tu.nl/articles/dataset/BPI_Challenge_2012/12689204

5. Dumas, M., Rosa, M.L., Mendling, J., Reijers, H.A.: Fundamentals of Business Process Management, Second Edition. Springer, Berlin, Heidelberg (2018). https://doi.org/10.1007/978-3-662-56509-4

6. Günther, C.: Process mining in flexible environments. Ph.D. thesis, Technische Universiteit Eindhoven (2009). https://doi.org/10.6100/IR644335

7. Ho, T.K., Basu, M.: Measuring the complexity of classification problems. In: 15th International Conference on Pattern Recognition, ICPR'00, Barcelona, Spain, 3–8 September 2000, pp. 2043–2047. IEEE Computer Society (2000). https://doi.org/10.1109/ICPR.2000.906015

8. Ho, T.K., Basu, M.: Complexity measures of supervised classification problems. IEEE Trans. Pattern Anal. Mach. Intell. **24**(3), 289–300 (2002). https://doi.org/10.1109/34.990132

9. Jain, S., Shukla, S., Wadhvani, R.: Dynamic selection of normalization techniques using data complexity measures. Expert Syst. Appl. **106**, 252–262 (2018). https://doi.org/10.1016/j.eswa.2018.04.008

10. Luengo, J., Fernández, A., García, S., Herrera, F.: Addressing data-complexity for imbalanced data-sets: a preliminary study on the use of preprocessing for C4.5. In: Ninth International Conference on Intelligent Systems Design and Applications, ISDA 2009, Pisa, Italy, November 30–2 December 2009, pp. 523–528. IEEE Computer Society (2009). https://doi.org/10.1109/ISDA.2009.233

11. Steeman, W.: BPI Challenge 2013, incidents, April 2013. https://doi.org/10.4121/uuid:500573e6-accc-4b0c-9576-aa5468b10cee, https://data.4tu.nl/articles/dataset/BPI_Challenge_2013_incidents/12693914

12. van der Aalst, W.M.: Process Mining: Data Science in Action, Second Edition. Springer, Berlin, Heidelberg (2016). https://doi.org/10.1007/978-3-662-49851-4

13. Wurm, B., Schmiedel, T., Mendling, J., Fleig, C.: Development of a measurement scale for business process standardization. In: European Conference on Information Systems (ECIS 2018). Association of Information Systems (2018)

3rd Workshop on Responsible Process Mining (RPM'22)

3rd Workshop on Responsible Process Mining (RPM)

Process mining has been successfully applied in analyzing and improving processes based on event logs in all kinds of environments. Responsible Process Mining (RPM) is highly relevant to our more and more data-driven society and has received less focus. FACT (Fair, Accurate, Confidential, and Transparent) and similar other principles for data science and machine learning have been proposed[1] to guide the development and application of data science. Issues such as lacking data quality in event logs, identifiable personal data in event logs, biased event logs, learning, discovery techniques with opaque parameters, uncertain event data, and many more aspects threaten compliance with these principles in process mining. However, process mining could also be applied to help with the "FACT-ful" application of machine learning and other data-driven techniques by bringing transparency. All such aspects of RPM were in the scope of the RPM workshop thereby covering a wide range of concepts and challenges such as fairness, accuracy, confidentiality, privacy, transparency, explainability, trust, data quality, ethics, security, and other related topics.

The main objective of the RPM workshop was to create a forum where researchers and practitioners can meet each other and start new collaboration points to promote responsible process analytics. We also considered topics from the ethics aspect to clarify real ethical issues for the process mining community with respect to the rules and regulations. We invited researchers and industry to share their research, ideas, experience reports, and challenges in this area.

For this year's edition, we received seven papers that cover all three topics and both perspectives. From them, we were able to accept three full papers for presentation and inclusion in the workshop proceedings. In addition, we invited one submission for a presentation-only session.

Our workshop program was joined together with the workshop on the related topic on Data Quality and Transformation in Process Mining (DQT-PM). We started with an inspiring keynote on "Sustainability at Celonis" by Janina Nakladal. "Discrimination-Aware Process Mining: a Discussion" was presented as the first paper in the workshop. It gave an overview on how fairness metrics can be applied in a process mining setting. The second paper "BERMUDA: Participatory Mapping of Domain Activities to Event Data via System Interfaces" proposes a solution for mapping domain activities to specific events. The full paper session was wrapped up with the paper "TraVaS: Differentially Private Trace Variant Selection for Process Mining" which is a novel approach for the differential private publication of trace-variant counts. Finally, we discussed the question "Can we trust Process Mining results?" for which we invited Anne Rozinat (Fluxicon) and Sander Leemans (RWTH Aachen) to bring their views from practice and research.

Around 30 attendees were present during the keynote, workshop presentations, and panel discussions. Due to the generous support of the ICPM organizers, we could award the best presentation. The Best Paper Award of the RPM workshop in 2022 went to

---

[1] https://redasci.org.

Majid Radfiei, Frederik Wangelik, and Wil M.P. van der Aalst for "TraVaS: Differentially Private Trace Variant Selection for Process Mining".

November 2022

Felix Mannhardt
Flavia Maria Santoro
Majid Rafiei
Stephan Fahrenkrog-Petersen

Organization

Organizing Committee

Felix Mannhardt	Eindhoven University of Technology, The Netherlands
Flavia Maria Santoro	University of the State of Rio de Janeiro, Brazil
Majid Rafiei	RWTH Aachen University, Germany
Stephan Fahrenkrog-Petersen	Humboldt-Universität zu Berlin, Germany

Program Committee

Agnes Koschmider	Kiel University, Germany
Alessandro Stefanini	University of Pisa, Italy
Florian Tschorsch	Technical University Berlin, Germany
Gamal Elkoumy	University of Tartu, Estonia
Luciano Garcia Bañuelos	Tecnologico de Monterrey, Mexico
Martin Kabierski	Humboldt-Universität zu Berlin, Germany
Moe Wynn	Queensland University of Technology, Australia
Nicola Zannone	Eindhoven University of Technology, The Netherlands
Renata de Carvalho	Eindhoven University of Technology, The Netherlands
Shangping Ren	San Diego State University, USA
Xixi Lu	Utrecht University, The Netherlands

Discrimination-Aware Process Mining: A Discussion

Timo Pohl, Mahnaz Sadat Qafari$^{(\boxtimes)}$, and Wil M. P. van der Aalst

Process and Data Science Chair (PADS), RWTH Aachen University,
Aachen, Germany
timo.pohl@rwth-aachen.de, {m.s.qafari,wvdaalst}@pads.rwth-aachen.de

Abstract. Organizations increasingly use process mining techniques to gain insight into their processes. Process mining techniques can be used to monitor and/or enhance processes. However, the impact of processes on the people involved, in terms of unfair discrimination, has not been studied. Another neglected area is the impact of applying process mining techniques on the fairness of processes. In this paper, we overview and categorize the existing fairness concepts in machine learning. Moreover, we summarize the areas where fairness is relevant to process mining and provide an approach to applying existing fairness definitions in process mining. Finally, we present some of the fairness-related challenges in processes.

Keywords: Process mining · Fairness · Discrimination

1 Introduction

Organizations interact with and affect people, such as customers, employees, or stockholders in many forms. They operate in various sensitive environments such as education, employment, healthcare, and finance. Processes taking place in such sensitive environments often have important and life-changing effects on the people involved. Moreover, such processes typically involve several decision-makings which are performed by human resources or (supported by) machine learning algorithms trained on historical data. These decision-makings are one of many factors that make processes vulnerable to various forms of discrimination. See [20] for real-life examples of discriminatory outcomes produced by algorithmic decision makers. As the impact of processes on the people involved can be very drastic, it is crucial to be able to identify instances of discrimination within processes in order to minimize negative impacts.

Process mining is a set of techniques that combine data science with model-based process analysis to enable the understanding and improvement of operational processes. Even though the concept of responsible data science has been investigated in process mining related literature, [2,4], to the best of our knowledge, in this area, [23] is the only work dedicated to fairness. In this work, making fair conclusions, which is one of the main aspects of fairness in process mining, is

© The Author(s) 2023
M. Montali et al. (Eds.): ICPM 2022 Workshops, LNBIP 468, pp. 101–113, 2023.
https://doi.org/10.1007/978-3-031-27815-0_8

investigated. Here, we mainly focus on another main aspect of fairness in process mining: detecting unfair discrimination against cases and resources. Intuitively, (unfair) discrimination is the act of treating similar individuals in the same situation differently based on one or more protected attributes, such as ethnicity, race, gender, (dis)ability, or sexual orientation [11].

Typically, process mining techniques are categorized into three types: process discovery, conformance checking, and process enhancement. Figure 1 (adapted from [1]) shows the interaction between the processes, the environment they take place in, and the process mining techniques. Processes impact their environment, which may intentionally or unintentionally pose discrimination towards the people in their environment. This discrimination might have stemmed from the process itself, its resource(s), or learned from the historical data. The interaction between the process and its environment is captured by the information systems and manifests itself in the event log. The discrimination level of the process can get aggravated by applying the results of process mining techniques on event logs containing discrimination.

Fairness is a context-sensitive concept. Consequently, there is a huge number of fairness definitions in the literature, some of which are in contradiction with each other [8]. Furthermore, there is a lack of consensus, both in academia and society, on which definition of fairness is the correct one [14, 16]. This makes it hard to decide on the proper definition of fairness to audit a process.

This issue is aggravated when there are multiple human entities with different roles and desires in an organization as each one may entail a different notion of fairness. Therefore, in this paper, we categorize the fairness concepts and definitions based on their properties such that it makes it easier for the user to select the appropriate one. We discuss some of the applications and challenges of applying fairness in process mining. Moreover, we elaborate on a mapping between the existing techniques to measure fairness and process mining.

The rest of the paper is organized as follows. In Sect. 2, we provide a brief overview of fairness considerations in literature and describe common fairness

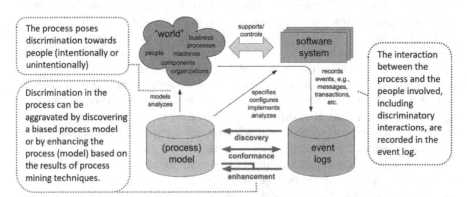

Fig. 1. Process evolution diagram; positioning of the three main types of process mining [1]. Some of the areas where discrimination can play a role in process mining are shown in this picture.

concepts and measures. In Sect. 3, we discuss the possible applications of fairness in process mining. In Sect. 4 we elaborate on mapping the existing fairness definitions to process mining. Finally, in Sect. 5, we conclude and provide directions for future work.

2   Literature Review

In this section, we provide an overview of the fairness understandings, concepts, and measures defined in the literature. We start by defining relevant terms and concepts. Then, we present a taxonomy that provides an overview of various fairness measures. Due to the extensive amount of fairness-related scientific literature, we present only concepts and measures potentially relevant to the area of process mining. For a comprehensive overview of fairness research, we refer interested readers to [8,16,20,25].

2.1   Relevant Terms

Here, we briefly discuss terms relevant to fairness. For a detailed discussion on such fairness fundamentals, we refer readers to Chap. 3 of [10].

- *Discrimination:* The word *discrimination* means "to divide", "separate", "distinguish", which is exactly the goal of classification. Therefore, discrimination itself is not necessarily unjust or unfair. However, discrimination is considered unfair if individuals receive harmful treatment based on their membership to a specific group [3].
- *Protected groups/Sensitive attributes.* A protected group is a subgroup of the population. The attributes indicating if an individual belongs to a protected group are called *sensitive attributes.*
- *Outcome.* Outcome is an attribute that captures an aspect of the system that is supposed to be fair. It is important to note that not just the outcome is context-dependent, but also its desirability. For example, in a hospital context, less waiting time for visiting a doctor is more desirable while more waiting time (up to a threshold) between an elaborate surgery and the discharge of a patient is more desirable.

2.2   Fairness Taxonomy

In this subsection, we present fairness concepts and measures defined in machine learning literature. We structure these measures in a taxonomy (Fig. 2), which is an extension of the fairness tree presented by Saleiro et al. in [25]. The fairness definitions in machine learning can be conceptually divided into *group fairness* definitions and *individual fairness* definitions [7,24,28].

Group Fairness assesses the (approximate) parity of some statistical measure across all demographic sub-populations [7,15]. The group fairness measures are further divided into three categories: disparate distribution, disparate representation, and disparate error.

1. *Distribution-based fairness.* Here, the main idea is that the distribution of the predictions should be similar across all subgroups [21]. Another example of distribution-based fairness measures is proposed in [9].
2. *Measures assessing representation.* The fairness measures in this category are based on the representation of the various subgroups in the outcome of a classifier or a subset selection method [13]. Based on the application and context, the measures are further divided into the following two categories.
    - *Coverage-based fairness.* In this category of measures, the main concern is either having the same number of people from each group or having a number proportional to their relative representation in the whole population in the selected/sampled groups [25].
    - *Ranking-based fairness* [17] defines measures for assessing representation tailored for scenarios in which individuals are ranked according to some predicted score. It also assumes a notion of ground truth which indicates the correct ordering. In essence, this definition requires that every subgroup has an equal representation in the top-n candidates in both rankings, one ranked by ground truth, the other by predicted score. Another example of ranking-based fairness is defined in [27]. Here, the fairness criterion is that the number of protected elements in the top-n candidates (for every n) is the same number that would be expected if the top-n candidates were picked at random from the overall population.
3. *Measures assessing error.* This group of measures assesses the discrimination made via errors made by the predictor and requires the existence of some predicted value, as well as a notion of ground truth [6,16]. These measures are further subdivided into three contextual categories: *assistive*, *punitive*, and *neutral.*
    - *Assistive context.* In this context, a positive classification is assumed to bring benefits to the individuals, therefore false negatives are more undesirable in terms of fairness than false positives.
    - *Punitive context.* This context is exactly the other way around, i.e., a positive classification is assumed to bring negative consequences for the individuals. Hence, false positives are more undesirable in terms of fairness than false negatives.
    - *Neutral contexts.* Here, we assume that false negatives and false positives are equally undesirable.

The main advantage of group fairness definitions is their simplicity. They can be easily explained and verified [8]. However, their main drawback comes from the fact that this category of fairness definitions provides guarantees only to "average" members of the protected groups. Consequently, they do not provide guarantees to individuals or subgroups within the protected groups. Moreover, some of these measures can be at odds with one another [8].

It is important to note, that group fairness measures based on parity require some assumptions. The main assumption is that differences between groups are due solely to unwarranted bias and that all warranted differences have been eliminated (for example by removing them from the data) [15]. This includes the assumption that the reasons for existing differences do not lie in the choices of individuals but in factors outside of their control [15]. If these assumptions apply, these measures can help in correcting the unjust bias. However, if these assumptions do not apply, enforcing them can lead to outcomes that are unfair from the perspective of an individual or it can lead to a form of reverse discrimination towards the rest of the population [16].

Individual Fairness assesses the similarity of the outcome of pairs of similar individuals ignoring their differences in terms of protected attributes [9]. Two main techniques for assessing individual fairness are *similarity-based fairness* and *counterfactual fairness* (highlighted in yellow in Fig. 2).

1. *Similarity-based fairness* assesses individual fairness by using two similarity metrics. The first metric estimates the similarity of two individuals. The second metric estimates the similarity of the outcomes that two individuals received. To assess the fairness from individual A's perspective, one simply matches A to the most similar individual(s) in the data. Then, the similarity of the two individuals is compared with the similarity of their outcomes. By doing this for every individual in our data, we can measure how similarly similar individuals are treated. Examples of similarity-based fairness measures can be found in [9, 28].
2. *Counterfactual fairness* is formulated in the context of fair classifications. The main idea is to investigate the question of "how would the prediction change if the protected attribute of an individual were different" [12]. Under this approach, a decision is considered fair towards an individual if the outcome of the decision is the same in (a) the actual world and (b) a counterfactual world where the individual belonged to a different demographic group [19]. Counterfactual fairness can also be used to assess group fairness. By studying in what direction the prediction changes when changing protected attributes, it is possible to infer which groups are given preferential outcome(s). For example, if by changing the group membership from G to G', the prediction always changes from a negative to a positive outcome, this indicates discrimination against either group G or G'.

The main advantage of individual fairness definitions is their semantics, as they provide guarantees to individuals and not average members. However, they require making significant assumptions. For example, similarity-based fairness measures are built on similarity measures, the definition of which can require a large amount of domain knowledge that even domain experts rarely possess.

3   Fairness Applications in Process Mining

Fairness has three key applications in process mining. In the following, we briefly discuss each application and provide promising lines of research for each one. It is worth noting that fairness is not relevant in all processes. For example, in fully automated processes with no human involvement, fairness does not play a

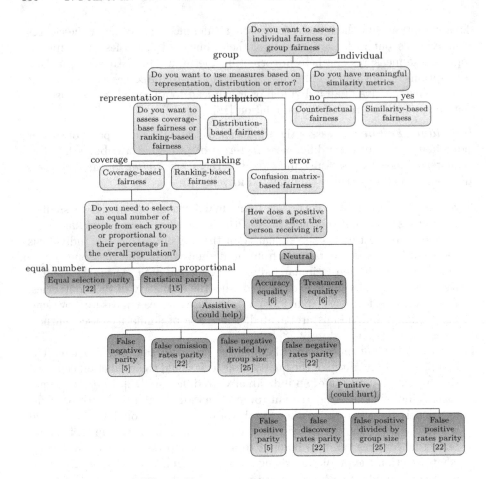

Fig. 2. Taxonomy of fairness measures

role. The relevance of fairness to a process depends on (1) how much it involves humans (for example, as cases or resources) and (2) how strong the impact of the process on the lives of the involved people is.

Discrimination in Processes. Processes involve at least two discrimination-relevant entities: *resources* and *cases*. The general idea is, that cases cannot directly influence the process but may suffer from discrimination. From a case perspective, waiting times in and between activities, the number of re-do's, the success rate, occurrences of deviations, and the allocation of resources are some examples of possible outcomes (as defined in Sect. 2). Resources, in turn, can cause discrimination by making biased decisions. However, they can also be affected by discrimination. From a resource perspective, possible outcomes include the assigned workload and the complexity of the assigned tasks. Some of the interesting lines of research concerned with discrimination in processes are:

- developing process mining specific measures to assess the level of discrimination in event logs and process models,
- developing methods for on-time monitoring of fairness in a process so that process owners can react on time and prevent unfair discrimination, and
- providing methods to improve/enhance fairness in a process by reducing the discrimination level in the event log or process model.

Making Fair Conclusions.[1] Root cause analysis is one of the main steps before designing re-engineering steps to enhance a process. Traditionally, root cause analysis is performed using machine learning techniques that are based on pattern recognition and correlation. However, correlation does not necessarily imply causation. Thus, applying these results, especially when affecting people (e.g., by blaming, firing, promoting), can result in unfairness. For example, in a hospital, is it fair to say that the cardiac surgeon with the highest mortality rate among his/her patients is the worst surgeon? Or is he/she the most experienced one who gets the hardest cases? Several factors must be considered to infer causal relationships. Possible reasons for situations where correlation does not imply causality include the Simpson-paradox [26] and (sampling) bias in the data. Two interesting lines of research for this application are:

- providing methods to distinguish causality from mere correlation, and
- providing methods for evaluating the extent to which a particular cause is responsible for an effect (outcome)

Impact of Process Mining Techniques on Fairness. There are several algorithms and heuristics for performing process mining tasks, each of which can be fine-tuned by adjusting various parameters. These methods have been developed to optimize various metrics, but not fairness. Moreover, some process mining techniques could distort the results of a fairness analysis. For example, it is a commonly used rule of thumb, that the discovered model should be able to explain 80% of the cases in the event log. However, how this filtering step affects the results of a fairness analysis, has not been studied. In general, any process mining technique that its process analysis pipeline involves filtering, ranking, or decision making (e.g., in the form of clustering or classification) is prone to causing or amplifying discrimination. Promising lines of research in this area include:

- investigating the effect of process mining techniques in terms of the possibility of causing/reinforcing discrimination,
- developing fairness-aware quality measures for process models and event logs,
- investigating the effect that applying confidentiality preserving techniques has on the fairness of event logs, and
- providing methods to find and remove the root cause of discrimination in processes.

---

[1] Even though this aspect of fairness is not the main focus of this paper, we mention it for completeness.

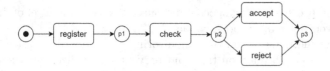

Fig. 3. An example of a simple process.

4   Mapping Existing Fairness Definitions to Process Mining

Many fairness definitions and measures in fair machine learning have been defined in the context of classification ([8,16], also see Table 2 in [20]). Most of these classification-based measures require the following inputs that are not always clearly defined in a process mining context:

1. a *dataset*, in tabular form, containing one or more sensitive attributes and possibly some descriptive attributes,
2. a *model* to analyze its outcome in terms of fairness. In a classification context, the outcome corresponds to the prediction made by the classifier.
3. a notion of *ground truth* is needed for measures assessing the errors made by the model. Such ground truth indicates how things should have been in a fair and ideal world, which in a classification context, corresponds to the ideal predictions.

To measure fairness in process mining, we are interested in assessing the fairness of the process (corresponding to model), in terms of its manifestation (analogous to outcome), compared to how it should have been (analogous to ground truth). We can assume that the ground truth is provided by a domain expert or can be computed (approximated) using a normative model. To be able to assess the discrimination level using the techniques mentioned in Sect. 2, we need to extract the data in a tabular form. Here, we briefly mention how to extract a data table from an event log. An event log is a collection of events, where each event refers to the occurrence of a specific activity at a specific point in time, for a specific case (identified with a specific case identifier). A *case* is defined as the chronologically ordered sequence of events with the same case identifier in the event log. An example of a simple process is shown in Fig. 3. Table 1 shows an event log with two cases $t_1 = \langle e_1, e_2, e_3 \rangle$ and $t_2 = \langle e_4, e_5, e_6 \rangle$ for the process in Fig. 3. To turn an event log to a tabular data, we use the method explained in [23]. This method involves three steps: 1) enriching the event log, 2) extracting a set of outcome-sensitive prefixes of the cases in the event log, and 3) extracting the tabular data called *situation feature table* (Fig. 4). In the following, we explain these three steps in more detail.

Enriching the Event Log. In this step, the event log is enriched with several derivative attributes extracted from the event log and possibly other sources. For example, we may add the decision made in a choice place as an attribute

Table 1. An event log with two cases for the process shown in Fig. 3.

Event identifier	Case id	Activity name	Timestamp	Resource	Gender
e_1	1	Register	19.03.3019	Alice	Female
e_2	1	Check	20.03.3019	Alice	Female
e_3	1	Reject	22.03.3019	Bob	Female
e_4	2	Register	22.03.3019	Sara	Male
e_5	2	Check	24.03.3019	Bob	Male
e_6	2	Accept	27.03.3019	Bob	Male

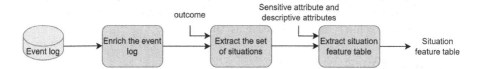

Fig. 4. The steps of extracting a situation feature table from an event log.

to the event that happened just before that choice place. More examples of attributes that can be used to enrich the event log include the event duration, waiting time for each event, throughput time of a case, the duration of a case on a normative model, or some ground truth indicated by a process expert.

Extracting the Set of Situations. In this step, we map each case to multiple prefixes of it, where each prefix ends with the occurrence of the outcome. These prefixes are called *situations*. Examples of situations include:

– If the outcome is a decision made in a choice place, each situation corresponds to the prefix of a case recorded before that place. For example, in the process of Fig. 3, if the outcome is the choice made in $p2$, then the two cases in Table 1 are mapped to the situations $s_1 = \langle e_1, e_2 \rangle$ and $s_2 = \langle e_4, e_5 \rangle$.
– If the outcome is an event attribute of a group of events, then each situation is a prefix of a case in the event log where the prefix ends with one of the events of that group. For example, in the process of Fig. 3, if the outcome is the duration of the event with activity name "check", then the two cases in the Table 1 are mapped to two situations $s_1 = \langle e_1 \rangle$ and $s_2 = \langle e_4 \rangle$.
– If the outcome is a case-level attribute, then each situation corresponds to a case. For example, in the process of Fig. 3, if the outcome is the "throughput time", then the two cases in the Table 1 are mapped to two situations $s_1 = \langle e_1, e_2, e_1 \rangle$ and $s_2 = \langle e_4, e_5, e_6 \rangle$.

Extracting the Situation Feature Table. In the third step, tabular data is extracted from the set of the situations in the previous step. The resulting table is called a *situation feature table*. The set of features extracted from the set of situations includes sensitive attributes and the outcome (and possibly the ground truth). This tabular data can be used to measure the level of discrimination. An

Table 2. A situation feature table extracted from the event log in Table 1 in which the outcome is the choice made at p2 and the sensitive attribute is "gender".

Duration-register	Resource-check	Gender	p2-choice
1 day	Alice	Female	Reject
2 days	Bob	Male	Accept

example of a situation feature table extracted from the event log in Table 1 is shown in Table 2 in which the outcome is the choice made in place $p2$ (Fig. 3) and the descriptive attributes are the duration of the event with activity name "register", the resource of the event with activity name "check", and the "gender". In this example "gender" is the sensitive attribute.

5   Conclusion

Organizations operate in many important areas of life, sometimes with a life-changing impact on people. This makes inspecting their impact in terms of discrimination (as one aspect of unfairness) an important topic. However, the fairness aspects of processes have rarely been considered in literature. In this paper, we discussed the placement of fairness in the process mining realm.

We discussed fairness primarily in terms of equal and non-discriminatory treatment of individuals and groups and provided an overview of various fairness definitions to detect discrimination. We presented these definitions in a structured way using a taxonomy. Furthermore, we discussed three potential key contributions that fairness can have in process mining, again with a focus on discrimination. We also provided an approach on how to map existing fairness definitions to process mining by using situation feature tables.

In conclusion, the main question one should ask before enhancing a process with fairness-related objectives is whether the differences between groups or individuals are the result of an unjust bias towards them and whether this bias needs to be corrected. Not all cases of discrimination are unfair. A methodology to quantify the explainable and illegal discrimination in data has been presented in [18]. Moreover, to assess the fairness of a system, it is crucial to be able to justify the selected fairness measurement from a moral perspective. Therefore, it is important to consider the assumptions behind each measure. For example, in similarity-based fairness measures, it is assumed that the similarity metric expresses ground truth (or the best available approximation of it) [9]. Also, the assumptions connected to statistical parity have been discussed in great detail in the academic literature [9,15,24]. Another point to note while planning to enhance a process with fairness objectives is that the costs (such as reduction in accuracy) are often immediately realized, whereas its benefits are usually not immediate and less tangible [8].

Acknowledgment. We thank Alexander von Humboldt (AvH) Stiftung for supporting our research.

References

1. van der Aalst, W.: Process Mining: Data Science in Action, vol. 2. Springer, Berlin, Heidelberg (2016). https://doi.org/10.1007/978-3-662-49851-4
2. van der Aalst, W.M.P.: Responsible data science: using event data in a people friendly manner. In: Hammoudi, S., Maciaszek, L., Missikoff, M., Camp, O., Cordeiro, J. (eds.) Enterprise Information Systems. ICEIS 2016. LNBIP, vol. 291, pp. 3–28. Springer, Cham (2017). https://doi.org/10.1007/978-3-319-62386-3_1
3. Aalst, W.M.P.: Responsible data science: using event data in a people friendly manner. In: Hammoudi, S., Maciaszek, L.A., Missikoff, M.M., Camp, O., Cordeiro, J. (eds.) ICEIS 2016. LNBIP, vol. 291, pp. 3–28. Springer, Cham (2017). https://doi.org/10.1007/978-3-319-62386-3_1
4. Aalst, W.M.P.: Responsible data science in a dynamic world. In: Strous, L., Cerf, V.G. (eds.) IFIPIoT 2018. IAICT, vol. 548, pp. 3–10. Springer, Cham (2019). https://doi.org/10.1007/978-3-030-15651-0_1
5. Angwin, J., Larson, J., Mattu, S., Kirchner, L.: Machine bias. In: Ethics of Data and Analytics, pp. 254–264. Auerbach Publications (2016)
6. Berk, R., Heidari, H., Jabbari, S., Kearns, M., Roth, A.: Fairness in criminal justice risk assessments: the state of the art. Sociol. Methods Res. **50**(1), 3–44 (2021)
7. Binns, R.: On the apparent conflict between individual and group fairness. In: Hildebrandt, M., Castillo, C., Celis, L.E., Ruggieri, S., Taylor, L., Zanfir-Fortuna, G. (eds.) FAT* 2020: Conference on Fairness, Accountability, and Transparency, Barcelona, Spain, 27–30 January 2020, pp. 514–524. ACM (2020)
8. Chouldechova, A., Roth, A.: A snapshot of the frontiers of fairness in machine learning. Commun. ACM **63**(5), 82–89 (2020)
9. Dwork, C., Hardt, M., Pitassi, T., Reingold, O., Zemel, R.: Fairness through awareness. In: Proceedings of the 3rd Innovations in Theoretical Computer Science Conference, pp. 214–226. ITCS 2012, Association for Computing Machinery, New York, NY, USA (2012)
10. Ekstrand, M.D., Das, A., Burke, R., Diaz, F.: Fairness and discrimination in information access systems. CoRR abs/2105.05779 (2021). https://arxiv.org/abs/2105.05779
11. Fibbi, R., Midtbøen, A.H., Simon, P.: Concepts of discrimination. In: Migration and Discrimination. IRS, pp. 13–20. Springer, Cham (2021). https://doi.org/10.1007/978-3-030-67281-2_2
12. Garg, S., Perot, V., Limtiaco, N., Taly, A., Chi, E.H., Beutel, A.: Counterfactual fairness in text classification through robustness. In: Conitzer, V., Hadfield, G.K., Vallor, S. (eds.) Proceedings of the 2019 AAAI/ACM Conference on AI, Ethics, and Society, AIES 2019, Honolulu, HI, USA, 27–28 January 2019, pp. 219–226. ACM (2019)
13. Grabowicz, P.A., Perello, N., Mishra, A.: Marrying fairness and explainability in supervised learning. In: 2022 ACM Conference on Fairness, Accountability, and Transparency, pp. 1905–1916. FAccT 2022, Association for Computing Machinery (2022)
14. Harrison, G., Hanson, J., Jacinto, C., Ramirez, J., Ur, B.: An empirical study on the perceived fairness of realistic, imperfect machine learning models. In: Proceedings of the 2020 Conference on Fairness, Accountability, and Transparency, pp. 392–402. FAT* 2020, Association for Computing Machinery, New York, NY, USA (2020)
15. Hertweck, C., Heitz, C., Loi, M.: On the moral justification of statistical parity. In: Proceedings of the 2021 ACM Conference on Fairness, Accountability, and

Transparency, pp. 747–757. FAccT 2021, Association for Computing Machinery, New York, NY, USA (2021)

16. Hutchinson, B., Mitchell, M.: 50 years of test (un)fairness: lessons for machine learning. In: Boyd, D., Morgenstern, J.H. (eds.) Proceedings of the Conference on Fairness, Accountability, and Transparency, FAT* 2019, Atlanta, GA, USA, 29–31 January 2019, pp. 49–58. ACM (2019)

17. Jones, M.B.: Moderated regression and equal opportunity. Educ. Psychol. Meas. **33**(3), 591–602 (1973)

18. Kamiran, F., Žliobaitė, I.: Explainable and non-explainable discrimination in classification. In: Custers, B., Calders, T., Schermer, B., Zarsky, T. (eds.) Discrimination and Privacy in the Information Society. Studies in Applied Philosophy, Epistemology and Rational Ethics, vol. 3, pp. 155–170. Springer, Berlin, Heidelberg (2013). https://doi.org/10.1007/978-3-642-30487-3_8

19. Kusner, M.J., Loftus, J.R., Russell, C., Silva, R.: Counterfactual fairness. In: Advances in Neural Information Processing Systems 30: Annual Conference on Neural Information Processing Systems 2017, 4–9 December 2017, Long Beach, CA, USA, pp. 4066–4076 (2017)

20. Mehrabi, N., Morstatter, F., Saxena, N., Lerman, K., Galstyan, A.: A survey on bias and fairness in machine learning. ACM Comput. Surv. (CSUR) **54**(6), 1–35 (2021)

21. Pfohl, S.R., Foryciarz, A., Shah, N.H.: An empirical characterization of fair machine learning for clinical risk prediction. J. Biomed. Inform. **113**, 103621 (2021)

22. Powers, D.M.: Evaluation: from precision, recall and f-measure to roc, informedness, markedness and correlation (2020). arXiv preprint arXiv:2010.16061

23. Qafari, M.S., van der Aalst, W.: Fairness-aware process mining. In: Panetto, H., Debruyne, C., Hepp, M., Lewis, D., Ardagna, C.A., Meersman, R. (eds.) OTM 2019. LNCS, vol. 11877, pp. 182–192. Springer, Cham (2019). https://doi.org/10.1007/978-3-030-33246-4_11

24. Räz, T.: Group fairness: independence revisited. In: Elish, M.C., Isaac, W., Zemel, R.S. (eds.) FAccT 2021: 2021 ACM Conference on Fairness, Accountability, and Transparency, Virtual Event/Toronto, Canada, 3–10 March 2021, pp. 129–137. ACM (2021)

25. Saleiro, P., et al.: Aequitas: a bias and fairness audit toolkit. CoRR abs/1811.05577 (2018)

26. Simpson, E.H.: The interpretation of interaction in contingency tables. J. R. Stat. Soc. Ser. B (Methodol.) **13**(2), 238–241 (1951)

27. Zehlike, M., Bonchi, F., Castillo, C., Hajian, S., Megahed, M., Baeza-Yates, R.: FA*IR: a fair top-k ranking algorithm, pp. 1569–1578. CoRR (2017)

28. Zemel, R., Wu, Y., Swersky, K., Pitassi, T., Dwork, C.: Learning fair representations. In: Proceedings of the 30th International Conference on International Conference on Machine Learning, vol. 28, pp. III-325-III-333. ICML 2013, JMLR.org (2013)

TraVaS: Differentially Private Trace Variant Selection for Process Mining

Majid Rafiei[✉][iD], Frederik Wangelik[iD], and Wil M. P. van der Aalst[iD]

Chair of Process and Data Science, RWTH Aachen University, Aachen, Germany
majid.rafiei@pads.rwth-aachen.de

Abstract. In the area of industrial process mining, privacy-preserving event data publication is becoming increasingly relevant. Consequently, the trade-off between high data utility and quantifiable privacy poses new challenges. State-of-the-art research mainly focuses on differentially private trace variant construction based on prefix expansion methods. However, these algorithms face several practical limitations such as high computational complexity, introducing fake variants, removing frequent variants, and a bounded variant length. In this paper, we introduce a new approach for direct differentially private trace variant release which uses anonymized *partition selection* strategies to overcome the aforementioned restraints. Experimental results on real-life event data show that our algorithm outperforms state-of-the-art methods in terms of both plain data utility and result utility preservation.

Keywords: Process mining · Differential privacy · Event data

1 Introduction

In recent years, process mining and event data analysis have been successfully deployed in many industries. The main objectives are to learn process models from event logs for further behavioral inference (so-called *process discovery*), to extend existing models using event logs (so-called *model enhancement*), or to assess the alignment between a process model and an event log (so-called *conformance checking*) [2]. However, often the underlying event data are bound to personal identifiers or other private information. A prominent example is the process management of hospitals where the cases are patients being treated by staff. Without means of privacy protection, any adversary is able to extract sensitive information about individuals and their properties. Thus, privacy regulations, such as GDPR [1], typically restrict data storage and access which motivates the development of privacy preservation techniques.

The majority of state-of-the-art privacy preservation techniques are built on Differential Privacy (DP), which offers a noise-based privacy definition. This is due to its important features, such as providing mathematical privacy guarantees and security against *predicate-singling-out* attacks [3]. The goal of techniques

Funded under the Excellence Strategy of the Federal Government and the Länder. We also thank the Alexander von Humboldt Stiftung for supporting our research.

M. Montali et al. (Eds.): ICPM 2022 Workshops, LNBIP 468, pp. 114–126, 2023.
https://doi.org/10.1007/978-3-031-27815-0_9

Table 1. A simple event log from the healthcare context including trace variants and their frequencies.

Trace variant	Frequency
$\langle register, visit, blood\text{-}test, release \rangle$	10
$\langle register, blood\text{-}test, visit, release \rangle$	8
$\langle register, visit, release \rangle$	20
$\langle register, visit, blood\text{-}test, blood\text{-}test, release \rangle$	5

based on DP is to hide the participation of an individual in the released output by injecting noise. The amount of noise is mainly determined by the privacy parameters, ϵ and δ, and the sensitivity of the underlying data. State-of-the-art research targeting (ϵ, δ)-DP methods in process mining focuses on releasing raw privatized activity sequences performed for cases, i.e., *trace variants*. Table 1 shows a sample of such event data in the healthcare context, where each trace variant belongs to a case, i.e., a patient, and one case cannot have more than one trace variant. This format describes the *control-flow* of event logs that is basis for the main process mining activities. The trace variant of a case is considered sensitive information because it contains the complete sequence of activities performed for the case that can be exploited to conclude private information, e.g., patient diseases in the healthcare context.

To achieve differential privacy for trace variants, the state-of-the-art approach [12] inserts noise drawn from a *Laplacian distribution* into the variant distribution obtained from an event log. This approach has several drawbacks including: (1) *introducing fake variants*, (2) *removing frequent true variants*, and (3) *limited length for generated trace variants*. A recent work called *SaCoFa* [9], attempts to mitigate drawbacks (1) and (2) by gaining knowledge regarding the underlying process semantics from original event data. However, the privacy quantification of all extra queries to gain knowledge regarding the underlying semantics is not discussed. Moreover, the third drawback still remains since this work, similar to [12], employs a *prefix-based* approach. The prefix-based approaches need to generate all possible unique variants based on a set of activities to provide differential privacy for the original distribution of variants. Since the set of possible trace variants that can be generated given a unique set of activities is infinite, the prefix-based techniques need to bound the length of generated sequences. Also, to limit the search space these approaches typically include a pruning parameter to exclude less frequent prefixes.

We introduce an (ϵ, δ)-DP approach for releasing the distribution of trace variants that focuses on the aforementioned drawbacks. In contrast to the prefix-based approaches, the underlying algorithm is based on (ϵ, δ)-DP for *partition selection* that allows for a direct publication of arbitrarily long sequences [4]. Employing differentially private partition selection techniques, the actual frequencies of all trace variants can directly be queried without guessing (generating) trace variants. Internally, random noise drawn from a specific geometric distribution is injected into the corresponding frequencies, and all variants whose privatized frequencies fall beyond a threshold are removed. Hence, no fake trace variants are introduced, and only some infrequent variants may disappear from the output. Moreover, no tedious fine-tuning has to be conducted and no computationally expensive search needs to be included. In Sect. 5, we introduce different metrics to evaluate the *data* and *result* utility preservation of our approach. We also run our experiments for the state-of-the-art prefix-based methods and show superior data and result utilities compared to these methods.

The remainder of this paper is structured as follows. In Sect. 2, we provide a summary of related work. Preliminaries and notations are provided in Sect. 3. Section 4 introduces the theoretical background of differentially private *partition selection*, and describes our *TraVaS* algorithm. In Sect. 5, the experimental results based on real-life event logs are shown. Section 6 concludes the paper.

2   Related Work

The research area of privacy and confidentiality in process mining is recently growing in importance. Several techniques have been proposed to address the privacy and confidentiality issues. In this paper, our focus is on the so-called *noise-based* techniques that are based on the notion of *differential privacy*. In [12], the authors apply an (ϵ, δ)-DP mechanism to event logs to privatize *directly-follows relations* and trace variants. The underlying principle uses a combination of an (ϵ, δ)-DP noise generator and an iterative query engine that allows an anonymized publication of trace variants with an upper bound for their length. *SaCoFa* [9] is the most recent extension of the aforementioned (ϵ, δ)-DP mechanism that attempts to optimize the query structures with the help of underlying semantics. Another extension of [12] is the *PRIPEL* approach, where more event attributes can be secured using the so-called *sequence enrichment* [8].

Whereas most of the aforementioned ideas target raw event logs, in [7], the focus is on *directly-follows graphs*. During the edge generation, connections are randomized using (ϵ, δ)-DP mechanisms to balance utility preservation and privacy risks. As the main benchmark model for our work, we choose the technique by Mannhardt et al. [12] since it focuses on trace variants and is the basis of most of the other techniques. Moreover, its privacy guarantees are directly proven by (ϵ, δ)-DP mechanisms, i.e., no extra privacy analysis is required. Nevertheless, we also compare our results with SaCoFa as the most recent extension of the benchmark to demonstrate the superior performance of our approach.

3   Preliminaries

In this section, we introduce the necessary mathematical concepts and definitions utilized throughout the remainder of the paper. Let A be a set. $B(A)$ is the set of all multisets over A. A multiset A can be represented as a set of tuples $\{(a, A(a)) | a \in A\}$ where $A(a)$ is the frequency of $a \in A$. Given A and B as two multisets, $A \uplus B$ is the sum over multisets, e.g., $[a^2, b^3] \uplus [b^2, c^2] = [a^2, b^5, c^2]$. We define a finite sequence over A of length n as $\sigma = \langle a_1, a_2, \ldots, a_n \rangle$ where $\sigma(i) = a_i \in A$ for all $i \in \{1, 2, \ldots, n\}$. The set of all finite sequences over A is denoted with A^*.

3.1 Event Data

The data used by *process mining* techniques are typically collections of unique events that are recorded per activity execution and characterized by their attributes. We denote $\mathcal{E}$ as the universe of events. Then, a *trace* σ, which is a single process execution, is represented as a sequence of events $\sigma = \langle e_1, e_2, ..., e_n \rangle \in \mathcal{E}^*$ belonging to the same case and having a fixed ordering based on timestamps. Note that events are unique and cannot appear in more than one trace. Moreover, each case (individual) contributes to only one trace. An event log L can be represented as a set of traces $L \subseteq \mathcal{E}^*$. Our work focuses on the control-flow aspect of an event log that only considers the activity attribute of events in traces. We define a simple event log based on activity sequences, so-called *trace variants*.

Definition 1 (Trace Variant). *Let $\mathcal{A}$ be the universe of activities. A trace variant $\sigma = \langle a_1, a_2, ..., a_n \rangle \in \mathcal{A}^*$ is a sequence of activities performed for a case.*

Definition 2 (Simple Event Log). *A simple event log L is defined as a multiset of trace variants $L \in B(\mathcal{A}^*)$. $\mathcal{L}$ denotes the universe of simple event logs.*

3.2 Differential Privacy

In the following, we introduce the necessary concepts of (ϵ, δ)-DP for our research. The main idea of DP is to inject noise into the original data in such a way that an observer who sees the randomized output cannot tell if the information of a specific individual is included in the data [6]. Considering simple event logs, i.e., the distribution of trace variants, as our sensitive event data, differential privacy can formally be defined as Definition 3.

Definition 3 ((ϵ, δ)-DP for Event Logs). *Let L_1 and L_2 be two neighbouring event logs that differ only in a single entry, e.g., $L_2 = L_1 \uplus [\sigma]$ for any $\sigma \in \mathcal{A}^*$. Also, let $\epsilon \in \mathbb{R}_{>0}$ and $\delta \in \mathbb{R}_{>0}$ be two privacy parameters. A randomized mechanism $\mathcal{M}_{\epsilon,\delta}: \mathcal{L} \to \mathcal{L}$ provides (ϵ, δ)-DP if for all $S \subseteq \mathcal{A}^* \times \mathbb{N}$: $Pr[\mathcal{M}_{\epsilon,\delta}(L_1) \in S] \leq e^{\epsilon} \times Pr[\mathcal{M}_{\epsilon,\delta}(L_2) \in S] + \delta$. Given $L \in \mathcal{L}$, $\mathcal{M}_{\epsilon,\delta}(L) \subseteq \{(\sigma, L'(\sigma)) \mid \sigma \in \mathcal{A}^* \wedge L'(\sigma) = L(\sigma) + x_\sigma\}$, with x_σ being realizations of i.i.d. random variables drawn from a probability distribution.*

In Definition 3, ϵ as the first privacy parameter specifies the probability ratio, and δ as the second privacy parameter allows for a linear violation. In the strict case of $\delta = 0$, $\mathcal{M}$ offers ϵ-DP. The randomness of respective mechanisms is typically ensured by the noise drawn from a probability distribution that perturbs original variant-frequency tuples and results in non-deterministic outputs. The smaller the privacy parameters are set, the more noise is injected into the mechanism outputs, entailing a decreasing likelihood of tracing back the instance existence based on outputs.

A commonly used $(\epsilon, 0)$-DP mechanism for real-valued statistical queries is the *Laplace* mechanism. This mechanism injects noise based on a Laplacian distribution with scale $\Delta f / \epsilon$. Δf is called the sensitivity of a statistical query f. Intuitively, Δf indicates the amount of uncertainty we must introduce into the output in order to hide the contribution of single instances at $(\epsilon, 0)$-level. In our context, f is the frequency of a trace variant. Since one individual, i.e., a case, contributes to only one trace, $\Delta f = 1$. In case an individual can appear in more than one trace, the sensitivity needs to be accordingly increased assuming the same value for the privacy parameter ϵ. State-of-the-art event data anonymization frameworks such as our benchmark often use the *Laplace mechanism*.

4   Partition Selection Algorithm

We first highlight the problem of *partition selection* and link it to event data release. Then, the algorithmic details are presented with a brief analysis.

4.1   Partition Selection

Many data analysis tasks can be expressed as per-partition aggregation operations after grouping the data into an unbounded set of partitions. When identifying the variants of a simple log L as categories, the transformation from L to pairs $(\sigma, L(\sigma))$ becomes a specific instance of these aggregation tasks. To render such queries differentially private, two distinct steps need to be executed. First, all aggregation results are perturbed by noise addition of suitable mechanisms. Next, the set of unique partitions must be modified to prevent leakage of information on the true data categories (*differentially private partition selection*) [4,6]. In case of publicly known partitions or bounded partitions from a familiar finite domain, the second step can be reduced to a direct unchanged release or a simple guessing-task, respectively. However, for the most general form of unknown and infinite category domains, guessing is not efficient anymore and an (ϵ, δ)-DP *partition selection* strategy can be used instead.

Recently, in [4], the authors proposed an (ϵ, δ)-DP *partition selection* approach, where they provided a proof of an optimal partition selection rule which maximizes the number of released category-aggregation pairs while preserving (ϵ, δ)-DP. In particular, the authors showed how the aforementioned anonymization steps can be combined into an explicit (ϵ, δ)-DP mechanism based on a k-Truncated Symmetric Geometric Distribution (k-TSGD), see Definition 4. We exploit the analogy between *partition selection* and simple event log publication and transfer this mechanism to the event data context. Definition 5 shows the respective definition based on a k-TSGD.[1]

Definition 4 (k-TSGD). *Given probability* $p \in (0,1)$, $m = p/(1+(1-p)-2(1-p)^{k+1})$, *and* $k \geq 1$, *the k-TSGD of* (p, k) *over* $\mathbb{Z}$ *formally reads as:*

$$k\text{-}TSGD[X = x \mid p, k] = \begin{cases} m \cdot (1-p)^{|x|} & \text{if } x \in [-k, k] \\ 0 & \text{otherwise} \end{cases} \quad (1)$$

Definition 5 ((ϵ, δ)-DP for Event Logs Based on k-TSGD). *Let* $\epsilon \in \mathbb{R}_{>0}$ *and* $\delta \in \mathbb{R}_{>0}$ *be the privacy parameters, and* $\mathcal{M}_{\epsilon, \delta}^{k-TSGD} : \mathcal{L} \to \mathcal{L}$ *be a randomized*

---

[1] A respective proof can be found in Sec. 3 of [4].

mechanism based on a *k-TSGD*. Given $L \in \mathcal{L}$ as an input of the randomized mechanism, an event log $L' = \{(\sigma, L'(\sigma)) \mid \sigma \in L \wedge L'(\sigma) > k\} \in rng(\mathcal{M}_{\epsilon,\delta}^{k-TSGD})$ is an (ϵ, δ)-DP representation of L if $L'(\sigma) = L(\sigma) + x_\sigma$ is the noisified frequency with x_σ being realization of i.i.d random variables drawn from a *k-TSGD* with parameters (p, k), where $p = 1 - e^{-\epsilon}$ and $k = \lceil 1/\epsilon \times ln((e^\epsilon + 2\delta - 1)/\delta(e^\epsilon + 1)) \rceil$.

Definition 5 shows the direct (ϵ, δ)-DP release of trace variants by first perturbing all variant frequencies and then truncating infrequent behavior. Additionally, optimality is guaranteed w.r.t. the number of variants being published due to the *k-TSGD* structure [4]. Note that the underlying *k-TSGD* mechanism assumes each case only contributes to one variant. In case this requirement needs to be violated, sensitivity considerations force a decrease in (ϵ, δ).

The development of differentially private *partition selection* enables significant performance improvements for private trace variant releases. As there are infinite activity sequences defining a variant, former approaches had to either guess or query all of these potentially non-existing sequences in a cumbersome fashion due to the ex-ante category anonymity in (ϵ, δ)-DP. On the contrary, *partition selection* only needs one noisified aggregation operation followed by a specific truncation. Hence, the output contains only existing variants that are independent of external parameters or query patterns.

4.2   Algorithm Design

Algorithm 1 presents the core idea of *TraVaS* which is based on Definition 5. We also propose a utility-aware extension of *TraVaS*, so-called *uTraVaS*, that utilizes the privacy budgets, i.e., ϵ and δ, by several queries w.r.t. data utility. In this paper, we focus on *TraVaS*, the details of *uTraVaS* are provided on GitHub.[2]

Algorithm 1 (TraVaS) allows to anonymize variant-frequency pairs by injecting *k-TSGD* noise within one run over the according simple log. After a simple log L and privacy parameters $(\epsilon > 0, \delta > 0)$ are provided, the *travas* function first transforms (ϵ, δ) into *k-TSGD* parameters (p, k). Then, each variant frequency $L(\sigma)$ becomes noisified using i.i.d *k-TSGD* noise x_σ (see Definition 5). Eventually, the function removes all modified infrequent variants where the perturbed frequencies yield numbers below or equal to k. Due to the partition

---

Algorithm 1: Differentially Private Trace Variant Selection (TraVaS)

Input: Event log L, DP-Parameters (ϵ, δ)
Output: (ϵ, δ)-DP log L'

```
1  function travas (L, ε, δ)
2      p = 1 − e^−ε                                              // compute probability
3      k = ⌈1/ε × ln ((e^ε + 2δ − 1)/(δ(e^ε + 1)))⌉             // compute threshold
4      forall (σ, L(σ)) ∈ L do
5          x_σ = rTSGD (p, k)                                    // generate i.i.d k-TSGD noise
6          if L(σ) + x_σ > k then
7              add (σ, L(σ) + x_σ) to L'
8      return L'
```

---

2 https://github.com/wangelik/TraVaS/tree/main/supplementary.

selection mechanism, the actual frequencies of all trace variants can directly be queried without guessing trace variants. Thus, *TraVaS* is considerably more efficient and easier to implement than current state-of-the-art prefix-based methods.

5   Experiments

We compare the performance of *TraVaS* against the state-of-the-art benchmark [12] and its extension (*SaCoFa* [9]) on real-life event logs. Due to algorithmic differences between our approach and the prefix-based approaches, it is particularly important to ensure a fair comparison. Hence, we employ divergently structured event logs and study a broad spectrum of privacy budgets (ϵ, δ). Moreover, the sequence cutoff for the benchmark and *SaCoFa* is set to the length that covers 80% of variants in each log, and the remaining pruning parameter is adjusted such that on average anonymized logs contain a comparable number of variants with the original log. Note that *TraVaS* guarantees the optimal number of output variants due to its underlying differentially private partition selection mechanism [4], and it does not need to limit the length of the released variants. Thus, the aforementioned settings consider the limitations of the prefix-based approaches to have a fair comparison.

We select two event logs of varying size and trace uniqueness. As we discussed in Sect. 4, and it is considered in other research such as [9,12], and [14], infrequent variants are challenging to privatize. Thus, trace uniqueness is an important analysis criterion. The Sepsis log describes hospital processes for Sepsis patients and contains many rare traces [11]. In contrast, BPIC13 has significantly more cases at a four times smaller trace uniqueness [5]. The events in BPIC13 belong to an incident and problem management system called VINST. Both logs are realistic examples of confidential human-centered information where the case identifiers refer to individuals. Detailed log statistics are shown in Table 2.

5.1   Evaluation Metrics

To assess the performance of an (ϵ, δ)-DP mechanism, suitable evaluation metrics are needed to determine how valuable the anonymized outputs are w.r.t. the original data. In this respect, we first consider a *data utility* perspective where the similarity between two logs is measured independent of future applications. For our experiments, two respective metrics are considered. From [13], we adopt *relative log similarity* that is based on the *earth mover's distance* between two trace variant distributions, where the normalized *Levenshtein* string edit distance is used as a similarity function between trace variants. The *relative log similarity*

Table 2. General statistics of the event logs used in our experiments.

Event log	#Events	#Cases	#Activities	#Variants	Trace uniqueness
Sepsis	15214	1050	16	846	80%
BPIC13	65533	7554	4	1511	20%

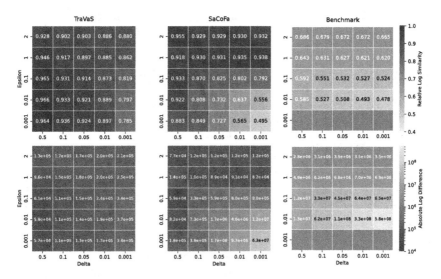

Fig. 1. The *relative log similarity* and *absolute log difference* results of anonymized BPIC13 logs generated by *TraVaS*, the benchmark, and *SaCoFa*. Each value represents the mean of 10 runs.

metric quantifies the degree to which the variant distribution of an anonymized log matches the original variant distribution on a scale from 0 to 1.

In addition, we introduce an *absolute log difference* metric to account for situations where distribution-based metrics provide only different expressiveness. Exemplary cases are event logs possessing similar variant distributions, but significantly different sizes. For such scenarios, the *relative log similarity* yields high similarity scores, whereas *absolute log difference* can detect these size disparities. To derive an absolute log difference value, we first transform both input logs into a *bipartite graph* of variant vertices. Then a *cost network flow* problem [15] is solved by setting demands and supplies to the absolute variant frequencies and utilizing a *Levenshtein* distance between variants as an edge cost. Hence, the resulting optimization value of an (ϵ, δ)-DP log resembles the number of *Levenshtein* operations to transform all respective variants into variants of the original log. In contrast to our *relative log similarity* metric, this approach can also penalize a potential matching impossibility. More information on the exact algorithms is provided on GitHub.[3]

Besides comparing event logs based on *data utility* measures, we additionally quantify the algorithm performance with *process discovery* oriented *result utilities*. We use the *inductive miner infrequent* [10] with default noise threshold of 20% to discover process models from the privatized event logs for all (ϵ, δ) settings under investigation. Then, we compare the models with the original event log to obtain token-based replay *fitness* and *precision* scores [2]. Due to the probabilistic nature of (ϵ, δ)-DP, we average all metrics over 10 anonymized logs for each setting, i.e., 10 separate algorithm runs per setting.

---

[3] https://github.com/wangelik/TraVaS/tree/main/supplementary.

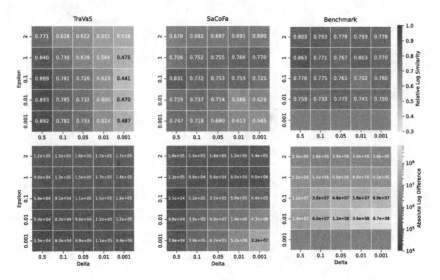

Fig. 2. The *relative log similarity* and *absolute log difference* results of anonymized Sepsis event logs generated by *TraVaS*, the benchmark, and *SaCoFa*. Each value represents the mean of 10 runs.

5.2   Data Utility Analysis

In this subsection, the results of the two aforementioned data utility metrics are presented for both real-life event logs. We compare the performance of *TraVaS* against our benchmark and *SaCoFa* based on the following privacy parameter values: $\epsilon \in \{2, 1, 0.1, 0.01, 0.001\}$ and $\delta \in \{0.5, 0.1, 0.05, 0.01, 0.001\}$.

Figure 1 shows the average results on BPIC13 in a four-fold heatmap. The grey fields represent a general unfeasibility of the strong privacy setting $\epsilon = 0.001$ for our benchmark method. Due to the intense noise perturbation, the corresponding variant generation process ncreased the number of artificial variant fluctuations to an extent that could not be averaged in a reasonable time. Apart from this artifact, both *relative log similarity* and *absolute log difference* show superior performance of *TraVaS* for most investigated (ϵ, δ) combinations. In particular, for stronger privacy settings, *TraVaS* provides a significant advantage over *SaCoFa* and benchmark. Whereas more noise, i.e., lower (ϵ, δ) values, generally decreases the output similarity to the original data, *TraVaS* results seem to particularly depend on δ. According to Definition 5, this observation can be explained by the stronger relation between k and δ compared to k and ϵ.

The evaluation of the Sepsis log is presented in Fig. 2. In contrast to BPIC13, Sepsis contains many variants occurring only once or twice. While our *absolute log difference* shows a similar expected trend with (ϵ, δ) as Fig. 1, the *relative log similarity* metric indicates almost constant values for the prefix-based techniques and a considerable δ-dependency for *TraVaS*. We explain the resulting patterns by examining the underlying data structure in more detail. As mentioned, the frequency threshold k of *TraVaS* strongly correlates with δ. Hence, event logs

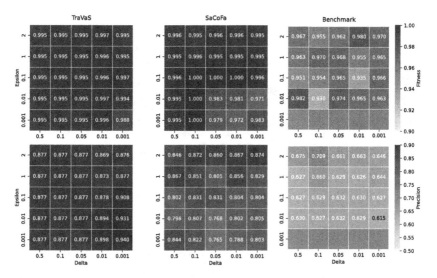

Fig. 3. The *fitness* and *precision* results of anonymized BPIC13 event logs generated by *TraVaS*, the benchmark, and *SaCoFa*. Each value represents the mean of 10 runs.

with prominent infrequent traces, e.g., Sepsis, are significantly truncated for strong (ϵ, δ)-DP. Since this variant removal leads to a distribution mismatch when being compared to the original log, the *relative log similarity* forms a step-wise pattern as in Fig. 2. In contrast, the prefix-based techniques iteratively generate variants that may or may not exist in the original log. In logs with high trace uniqueness, there exist many unique variants that are treated similarly to non-existing variants due to close frequency values, i.e., 0 and 1. Thus, in the anonymized logs, unique variants either appear with larger noisified frequencies or are replaced with fake variants having larger noisified frequencies. This process remains the same for different privacy settings but with larger frequencies for stronger privacy guarantees. Hence, the *relative log similarity* metric stays almost constant although the noise increases with stronger privacy settings. However, the *absolute log difference* metric can show differences. *uTraVaS* shows even better performance w.r.t. the data utility metrics.[4]

5.3 Process Discovery Analysis

We conduct a *process discovery* investigation based on *fitness* and *precision* scores. For the sake of comparability, the experimental setup remains unchanged. Figure 3 shows the results for BPIC13, where the original fitness and precision values are 0.995 and 0.877, respectively. *TraVaS* provides almost perfect replay behavior w.r.t. *fitness* while the prefix-based alternatives show lower values. This observation can be explained by the different algorithmic approach of *TraVaS* and some characteristics of BPIC13. *TraVaS* only adopts true behavior that

---

[4] https://github.com/wangelik/TraVaS/tree/main/experiments.

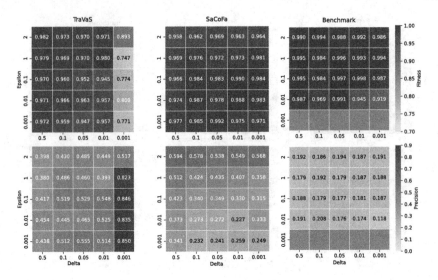

Fig. 4. The *fitness* and *precision* results of anonymized Sepsis event logs generated by *TraVaS*, the benchmark, and *SaCoFa*. Each value represents the mean of 10 algorithm runs.

results in a simplified representation of the original process model. Due to the rather low trace uniqueness and comparably large log-size of BPIC13, this simplification is minor enough to allow an almost perfect fitness. In contrast, the fake variants generated by prefix-based approaches negatively affect their fitness scores. The precision metric evaluates the fraction of behavior in a model discovered from an anonymized log that is not included in the original log. Due to the direct release mechanism of *TraVaS* that only removes infrequent variants, we achieve more precise process models than the alternatives. Furthermore, the correlation between threshold k and noise intensity enables *TraVaS* to even rise precision for stronger privacy guarantees. Conversely, the fake variants generated by prefix-based approaches can lead to inverse behavior.

Figure 4 shows the *fitness* and *precision* results for Sepsis, where the original fitness and precision values are 0.952 and 0.489, respectively. Whereas *TraVaS* dominates the prefix-based approaches w.r.t. *precision* as in Fig. 3, our fitness score shows a slight under-performance. Unlike BPIC13, the high trace uniqueness and smaller log-size prohibit the underlying *partition selection* mechanism to achieve negligible threshold for infrequent variant removal. Thus, the discovered process models from anonymized logs miss parts of the original behavior. This shows that carefully tuned prefix-based mechanisms might have an advantage in terms of fitness for small logs with many unique traces. We particularly note that this limitation of *TraVaS* vanishes as soon as the overall log-size grows. The reason lies in the size-independent threshold k while the pruning parameter of prefix-based approaches intensifies with the data size. The process discovery analyses for *uTraVaS*, available on GitHub, show even better performance.

6   Discussion and Conclusion

In this paper, we demonstrated a novel approach to release anonymized distributions of trace variants based on (ϵ, δ)-DP mechanisms. The corresponding algorithm (*TraVaS*) overcomes the variant generation problems of prefix-based mechanisms (see Sect. 1) and directly queries all true variants. Our experiments with two differently structured event logs showed that *TraVaS* outperforms the state-of-the-art approaches in terms of *data utility* metrics and process-discovery-based *result utility* for most of the privacy settings. In particular, for large event logs containing many long trace variants, our implementation has no efficient alternative. Regarding limitations and future improvements, we generally note that the differentially private partition selection mechanism only works for $\delta > 0$, whereby limits of small values can be problematic on large collections of infrequent variants. Thus, all use cases that require strict ϵ-DP still need to apply prefix-based mechanisms. Finding a more efficient solution for $\delta = 0$ seems to be a valuable and interesting future research topic.

References

1. GDPR. https://data.europa.eu/eli/reg/2016/679/oj. Accessed 15 May 2021
2. van der Aalst, W.M.P.: Process Mining - Data Science in Action, 2nd edn. Springer, Cham (2016)
3. Cohen, A., Nissim, K.: Towards formalizing the GDPR's notion of singling out. Proc. Natl. Acad. Sci. U.S.A. **117**(15), 8344–8352 (2020)
4. Desfontaines, D., Voss, J., Gipson, B., Mandayam, C.: Differentially private partition selection. Proc. Priv. Enhancing Technol. **2022**(1), 339–352 (2022)
5. van Dongen, B.F., Weber, B., Ferreira, D.R., Weerdt, J.D.: BPI challenge 2013. In: Proceedings of the 3rd Business Process Intelligence Challenge (2013)
6. Dwork, C.: Differential privacy: a survey of results. In: Agrawal, M., Du, D., Duan, Z., Li, A. (eds.) TAMC 2008. LNCS, vol. 4978, pp. 1–19. Springer, Heidelberg (2008). https://doi.org/10.1007/978-3-540-79228-4_1
7. Elkoumy, G., Pankova, A., Dumas, M.: Privacy-preserving directly-follows graphs: balancing risk and utility in process mining. CoRR abs/2012.01119 (2020)
8. Fahrenkrog-Petersen, S.A., van der Aa, H., Weidlich, M.: PRIPEL: privacy-preserving event log publishing including contextual information. In: Fahland, D., Ghidini, C., Becker, J., Dumas, M. (eds.) BPM 2020. LNCS, vol. 12168, pp. 111–128. Springer, Cham (2020). https://doi.org/10.1007/978-3-030-58666-9_7
9. Fahrenkrog-Petersen, S.A., Kabierski, M., Rösel, F., van der Aa, H., Weidlich, M.: Sacofa: semantics-aware control-flow anonymization for process mining. In: 3rd International Conference on Process Mining, ICPM. IEEE (2021)
10. Leemans, S.J.J., Fahland, D., van der Aalst, W.M.P.: Discovering block-structured process models from event logs containing infrequent behaviour. In: Lohmann, N., Song, M., Wohed, P. (eds.) BPM 2013. LNBIP, vol. 171, pp. 66–78. Springer, Cham (2014). https://doi.org/10.1007/978-3-319-06257-0_6
11. Mannhardt, F.: Sepsis Cases (2016). https://doi.org/10.4121/uuid:915d2bfb-7e84-49ad-a286-dc35f063a460
12. Mannhardt, F., Koschmider, A., Baracaldo, N., Weidlich, M., Michael, J.: Privacy-preserving process mining - differential privacy for event logs. Bus. Inf. Syst. Eng. **61**(5), 595–614 (2019)

13. Rafiei, M., van der Aalst, W.M.P.: Towards quantifying privacy in process mining. In: Leemans, S., Leopold, H. (eds.) ICPM 2020. LNBIP, vol. 406, pp. 385–397. Springer, Cham (2021). https://doi.org/10.1007/978-3-030-72693-5_29
14. Rafiei, M., van der Aalst, W.M.P.: Group-based privacy preservation techniques for process mining. Data Knowl. Eng. **134**, 101908 (2021)
15. Tomlin, J.A.: Minimum-cost multicommodity network flows. Oper. Res. **14**, 45–51 (1966)

BERMUDA: Participatory Mapping of Domain Activities to Event Data via System Interfaces

Vlad P. Cosma[1,2], Thomas T. Hildebrandt[1(✉)],
Christopher H. Gyldenkærne[3], and Tijs Slaats[1]

[1] Copenhagen University, Copenhagen 2200, Denmark
{vco,hilde,slaats}@di.ku.dk
[2] KMD ApS, Ballerup 2750, Denmark
vco@kmd.dk
[3] Roskilde University, Roskilde, Denmark
chrgyl@ruc.dk

Abstract. We present a method and prototype tool supporting participatory mapping of domain activities to event data recorded in information systems via the system interfaces. The aim is to facilitate responsible secondary use of event data recorded in information systems, such as process mining and the construction of predictive AI models. Another identified possible benefit is the support for increasing the quality of data by using the mapping to support educating new users in how to register data, thereby increasing the consistency in how domain activities are recorded. We illustrate the method on two cases, one from a job center in a danish municipality and another from a danish hospital using the healthcare platform from Epic.

Keywords: Data quality · Secondary use · Event extraction · Event matching · Participatory design

1 Introduction

The abundance of data recorded in information systems and easily accessible technologies for data processing, such as predictive AI models and process mining [1,2], have created huge expectations of how data science can improve the society.

However, there has also been an increasing voicing of concerns [3,11,18,39], pointing out that merely having access to data and technologies is not sufficient to guarantee improvements. In the present paper we focus on data quality and responsible event extraction in the context of secondary use of event data [34] recorded in information systems. That is, data representing events in the domain of use, such as the start and completion of work tasks which has as primary use to support case workers and document the progress of a case, but is intended

---

A 2-page extended abstract presenting early ideas of the paper was published in [13].

M. Montali et al. (Eds.): ICPM 2022 Workshops, LNBIP 468, pp. 127–139, 2023.
https://doi.org/10.1007/978-3-031-27815-0_10

to be used for secondary purposes, such as building predictive AI models or the discovery of processes using process mining tools.

The challenges of event data quality are manifold [9], including handling event granularity, incorrect or missing data and incorrect timestamps of events [17]. A more fundamental problem in the context of secondary use of event-data is that of ensuring a consistent and correct matching of event data to business activities [7].

The lack of research in the area of event log creation has been pointed out in several papers [2,7,9,16,21,26,29,30,36,38]. This task is in general associated with words and expressions like: costly, time consuming, tedious, unstructured, complex, garbage-in garbage-out. Historically, research for data-driven innovation and improving productivity has shown to pay little to no attention to how data is created and by who. Data is often created within a system and its user interface where a given context for capturing and using data has been established through continuous sense-making between people that have local and often individual understanding of why data is generated and for what. Studies claim [22,41] that data science initiatives are often initiated at high-level and allocated from domain of data creation while the data science product is re-introduced as a model that needs to be adapted by the practice where data is created. While data driven systems can be evaluated with good results on artificial data from the data domain, it is often a struggle to create value for the domain users. This is due to trust of data origin, what it represents and how new intents for its purpose comes through what could be considered a back-door top-down method. A Participatory Design(PD)-study [18] investigated a mismatch between data extraction findings at an administration level of cross-hospital management and how doctors and clinical secretaries represented their ways of submitting data, highlighting a need for re-negotiating data creation and its purpose in a way so data scientists can contribute to better data capture infrastructures as well as giving health-care workers a saying in how such data capture infrastructures are prioritized in their given domains of non-digital work. In PD [8,23,32] as a field such presented tensions are not new. Here PD as a design method and practice has sought to create alignment between workers existing understanding of own work and emerging systems through design as a practice for visualising such tensions across actors of an innovation or IT project. PD is from here seeking, in a democratic manner, to find solutions and interests that can match partners across hierarchies.

As a means to facilitate responsible secondary use of event data, we propose in this paper the BERMUDA (*Business Event Relation Map via User-interface to Data for Analysis*) method to capture and maintain the link between domain knowledge and the data in the information system. The method supports involvement of domain experts in the mapping of activities or events in the business domain to user-interface elements, and of system engineers in the mapping of user-interface elements to database records used by data scientists. In other words, the method helps documenting the inter-relationship in the "BERMUDA triangle" between the domain concepts, the user interface and the database, which often disappears. We see that by breaking down the barrier between data-creators and data scientists and building tools for involvement and iterative feedback of data infrastructures and their user front-end, new discussions for data cooperation can occur. The mapping is independent of any specific data analysis, but should of course include the activities and events of relevance for the analysis at hand. In particular, the method contributes to the responsible application of process mining [27] by supporting a collaborative creation of event logs.

The motivation for the method came from research into the responsible engineering of AI-based decision support tools in Danish municipalities within the EcoKnow [19] research project and later the use of the method was also found relevant in a study of a Danish hospital wanting to create an AI-based predictive model for clinical no-shows. The method and prototype were initially evaluated by a consultant employed in a process mining company and a municipal case worker collaborating with the authors in the EcoKnow research project.

The paper is structured as follows. Prior and related work is discussed in Sect. 2. Sect. 3 explains our proposed BERMUDA method, where we also show a prototype tool. Sect. 4 introduces two specific case studies in a job center and a danish hospital. A brief evaluation of the use of the method in the first case along with a discussion on the results is made in Sect. 5. Lastly, in Sect. 6 we conclude and discuss future work.

2   Prior and Related Work

Within health-care informatics, problems arising from having a primary use of data (original intend of health-care delivery and services) and different, secondary use of data (emergence of new possibilities through statistics and data science) has been highlighted in several studies [5,28,37]. The authors of [5] found that underlying issues for data quality and reuse was attributed to differential incentives for the accuracy of the data; flexibility in system software that allowed multiple routes to documenting the same tasks; variability in documentation practices among different personnel documenting the same task; variability in use of standardized vocabulary, specifically, the internally developed standardized vocabulary of practice names; and changes in project procedures and electronic system configuration over time, as when a paper questionnaire was replaced with an electronic version.

Such underlying socio-technical issues to data capturing can attribute to an overall lower degree of data integrity resulting in little to no secondary usefulness of data representing health-care events. A similar [18] study conducted by this papers co-authors highlighted the need for iteratively aligning data creation and use with domain experts and data creators (i.e. doctors, nurses, secretaries, etc.) when conducting data science on operational data from hospitals.

We see event abstraction [40] as a related topic to our paper, however we approach the problem in a top-down manner i.e. from domain knowledge down to the data source. A similar top-down approach exists in database systems [12] where an ontology of domain concepts is used to query the databases. We do not aim to propose techniques for process discovery as there are a plethora of tools already in use for this task, some of which [35] also allow for domain expert interventions. We propose BERMUDA both for pre-processing of data before moving to process discovery or building predictive models, and for training of new users in how to consistently record data suitable for the secondary uses.

The paper [21] provides a procedure for extracting event logs from databases that makes explicit the decisions taken during event log building and demonstrates it through a running example instead of providing tool support. The paper [7] present a semi-automatic approach that maps events to activities by transforming the mapping problem into the a constraint satisfaction problem, but it does not directly handle the event log extraction.

In [29] the authors describe a meta model that separates the extraction and analysis phases and makes it easy to connect event logs with SQL queries. In [30] they associate events from different databases into a single trace and propose an automated event log building algorithm. They point towards the lack of domain knowledge as a driving force for an automated and efficient approach. They discuss that their definition of event log "interestingness" as an objective score ignores aspects of domain level relevance. Both papers bind database scripts and event log concepts in order to build ontologies/meta-models, but do not link to domain knowledge in order to provide traceability to domain experts, such that the limitations of the "interestingness" score may be overcome.

To summarize, most work [6,9,10,16,17,24,25,33,38] on event data quality so far has focused on technical means to repair and maintain the quality of event logs [15]. Our approach complements these approaches by focusing on the socio-technical problem of aligning what is done in practice by the users of the information systems, i.e. how is a domain activity registered within the system, and at the other hand, where is this event stored in the database.

3   BERMUDA: Mapping Domain Events to Data

Our method relies on so-called BERMUDA triples (**e, i, d**) as illustrated in Fig. 1, recording the relation between respectively a domain event **e**, a user interface element **i** of the information system in which the domain event is registered and the location of the resulting data element **d** in the database. A concrete example from one of our case studies can be seen in Fig. 2. Here a domain event "Register ... during the first interview" is described in a textual audit schema. This is linked by a screen shot to the drop down menu in the user interface, where the case worker performs this concrete registration. And finally, the location of the resulting data element is recorded by an SQL statement that extracts the event.

There are typically three roles involved in the recording such BERMUDA triples: Data scientist (or analyst), domain expert and system engineer. As guidance towards applying our method we recommend following these steps:

1. **Domain to user interface**. For each domain event **e**, the domain experts record an association (**e, i**) between the domain event **e** and an (user or system) interface element **i**.

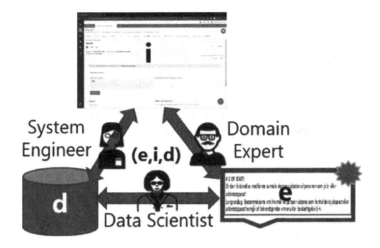

Fig. 1. BERMUDA method

2. **User interface to data**. Through code inspection or simulation, system engineers develop the correct database query **d** to extract the data recording the event **e** created via the interface element **i** resulting in a triple **(e, i, d)**.
3. **Triples to event log**. The data scientist merges and refines the database queries and creates the initial version of the event log. The event log entries are enriched with extra attributes that hold a reference to the domain event, the interface element and the data source from where the entry originated.

Prototype Tool. To facilitate the adoption of the BERMUDA method we present a prototype tool to illustrate how the triples can be created and an event log extracted. A screenshot from the prototype is shown in Fig. 2. Briefly, the UI consists of 3 input areas in the top for documenting the individual parts of triples (description of domain event, system interface, script for extracting the event from the system), an input area at the bottom for adding and selecting a

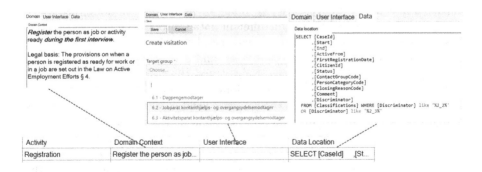

Fig. 2. BERMUDA method Prototype

triple to document, and a display area (not shown in the figure) for the resulting event log.[1]

The prototype has a simple role base access control supporting the use of the method in practice. All roles have access to the description of domain events, in order to build trust through a common domain understanding. Domain experts have access to domain events and the user interface input areas. System engineers need access to all areas, but not the production data in the information system. Data scientists are allowed access to all areas except they can not see the data extraction scripts, if they are covered by intellectual propriety rights. They can however run the scripts on the production system, to extract the event data.

4   Cases: Secondary Use of Municipal and Health Data

We discuss the method in relation to two concrete cases from Denmark where data in respectively a municipality and a hospital were intended to be used for AI-based decision support. Case 1 is elicited at a municipal job center in Denmark and case 2 covers our work with a regional research hospital where a project aiming for producing and using an AI model for no-shows. Both cases unveiled a gap between how data is produced in a local context for its primary purpose of case management and what it represents when extracted and used for decision support. We made an evaluation of our BERMUDA prototype for case one and speculate how it could be used in case two.

Case 1: As part of the EcoKnow research project [19], we had by the software vendor KMD (kmd.dk), been given access to interact with the system engineers that developed the case management system used in danish job centers. Collaborating with colleagues in the EcoKnow research project performing field studies at the job center [4, 20, 31], we also had the opportunity to gather domain knowledge through workshops, semi-structured interviews and informal methods from job center employees. Finally, we had access to historical data from about 16000 citizens with the purpose of researching the possibilities for improving compliance and the experienced quality of case management in municipalities.

In addition to our case we interviewed a consultant at a process mining company Infoventure (infoventure.dk), doing conformance checking, using the same case management system but a different data source. Their current practice relies on first co-creating a document with employees at the job center, which contained the necessary domain knowledge and screenshots of user interface elements with relevant explanations. Next it was the task of the consultant to build extraction scripts for the identified domain events. During this phase there was ongoing communication with the software vendor and job center employees through meetings, calls or emails, in order to build up the necessary domain and system knowledge. Often he would observe specific data (an exact timestamp or citizen registration number) in the user interface and proceed to search for that exact information in the database. This process was done either offline, with the

---

[1] The prototype is available at: https://github.com/paul-cvp/bermuda-method.

aid of screenshots, or on site by sitting next to a case worker. The links between domain events and the data extracted from the database was recorded in an ad-hoc way and only available to the consultant.

Domain Activities/Events: We used a management audit schema comprised of 21 questions. From these questions we define the domain activities/events relevant for the case compliance analysis. For example: From the audit question "Is the first job interview held within one week of the first request? Legal basis: LAB §31(3)" we can identify several domain event data of interest: first request, first job interview, first week passed.

Graphical User Interface (GUI) Areas for Recording Domain Events. A case-worker employed at the job center associated the domain events identified in the audit questions with areas of the user interface where caseworkers record the event. From the 21 questions, 11 domain events could be identified that could be given a user interface association. For 3 of the domain events, the caseworker was unsure where to record it. A data scientist was able to associate 12 of the 21 domain events to a field in the user interface. This relatively low number of associations can be explained by the fact that the audit schema was created by the municipality and not the vendor of the it-system, and thus, some of the domain events relevant for the audit did not have a direct representation in the user interface. Therefore certain events were completely missing or documented in free text fields, while others require access to other systems used by the municipality. In particular, as also observed in [4], the free text field was sometimes used to describe the categorisation of the unemployed citizen (as activity or job ready) or the reason for the choice of categorisation, by selecting the reason "other", instead of using one of the specific predefined values available in the system interface.

Data and Database Organization. The database contains 133 tables with 1472 columns in total. By having access to source code and the system engineers, we mapped the identified GUI elements to the database. Furthermore this limited our inspection to 8 main tables from which the data was extracted and 4 tables used for mapping table relations, thus ensuring data minimisation as specified in the General Data Protection Regulation (GDPR) [14].

Case 2: In the wake of a grand scale implementation of an EPIC[2] Regional Electronic Health Record-system (EHR-system) purchase and implementation, we have since 2017 been engaged in a longitudinal case-study of facilitating and developing an AI-model for predicting patient no-shows based on clinical event and demographic data. The project was pioneering as the first test of the models developed from local data and appointed a small endoscopy unit at Bispebjerg hospital (a research hospital in the capital region of Denmark). The project have a foundation in participatory design and end-user involvement in pursuit

---

[2] epic.com.

of creating visions for use of data and AI, as well as creating synergy effects for data creation among clinicians, nurses and clinical secretaries as domain experts creating clinical event data used to predict future no-shows.

We extracted 8 different data sets together with the regional data team to learn about implications for applying such data for machine-learning purposes. We here learned, that missing data values and incomplete submissions were largely representing the first data sets and that due to missing guidelines and coordinated workflows each individual health care person had different understanding of the categories used to report clinical appointment statuses.

Domain Events: Interpretations of the events. We conducted 2 follow-up interviews with clinical secretaries to understand the local flow of data submission into the EHR-system. The clinical secretaries demonstrated their data submission practices and their understanding of how to document clinical appointment statuses into the EHR-system. We further conducted four 2-h workshops involving the clinical secretaries in putting context to their workflow and use of categories to assign meaning to no-show categories. In the same period, we invited Regional data management and extraction teams to learn from practices and iteratively extract data sets with no-show data.

Data and Database Organization. 8 data sets were extracted in total over a period of 3 months before a machine learning algorithm could be fed with a data set with sufficient domain contexts to remove categories that didn't have meaning for secondary use. The best example of this was again the free text category "other" as a category for assigning reason for no-shows or cancellations of appointments. This category was heavily used by all clinical staff due to its ability to avoid reading through 16 other categories of reason for mentioned outcome. The first data set had 81.000 rows and observations with 2/3 of those past appointments being assigned "other" with text-field inputs sometimes representing the same categories as suggested in the drop-down menu and sometimes left empty or with "other" written in the text-field. A further 11.000 appointments were deemed incomplete or "in process" several months after appointment date. When sorting out unassigned events for appointment status the department only had 2880 observations left for the machine learning algorithm.

5   Initial Evaluation

As an initial qualitative evaluation of the usefulness of the method, we conducted two semi-structured interviews, one with a municipal case worker acting as a domain expert and another with a data scientist working as consultant in the process analysis company Infoventure. Both interview respondents collaborated with the authors in the Ecoknow research project. The municipal case worker was given the task of mapping business activities to user-interface elements of a case and document management system. The consultant was asked about the current practice of documenting event log extraction for process mining, illustrated by a concrete case, and how the Bermuda prototype could support or improve this practice.

Overall, the evaluation indicated, that the BERMUDA method exhibits the following positive proprieties:

- **Transparency, Accountability, and Traceablity.** The BERMUDA triples make it possible to trace the relation between events extracted from a data base, e.g. for the creation of an event log, and domain events. Both interviewees saw the advantage in unambiguously referencing domain events across different roles of a data science project (domain expert, software engineer, data scientist), thereby providing accountability for the data provenance/lineage, while also building trust across different roles.
- **Accuracy.** Through the participatory co-creation of the event log it is possible to observe that the event log correctly captures the relevant domain knowledge. As each of the roles interact with each other, they can observe that the correct steps were taken in the extraction of event data for secondary use. This was already to some extend part of the current practices, but BERMUDA supported the consistent documentation.
- **Maintainability and Training.** The interview participants indicated that the Bermuda method is useful for maintaining event logs over time when changes happen in the domain or system, because the information is documented consistently in one place. They also pointed out, that the method and tool for the same reason could be valuable both in training new data scientists and new case workers.
- **Protection of Intellectual Property.** Since each link in the BERMUDA triangle can be defined independently, the system engineers can provide mappings that can be used to extract events without revealing the code of the system. We observed this in the interaction between the data science consultant and the system engineers developing the job center solution.

Limitations. Firstly, the tool is not mature enough to replace a general SQL scripting environment. Secondly, it does not yet account for data that are not stored in an SQL database, nor for data that is not recorded via user interface, as for instance data recorded automatically by system events.

6   Conclusion and Future Work

In this paper we presented BERMUDA, a method for facilitating the responsible secondary use of event data in data science projects by supporting the collaboration between domain experts, system engineers and data scientists on associating domain events, via user interfaces to data in the database. This facilitates transparent extraction of event logs for analysis and thereby accountable data lineage. We discussed its use through cases of data science projects at a job center in a Danish municipality and a Danish hospital. In particular, both cases highlight the frequent use of the category "other" in the registration of reasons for domain events, instead of using pre-defined values in drop down menus. We showed through a prototype tool how BERMUDA can facilitate the interactions between domain experts, system engineers and data scientists. Furthermore we conducted interviews in order to lightly evaluate its usefulness and limitations.

In the future we expect to conduct more field trials of the method and interview more practitioners in order to do a thematic analysis for better qualitative feedback. We aim to investigate how the results of applying BERMUDA can be used when training domain experts to use the appropriate categories instead of"other". We also aim to extend the tool with an automatic signaling system to monitor for changes in the user interface and in the database structure to notify the data scientist of possible misalignment in existing processes. We hope to increase the robustness of the tool and its compatibility with existing process mining tools. We also aim to provide the prototype as an online tool in order to facilitate remote cooperative work. Finally we aim to support a broader range of input and output formats by applying the method on diverse data sources from information systems in relevant domains.

Acknowledgements. Thanks to Infoventure, KMD Momentum, Bispebjerg Hospital, The Capital Region of Denmark, Gladsaxe and Syddjurs municipalities, and the reviewers.

References

1. van der Aalst, W.M.P.: Process Mining - Data Science in Action, 2nd edn. Springer, Cham (2016)
2. van der Aalst, W., et al.: Process mining manifesto. In: Daniel, F., Barkaoui, K., Dustdar, S. (eds.) BPM 2011. LNBIP, vol. 99, pp. 169–194. Springer, Heidelberg (2012). https://doi.org/10.1007/978-3-642-28108-2_19
3. On AI, H.L.E.G.: Ethics guidelines for trustworthy AI. https://digital-strategy.ec.europa.eu/en/library/ethics-guidelines-trustworthy-ai
4. Ammitzbøll Flügge, A., Hildebrandt, T., Møller, N.H.: Street-level algorithms and AI in bureaucratic decision-making: a caseworker perspective. Proc. ACM Hum.-Comput. Interact. 5(CSCW1), 1–23 (2021). https://doi.org/10.1145/3449114
5. Ancker, J.S., et al.: Root causes underlying challenges to secondary use of data. In: AMIA Annual Symposium Proceedings, vol. 2011, p. 57. American Medical Informatics Association (2011)
6. Andrews, R., Emamjome, F., ter Hofstede, A.H.M., Reijers, H.A.: An expert lens on data quality in process mining. In: ICPM, pp. 49–56. IEEE (2020)
7. Baier, T., Rogge-Solti, A., Weske, M., Mendling, J.: Matching of events and activities - an approach based on constraint satisfaction. In: Frank, U., Loucopoulos, P., Pastor, Ó., Petrounias, I. (eds.) PoEM 2014. LNBIP, pp. 58–72. Springer, Heidelberg (2014). https://doi.org/10.1007/978-3-662-45501-2_5
8. Björgvinsson, E., Ehn, P., Hillgren, P.A.: Participatory design and democratizing innovation. In: Proceedings of the 11th Biennial Participatory Design Conference, pp. 41–50 (2010)
9. Bose, J.C.J.C., Mans, R.S., van der Aalst, W.M.P.: Wanna improve process mining results? In: CIDM, pp. 127–134. IEEE (2013)

10. Bose, R.P.J.C., van der Aalst, W.M.P., Žliobaitė, I., Pechenizkiy, M.: Handling concept drift in process mining. In: Mouratidis, H., Rolland, C. (eds.) CAiSE 2011. LNCS, vol. 6741, pp. 391–405. Springer, Heidelberg (2011). https://doi.org/10. 1007/978-3-642-21640-4_30

11. Cabitza, F., Campagner, A., Balsano, C.: Bridging the "last mile" gap between AI implementation and operation:"data awareness" that matters. Ann. Transl. Med. **8**(7), 501 (2020)

12. Calvanese, D., Giacomo, G.D., Lembo, D., Lenzerini, M., Rosati, R.: Ontology-based data access and integration. In: Liu, L., Özsu, M.T. (eds.) Encyclopedia of Database Systems, pp. 2590–2596. Springer, New York (2018). https://doi.org/10. 1007/978-1-4614-8265-9_80667

13. Cosma, V.P., Hildebrandt, T.T., Slaats, T.: BERMUDA: towards maintainable traceability of events for trustworthy analysis of non-process-aware information systems. In: EMISA Forum, vol. 41, no. 1. De Gruyter (2021)

14. Council of European Union: Regulation (EU) 2016/679 of the European parliament and of the council of 27 April 2016 on the protection of natural persons with regard to the processing of personal data and on the free movement of such data (2016) https://publications.europa.eu/s/llVw

15. De Weerdt, J., Wynn, M.T.: Foundations of process event data. Process Min. Handb. LNBIP **448**, 193–211 (2022)

16. Emamjome, F., Andrews, R., ter Hofstede, A.H.M., Reijers, H.A.: Alohomora: unlocking data quality causes through event log context. In: ECIS (2020)

17. Fischer, D.A., Goel, K., Andrews, R., van Dun, C.G.J., Wynn, M.T., Röglinger, M.: Enhancing event log quality: detecting and quantifying timestamp imperfections. In: Fahland, D., Ghidini, C., Becker, J., Dumas, M. (eds.) BPM 2020. LNCS, pp. 309–326. Springer International Publishing, Cham (2020). https://doi.org/10. 1007/978-3-030-58666-9_18

18. H. Gyldenkaerne, C., From, G., Mønsted, T., Simonsen, J.: PD and the challenge of AI in health-care. In: Proceedings of the 16th Participatory Design Conference 2020-Participation (s) Otherwise, vol. 2, pp. 26–29 (2020)

19. Hildebrandt, T.T., et. al.: EcoKnow: engineering effective, co-created and compliant adaptive case management systems for knowledge workers, pp. 155–164. Association for Computing Machinery, New York, (2020). https://doi.org/10.1145/ 3379177.3388908

20. Holten Møller, N., Shklovski, I., Hildebrandt, T.T.: Shifting concepts of value: designing algorithmic decision-support systems for public services. In: Proceedings of the 11th Nordic Conference on Human-Computer Interaction: Shaping Experiences, Shaping Society. NordiCHI 2020, Association for Computing Machinery, New York (2020). https://doi.org/10.1145/3419249.3420149

21. Jans, M., Soffer, P.: From relational database to event log: decisions with quality impact. In: Teniente, E., Weidlich, M. (eds.) BPM 2017. LNBIP, vol. 308, pp. 588–599. Springer, Cham (2018). https://doi.org/10.1007/978-3-319-74030-0_46

22. Jung, J.Y., Steinberger, T., So, C.: Domain experts as owners of data: towards sustainable data science (2022)

23. Kensing, F., Simonsen, J., Bodker, K.: Must: a method for participatory design. Human Comput. Interact. **13**(2), 167–198 (1998)

24. Leopold, H., van der Aa, H., Pittke, F., Raffel, M., Mendling, J., Reijers, H.A.: Searching textual and model-based process descriptions based on a unified data format. Softw. Syst. Model. **18**(2), 1179–1194 (2019)

25. Li, G., de Murillas, E.G.L., de Carvalho, R.M., van der Aalst, W.M.P.: Extracting object-centric event logs to support process mining on databases. In: Mendling, J., Mouratidis, H. (eds.) CAiSE 2018. LNBIP, vol. 317, pp. 182–199. Springer, Cham (2018). https://doi.org/10.1007/978-3-319-92901-9_16

26. Lux, M., Rinderle-Ma, S.: Problems and challenges when implementing a best practice approach for process mining in a tourist information system. In: BPM (Industry Track). CEUR Workshop Proceedings, vol. 1985, pp. 1–12. CEUR-WS.org (2017)

27. Mannhardt, F.: Responsible process mining. Process Min. Handb. LNBIP **448**, 373–401 (2022)

28. Meystre, S.M., Lovis, C., Bürkle, T., Tognola, G., Budrionis, A., Lehmann, C.U.: Clinical data reuse or secondary use: current status and potential future progress. Yearb. Med. Inform. **26**(01), 38–52 (2017)

29. de Murillas, E.G.L., Reijers, H.A., van der Aalst, W.M.P.: Connecting databases with process mining: a meta model and toolset. Softw. Syst. Model. **18**(2), 1209–1247 (2019)

30. de Murillas, E.G.L., Reijers, H.A., van der Aalst, W.M.P.: Case notion discovery and recommendation: automated event log building on databases. Knowl. Inf. Syst. **62**(7), 2539–2575 (2020)

31. Petersen, A.C.M., Christensen, L.R., Harper, R., Hildebrandt, T.: "We would never write that down": classifications of unemployed and data challenges for AI. Proc. ACM Hum. Comput. Interact. **5**(CSCW1), 1–26 (2021). https://doi.org/10.1145/3449176

32. Robertson, T., Simonsen, J.: Participatory design: an introduction. In: Routledge International Handbook of Participatory Design, pp. 1–17. Routledge (2012)

33. Sànchez-Ferreres, J., van der Aa, H., Carmona, J., Padró, L.: Aligning textual and model-based process descriptions. Data Knowl. Eng. **118**, 25–40 (2018)

34. Schrodt, P.A.: The statistical characteristics of event data. Int. Interact. **20**(1–2), 35–53 (1994)

35. Schuster, D., van Zelst, S.J., van der Aalst, W.M.P.: Cortado–an interactive tool for data-driven process discovery and modeling. In: Buchs, D., Carmona, J. (eds.) PETRI NETS 2021. LNCS, pp. 465–475. Springer International Publishing, Cham (2021). https://doi.org/10.1007/978-3-030-76983-3_23

36. Slaats, T.: Declarative and hybrid process discovery: recent advances and open challenges. J. Data Semant. **9**(1), 3–20 (2020). https://doi.org/10.1007/s13740-020-00112-9

37. Smylie, J., Firestone, M.: Back to the basics: identifying and addressing underlying challenges in achieving high quality and relevant health statistics for indigenous populations in canada. Stat. J. IAOS **31**(1), 67–87 (2015)

38. Suriadi, S., Andrews, R., ter Hofstede, A.H.M., Wynn, M.T.: Event log imperfection patterns for process mining: towards a systematic approach to cleaning event logs. Inf. Syst. **64**, 132–150 (2017)

39. Team, R.: Responsible data science. https://redasci.org/

40. van Zelst, S.J., Mannhardt, F., de Leoni, M., Koschmider, A.: Event abstraction in process mining: literature review and taxonomy. Granular Comput. **6**(3), 719–736 (2020). https://doi.org/10.1007/s41066-020-00226-2

41. Zhang, A.X., Muller, M., Wang, D.: How do data science workers collaborate? roles, workflows, and tools. Proc. ACM on Hum. Comput. Interact. **4**(CSCW1), 1–23 (2020)

3rd International Workshop on Streaming Analytics for Process Mining (SA4PM'22)

3rd International Workshop on Streaming Analytics for Process Mining (SA4PM'22)

Streaming Process Mining is an emerging area in process mining that spans data mining (e.g. stream data mining; mining time series; evolving graph mining), process mining (e.g. process discovery; conformance checking; predictive analytics; efficient mining of big log data; online feature selection; online outlier detection; concept drift detection; online recommender systems for processes), scalable big data solutions for process mining and the general scope of online event mining. In addition to many other techniques that are all gaining interest and importance in industry and academia. The SA4PM workshop aims at promoting the use and the development of new techniques to support the analysis of streaming-based processes. We aim at bringing together practitioners and researchers from different communities, e.g., Process Mining, Stream Data Mining, Case Management, Business Process Management, Database Systems, and Information Systems, who share an interest in online analysis and optimization of business processes and process-aware information systems with time, storage, or complexity restrictions. Additionally, SA4PM aims to attract research results on scalable algorithmic process mining solutions in general, given that the work addresses how such efficient solutions would function under streaming settings. The workshop aims at discussing the current state of ongoing research and sharing practical experiences, exchanging ideas, and setting up future research directions.

This third edition of the workshop attracted 4 international submissions, one of which was redirected to another workshop before the reviewing due to relevance. Each paper was reviewed by at least three members of the Program Committee. From these submissions, the top 2 were accepted as full papers for presentation at the workshop. Both presenters got the chance to interact with the audience through panel discussions. The SA4PM'22 workshop shared the program this year with the EdBA'22 workshop, which further enriched the discussions among various audience members. The papers presented at SA4PM'22 provided a mix of novel research ideas and focused on online the customer journey optimization and streaming declarative processes.

Lisan Wolters et al. focus on online process predictions by introducing a framework that continuously retrains machine learning models to predict the occurence of activities of interest in the remainder of the customer journey. The proposed framework, called HIAP, uses process mining techniques to analyze the customer journeys. Different prediction models are researched to investigate which model is most suitable for high importance activity prediction. Furthermore the effect of using a sliding window or landmark model for (re)training a model is investigated. The framework is evaluated using a health insurance real dataset and a benchmark data set. The efficiency and prediction quality results highlight the usefulness of the framework under various realistic online business settings.

Next, Andrea Burattin et al. addressed the problem of online process discovery through an algorithm that extracts declarative processes as dynamic condition graphs from event streams. Streams are monitored to generate temporal representations of the process, later processed to create declarative models. The authors validated the technique by identifying drifts in a publicly available dataset of event streams. The used metrics extend the Jaccard similarity measure to account for process change in a declarative setting. The technique and the data used for testing are available online.

We hope that the reader will find this selection of papers useful to keep track of the latest advances in the stream process mining area. We are looking forward to showing new advances in future editions of the SA4PM workshop.

November 2022   Marwan Hassani
                                                                       Andrea Burattin
                                                                   Sebastiaan van Zelst
                                                                       Thomas Seidl

Organization

Workshop Chairs

Marwan Hassani — Eindhoven University of Technology, The Netherlands

Andrea Burattin — Technical University of Denmark, Denmark

Sebastiaan van Zelst — Fraunhofer Institute for Applied Information Technology / RWTH Aachen University, Germany

Thomas Seidl — Ludwig-Maximilians-Univ. München, Germany

Program Committee

Ahmed Awad — University of Tartu, Estonia

Marco Comuzzi — Ulsan National Institute of Science and Technology, South Korea

Massimiliano de Leoni — University of Padua, Italy

Jochen De Weerdt — Katholieke Universiteit Leuven, Belgium

Agnes Koschmider — Kiel University, Germany

Xixi Lu — Utrecht University, The Netherlands

Yorick Spenrath — Eindoven University of Technology, The Netherlands

Boudewijn Van Dongen — Eindhoven University of Technology, The Netherlands

Eric Verbeek — Eindhoven University of Technology, The Netherlands

Predicting Activities of Interest in the Remainder of Customer Journeys Under Online Settings

Lisan Wolters[✉] and Marwan Hassani[iD]

Eindhoven University of Technology, Eindhoven, The Netherlands
lisanwolters@outlook.com, m.hassani@tue.nl

Abstract. Customer journey analysis is important for organizations to get to know as much as possible about the main behavior of their customers. This provides the basis to improve the customer experience within their organization. This paper addresses the problem of predicting the occurrence of a certain activity of interest in the remainder of the customer journey that follows the occurrence of another specific activity. For this, we propose the HIAP framework which uses process mining techniques to analyze customer journeys. Different prediction models are researched to investigate which model is most suitable for high importance activity prediction. Furthermore the effect of using a sliding window or landmark model for (re)training a model is investigated. The framework is evaluated using a health insurance real dataset and a benchmark data set. The efficiency and prediction quality results highlight the usefulness of the framework under various realistic online business settings.

Keywords: Process mining · Process prediction · Customer journey analysis · Streaming data · Machine learning · Deep learning

1 Introduction

Customer journey analysis is useful for companies trying to understand how the customer interacts with the company. Next to understanding the customer journey it can also be used to improve the customer experience [1]. Customers can interact with a company over multiple channels, such as website visits, phone calls, physical presence at stores, etc. Not all interactions (or touchpoints) provide the same customer experience and satisfaction [2]. Next to understanding current customer journeys, it is also interesting for companies to predict whether customers will interact with a certain touchpoint on a later moment in their journey. Knowing in advance which customer will encounter certain touchpoints, might provide the option to prevent the occurrence of touchpoints that often indicate a negative feeling towards the journey which in turn might result with saving resources. Current research has already shown interest in next event prediction and final outcome prediction for running customer cases [3,6]. In this paper, the research conducted will investigate whether the customer will interact

© The Author(s) 2023
M. Montali et al. (Eds.): ICPM 2022 Workshops, LNBIP 468, pp. 145–157, 2023.
https://doi.org/10.1007/978-3-031-27815-0_11

with a certain activity in the remainder of its journey. Therefore, neither next activity prediction nor final outcome prediction will alone be sufficient. Filling the gap in future touchpoint of interest prediction is achieved by providing a repeatable framework for future high importance activity prediction (HIAP). The main use case of this work comes from a health insurer company that we will refer to as Yhealth. Yhealth wants to retrieve insights in which customers are most likely to call Yhealth. Performing a call is often experienced bad; therefore, it is interesting to prevent such interactions. A first step in prevention is knowing which customer will call. For this purpose, a data set containing declaration data of the customer is provided. The goal is to predict at a certain moment in the customer journey which customers will call Yhealth in the remainder of their journey. The solution proposed in this paper uses online process mining techniques to analyze the current customer journeys. The insights gathered serve as basis to indicate the decision moment (DeM) and potential activity (PoAc). For customer journeys reaching the DeM it should be predicted whether the customer will interact with the PoAc in the remainder of its journey. Machine and deep learning models are trained to perform predictions. The solution provides a repeatable framework to predict the occurrence of a PoAc in a customer journey. The performance of the different prediction models is evaluated. Next, research is conducted in the resources needed to keep a model up to date to recent customer journeys with respect to the quality gain, using online settings with a sliding window model and a landmark window model. This research shows that it is important to focus on recent traces to observe and react on changing behaviour of the customer.

The paper is structured as follows: Sect. 2 provides an overview of related work. Section 3 contains notations used in the paper and explains the research problem in more details. Section 4 defines the proposed framework, which is then evaluated in Sect. 5. Section 6 concludes the paper with an outlook.

2   Related Work

Predicting next events and timestamps in a running trace is discussed in several works. Though none of these works have the same assumptions, data or goal. In [7] a technique to analyze and optimize the customer journey by applying process mining and sequence-aware recommendations is proposed. These techniques are used to optimize key performance indicators to improve the customer journey by providing personalized recommendations. The goal of predicting what a customer will like differs from predicting what a customer will do. Especially predicting whether a customer will encounter an action that is often experienced badly is a different goal. Therefore, the second phase of sequence-aware recommendations is not applicable in the current context. Predicting a next event and its associated timestamp in a customer journey is discussed in [6]. They propose a RNN with the LSTM architecture for both next event and suffix prediction. Suffix prediction is applied by iteratively predicting the next event. This may result in a poor suffix quality as an error in a previous prediction is propagated to the next prediction. This approach encounters difficulties with traces in which the same event occurs multiple times as in that case the model will predict overly long sequences of that event. In the case of a health insurer, some events are expected to reoccur. Therefore, a solution for this limitation should be implemented to be applicable in the current context. Another approach on suffix prediction is applied in [5] by using an encoder-decoder GAN. The encoder and decoder are both represented by an LSTM network and allow the creation of variable length suffixes. This technique is used to predict suffixes up to the end of the trace. Furthermore, a suffix is not generated at a certain point in the customer journey, which is of high importance in the current research. Different ML and DL techniques for outcome predictions are evaluated in [4]. The outcome of a trace is predicted for a journey up to x events in which x has values from 1 to 10. Predicting the final outcome of a case is not the same as predicting whether a certain activity will occur. However, it should be possible to adapt the final outcome to high importance activity prediction. But nonetheless the technique is not applicable in the current research as a prediction should be provided as soon as a certain proposition holds for that trace, instead of after x events. In [8], the authors propose a framework for online prediction of the final outcome of retailer consumer behaviour using several aggregation methods.

3   Problem Exposition

This section defines the notation needed to understand the HIAP framework and describes the research problem in more details. Let $\mathcal{CJ} = (cj_1, cj_2, ..., cj_n)$ be a log containing the customer interactions. Each row in the log $cj_r = (cu_j, t, i, ia_1, ..ia_m)$ defines a single interaction of customer cu_j. The customer conducted touchpoint i at time t. The interaction of the customer may have interaction attributes $(ia_1, ...ia_m)$. Later, $\mathcal{CJ}$ is converted into an event log. Let $\mathcal{L} = (e_1, e_2, ...e_n)$ be the event log of the customer journey. Each row in the log $e_r = (c_i, t, a, d_1, ..d_k)$ defines a single event performed by one case identifier c_i. Each customer cu_j can be mapped to a c_i. The touchpoint of the interaction of the customer is renamed to an activity a and the activity is performed at time t. Each touchpoint i will be mapped to an activity a, but multiple touchpoints might be mapped to the same activity a. Furthermore, events can have attributes $d_1, ...d_k$, extracted from the interaction attributes. The log $\mathcal{L}$ contains all traces of the customers in CJ. Let $\sigma_i = <e_1, e_2, ..., e_{|\sigma_i|}>$ define the trace of case identifier c_i. The α-prefix is the trace up to and including the first α events. The suffix is defined as event $(\alpha + 1)$ until the end of the trace.

This work aims to use process mining techniques to improve customer journey analysis and use the insights to improve the customer experience. A repeatable framework for future touchpoint prediction in a customer journey is proposed. The result can be used to make the customer journey smoother, which will result in a more satisfied customer. For a customer journey a PoAc and DeM in the trace will be defined. Based on DeM x, we know the x-prefix $<e_1, ...e_x>$ of a customer journey. Using the information in the x-prefix, the goal is to predict whether PoAc y will occur in the x-suffix of the customer. Where the x-suffix is $<e_{x+1}, ..., e_{|trace|}>$. Customer journeys may change rapidly, therefore the prediction models should facilitate updates and the framework is tested by means of data streams. Using data streams stresses the effect of incorporating changing behaviour of customers. Without using data streams, models are based on older customer data and in the case of changing customer behaviour the prediction will become unreliable. When models are retrained over time the recent changes in customer behaviour is still considered and models will provide predictions with a higher performance.

4   High Importance Activity Prediction Framework

This chapter introduces the high importance activity prediction (HIAP) framework to predict the occurrence of an interesting touchpoint in the remainder of the customer journey based on the journey up to a specific point in time. The prediction uses information of the event log prefixes and possible customer information to predict for a specific customer whether (s)he will have a specific interaction in the future. Figure 1 shows an overview of the framework. This chapter explains the steps of the framework.

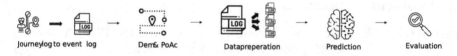

Journeylog to event log   Dem& PoAc   Datapreperation   Prediction   Evaluation

Fig. 1. Schematic overview of the proposed framework

The goal of the first step is to create a preprocessed event log $\mathcal{L}$ that can be used for the research. Preprocessing is needed to combine data of different sources, infer missing data and remove unnecessary data [9]. Different scenarios require different data harmonization techniques. Examples are data cleaning, transforming interactions and transforming a customer journey to an event log.

4.1   Critical Moments

The process model of event log $\mathcal{L}$ is used for defining critical moments. The critical moments are the decision moment(DeM) and the potential activity (PoAc).

Decision Moment Definition. The goal of HIAP is to predict whether a certain activity will occur based on a predefined moment in the trace. This specific moment can be defined either by a specific activity or by a proposition based on the events in the trace. The first time that such an activity occurs or the proposition holds will be taken as the DeM of the trace. When determining the DeM two criteria should be considered. First, the goal of the prediction is to be able to adjust the remainder of the trace and prevent the occurrence of a certain activity or to be able to save resources. As a result, the prediction should be early in the process. Second, the prediction should be as accurate as possible. In general, more accurate predictions can be provided at the moment that more information is available about the current process. Therefore, a balance should be found between choosing an early DeM and the quality of the prediction [10]. As the prediction takes place at a certain moment, only the traces in $\mathcal{L}$ that at some moment satisfy the condition of a DeM should be considered. The traces that do not satisfy the DeM should be removed from the log.

Potential Activity Definition. The PoAc is the activity of which it is preferred to know whether it will occur in the remainder of the customer journey. The DeM should be a proposition that is met earlier in the trace than that the PoAc occurs. However, the PoAc may be an activity that is occurring at a random moment in the suffix of the trace with respect to the DeM.

4.2 Data Preparation

Prior to the prediction phase a training, a validation and a test set should be created. Two methods are used to create those sets, one being a static method and the second method a streaming setting. Method one uses chronological in time the first 70% of the data as training data, the next 10% as validation data and the last 20% as test data. For the second method, a sliding window and a landmark model are used to investigate the effect on the training time and prediction performance. These results provide insights in the need to use all historical data or only recent historical data to keep the prediction models up to date. Using a wider period of time results in a considering more customer journeys and more likely a wider spectrum of use cases. While narrowing the time window provides a more detailed focus on recent customer journeys and provides more details on recent behaviour. In this case, a start date and end date of the window is defined. The training and the validation sets are composed of the traces that are completed in this window. The test set is constructed of the set of traces of which the proposition defining the DeM is satisfied in this time window, but that are not yet completed.

4.3 Prediction of the Potential Activity

In this paper three models are considered for the prediction of the PoAc to determine which model is most suited. The possible methods for prediction are not limited to these models; therefore, it is possible to consider other models too.

Random Forest Classifier. In order to train a RFC, the traces first need to be represented as a set of features [11]. These features consist of a set of independent variables and one dependent variable. This set of independent variables should be deduced from the trace that is available up to the DeM as well as available customer details. The dependent variable represents the occurrence of the PoAc in the suffix of the trace. Resulting in a binary decision.

Long-Short-Term-Memory Network. The LSTM used in the research is inspired on the implementation of [4] for final outcome prediction. Their preprocessing entails multiple steps. First, they defined the number x of events which should be considered while creating the feature vector. The feature vectors only entail information of the event and trace attributes that are available up to that moment of the trace. The traces that did not contain at least x events are removed from the log. Last, the label indicating the final outcome of the current trace is assigned to the feature vector. This part of the feature vector is used to compare the prediction with the ground truth and to train model parameters. This preprocessing is not directly applicable in the current research. The event number of the DeM may differ from one trace to another, but for each trace the prediction should be provided at the DeM. For each trace, the number of events prior to the DeM can be extracted. Furthermore, a number y of events is defined, defining the preferred prefix length for each trace. Traces containing more than y events up to the DeM, should be shortened. Only the last y events up to the DeM should be kept. Traces that have less than y events up to the DeM should lengthened with artificial events, added to the start of the trace. The events occurring later than the DeM, should still be preserved. The trace suffix will be used to determine the dependent variable, indicating whether the PoAc occurs. The feature vectors are used as input to a LSTM network classifier. The model is trained with a two-stage learning strategy as explained in [4].

Generative Adversarial Network. The GAN described is an adaption of the model in [5] for suffix prediction. The implementation needed some modification regarding the creation of the training, the validation and the test set and the number of prefix and suffixes created for each trace. [5] created the training, the validation and the test sets by randomly selecting instances from the complete log. In this research those are defined based on the timestamp of the DeM or based on the timeframe. Secondly, one prefix-suffix combination should be created per trace based on the DeM. The PoAc activity prediction could be determined by the occurrence of the PoAc in the suffix returned by the model.

4.4 Model Comparison and Future Model Use

The next step is to evaluate the performance of each classifier to judge the trustworthiness of the classifiers and to compare the different models. Depending on the research field and goal of the research the quality of each model will be accessed by the F1-score and/or recall. Generally, a higher score implies that the model is outperforming the other models [9]. Furthermore, the three models should also be compared to a baseline model. As baseline model a random predictor is used. The random predictor uses the distribution of the occurrence of the PoAc in the training set and predicts for the test set that the PoAc will occur in the same percentage of cases. The average prediction performance over 1000 runs is used as result for the baseline model. After training a model, the goal is to predict for new cases, as soon as the DeM property holds, whether the PoAc will occur. Predictions should be as reliable as possible in such cases; therefore, the model that is expected to be most trustworthy should be used.

The model that is evaluated to be the best model, can be used for future instance predictions. After training a model, the model can be stored, such that the model can be used for future predictions of the PoAc. At the moment that the proposition defining the DeM holds for a new customer journey, it can be represented with the same feature representation as the original data. A prediction on the occurrence of the PoAc will be provided by the model. The prediction can be used to act upon to improve the customer experience.

5 Experimental Evaluation

This section evaluates the application of the HIAP research on the Yhealth and benchmark BPI 2012 dataset.

5.1 Health Insurer Data Set

The Dutch health insurer data set contains details about the declaration process for customers. The log $\mathcal{CJ}$ covers a time period of two months, recording for all interactions cj_r the touchpoint i, its timestamp t and the customer identifier cu_j. In addition, anonymized customer details are available and touchpoints are related to further attributes, for example for a call the question is recorded. The data harmonization is conducted with the help of Yhealth. Steps taken are filtering of phone calls based on the subject, mapping of touchpoints to belong to a declaration and filtering incomplete traces. This resulted in an event log $\mathcal{L}$ consisting of 95,457 traces accounting for nearly 400,000 events. Most traces are relatively short as 95% of the traces had less than 10 events. The goal for Yhealth is to determine whether a customer will call as a follow-up to obtaining the result of the declaration. Calling is often perceived negatively by the customer; therefore, Yhealth would like to prevent the occurrence of a call. The first step to prevent the call is to know who will call. For that reason, the PoAc is defined as a call. The DeM is the moment that the result of a declaration is sent to the customer. This moment is chosen as earlier in the trace, for a lot of traces not enough information is available for the prediction and the result of the declaration will provide valuable information for the prediction. The log is imbalanced, as only 3.5% of the traces contain a call event on a later moment than receiving the result on a declaration. The set is used to create a training, a validation and a test set. The training set is undersampled such that the occurrence of the PoAc is more evenly distributed in the suffix with respect to the DeM.

The next step is to convert the traces to input for the RFC, LSTM and GAN. For all three models the traces up to the moment that the customer receives the results of a declaration is used as input to train a model for predictions. In the case of the RFC the traces have to be converted in a set of independent decision variables and one dependent variable which is the PoAc. The independent variables contain information of trace and event attributes. The input features of the LSTM network contain information on trace attributes and event attributes. All input features should have the same length; therefore, each trace is preprocessed such that it contains 5 events up to the DeM. The preprocessing of [4] is used to create the feature representation. The GAN network uses the original prefixes up to the DeM. The input of the training set also contains the suffixes which are either the suffix up to the PoAc or the complete suffix when PoAc is not in the suffix. The feature representation as proposed in [7] is the input for the encoder-decoder GAN.

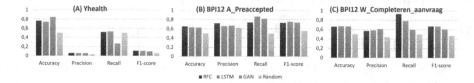

Fig. 2. Performance measures of the prediction models in offline setting

To determine which model can be used best, the three models and baseline model should be compared. The result is shown in Fig. 2(A). None of the models is performing best on all four performance measures. For the case of Yhealth it is most important to know whether a customer is likely to call. Therefore recall together with F1-score are the most import performance measures. On these two measures the LSTM and RFC model are performing best. The F1 score of both these models is doubled with respect to the random classifier; therefore, outperforming the baseline model. Without affecting the quality of the model, LSTM networks usually require a higher hardware requirement to train and use the model [4], which is not always available. Furthermore, RFC models are easier to understand and explain for humans. Accordingly, the RFC might be selected as the best prediction model for Yhealth.

Next to comparing the three prediction models on the complete data set, research is conducted in applying a sliding window and landmark model. A sliding window model only trains over the most recent instances, while a landmark model trains on the complete history of available data. Therefore, it is expected that a landmark model needs more resources to train a model. However, it is also expected that the quality of the predictions will be higher, as more training data is available. For this purpose, sub windows of the complete data are used to create the training, the validation and the test set for the sliding window and landmark model. In the current research, all models are trained on a CPU. If a GPU would be available the models could benefit from improved parallel computations. A GAN and LSTM network are expected to benefit more from a GPU, while the RFC is expected to be faster on a CPU.

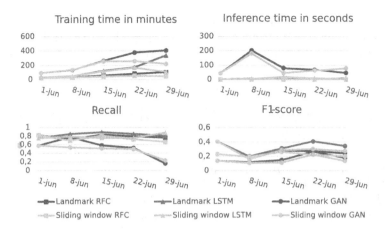

Fig. 3. Sliding window and landmark model results for the Yhealth data set.

The results of using a sliding window and landmark model on the Yhealth data set is shown in Fig. 3. For the sliding window, each window contains two weeks of data and the window shifts with one week for each new window. For the landmark model the first window contains two weeks of data, the next windows each increase with the data of one extra week. As can be seen in Fig. 3 the training time of the landmark model increases as the window size increases. Considering the same window, the RFC model is trained faster than the LSTM model and the LSTM models is faster than the GAN model. The inference time for the RFC and LSTM model is similar, but the GAN model is slower. For each model, the precision and F1-score of the landmark model is at least as high as their counterparts of the sliding window. This shows that the landmark model is eager to learn using more journeys, even if these journey are already a little older. Considering the recall score, up to the window ending at June 22, the landmark model is performing better than the sliding window for each prediction model. For the window ending at June 29, the GAN and the LSTM models trained over the sliding window have higher recall scores than the two models trained over the landmark model. The GAN model is performing worst for almost all windows. As of the window ending at June 15, the LSTM model on the sliding window and landmark model scores are slightly higher than the RFC model. However, the training time of the RFC model is considerably shorter. For a model to provide predictions, it is important to regularly update the model to new instances. Updating a model is easiest if training takes as less time as possible, but the results should not be affected by the reduction of the training time. Especially the time to train the LSTM model on the landmark model is too long for the last window. Therefore, the landmark LSTM model is not the most preferred model. The gain in performance for the LSTM sliding window model is small with respect to the RFC model on the landmark model. The performance of the RFC model with the sliding window is again slightly lower. However, the model with the lowest performance requires the shortest training time. As the RFC model is easier to understand, the RFC model is the preferred model to use. The running time of the landmark model of the RFC is not yet too long; therefore, the landmark model is preferred over the sliding window.

5.2   BPI 2012 Data Set

Since the data of Yhealth is confidential, the HIAP framework is replicated on the public available BPI 2012 event log. The BPI 2012 challenge event log contains data of the application process for a personal loan or overdraft within a Dutch financial institute. Only events with the life cycle attribute value 'complete' are considered and only traces that either have an approved, cancelled or declined application. The event log covers a time period of 6 months and contains around 12,700 cases and 156,000 events. The process model of the event log is used to determine the critical moments. A new sub-process in the log is initiated if a customer requests a loan, in that case the Dutch financial institute determines whether an offer will be sent to the customer. In order to determine whether an offer will be sent, human resources are needed to complete the application and to create an offer. If it is known early enough whether an offer will be sent, the resources could be used only for cases in which indeed an offer will be provided to the customer. Therefore, the PoAc is the activity 'O_SENT'. At the activities of 'W_Completeren_aanvraag' (Complete application,W_C_a) and 'A_PREACCEPTED' (A_p) the remainder of the process can still contain the activity 'O_SENT', but the process might also finish without the activity 'O_SENT'. Accordingly, two DeMs are defined, 1) the moment at which 'A_p' occurs and 2) the moment at which 'W_C_a' occurs. For the prediction task on the DeM of 'A_p' only traces in which the activity 'A_p' occurs are considered. Resulting in 6968 traces. For the activity 'W_C_a' the event log also consist of 6968 traces. The occurrence of 'O_SENT' is 67, 2% and 44, 1% respectively. After creating a training, a validation and a test set for both DeMs, the training set is balanced on the occurrence of 'O_SENT'.

The next step is to convert the traces to inputs for the RFC, LSTM and GAN for both DeMs. For all three models the traces up to the moment 'A_p' as well as the moment 'W_C_a' are used separately as input to train a model for predictions. In the case of the RFC the traces have to be converted to a feature representation. The independent variables contain information of trace and event attributes. The input features of the LSTM network contain similarly information on trace attributes and event attributes. The trace length is set to 3 for 'A_p' and 6 for 'W_C_a' up to the DeM. The preprocessing of [4] is used to create the feature representation. For each trace, additional independent variables are created, which are the amount of loan or overdraft requested by the customer, the number of activities so far, the types of these activities and time between them. The GAN network uses the original prefixes up to the DeM. The input of the training set also contains the suffixes which are either the suffix up to the PoAc or the complete suffix when PoAc is not in the suffix. The feature representation as proposed in [7] is the input for the encoder-decoder GAN.

To determine the best prediction model, the three models and the baseline model should be compared. The result is shown Fig. 2(B) and (C). For both DeMs the three models are outperforming the baseline model, as the models score higher on all performance measures. For DeM 'A_p' the F1-score for all three models is comparable. The recall is best on the LSTM model. Therefore, the LSTM model is preferred in predicting 'O_SENT'. For DeM 'W_C_a' the RFC and LSTM model score equally on the F1-score and slightly better than the GAN model. The recall score of the RFC is outperforming those of the LSTM and GAN model. The RFC model is best for the current prediction task.

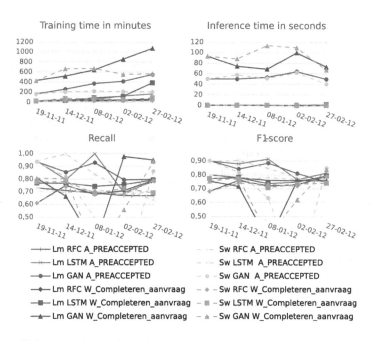

Fig. 4. Sliding window and landmark model results on the BPI 2012 data set.

Next the results of using a sliding window and a landmark model are discussed. The first window consists of 50 days and for each timeframe it either shifts by 25 days (Sw) or 25 days of data are added (Lm). The results for both 'A_p' and 'W_C_a' are shown in Fig. 4. For both DeMs it is the case that the training time of the sliding window models is relatively consistent over the different windows, while the training time of the landmark model increases. Resulting in a longer training time for the landmark model for later windows. Furthermore the training time and the inference time of the GAN is longer than the counterparts of the LSTM and RFC model. Considering the performance measure, the GAN model shows some poor performance results for some of the windows. This might be caused by the goal of training for suffix prediction, which is a different goal than predicting a PoAc. For both the RFC and LSTM model the performance (recall and F1-score) for the landmark model are comparable to the sliding window results. Therefore models are not learning form more data and only retraining on the most recent data is needed. For prediction moment 'A_p' the LSTM model is performing better than the RFC model on most windows. Therefore, considering training time, inference time, recall and F1-score the LSTM model with sliding window is preferred. On the other hand, for prediction moment 'W_C_a' the RFC on both windows and the LSTM model on the landmark window perform better than the LSTM with the sliding window. Considering the training time, inference time, recall and F1-score the RFC on the sliding window is preferred.

6   Conclusion

In this paper the HIAP framework is proposed as a repeatable framework for predicting the occurrence of a PoAc at a DeM in the customer journey. Different machine and deep learning models are compared for future predictions of touchpoint of interest using two windowing methods. To show the relevance of the framework, we tested it using two datasets showing the prediction power and the impact of using a sliding window or a landmark window. Showing that the preferred prediction model and windowing technique depends the type of customer journey data. Interesting future research is to predict the moment at which the expected activity is expected to occur [6]. This provides information on the possibility to prevent the activity to occur.

References

1. Bernard, G., Andritsos, P.: Contextual and behavioral customer journey discovery using a genetic approach. In: Welzer, T., Eder, J., Podgorelec, V., Kamišalić Latifić, A. (eds.) ADBIS 2019. LNCS, vol. 11695, pp. 251–266. Springer, Cham (2019). https://doi.org/10.1007/978-3-030-28730-6_16
2. van der Veen, G., Ossenbruggen, R.: Mapping out the customer's journey: customer search strategy as a basis for channel management. J. Mark. Channelsl **22**, 202–213 (2015)
3. Hassani, M., Habets, S.: Predicting next touch point in a customer journey: a use case in telecommunication. In: ECMS 2021 Proceedings, vol. 35 (2021)
4. Kratsch, W., Manderscheid, J., Roeglinger, M., Seyfried, J.: Machine learning in business process monitoring: a comparison of deep learning and classical approaches used for outcome prediction. Bus. Inf. Syst. Eng. **63**, 261–276 (2021). https://doi.org/10.1007/s12599-020-00645-0
5. Taymouri, F., La Rosa, M.: Encoder-decoder generative adversarial nets for suffix generation and remaining time prediction of business process models (2020). arXiv:2007.16030
6. Tax, N., Verenich, I., La Rosa, M., Dumas, M.: Predictive business process monitoring with LSTM neural networks. In: CAiSE, pp. 477–492 (2017)
7. Terragni, A., Hassani, M.: Optimizing customer journey using process mining and sequence-aware recommendation. In: ACM/SIGAPP (SAC), pp. 57–65 (2019)

8. Spenrath, Y., Hassani, M., van Dongen, B.F.: Online prediction of aggregated retailer consumer behaviour. In: Munoz-Gama, J., Lu, X. (eds.) ICPM 2021. LNBIP, vol. 433, pp. 211–223. Springer, Cham (2022). https://doi.org/10.1007/978-3-030-98581-3_16
9. van der Aalst, W.: Process Mining: Data Science in Action. Springer, Cham (2016)
10. Metzger, A., Neubauer, A., Bohn, P., Pohl, K.: Proactive process adaptation using deep learning ensembles. In: Giorgini, P., Weber, B. (eds.) CAiSE 2019. LNCS, vol. 11483, pp. 547–562. Springer, Cham (2019). https://doi.org/10.1007/978-3-030-21290-2_34
11. Breiman, L.: Random forests. Mach. Learn. **45**, 5–32 (2001)

Uncovering Change: A Streaming Approach for Declarative Processes

Andrea Burattin[1], Hugo A. López[1(✉)], and Lasse Starklit[2]

[1] Technical University of Denmark, Kgs. Lyngby, Denmark
hulo@dtu.dk
[2] Netcompany A/S, Copenhagen, Denmark

Abstract. Process discovery is a family of techniques that helps to comprehend processes from their data footprints. Yet, as processes change over time so should their corresponding models, and failure to do so will lead to models that under- or over-approximate behaviour. We present a discovery algorithm that extracts declarative processes as Dynamic Condition Response (DCR) graphs from event streams. Streams are monitored to generate temporal representations of the process, later processed to create declarative models. We validated the technique by identifying drifts in a publicly available dataset of event streams. The metrics extend the Jaccard similarity measure to account for process change in a declarative setting. The technique and the data used for testing are available online.

Keywords: Streaming process discovery · Declarative processes · DCR graphs

1 Introduction

Process discovery techniques promise that given enough data, it is possible to output a realistic model of the process as is. This evidence-based approach has a caveat: one needs to assume that inputs belong to the same process. Not considering process variance over time might end in under- or over-constrained models that do not represent reality. The second assumption is that it is possible to identify full traces from the event log. This requirement indeed presents considerable obstacles in organizations where processes are constantly evolving, either because the starting events are located in legacy systems no longer in use, or because current traces have not finished yet. Accounting for change is particularly important in declarative processes. Based on a "outside-in" approach, declarative processes describe the minimal set of rules that generate accepting traces. For process mining, the simplicity of declarative processes has been demonstrated to fit well with real process executions, and declarative miners are currently the most precise miners in use[1]. However, little research exists regarding how declarative miners are sensitive to process change. The objective of this paper is to study how declarative miners can give accurate and timely views of partial traces (so-called *event streams*). We integrate techniques of streaming process mining to declarative

---

[1] See https://icpmconference.org/2021/process-discovery-contest/.

Alphabetical order, equal authors contribution.

© The Author(s) 2023
M. Montali et al. (Eds.): ICPM 2022 Workshops, LNBIP 468, pp. 158–170, 2023.
https://doi.org/10.1007/978-3-031-27815-0_12

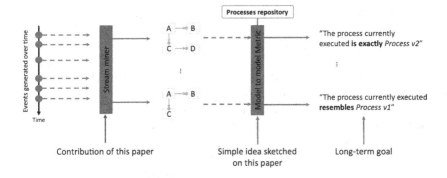

Fig. 1. Contribution of the paper

modelling notations, in particular, DCR graphs [14]. While previous works of streaming conformance checking have addressed other declarative languages (e.g.: Declare [23]), these languages are fundamentally different. Declare provides a predefined set of 18 constraint templates with an underlying semantics based on LTL formulae on finite traces [12]. Instead, DCR is based on a minimal set of 5 constraints, being able to capture regular and omega-regular languages [13]. In comparison with Declare, DCR is a language adopted by the industry: DCR is integrated into KMD Workzone, a case management solution used by 70% of central government institutions in Denmark [22]. Event streams present challenges for discovery. Streams are potentially infinite, making memory and time computation complexities major issues. Our technique optimizes these aspects by relying on intermediate representations that are updated at runtime. Another aspect is *extensibility*: our technique can be extended to more complex workflow patterns via the combination of atomic DCR constraints. Figure 1 illustrates our contribution: a streaming mining component, capable of continuously generating DCR graphs from an event stream (here we use the plural *graphs* to indicate that the DCR model could evolve over time, to accommodate drifts in the model that might occur). Towards the long-term goal of a system capable of spotting changes in a detailed fashion, we will also sketch a simple model-to-model metric for DCR, which can be used to compare the results of stream mining with a catalogue or repository of processes. An implementation of our techniques together with tests and datasets is available in Beamline[2] [6].

The rest of the paper is structured as follows: related works are presented in Sect. 2; theoretical background is covered in Sect. 3. The streaming discovery is presented in Sect. 4 and the approach is validated in Sect. 5. Section 6 concludes.

2   Related Work

This is the first work aiming at discovering DCR graphs from event streams. We find related work in offline discovery of DCR graphs and stream process mining for Declare.

Offline Process Discovery Techniques. The most current discovery technique for DCR graphs is the DisCoveR algorithm [4]. In their paper, the authors claim an accuracy of

---

[2] See https://github.com/beamline/discovery-dcr.

96,1% with linear time complexity (in PDC 2021 the algorithm achieved 96.2%). The algorithm is an extension of the ParNek algorithm [21] using an efficient implementation of DCR mapping via bit vectors. In its most recent version [24], DisCoveR has been extended with the idea of having both positive and negative examples to produce a more precise process model. Other related works derive from conformance checking [10] and process repair [1] techniques. Both fields aim at understanding whether executions can be replayed on top of an existing processes model. However, in our case, we wanted to separate the identification of the processes (i.e., control-flow discovery) from the calculation of their similarity (i.e., the model-to-model metric) so that these two contributions can be used independently from each other. Conformance checking and process repair, on the other hand, embed the evaluation and the improvement into one "activity".

Online Discovery for Declarative Models. In [7] a framework for the discovery of Declare models from streams was introduced as a way to deal with large collections of datasets that are impossible to store and process altogether. In [20] this work was generalized to handle the mining of data constraints, leveraging the MP-Declare notation [9].

Streaming Process Mining in General. In his PhD thesis [29], van Zelst proposes process mining techniques applicable to process discovery, conformance checking, and process enhancement from event streams. An important conclusion from his research consists of the idea of building intermediate models that capture the knowledge observed in the stream before creating the final process model. In [5] the author presents a taxonomy for the classification of streaming process mining techniques. Our techniques constitute a hybrid approach in the categories in [5], mixing a smart window-based model which is used to construct and maintain an intermediate structure updated, and a problem reduction technique used to transform the such structure into a DCR graph.

3   Background

In the following section, we recall basic notions of Directly Follows Graphs [1] and the Dynamic Condition Response (DCR) graphs [14]. While, in general, DCR is expressive to capture multi-perspective constraints such as time and data [15, 26], in this paper we use the classical, set-based formulation first presented in [14] that contains only four most basic behavioural relations: conditions, responses, inclusions and exclusions.

Definition 1 (Sets, Events and Sequences). *Let C denote the set of possible case identifiers and let A denote the set of possible activity names. The event universe is the set of all possible events $\mathcal{E} = C \times A$ and an event is an element $e = (c, a) \in \mathcal{E}$. Given a set $\mathbb{N}_n^+ = 1, 2, \ldots, n$ and a target set A, a sequence $\sigma : \mathbb{N}_n^+ \mapsto A$ maps index values to elements in A. For simplicity, we can consider sequences using a string interpretation: $\sigma = \langle a_1, \ldots, a_n \rangle$ where $\sigma(i) = a_i \in A$.*

We can now formally characterize an event stream:

Definition 2 (Event stream). *An event stream is an unbounded sequence mapping indexes to events: $S : \mathbb{N}^+ \to \mathcal{E}$.*

Definition 3 (Directly Follows Graph (DFG)). *A DFG is a graph $G = (V, R)$ where nodes represent activities (i.e., $V \subseteq A$), and edges indicate directly follows relations from source to target activities (i.e., $(a_s, a_t) \in R$ with $a_s, a_t \in V$, so $R \subseteq V \times V$).*

Definition 4 (Extended DFG). *An extended DFG is a graph $G_x = (V, R, X)$ where (V, R) is a DFG and X contains additional numerical attributes referring to the nodes: $X : V \times Attrs \rightarrow \mathbb{R}$, where Attrs is the set of all attribute names. To access attribute α_1 for node v we use the notation $X(v, \alpha_1)$.*

We use the following attributes: avgFO: average index of the first appearance of an activity in a trace; noTraceApp: current number of traces containing the activity; avgIdx: average index of the activity in a trace; and noOccur: number of activity occurrences.

Definition 5 (DCR Graph). *A DCR graph is a tuple $\langle \mathcal{A}, M, \rightarrow\bullet, \bullet\rightarrow, \rightarrow+, \rightarrow\% \rangle$, where $\mathcal{A}$ is a set of activities, $M \subseteq \mathcal{P}(\mathcal{A}) \times \mathcal{P}(\mathcal{A}) \times \mathcal{P}(\mathcal{A})$ is a marking, and $\phi \subseteq \mathcal{A} \times \mathcal{A}$ for $\phi \in \{\rightarrow\bullet, \bullet\rightarrow, \rightarrow+, \rightarrow\%\}$ are relations between activities.*

A DCR graph defines processes whose executions are finite and infinite sequences of activities. An activity may be executed several times. The three sets of activities in the marking $M = (\mathsf{Ex}, \mathsf{Re}, \mathsf{In})$ define the state of a process, and they are referred to as the *executed* activities (Ex), the *pending* response (Re)[3] and the *included* activities (In). DCR relations define what is the effect of executing one activity in the graph. Briefly: Condition relations $a \rightarrow\bullet a'$ say that the execution of a is a prerequisite for a', i.e. if a is included, then a must have been executed for a' to be enabled for execution. Response relations $a\bullet\rightarrow a'$ say that whenever a is executed, a' becomes pending. In a run, a pending event must eventually be executed or be excluded. We refer to a' as a response to a. An inclusion (respectively exclusion) relation $a \rightarrow+a'$ (respectively $a \rightarrow\% a'$) means that if a is executed, then a' is included (respectively excluded).

For a DCR graph[4] P with activities $\mathcal{A}$ and marking $M = (\mathsf{Ex}, \mathsf{Re}, \mathsf{In})$ we write $P_{\bullet\rightarrow}$ for the set of pairs $\{(x, y) \mid x \in \mathcal{A} \wedge y \in \mathcal{A} \wedge (x, y) \in \bullet\rightarrow\}$ (similarly for any of the relations in ϕ) and we write $P_{\mathcal{A}}$ for the set of activities. Definition 5 omits the existence of a set of labels and labelling function present in [14]. This has a consequence in the set of observable traces: Assume a graph $G = \langle \{a, b\}, (\emptyset, \{a, b\}, \{a, b\}), \emptyset, \emptyset, \emptyset, \emptyset \rangle$ as well as a set of labels $L = \{p\}$ and a labelling function $l = \{(a, p), (b, p)\}$. A possible run of G has the shape $\sigma = \langle p, p \rangle$, which can be generated from 1) two executions of a, 2) two executions of b or 3) an interleaved execution of a and b. By removing the labels from the events (or alternatively, assuming an injective surjective labelling function in [14]), we assume that two occurrences of the event in the stream imply event repetition.

4   Streaming DCR Miner

This section presents the general structure of the stream mining algorithm for DCR graphs. The general idea of the approach presented in this paper is depicted in Fig. 2: constructing and maintaining an extended DFG structure (cf. Definition 4) starting from the stream and then, periodically, a new DCR graph is extracted from the most recent version of the extended DFG available. The extraction of the different DCR rules starts from the same extended DFG instance. For readability purposes, we split the approach

---

[3] We might simply say pending when it is clear from the context.
[4] We will use "DCR graph" and "DCR model" interchangeably in this paper.

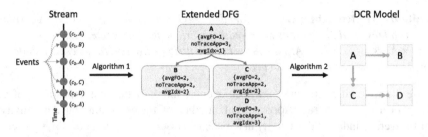

Fig. 2. Conceptual representation of the discovery strategy in this paper.

Algorithm 1: General structure of Streaming DCR Miner

Input: S: stream of events; m_t: maximum number of traces to store; m_e: maximum number of events per trace to store; $\langle T, \leq \rangle$: Pattern poset

1 Initialize map obs ▷ Maps case ids to the sequence of activities
2 Initialize map deps ▷ Maps case ids to one activity name
3 Initialize extended DFG $G_X = (V, R, X)$
4 **forever do**
       ▷ Step 0: Observe new activity a for case c
5 | $(c, a) \leftarrow observe(S)$
       ▷ Step 1: Update of the extended DFG
6 | **if** $c \in obs$ **then**
7 | | Refresh the update time of c
8 | | **if** $|obs(c)| \geq m_e$ **then**
9 | | | Remove oldest (i.e., earliest update time) event from list $obs(c)$
10 | | | Update V and X of G_X to be consistent with the event just removed
11 | **else**
12 | | **if** $|obs| \geq m_t$ **then**
13 | | | Remove the oldest (i.e., earliest update time) trace from obs and all its events
14 | | | Update V and X of G_X to be consistent with the events just removed
15 | | obs$(c) \leftarrow \langle \rangle$ ▷ Create empty list for obs(c)
16 | obs$(c) \leftarrow$ obs$(c) \cdot \langle a \rangle$ ▷ Append a to obs(c)
17 | $V \leftarrow V \cup \{a\}$
18 | Update frequency and avg appearance index in X component of G_X ▷ The average appearance index is updated considering the new position given by $|obs(c)|$
19 | **if** $c \in deps$ **then**
20 | | $R \leftarrow R \cup \{(deps(c), a)\}$
21 | deps$(c) \leftarrow a$
22 | **if** *trigger periodic cleanup* **then** ▷ Periodic cleanup of deps
23 | | Remove the oldest cases from deps
       ▷ Step 2: Periodic update of the DCR model (enough time/new behaviour)
24 | **if** *trigger periodic update of the model* **then**
25 | | $M \leftarrow$ mine$(\langle T, \leq \rangle, G_X)$ ▷ See Algorithm 2
26 | | Notify about new model M

---

into two phases. The former (Algorithm 1) is in charge of extracting the extended DFG, the latter (Algorithms. 2, 3, 4) focuses on the extraction of DCR rules from the extended DFG.

Algorithm 1 takes as input a stream of events S, two parameters referring to the maximum number of traces m_t and events to store m_e and a set of DCR patterns to mine. The algorithm starts by initializing two supporting map data structures obs and deps as well as an empty extended DCR graph G_X (lines 1–3). obs is a map associating

---

Algorithm 2: Mining of rules starting from the extended DFG

Input: $\langle T, \leq \rangle$: Pattern poset, $G_X = (V, R, X)$: extended DFG

1 $P \leftarrow \langle V, M_{init}, \rightarrow\bullet = \emptyset, \bullet\rightarrow = \emptyset, \rightarrow+ = \emptyset, \rightarrow\% = \emptyset \rangle \triangleright$ Initial DCR graph
2 $Rels, CompRels \leftarrow \emptyset, \emptyset$
3 **foreach** $t \in MinimalElements(\langle T, \leq \rangle)$ **do** $\triangleright$ Baseline for atomic patterns
4 $\quad \lfloor \; Rels \leftarrow Rels \cup MineAtomic(G_X, t)$
5 **foreach** $t \in T \backslash MinimalElements(\langle T \leq \rangle)$ **do** $\triangleright$ Composite case
6 $\quad \lfloor \; CompRels \leftarrow CompRels \cup MineComposite(G_X, t, Rels)$
7 **if** $CompRels \neq \emptyset$ **then**
8 $\quad \mid \; P \leftarrow P \oplus CompRels$
9 **else**
10 $\quad \lfloor \; P \leftarrow P \oplus Rels$
11 **return** $RemoveRedundancies(P) \triangleright$ Apply transitive reduction

---

case ids to sequences of partial traces; deps is a map associating case ids to activity names. After initialization, the algorithm starts consuming the actual events in a never-ending loop (line 4). The initial step consists of receiving a new event (line 5). Then, two major steps take place: the first step consists of updating the extended DFG; the second consists of transforming the extended DFG into a DCR model. To update the extended DFG the algorithm first updates the set of nodes and extra attributes. If the case id c of the new event has been seen before (line 6), then the algorithm refreshes the update time of the case id (line 7, useful to keep track of which cases are the most recent ones) and checks whether the maximum length of the partial trace for that case id has been reached (line 8). If that is the case, then the oldest event is removed and the G_X is updated to incorporate the removal of the event. If this is the first time this case id is seen (line 11), then it is first necessary to verify that the new case can be accommodated (line 12) and, if there is no room, then first some space needs to be created by removing oldest cases and propagating corresponding changes (lines 13–14) and then a new empty list can be created to host the partial trace (line 15). In either situation, the new event is added to the partial trace (line 16) and, if needed, a new node is added to the set of vertices V (line 17). The X data structure can be refreshed by leveraging the properties of the partial trace seen so far (line 18). To update the relations in the extended DFG (i.e., the R component of G_X), the algorithm checks whether an activity was seen previously for the given case id c and, if that is the case, the relation from such activity (i.e., deps(c)) to the new activity just seen (i.e., a) is added (lines 19–20). In any case, the activity just observed is now the latest activity for case id c (line 21) and oldest cases (i.e., cases not likely to receive any further events) are removed from deps (line 23). Finally, the algorithm refreshes the DCR model by calling the procedure that transforms (lines 25-26) the extended DFG into a DCR model (cf. Algorithm 2). Updates can be triggered based on some periodicity (line 24) or based on the amount of behaviour seen. The mechanics of such periodicity are beyond the scope of the paper.

Algorithm 2 generates a DCR graph from an extended DFG. First, it (1) defines patterns that describe occurrences of atomic DCR constraints in the extended DFG, and then it (2) defines composite patterns that describe the most common behaviour. Given a set of relation patterns T, $\langle T, \leq \rangle$ denotes a pattern dependency poset with $\leq$ a partial order over T. Similarly $MinimalElements(\langle T, \leq \rangle) = \{x \in T \mid \nexists y \in T.y \leq x\}$. Patterns as posets allow us to reuse and simplify the outputs from the discovery algorithm. Consider a pattern describing a sequential composition from a to b (similar to a flow

---

Algorithm 3: Atomic miner

Input: $G_X = (V, R, X)$: extended DFG, u: DCR Pattern

1 $Rels \leftarrow \emptyset$ ▷ Empty dictionary of mined relations
2 **foreach** $(s, t) \in R$ **do**
3   **switch** u ▷ Pattern match with each atomic pattern
4   **do**
5   **case** *RESPONSE*
6   **if** $X(s, avgIdx) < X(t, avgIdx)$ **then**
7              $Rels[u] \leftarrow Rels[u] \cup (s, t, \bullet\rightarrow)$
8   **case** *CONDITION*
9   **if** $X(s, avgFO) < X(t, avgFO) \wedge X(s, noTraceApp) \geq X(t, noTraceApp)$ **then**
10              $Rels[u] \leftarrow Rels[u] \cup (s, t, \rightarrow\bullet)$
11   **case** *SELFEXCLUDE*
12   **if** $X(s, noOccur) = 1$ **then**
13              $Rels[u] \leftarrow Rels[u] \cup (s, s, \rightarrow\%)$

      ▷ Further patterns here...
14   **return** $Rels$

Algorithm 4: Composite miner

Input: $G_X = (V, R, X)$: extended DFG, u: DCR Pattern, $Rels$: Mined Relations

1 **switch** u **do**
2   **case** *EXCLUDEINCLUDE*
3   **return** $Rels[SELFEXCLUDE] \cup Rels[PRECEDENCE] \cup Rels[NOTCHAINSUCCESION]$ ▷ Removes
          redundant relations
4   ▷ Further patterns here

---

in BPMN). A DCR model that captures a sequential behaviour will need 4 constraints: $\{a\rightarrow\bullet b, a\bullet\rightarrow b, a\rightarrow\%a, b\rightarrow\%b\}$. Consider $T = \{T_1 : Condition, T_2 : Response, T_3 : Exclusion, T_4 : Sequence\}$. The pattern poset $\langle T, \{(T_4, T_1), (T_4, T_2), (T_4, T_3)\}\rangle$ defines the dependency relations for a miner capable of mining sequential patterns. Additional patterns (e.g. exclusive choices, escalation patterns, etc.), can be modelled similarly. Pattern posets are finite, thus there exist minimal elements. The generation of a DCR model from an extended DFG is described in Algorithm 2. We illustrate the mining of DCR *conditions*, *responses* and *self-responses*, but more patterns are available in [25]. The algorithm takes as input an extended DFG G_X and a pattern poset. It starts by creating an empty DCR graph P with activities equal to the nodes in G_X and initial marking $M_{init} = \{\emptyset, \emptyset, V\}$, that is, all events are included, not pending and not executed. We then split the processing between atomic patterns (those with no dependencies) and composite patterns. The map Rel stores the relations from atomic patterns, that will be used for the composite miner. We use the merge notation $P \oplus Rels$ to denote the result of the creation of a DCR graph whose activities and markings are the same as P, and whose relations are the pairwise union of the range of $Rels$ and its corresponding relational structure in P. Line 11 applies a transitive reduction strategy [4], reducing the number of relations while maintaining identical reachability properties.

The atomic and composite miners are described in Algorithms 3, and 4. The atomic miner in Algorithm 3 iterates over all node dependencies in the DFG and the pattern matches with the existing set of implemented patterns. Take the case of a response constraint. We will identify it if the average occurrence of s is before t (line 6). This condition, together with the dependency between s and t in G_X is sufficient to infer a response constraint from s to t. To detect conditions, the algorithm verifies another set of properties: given a dependency between s and t, it checks that the first occurrence of s precedes t and that s and t appeared in the same traces (approximated by counting the number of traces containing both activities, line 9). The composite miner in Algorithm 4 receives the DFG, a pattern, and the list of mined relations from atomic patterns. We provide an example for the case of include and exclude relations. This pattern is built as a combination of self-exclusions, precedence, and not chain successions. As these atomic patterns generate each set of include/exclude relations, the pattern just takes the set union construction.

Suitability of the Algorithms for Streaming Settings. Whenever discussing algorithms that can tackle the streaming process mining problem [5], it is important to keep in mind that while a stream is assumed to be infinite, only a finite amount of memory can be used to store all information and that the time complexity for processing each event must be constant. Concerning the memory, an upper bound on the number of stored events in Algorithm 1 is given by $m_t \cdot m_e$ where m_e is the number of unique events and m_t is the number of parallel traces. Moreover, note that the extended DFG is also finite since there is a node for each activity contained in the memory. Concerning the time complexity, Algorithm 1 does not perform any unbounded backtracking. Instead, for each event, it operates using just maps that have amortized constant complexity or on the extended DFG (which has finite, controlled size). The same observation holds for Algorithm 2 as it iterates on the extended DFG which has a size bounded by the provided parameters (and hence, can be considered constant).

5   Experimental Evaluation

To validate our approach we executed several tests, first to validate quantitatively the streaming discovery on synthetic data, then to qualitatively evaluate the whole approach on a real dataset. Due to lack of space, we only report quantitative tests, while performance and the qualitative evaluation can be found in a separate technical report [8].

5.1   Quantitative Evaluation of Streaming Discovery

Recall from the previous section that time/space complexity are constant for streaming settings. Thus, our analysis will focus on studying how the algorithm behaves when encountering sudden changes in a stream. We compare with other process discovery algorithms for DCR graphs, in this case, the DisCoveR miner [4]. The tests are performed against a publicly available dataset of events streams [11]. This dataset includes (1) a synthetic stream inspired by a loan application process, and (2) perturbations to the original stream using change patterns [28]. Recall that the DisCoveR miner is an *offline* miner, thus it assumes an infinite memory model. To provide a fair evaluation we need to parameterize DisCoveR with the same amount of available memory. We divided the experiment into two parts: a simple stream where the observations of each process instance arrive in an ordered manner (i.e., one complete process instance at a

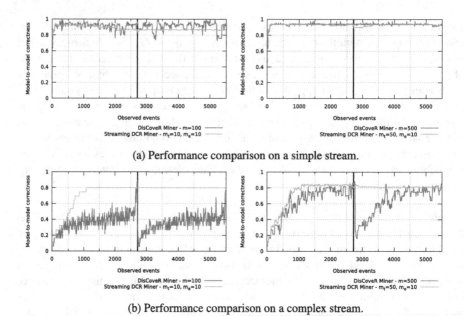

(a) Performance comparison on a simple stream.

(b) Performance comparison on a complex stream.

Fig. 3. Performance comparison between the offline DisCoveR miner and the streaming DCR Miner with equal storage available (capacity of up to 100 and 500 events).

time) and a complex stream where observations from many instances arrive intertwined. As no initial DCR graph exists for this process, and no streaming DCR miner exists, we used the DisCoveR miner in its original (offline) setting to generate a baseline graph using the entire dataset. This model (the one calculated with offline DisCoveR) was used to calculate the model-to-model similarity between the DCR stream miner and the DisCoveR miner with memory limits. For the sake of simplicity, in this paper, we considered only the case of sudden drifts, while we discuss other types of drift in future work.

We introduce a metric that quantifies the similarity between two DCR graphs. It can be used, for example, to identify which process is being executed with respect to a model repository, or by quantifying the *change rate* of one process over time. The metric takes as input two DCR graphs P and Q as well as a weight relation W that associates each DCR relation in ϕ (cf. Definition 5) with a weight, plus one additional weight for the activities. Then it computes the weighted Jaccard similarity [17] of the sets of relations and the set of activities, similarly to what happens in [2] imperative models:

Definition 6 (DCR Model-to-Model metric). *Given P and Q two DCR graphs, and $W : \phi \cup \{act\} \to \mathbb{R}$ a weight function in the range $[0, 1]$ such that $\sum_{r \in \phi \cup \{act\}} W(r) = 1$. The model-to-model similarity metric is defined as:*

$$S(P, Q, W) = W(act) \cdot \frac{|P_A \cap Q_A|}{|P_A \cup Q_A|} + \sum_{r \in \phi} W(r) \cdot \frac{|P_r \cap Q_r|}{|P_r \cup Q_r|} \qquad (1)$$

The similarity metric compares the relations in each of the two DCR graphs, thus returning a value between 0 and 1, where 1 indicates a perfect match and 0 stands for no match at all. A brief evaluation of the metric is reported in Appendix A.

The results of the quantitative evaluation are reported in Fig. 3. Each figure shows the performance of the incremental version of DisCoveR and the streaming DCR miner against 2 different configurations over time. The vertical black bars indicate where a sudden drift occurred in the stream. While the performance for the simple stream is very good for both the DisCoveR and the streaming DCR miners, when the stream becomes more complicated (i.e., Fig. 3b), DisCoveR becomes less effective, and, though its average performance increases over time, the presence of the drift completely disrupt the accuracy. In contrast, our approach is more robust to the drift and more stable over time, proving its ability at managing the available memory in a more effective way.

5.2 Discussion

One of the limitations of the approach regards precision with respect to offline miners. A limiting aspect of our work is the choice of the intermediate structure. A DFG representation may report confusing model behaviour as it simplifies the observations using purely a frequency-based threshold [27]. A DFG is in essence an imperative data structure that captures the most common flows that appear in a stream. This, in a sense, goes against the declarative paradigm as a second-class citizen with respect to declarative constraints. We believe that the choice of the DFG as an intermediate data structure carries out a loss of precision with respect to the DisCoveR miner in offline settings. However, in an online setting, the DFG still provides a valid approximation to observations of streams where we do not have complete traces. This is far from an abnormal situation: IoT communication protocols such as MQTT [16] assume that subscriber nodes might connect to the network *after* the communications have started, not being able to identify starting nodes. Specifically, in a streaming setting it is impossible to know exactly when a certain execution is complete and, especially in declarative settings, certain constraints describe liveness behaviours that can only be verified after a whole trace has been completely inspected. While watermarking techniques [3] could be employed to cope with *lateness* issues, we have decided to favour self-contained approaches in this paper, leaving for future work the exploration of watermarking techniques.

6 Conclusion and Future Work

This paper presented a novel streaming discovery technique capable of extracting declarative models expressed using the DCR language, from event streams. Additionally, a model-to-model metric is reported which allows understanding if and to what extent two DCR models are the same. An experimental evaluation, comprising both synthetic and real data, validated the two contributions separately as well as their combination in a qualitative fashion, which included interviews with the process owner.

We plan to explore several directions in future work. Regarding the miner, we plan to extend its capabilities to the identification of sub-processes, nesting, and data constraints. Regarding the model-to-model similarity, we would like to embed more semantic aspects, such as mentioned in [18]. A possible limitation of the streaming miner algorithm approach followed here relates to the updating mechanism. Currently lines 22–24 of Algorithm 1 perform updates based entirely on periodic updates triggered by time, which will generate notifications even when no potential changes in the model have been identified. A possibility to extend the algorithm will be to integrate the model-to-model similarity as a parameter to the discovery algorithm, so models only get updated after a given change threshold (a similarity value specified by the user) is reached.

A   Quantitative Evaluation of Model-to-Model Metric

To validate our metric we used a dataset of 28 DCR process models collected from previous mapping efforts [19]. For each model, we randomly introduced variations such as: adding new activities connected to the existing fragments, adding disconnected activities, deleting existing activities, adding and removing constraints, and swapping activity labels in the process. By systematically applying all possible combinations of variations in a different amount (e.g., adding 1/2/3 activities and nothing else; adding 1/2/3 activities and removing 1/2/3 con-

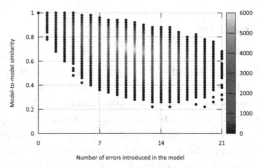

Fig. 4. Correlation between the model-to-model metric and the number of model changes. The colour indicates the density of observations. (Color figure online)

straints) we ended up with a total of 455,826 process models with a quantifiable amount of variation from the 28 starting processes. Figure 4 shows each variation on a scatter plot where the x axis refers to the number of introduced variations and the y axis refers to the model-to-model similarity. The colour indicates the number of models in the proximity of each point (since multiple processes have very close similarity scores). For identifying the optimal weights we solve an optimization problem, aiming at finding the highest correlation between the points, ending up with: $W = \{(\rightarrow\bullet, 0.06), (\bullet\rightarrow, 0.07), (\rightarrow\diamond, 0.06), (\rightarrow+, 0.07), (\rightarrow\%, 0.13), (\mathsf{act}, 0.61)\}$ leading to a Pearson's correlation of -0.56 and a Spearman's correlation of -0.55. These values indicate that our metric is indeed capable of capturing the changes. As the metric is very compact (value in $[0, 1]$) and operates just on the topological structure of the model, it cannot identify all details. However, the metric benefits from a fast computation.

References

1. van der Aalst, W.: Process Mining. Springer, Berlin Heidelberg (2016)
2. Aiolli, F., Burattin, A., Sperduti, A.: A business process metric based on the alpha algorithm relations. In: Daniel, F., Barkaoui, K., Dustdar, S. (eds.) BPM 2011. LNBIP, vol. 99, pp. 141–146. Springer, Heidelberg (2012). https://doi.org/10.1007/978-3-642-28108-2_13
3. Akidau, T., et al.: Watermarks in stream processing systems: semantics and comparative analysis of apache Fink and google cloud dataflow. VLDB (2021)
4. Back, C.O., Slaats, T., Hildebrandt, T.T., Marquard, M.: DisCoveR: accurate and efficient discovery of declarative process models. Int. J. Softw. Tools Technol. Transfer **24**, 563–587 (2021). https://doi.org/10.1007/s10009-021-00616-0
5. Burattin, A.: Streaming process discovery and conformance checking. In: Encyclopedia of Big Data Technologies. Springer, Cham (2019)
6. Burattin, A.: Streaming process mining with beamline. In: ICPM Demos (2022)
7. Burattin, A., Cimitile, M., Maggi, F.M., Sperduti, A.: Online discovery of declarative process models from event streams. IEEE Trans. Serv. Comput. **8**(6), 833–846 (2015)
8. Burattin, A., López, H.A., Starklit, L.: A monitoring and discovery approach for declarative processes based on streams (2022). https://doi.org/10.48550/arXiv.2208.05364
9. Burattin, A., Maggi, F.M., Sperduti, A.: Conformance checking based on multi-perspective declarative process models. Expert Syst. Appl. **65**, 194–211 (2016)
10. Carmona, J., van Dongen, B., Solti, A., Weidlich, M.: Conformance Checking. Springer, Cham (2018)
11. Ceravolo, P., Tavares, G.M., Junior, S.B., Damiani, E.: Evaluation goals for online process mining: a concept drift perspective. IEEE Trans. Serv. Comput. **15**, 2473–2489 (2020)
12. De Giacomo, G., De Masellis, R., Montali, M.: Reasoning on LTL on finite traces: insensitivity to infiniteness. In: AAAI Conference on Artificial Intelligence (2014)
13. Debois, S., Hildebrandt, T.T., Slaats, T.: Replication, refinement & reachability: complexity in dynamic condition-response graphs. Acta Informatica **55**(6), 489–520 (2018). https://doi.org/10.1007/s00236-017-0303-8
14. Hildebrandt, T., Mukkamala, R.R.: Declarative event-based workflow as distributed dynamic condition response graphs. In: PLACES, vol. 69 (2010)
15. Hildebrandt, T.T., Mukkamala, R.R., Slaats, T., Zanitti, F.: Contracts for cross-organizational workflows as timed dynamic condition response graphs. JLAMP **82**(5–7), 164–185 (2013)
16. Hunkeler, U., Truong, H.L., Stanford-Clark, A.: MQTT-S-a publish/subscribe protocol for wireless sensor networks. In: Proceedings of COMSWARE. IEEE (2008)
17. Jaccard, P.: The distribution of the flora of the alpine zone. New Phytol. **11**(2), 37–50 (1912)
18. López, H.A., Debois, S., Slaats, T., Hildebrandt, T.T.: Business process compliance using reference models of law. In: FASE 2020. LNCS, vol. 12076, pp. 378–399. Springer, Cham (2020). https://doi.org/10.1007/978-3-030-45234-6_19
19. López, H.A., Strømsted, R., Niyodusenga, J.-M., Marquard, M.: Declarative process discovery: linking process and textual views. In: Nurcan, S., Korthaus, A. (eds.) CAiSE 2021. LNBIP, vol. 424, pp. 109–117. Springer, Cham (2021). https://doi.org/10.1007/978-3-030-79108-7_13
20. Navarin, N., Cambiaso, M., Burattin, A., Maggi, F.M., Oneto, L., Sperduti, A.: Towards online discovery of data-aware declarative process models from event streams. In: IJCNN (2020)
21. Nekrasaite, V., Parli, A.T., Back, C.O., Slaats, T.: Discovering responsibilities with dynamic condition response graphs. In: Giorgini, P., Weber, B. (eds.) CAiSE 2019. LNCS, vol. 11483, pp. 595–610. Springer, Cham (2019). https://doi.org/10.1007/978-3-030-21290-2_37

22. Norgaard, L.H., et al.: Declarative process models in government centric case and document management. In: BPM (Industry Track). CEUR, vol. 1985, pp. 38–51. CEUR-WS.org (2017)

23. Pesic, M., van der Aalst, W.M.P.: A declarative approach for flexible business processes management. In: Eder, J., Dustdar, S. (eds.) BPM 2006. LNCS, vol. 4103, pp. 169–180. Springer, Heidelberg (2006). https://doi.org/10.1007/11837862_18

24. Slaats, T., Debois, S., Back, C.O.: Weighing the pros and cons: process discovery with negative examples. In: Polyvyanyy, A., Wynn, M.T., Van Looy, A., Reichert, M. (eds.) BPM 2021. LNCS, vol. 12875, pp. 47–64. Springer, Cham (2021). https://doi.org/10.1007/978-3-030-85469-0_6

25. Starklit, L.: Online Discovery and Comparison of DCR models from Event Streams using Beamline. Master's thesis, DTU (2021)

26. Strømsted, R., López, H.A., Debois, S., Marquard, M.: Dynamic evaluation forms using declarative modeling. In: BPM (Demos/Industry), pp. 172–179 (2018)

27. van der Aalst, W.M.: A practitioner's guide to process mining: limitations of the directly-follows graph. Procedia Comput. Sci. **164**, 321–328 (2019)

28. Weber, B., Reichert, M., Rinderle-Ma, S.: Change patterns and change support features-enhancing flexibility in process-aware information systems. Data Knowl. Eng. **66**(3), 438–466 (2008)

29. van Zelst, S.J.: Process mining with streaming data. Ph.D. thesis, Technische Universiteit Eindhoven (2019)

3rd International Workshop in Leveraging Machine Learning for Process Mining (ML4PM'22)

3rd International Workshop in Leveraging Machine Learning for Process Mining (ML4PM 2022)

Over the past several years, interest in combining Machine Learning (ML) and Process Mining (PM) methods has grown, as well as the challenges posed by using properly both methods. It is becoming more and more popular to apply ML to PM and to automate PM tasks, which is fostering a new research area.

By bringing together practitioners and researchers from both communities, the 3rd International Workshop on Leveraging Machine Learning for Process Mining aimed to discuss recent research developments at the intersection of ML and PM. The open call for contributions solicited submissions in the areas of outcome and time prediction, classification and clusterization of business processes, application of Deep Learning for PM, Anomaly detection for PM, Natural Language Processing and Text Mining for PM, Multi-perspective analysis of processes, ML for robot process automation, Automated process modeling and updating, ML-based Conformance checking, Transfer Learning applied to business processes, IoT business services leveraged by ML, Multidimensional PM, Predictive Process Monitoring, Prescriptive Learning in PM and Convergence of ML and Blockchain in Process Management.

The workshop attracted sixteen submissions confirming the liveliness of the field. Of the received sixteen submissions, eight submissions passed through the review process and were accepted for presentation at the workshop. Each paper was reviewed by three or four members of the program committee. Papers presented at the workshop were also selected for inclusion in the post-proceedings. These articles are briefly summarised below.

The paper of Kwon and Comuzzi presented a framework for AutoML in Predictive Process Monitoring (PPM). Through genetic algorithms, PPM-specific parameters and traditional hyperparameters for machine learning models have been explored creating a rich configuration space to provide pipeline recommendations.

The paper of Peeperkorn et al. discusses the negative impact of mislabelling cases as negative, particularly using XGBoost and LSTM neural networks. Promising results have been presented by changing the loss function used by a set of models during training to those of unbiased Positive-Unlabelled or non-negative Positive-Unlabelled learning.

The paper of Warmuth and Leopold, another regarding PPM, focuses on eXplainable Artificial Intelligence (XAI). The authors investigated the combination of textual and non-textual data used for explainable PPM. Furthermore, they analyzed the trade-off regarding the incorporation of textual data in predictive performance and explainability.

The paper of Faria Junior et al. presented an exploratory study based on frequent mining and trace clustering analysis as a mechanism for profile characterization. The clustering method has been fashioned over a vector representation from an object-centric event log.

The paper of Lahann et al. compared deep learning-based anomaly detection of process instances, creating a baseline and providing insights. They suggested minor refinement to build a simple LSTM detector capable of outperforming the existing approaches on several event log scenarios.

The paper of Grohs and Rehse proposed the attribute-based conformance diagnosis (ABCD) method. ABCD is a novel approach for correlating process conformance with trace attributes based on ML. The idea is grounded on identifying trace attributes that potentially impact the process conformance allowing proper processing.

The paper of Zbikowski et al. proposed a new representation for modelling multi-process environment with different process-based rewards. The proposal is based on Deep Reinforcement Learning to reach an optimal resource allocation policy based on a representation of a business process.

The paper of Kohlschmidt et al. shared some assumptions regarding those areas where a process enhancement is possible but the process presents a significantly different performance from their similar situations. They have defined a process enhancement area as a set of situations where the process performance is surprising.

In addition to these eight papers, the program of the workshop included the technical talk "Process Mining in Python: Basics and Integrations to Other Python Libraries" presented by Sebastiaan van Zelst.

We would like to thank all the authors submitted papers for publication in this book. We are also grateful to the members of the Program Committee and external referees for their excellent work in reviewing submitted and revised contributions with expertise and patience.

November 2022   Paolo Ceravolo
Sylvio Barbon Jr.
Annalisa Appice

Organization

Workshop Chairs

Paolo Ceravolo — Università degli Studi di Milano, Italy
Sylvio Barbon Junior — Università degli Studi di Trieste, Italy
Annalisa Appice — Università degli Studi di Bari Aldo Moro, Italy

Program Committee

Annalisa Appice — University of Bari Aldo Moro, Italy
Sylvio Barbon Junior — Univerity of Trieste, Italy
Mario Luca Bernardi — University of Sannio, Italy
Michelangelo Ceci — University of Bari, Italy
Paolo Ceravolo — University of Milan, Italy
Marco Comuzzi — Ulsan National Institute of Science and Technology, South Korea
Carl Corea — University of Koblenz-Landau, Germany
Riccardo De Masellis — Uppsala University, Sweden
Jochen De Weerdt — Katholieke Universiteit Leuven, Belgium
Shridhar Devamane — APS College of Engineering, India
Chiara Di Francescomarino — University of Trento, Italy
Matthias Ehrendorfer — University of Vienna, Austria
Maria Teresa Gómez López — University of Seville, Spain
Mariangela Lazoi — Università del Salento, Italy
Fabrizio Maria Maggi — Free University of Bozen-Bolzano, Italy
Gabriel Marques Tavares — Università degli Studi di Milano, Italy
Rafael Oyamada — State University of Londrina, Brazil
Emerson Paraiso — PUCPR - Pontificia Universidade Catolica do Parana, Brazil
Vincenzo Pasquadibisceglie — University of Bari Aldo Moro, Italy
Marco Pegoraro — RWTH Aachen University, Germany
Sarajane M. Peres — University of São Paulo, Brazil
Luigi Pontieri — ICAR, National Research Council of Italy (CNR), Italy
Domenico Potena — Università Politecnica delle Marche, Italy
Flavia Maria Santoro — University of Rio de Janeiro, Brazil
Natalia Sidorova — Eindhoven University of Technology, The Netherlands

Boudewijn Van Dongen   Eindhoven University of Technology,
     The Netherlands

Maurice van Keulen   University of Twente, The Netherlands

Bruno Zarpelao   State University of Londrina, Brazil

Deep Reinforcement Learning for Resource Allocation in Business Processes

Kamil Żbikowski, Michał Ostapowicz[✉], and Piotr Gawrysiak

Warsaw University of Technology, ul. Nowowiejska 15/19, 00-665 Warsaw, Poland
{kamil.zbikowski,michal.ostapowicz,piotr.gawrysiak}@pw.edu.pl

Abstract. Assigning resources in business processes execution is a repetitive task that can be effectively automated. However, different automation methods may give varying results that may not be optimal. Proper resource allocation is crucial as it may lead to significant cost reductions or increased effectiveness that results in increased revenues.

In this work, we first propose a novel representation that allows the modeling of a multi-process environment with different process-based rewards. These processes can share resources that differ in their eligibility. Then, we use double deep reinforcement learning to look for an optimal resource allocation policy. We compare those results with two popular strategies that are widely used in the industry. Learning optimal policy through reinforcement learning requires frequent interactions with the environment, so we also designed and developed a simulation engine that can mimic real-world processes.

The results obtained are promising. Deep reinforcement learning based resource allocation achieved significantly better results compared to two commonly used techniques.

Keywords: Resource allocation · Deep reinforcement learning · Double DQN · Process optimization

1 Introduction

In process science, there is a wide range of approaches that are employed in different stages of operational processes' life cycles. Following [1], these include, among others, optimization and stochastic techniques. Business processes can be also categorized according to the following perspectives: control-flow, organizational, data, and time perspective [2]. Resource allocation is focused on the organizational perspective utilizing optimization and stochastic approaches.

As it was emphasized in [3] resource allocation, while being important from the perspective of processes improvement, did not receive much attention at the time. However, as it was demonstrated in [4] the problem received much more attention in the last decade, which was reflected in the number of published scientific papers.

© The Author(s) 2023
M. Montali et al. (Eds.): ICPM 2022 Workshops, LNBIP 468, pp. 177–189, 2023.
https://doi.org/10.1007/978-3-031-27815-0_13

This paper addresses the problem of resource allocation with the use of methods known as approximate reinforcement learning. We specifically applied recent advancements in deep reinforcement learning such as double deep q-networks (double DQN) described in [5]. To use those methods we firstly propose a representation of a business processes suite that helps to design the architecture of neural networks in terms of appropriate inputs and outputs.

To the best of our knowledge, this is the first work that proposes a method utilizing double deep reinforcement learning for an on-line resource allocation for a multiple-process and multi-resource environment. Previous approaches either used so-called "post mortem" data in the form of event logs (e.g. [6]), or applied on-line learning, but due to the usage of tabular algorithms were limited by the exploding computational complexity when the number of possible states increased.

In the next section, we provide an overview of reinforcement learning methods and outline improvements of deep learning approaches over existing solutions. Then we analyze and discuss different approaches to resources allocation. In Sect. 3 we outline our approach for modeling operational processes for the purpose of training resource allocation agents. In Sect. 4 we describe the simulation engine used in training and its experimental setup. In Sect. 5 we evaluate the proposed approach and present outcomes of the experiments. In Sect. 6 we summarize the results and sketch potential future research directions.

2 Background and Related Work

2.1 Deep Reinforcement Learning

Following [7], reinforcement learning is "learning what to do – how to map situations to actions – so as to maximize a numerical reward signal". There are two main branches of reinforcement learning, namely tabular and approximate methods. The former provide a consistent theoretical framework that under certain conditions guarantees convergence. Their disadvantage is increasing computational complexity and memory requirements when the number of states grows. The latter are able to generalize over a large number of states but do not provide any guarantee of convergence.

The methods that we use in this work find optimal actions indirectly, identifying optimal action values for each state-action pair. Following recursive Bellman equation for the state-action pair [7], where $p(s', r|s, a)$ is a conditional probability of moving to state s' and receiving reward r after taking action a in state s; $\pi(a|s)$ is the probability of taking action a in state s; $\gamma \in [0, 1]$ is a discount factor:

$$q_\pi(s, a) = \sum_{s', r} p(s', r|s, a)[r + \gamma \sum_{a'} \pi(a'|s')q_\pi(s', a')], \tag{1}$$

an optimal policy is a policy that at each subsequent step takes an action that maximizes state-action value, that is $q_*(s, a) = max_\pi q_\pi(s, a)$.

When we analyze Eq. 1 we can intuitively understand problems with iterative tabular methods for finding optimal policy π^* for high-dimensional state spaces.

Fortunately, recent advancements in deep learning methods allow for further enhancement of approximate reinforcement learning methods with a most visible example being human-level results for Atari suite [8] obtained with the use of double deep Q-network [9].

2.2 Resource Allocation

In [4] we can find a survey of human resource allocation methods. The spectrum of approaches is wide. In [10–14] we can find solutions based on static, rule based algorithms.

There is a number of approaches for resource allocation that rely on applying predictive models. In [15] an offline prediction model based on LSTM is combined with extended minimum cost and maximum flow algorithms.

In [16] authors introduce Reinforcement Learning Based Resource Allocation Mechanism that utilizes Q-learning for the purpose of resource allocation. For handling multiple business processes, the queuing mechanism is applied.

Reinforcement learning has been also used for the task of proactive business process adaptation [17,18]. The goal there is to monitor the particular business process case while it is running and intervene in case of any detected upcoming problems.

The evaluations conducted in the aforementioned works are either based on simulations [16,18] or on analysis of historical data, mostly from Business Process Intelligence Challenge [15,17,19]. The latter has the obvious advantage of being real-world based dataset while simultaneously being limited by the number of available cases. The former offers a potentially infinite number of cases, but alignment between simulated data and real business processes is hard to achieve.

In [20] authors proposed a deep reinforcement learning method for business process optimization. However, their research objective is concentrated on analyzing which parameters of DQN are optimal.

3 Approach

This section describes the methods that we used to conduct the experiment. First, we will introduce concepts related to business process resource allocation. Then we will present double deep reinforcement learning [21] for finding optimal resource allocation policy. By optimal resource allocation policy, we mean such that maximizes the number of completed business process cases in a given period.

As it was pointed out earlier, both tabular and approximate algorithms in the area of reinforcement learning require frequent interaction with the execution environment. For the purpose of this work, we designed and developed a dedicated simulation environment that we call Simulation Engine. However, it can serve as a general-purpose framework for testing resource allocation algorithms as well. Concepts that we use for defining the business process environment assume the existence of such an engine. They incorporate parameters describing the level of uncertainty regarding their instances. The purpose here is to replicate stochastic behavior during process execution in real-world scenarios.

We imagine a business process workflow as a sequence of tasks[1] that are drawn from the queue and are being executed by adequate resources (both human and non-human). Each task realization is in fact an instance of a task specification described below. The task here is considered as an unbreakable unit of work that a resource can be assigned to and works on for a specified amount of time.

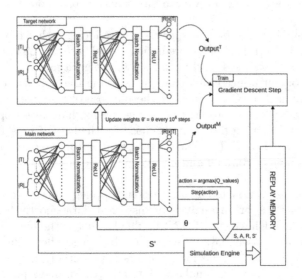

Fig. 1. Training architecture diagram. The learning process is centered around Simulation Engine that takes action from the main network and returns the reward and the next state. The architecture above follows the double deep Q-network (DDQN) approach [21].

Definition 1 (Task). *Let the tuple* (i, C^i, d, s, b) *define a task* t_i *that is a single work unit represented in the business process environment where:*

- *i is a unique task identifier where $i \in \{0, 1, 2, ...\}$,*
- *C^i is a set of transitions from a given task i,*
- *$d \in \mathbb{R}^+$ is a mean task duration with s being its standard deviation and*
- *$b \in \{0, 1\}$ indicates whether it is a starting task for a particular business process.*

Each task in the business process (see e.g. Figure 2a) may have zero or more connections from itself to other tasks.

---

[1] Task here should not be confused with the task definition used in reinforcement learning literature where it actually means the objective of the whole learning process. In the RL sense, our task would be to "solve" Business Process Suite (meaning obtaining as much cumulative reward as possible) in the form of Definition 6.

Definition 2 (Task Transition). *For a given task t_i a task transition c_j^i is a tuple (j, p) where j is a unique identifier of a task that this transition refers to and p is a probability of this transition. If $i = j$ it is a transition to itself.*

Definition 3 (Resource). *Let the tuple (k) define a single resource r_k where $k \in \{0, 1, 2, ...\}$ is a unique resources identifier. To refer to the set of all resources, we use $\hat{R}$.*

Definition 4 (Resource Eligibility). *If a resource r_k can be assigned to a task t_i it is said it is eligible for this task. Set $\mathcal{E}^i = \{e_k^i : e_k^i \in R^+\}$ contains all resource eligibility modifiers for a given task i. The lower the e_k^i, the shorter is the expected execution of task t_i. To refer to the set of all properties of eligibility for all defined resources $\hat{R}$ we use $\hat{E}$.*

The expected execution time of a task t_i is calculated by multiplying its duration by the resource eligibility modifier e_k^i.

Definition 5 (Business Process). *Let a tuple $(m, f_m, \mathbb{R}_m, \mathcal{T}_m)$ define a business process $\mathcal{P}_m$ where m is a unique identifier of a process $\mathcal{P}_m$ and $\mathcal{T}_m$ is a set of tasks belonging to the process $\mathcal{P}_m$ and $t_i \in \mathcal{T}_m \implies \neg \exists n : n \neq m \wedge t_i \in \mathcal{T}_n$. The relative frequency of a particular business process is defined by f_m. By $\mathbb{R}_m$ we refer to the reward that is received by finishing this business process instance. To refer to the set of all defined business processes, we use $\hat{P}$.*

An example of a business process can be found in Fig. 2a. Nodes represent tasks and their identifiers. Arrows define possible task transitions from particular nodes. The numbers on the arrows represent transition probabilities to other tasks.

Definition 6 (Business Process Suite). *Let a tuple $(\hat{R}, \hat{E}, \hat{P})$ define a Business Process Suite that consists of a resources set $\hat{R}$, resources eligibility set $\hat{E}$ and business processes set $\hat{P}$ such that: $\forall r_k \in \hat{R} \; \exists m, i \; e_k^i \in \hat{E} \wedge t_i \in \mathcal{T}_m \wedge \mathcal{P}_m \in \hat{P}$*

Business Process Suite is a meta definition of the whole business processes execution environment that consists of tasks that aggregate to business processes and resources that can execute tasks in accordance with the defined eligibility. We will refer to the instances of business processes as business process cases.

Definition 7 (Business Process Case). *Let a tuple $(\mathcal{P}_m, i, o)$ define a business process case $\tilde{\mathcal{P}}_m$ where $\mathcal{P}_m$ is a business process definition, i is a current task that is being executed and $o \in \{0, 1\}$ is information whether it is running (0) or was completed (1).*

Definition 8 (Task Instance). *Let a tuple (i, r_k) be a task instance $\tilde{t}_i$. At a particular moment of execution, there exists exactly one task instance matching business process case property i. The exact duration is determined by properties d and s of task definition t_i.*

Definition 9 (Task Queue). *Let the ordered list $(\mathcal{N}^{t_0}, \mathcal{N}^{t_1}, \mathcal{N}^{t_2}, ..., \mathcal{N}^{t_i})$ define a task queue that stores information about the number of task instances $\mathcal{N}^{t_i}$ for a given task t_i.*

Property 1. Direct consequence of Definitions 5, 7, 8 and 9 is that number of task instances in the task queue matching the definition of task with identifiers from particular business processes is equal to the number of business process cases.

The process of learning follows the schema defined in [5] and [9]. We use two sets of weights θ and θ'. The former is used for online learning with random mini-batches sampled from a dedicated experience replay queue $\mathcal{D}$. The latter is updated periodically to the weights of the more frequently changing counterpart. The update period used in tests was 10^4 steps. The detailed algorithm, based on [21], is outlined in Listing 1.

Algorithm 1. Double DQN training loop

1: Initialize number of episodes E, and number of steps in episode M
2: Initialize batch size β ▷ Set to 32 in tests
3: Initialize randomly two sets of neural network weights θ and θ'
4: $\mathcal{D} := \{\}$ ▷ Replay memory of size $E * M * 0.1$
5: Initialize environment $\mathcal{E}$
6: **for** e=0 in E **do**
7:     S := RESET($\mathcal{E}$)
8:     **for** m=0 in M **do**
9:         **if** RANDOM() $< \epsilon$ **then**
10:            a := SELECTRANDOMACTION()
11:        **else**
12:            a := $argmax_a Q(S, a; \theta)$
13:        **end if**
14:        $\mathbb{S}', \mathbb{R}$:= STEP($\mathcal{E}$, a)
15:        Put a tuple (S, a, R, S') in $\mathcal{D}$
16:        Sample β experiences from $\mathcal{D}$ to $(\mathbb{S}, \mathbb{A}, \mathbb{R}, \mathbb{S}')$
17:        $Q_{target} := \mathbb{R} + \delta * Q(\mathbb{S}', argmax_a Q(\mathbb{S}', a; \theta); \theta')$
18:        $Q_{current} := Q(\mathbb{S}, a; \theta)$
19:        $\theta_{t+1} = \theta_t + \nabla_{\theta_t}(Q_{target} - Q_{current})^2$
20:        Each 10^4 steps update $\theta' := \theta$
21:    **end for**
22: **end for**

In Fig. 1 an architecture of a system used in the experiment is presented in accordance with main data flows. It is a direct implementation of the training algorithm described in Algorithm 1. We used two neural networks: main and target. Both had the same architecture consisting of one input layer with $|\mathcal{R}| + |\mathcal{T}|$ inputs, two densely connected hidden layers containing 32 neurons each, and one output layer with $|\mathcal{R}|x|\mathcal{T}|$ outputs. After each hidden layer, there is a Batch Normalization layer [22]. Its purpose is to scale each output from the hidden neuron layer before computing the activation function. This operation improves training speed by reducing undesirable effects such as vanishing/exploding gradient updates.

The input configuration we used is defined as follows:

$$\mathbb{S} = [\rho_0, \rho_1, ...\rho_{|\mathcal{R}|-1}, \zeta_0, \zeta_1, ..., \zeta_{|\mathcal{T}|-1}] \qquad (2)$$

where $\rho_k = i$ refers to the resource assignment to one of its eligible tasks, and $\zeta_i = \mathcal{N}^{t_i} / \sum_{l=0}^{|\mathcal{T}|-1} \mathcal{N}^{t_l}$ is a relative load of a a given task with respect to all the tasks present in the task queue.

Outputs of the neural network are an approximation of a q-value for each of the available actions. The action here is assigning a particular resource to a particular task or taking no action for a current time step. Thus, number of outputs equals $|\mathcal{R}||\mathcal{T}| + 1$. This number grows quickly with the number of resources and tasks. This, in turn, may lead to a significant increase in training time or even an inability to obtain adequate q-value estimation.

In RL there exists a separation between continuing and episodic RL tasks [7]. The former are ending in a terminal state and differ in the rewards for the different outcomes. The latter are running infinitely and accumulate rewards over time. The business processes suite is a continuing RL task in its nature. However, in our work, we artificially terminate each execution after M steps simulating an episodic environment. We observed that it gave much better results than treating the whole set of business processes as a continuing learning task. As it is shown in Sect. 4 agents trained in such a way can be used in a continuing setup without loss of their performance.

4   Experimental Setup

This section briefly describes the setup of the experiments that we have conducted to assess the proposed methods and parametrization of a business process suite used for the evaluation.

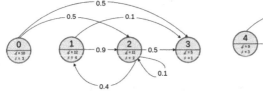

(a) Graph of a first business process.

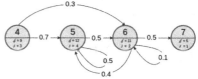

(b) Graph of a second business process.

Fig. 2. Business processes used in the evaluation.

To evaluate the proposed method we devised a business processes suite containing two business processes $m = 0$ and $m = 1$. Although they are quite small in terms of the number of tasks, the tasks transitions are nondeterministic which intuitively makes the learning process harder.

In Figs. 2a and 2b we can see both processes' graphs along with information about their tasks' parametrization. In Table 1 we can see available resources from the testing suite along with the information about their eligibility in regard to particular tasks.

Both processes have the same reward $R_0 = R_1 = 1$, which is received for each completed business process case. They differ in their relative frequency, which for the first process is $f_0 = 1$ and $f_1 = 6$ for the second one.

The resources we use in our experimental setup are of the same type, differing only in their eligibility in regard to the tasks.

Table 1. Resource eligibility. Values in cells define resource efficiency that is used in Simulation Engine. Final duration is obtained by multiplying duration d of a particular task by the adequate value from the table. A lack of value indicates that a particular resource is not eligible for a given task.

Task ID	Resources		
	0	1	2
0	–	0.75	2.8
1	1.4	0.3	–
2	0.3	–	2.7
3	–	2.7	0.1
4	0.6	2.6	–
5	0.4	–	10.5
6	1.1	–	1.7
7	0.4	0.6	2.5

In terms of algorithm parametrization, we set the number of episodes E to 600 and the number of steps in a single episode to 400. ϵ according to [5] was linearly annealed from 1 to 0.1 over first $E*M*0.1$ steps. The size of the memory buffer was set to $E*M*0.1$ elements.

5   Results and Discussion

We run 30 tests for the test suite. The results are presented in Fig. 3a. We can see that the variance in the cumulative sum of rewards is tremendous. Best models achieve up to 20 units of reward while the worst keep their score around zero.

Our findings are consistent with the general perception of how deep reinforcement learning works [23]. In particular, a training model that achieves satisfactory results strongly depends on weights initialization.

As we can see in Fig. 3b the value of a loss function also varies significantly. Moreover, its value after the initial drop steadily increases with subsequent

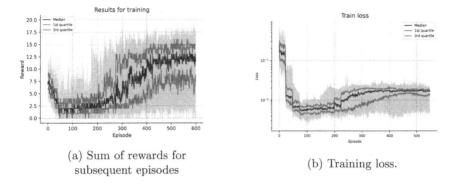

(a) Sum of rewards for
subsequent episodes

(b) Training loss.

Fig. 3. Training on the test suite over 30 training runs.

episodes. This is a phenomenon that is characteristic of DQN. The error measures the difference between training and main network outputs. This value is not directly connected with the optimization target - maximizing the cumulative reward over all steps.

In [5] authors recommend saving model parameters if they are better than the best previously seen (in terms of cumulative reward) during the current training run. This approach allows addressing - to some extent - a catastrophic forgetting effect and overall instability of approximate methods. For each run we save both the best and last episode's weights. After the training phase, we got 30 models as a result of keeping parameters giving the highest rewards during learning and 30 models with parameters obtained at the end of training. The distribution over all runs can be seen in Fig. 4a. We can see that the models with the best parameters achieve significantly higher cumulative rewards. The median averaged over 100 episodes was 14.04 for the best set of parameters and 12.07 for the last set.

To assess the results obtained by the deep learning agent we implemented two commonly used heuristics:

- FIFO (first in, first out) - the first-in-first-out policy was implemented in an attempt to avoid any potential bias while resolving conflicts in resource allocation. In our case, instead of considering task instances themselves, we try to allocate resources to the business process cases that arrived the earliest.
- SPT (shortest processing time) - our implementation of the shortest processing time algorithm tries to allocate resources to the task instances that take the shortest time to complete (without taking into account resource efficiencies for tasks). Thanks to this policy, we are able to prevent the longest tasks from occupying resources when these resources could be used to complete other, much shorter tasks and therefore shorten the task queue.

We conducted the same test lasting 100 episodes for both heuristics. Results are presented in Fig. 4b. The median averaged over 100 episodes was 11.54 for FIFO and 3.88 for SPT. SPT results were far below the FIFO. Comparing the

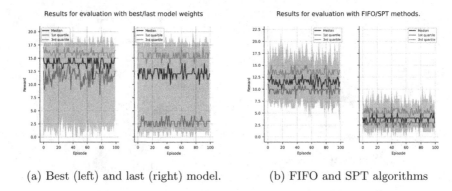

(a) Best (left) and last (right) model.   (b) FIFO and SPT algorithms

Fig. 4. Results over 30 runs.

results of the best model from the left side of Fig. 4a with results for FIFO from the left side of Fig. 4b, we can see that the cumulative reward for deep learning models is larger in the majority of episodes.

The improvement achieved by the deep RL model with each episode lasting 400 steps is not large considering its absolute value. The median FIFO agent's reward oscillates around 11, while the median deep RL's around 14. The question that arises here is whether this relation will hold with long (potentially infinitely) lasting episodes? To answer it, we conducted an experiment with 100 episodes with 5000 steps each. The results are presented in Fig. 5. We can see that the gap between rewards for DQN model and for FIFO increased. The average episode reward for DQN was 210.52, while for FIFO 145.84 and 80.2 for SPT.

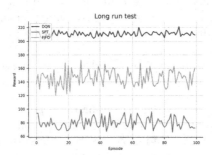

Fig. 5. Long run test for best model achieved during training compared to FIFO and SPT approaches. Each episode lasted 5000 time steps.

6   Conclusions and Future Work

In this paper, we applied double deep reinforcement learning for the purpose of resource allocation in business processes. Our goal was to simultaneously optimize resource allocation for multiple processes and resources in the same way as it has to be done in real-world scenarios.

We proposed and implemented a dedicated simulation environment that enables an agent to improve its policy in an iterative manner obtaining information about the next states and rewards. Our environment is thus similar to OpenAI's Gym. We believe that along with processes' definitions, it may serve as a universal testing suite improving the reproducibility of the results for different resource allocation strategies.

We proposed a set of rules for defining business processes suites. They are the formal representation of real-world business process environments.

The results of the double DQN algorithm for resources allocation were compared with two strategies based on common heuristics: FIFO and SPT. The deep RL approach obtained results that are 44% better than FIFO and 162% better than SPT. We were not able to directly compare our results to previously published studies as they are relatively hard to reproduce. This was one of the main reasons for publishing the code of both our simulation engine and training algorithm. We can see this as a first step toward a common platform that will allow different resource allocation methods to be reliably compared and assessed.

As for future work, it would be very interesting to train a resource allocation agent for a business process suite with a larger number of business processes that would be more deterministic compared to those used in this study. Such a setup would put some light on a source of complexity in the training process.

The number of potential actions and neural networks' outputs is a significant obstacle in applying the proposed method for complex business process suites with many processes and resources. In our future work, we plan to investigate other deep reinforcement learning approaches, such as proximal policy optimization, which tend to be more sample efficient than standard double DQN.

Reproducibility. Source code: https://github.com/kzbikowski/ProcessGym

References

1. Aalst, W.: Data science in action. In: Process Mining, pp. 3–23. Springer, Heidelberg (2016). https://doi.org/10.1007/978-3-662-49851-4_1
2. Van der Aalst, W.M.: Business process management: a comprehensive survey. Int. Sch. Res. Not. **2013** (2013)
3. Huang, Z., Xudong, L., Duan, H.: Mining association rules to support resource allocation in business process management. Expert Syst. Appl. **38**(8), 9483–9490 (2011)
4. Arias, M., Saavedra, R., Marques, M.R., Munoz-Gama, J., Sepulveda, M.: Human resource allocation in business process management and process mining. Manage. Decis. (2018)
5. Mnih, V., et al.: Human-level control through deep reinforcement learning. Nature **518**(7540), 529–533 (2015)
6. Liu, T., Cheng, Y., Ni, Z.: Mining event logs to support workflow resource allocation. Knowl.-Based Syst. **35**, 320–331 (2012)
7. Sutton, R.S., Barto, A.G.: Reinforcement Learning: An Introduction. MIT press, Cambridge (2018)
8. Bellemare, M.G., Naddaf, Y., Veness, J., Bowling, M.: The arcade learning environment: an evaluation platform for general agents. J. Artif. Intell. Res. **47**, 253–279 (2013)

9. Mnih, V., et al.: Playing Atari with deep reinforcement learning. arXiv preprint arXiv:1312.5602 (2013)
10. Huang, Z., Xudong, L., Duan, H.: Resource behavior measure and application in business process management. Expert Syst. Appl. **39**(7), 6458–6468 (2012)
11. Zhao, W., Yang, L., Liu, H., Wu, R.: The optimization of resource allocation based on process mining. In: Huang, D.-S., Han, K. (eds.) ICIC 2015. LNCS (LNAI), vol. 9227, pp. 341–353. Springer, Cham (2015). https://doi.org/10.1007/978-3-319-22053-6_38
12. Arias, M., Rojas, E., Munoz-Gama, J., Sepúlveda, M.: A framework for recommending resource allocation based on process mining. In: Reichert, M., Reijers, H.A. (eds.) BPM 2015. LNBIP, vol. 256, pp. 458–470. Springer, Cham (2016). https://doi.org/10.1007/978-3-319-42887-1_37
13. Havur, G., Cabanillas, C., Mendling, J., Polleres, A.: Resource allocation with dependencies in business process management systems. In: La Rosa, M., Loos, P., Pastor, O. (eds.) BPM 2016. LNBIP, vol. 260, pp. 3–19. Springer, Cham (2016). https://doi.org/10.1007/978-3-319-45468-9_1
14. Xu, J., Liu, C., Zhao, X.: Resource allocation vs. business process improvement: how they impact on each other. In: Dumas, M., Reichert, M., Shan, M.-C. (eds.) BPM 2008. LNCS, vol. 5240, pp. 228–243. Springer, Heidelberg (2008). https://doi.org/10.1007/978-3-540-85758-7_18
15. Park, G., Song, M.: Prediction-based resource allocation using LSTM and minimum cost and maximum flow algorithm. In: 2019 International Conference on Process Mining (ICPM), pp. 121–128. IEEE (2019)
16. Huang, Z., van der Aalst, W.M., Lu, X., Duan, H.: Reinforcement learning based resource allocation in business process management. Data Knowl. Eng. **70**(1), 127–145 (2011)
17. Metzger, A., Kley, T., Palm, A.: Triggering proactive business process adaptations via online reinforcement learning. In: Fahland, D., Ghidini, C., Becker, J., Dumas, M. (eds.) BPM 2020. LNCS, vol. 12168, pp. 273–290. Springer, Cham (2020). https://doi.org/10.1007/978-3-030-58666-9_16
18. Huang, Z., van der Aalst, W.M., Lu, X., Duan, H.: An adaptive work distribution mechanism based on reinforcement learning. Expert Syst. Appl. **37**(12), 7533–7541 (2010)
19. Palm, A., Metzger, A., Pohl, K.: Online reinforcement learning for self-adaptive information systems. In: Dustdar, S., Yu, E., Salinesi, C., Rieu, D., Pant, V. (eds.) CAiSE 2020. LNCS, vol. 12127, pp. 169–184. Springer, Cham (2020). https://doi.org/10.1007/978-3-030-49435-3_11
20. Silvander, J.: Business process optimization with reinforcement learning. In: Shishkov, B. (ed.) BMSD 2019. LNBIP, vol. 356, pp. 203–212. Springer, Cham (2019). https://doi.org/10.1007/978-3-030-24854-3_13
21. Van Hasselt, H., Guez, A., Silver, D.: Deep reinforcement learning with double q-learning. In: Proceedings of the AAAI Conference on Artificial Intelligence, vol. 30 (2016)
22. Ioffe, S., Szegedy, C.: Batch normalization: accelerating deep network training by reducing internal covariate shift. In: International Conference on Machine Learning, pp. 448–456. PMLR (2015)
23. Irpan, A.: Deep reinforcement learning doesn't work yet (2018). https://www.alexirpan.com/2018/02/14/rl-hard.html

On the Potential of Textual Data for Explainable Predictive Process Monitoring

Christian Warmuth[1,2(✉)] and Henrik Leopold[1,3]

[1] Hasso Plattner Institute, University of Potsdam, Potsdam, Germany
[2] SAP Signavio, Berlin, Germany
christian.warmuth@sap.com
[3] Kühne Logistics University, Hamburg, Germany
henrik.leopold@the-klu.org

Abstract. Predictive process monitoring techniques leverage machine learning (ML) to predict future characteristics of a case, such as the process outcome or the remaining run time. Available techniques employ various models and different types of input data to produce accurate predictions. However, from a practical perspective, explainability is another important requirement besides accuracy since predictive process monitoring techniques frequently support decision-making in critical domains. Techniques from the area of explainable artificial intelligence (XAI) aim to provide this capability and create transparency and interpretability for black-box ML models. While several explainable predictive process monitoring techniques exist, none of them leverages textual data. This is surprising since textual data can provide a rich context to a process that numerical features cannot capture. Recognizing this, we use this paper to investigate how the combination of textual and non-textual data can be used for explainable predictive process monitoring and analyze how the incorporation of textual data affects both the predictions and the explainability. Our experiments show that using textual data requires more computation time but can lead to a notable improvement in prediction quality with comparable results for explainability.

Keywords: Predictive process monitoring · Explainable Artificial Intelligence (XAI) · Natural language processing · Machine learning

1 Introduction

In recent years, machine learning (ML) techniques have become a key enabler for automating data-driven decision-making [14]. Machine learning has also found its way into the broader context of business process management. Here, an important application is to predict the future of business process executions - commonly known as predictive business process monitoring [7]. For example, a machine learning model can be used to predict the process outcome [20], the next activity [9] or the remaining time of a running process [21].

From a practical point of view, one of the critical shortcomings of many existing predictive process monitoring techniques is that their results are not

© The Author(s) 2023
M. Montali et al. (Eds.): ICPM 2022 Workshops, LNBIP 468, pp. 190–202, 2023.
https://doi.org/10.1007/978-3-031-27815-0_14

explainable, i.e., it remains unclear to the user how or why a certain prediction was made [17]. Especially in critical domains, such as healthcare, explainability, therefore, has become a central concern. Techniques in the area of explainable artificial intelligence (XAI) aim to shed light on black box ML models and provide transparency and interpretability [1]. Recognizing this, several so-called explainable predictive process monitoring techniques have been proposed [10,14,18]. They rely on well-established explainability approaches such as SHAP [12] and LIME [16] to support users in better understanding the predictions of the employed techniques.

What existing explainable predictive process monitoring techniques have in common is that they solely rely on numerical and categorical attributes and do not leverage textual data. This is surprising given that textual data often provides rich context to a process. Recognizing the potential value of textual data for explainable predictive process monitoring, we use this paper to empirically explore how the combination of textual and non-textual data affects the prediction quality, the explainability analysis, and the computational effort. To this end, we propose two novel strategies to combine textual and non-textual data for explainable predictive process monitoring and conduct extensive experiments based on an artificial dataset.

The remainder of this paper is organized as follows: Sect. 2 illustrates the problem and the potential of using textual data for explainable predictive process monitoring. Section 3 elaborates on our study design. The code for all experiments can be found on GitHub[1]. Section 4 presents the results. Section 5 discusses related work before Sect. 6 concludes our paper.

2   Problem Illustration

Predictive process monitoring techniques aim to predict the future state of current process executions based on the activities performed so far and process executions in the past [7]. Given a trace, we might, for instance, aim to predict the outcome of a trace [20]. Depending on the context, such an outcome could relate to the successful completion of a production process or the successful curing of a patient. Predicting the outcome of a process execution at an early stage enables early interventions, such as allocating additional resources or taking a different course of action still to reach the desired process outcome [22].

A central problem in process monitoring techniques leveraging ML is that it is nearly impossible for humans to understand why a particular prediction was made. This led to the development of techniques for explainable artificial intelligence, which aim to produce more explainable models without deterioration of the predictive performance. The goal is to help humans comprehend, effectively use, and trust artificial intelligence systems [1]. One widely employed XAI strategy is to produce a simpler, understandable model that approximates the results of the original prediction model [12] such as SHAP [10,18] or LIME [14] which are commonly used in the context of predictive process monitoring.

---

[1] https://github.com/christianwarmuth/explainable-predictive-process-monitoring-with-text.

All existing techniques for explainable predictive process monitoring have in common that they rely on numerical and categorical features only and do not consider textual data. This is surprising since textual data often can provide rich insights into the context of a process execution.

For example, consider a loan application process where customers may provide written statements about their financial situation, the purpose of the requested loan, and details of the repayment plan. This data might allow to more accurately predict whether the customer will pay back the loan and explain that prediction better. Figure 1 illustrates such a setting using an exemplary event log. We can see two cases where one applicant intends to spend the money on a wedding and the other on a new car. From the bank's perspective, this might make quite a difference since purchasing a car results in a physical asset that can be resold if the customer cannot pay it back.

case_id	activity	timestamp	loan amount	credit score	loan goal description
1566432	Create Application	15.03.2022 15:04	1.000$	0.93	I recently proposed to my wife so I ...
1566432	Review Application	17.03.2022 13:18	1.000$	0.93	/
1566432	Re-Negotiate Terms	17.03.2022 16:21	900$	0.93	/
1566432	Application Accepted	23.03.2022 09:15	900$	0.93	/
1748744	Create Application	16.03.2022 10:20	3.000$	0.87	I am planning to buy a new car and...
1748744	Review Application	17.03.2022 17:04	3.000$	0.87	/

Fig. 1. Exemplary eventlog with textual context data

Recognizing the potential value of textual data in the context of explainable predictive process monitoring, we use this paper to investigate how the combination of textual and non-textual data can be used for explainable predictive business process monitoring and analyze how the incorporation of textual data affects both the prediction quality and the explainability.

3   Study on the Impact of Textual Data on Explainable Predictive Process Monitoring

In this section, we describe the design of our study to investigate the potential of textual data for explainable predictive process monitoring. In Sect. 3.1, we first explain the different strategies we use for combining textual and non-textual data and the models chosen for their instantiation. In Sect. 3.2, we introduce the dataset and its creation. In Sect. 3.3, we elaborate on the preprocessing and in Sect. 3.4 we explain the training and explanation setup for the experiments.

3.1   Strategies and Models

Combining textual and non-textual data for explainable predictive process monitoring is not trivial. That is because these different types of input data must be combined in a useful way for both model building and inference and the explainability analysis. We propose two novel strategies:

Class Label or Probability Combination. Strategy one is to have two models (one for the textual data and one specific for the non-textual data). For inference, we can combine the class labels or the class probabilities output by the different models for prediction on real input. We have two separate explainability analyses as we have two individual models (Fig. 2).

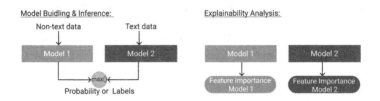

Fig. 2. Conceptual architecture strategy 1

Two-Stage Model. In a two-stage model approach, we have one model using solely textual information as stage 1. We then filter out the n most important features (e.g., words or smaller parts of a sentence) and feed them into the stage 2 model alongside non-textual information. The explainability analysis would be performed on the second-stage model, considering both data sources (Fig. 3).

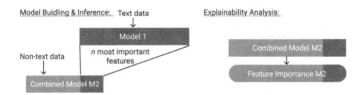

Fig. 3. Conceptual architecture strategy 2

We needed to choose a model for each input type to instantiate these strategies. For *non-textual data*, i.e., categorical and numerical input, we selected the XGBoost model since it has been found to deliver the best average performance in predictive process monitoring across various datasets with good scalability for large datasets [20]. XGBoost uses gradient tree boosting, a common ensemble learning technique (i.e., combining multiple machine learning models to derive a prediction) which performs boosting on decision trees [4]. For *textual data*, we use BERT (Bidirectional Encoder Representations from Transformers), a state-of-the-art NLP model introduced by Devlin et al., which outperforms previous methods on various NLP tasks and datasets. BERT can be described as a large language model and belongs to the family of transformer models, the current state-of-the-art models dealing with sequences [6].

3.2 Dataset

There is no public event log dataset available that contains rich textual context data. We, therefore, artificially augment an existing event log with textual data. We chose to augment the BPIC17 dataset with textual context data on case level in a parameterizable fashion with the LendingClub dataset. The BPI Challenge dataset from 2017 refers to a credit application process filed by customers of a Dutch financial institution through an online system [8]. Overall, 12792 of the 31413 loans were granted, which leaves us with a 0.41 minority class ratio for this binary process outcome prediction problem on loan acceptance. The Lending-Club dataset we use for dataset augmentation only includes textual descriptions of accepted loan applications, and we therefore have to redistribute the existing textual loan goal descriptions [11]. The redistribution is based on the topics discussed by the loan applicants in their loan goal description. In an initial data analysis, we identified the dominant topics using Latent Dirichlet Allocation, an NLP technique to retrieve topics in text corpora [2]. We assigned multiple topics to the two process outcomes and thus introduced in a controlled fashion, for example, that people who talk about medical issues in their loan goal description tend to be less likely to receive a loan offer. This approach creates a latent structure for the machine learning model to pick up in the prediction process. The topic attribution is performed based on the word occurrences per topic in the document. After determining the topic memberships, the dataset is augmented with the schematic depicted in Fig. 4 with a varying parameter of impurity, which adjusts the proportion of randomly assigned texts samples from the dataset during the data augmentation process. The loan goal descriptions are added to the original BPIC17 event log as an additional feature in the first event for each case (the filing of the loan application).

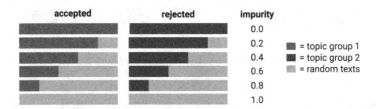

Fig. 4. Dataset augmentation strategy with impurity parameter

With an impurity of zero, the accepted cases are solely assigned the textual descriptions talking about topics in topic group 1. As the newly introduced textual features do not correlate with existing features, we thus introduce an additional dimension to differentiate between accepted and rejected cases. An impurity of 0.0 allows for an apparent differentiation in textual features. In contrast, an impurity of 1.0 would be a baseline with purely randomly sampled text for both outcomes, so there is no way to differentiate between the outcomes on the textual data. We henceforward define $purity = 1 - impurity$. For all experiments described in the following, we create 11 synthetically augmented dataset variants with an impurity ranging from 0.0 to 1.0 in steps of 0.1. We reduce measurement deviations by running each experiment 10 times and taking the arithmetic mean.

3.3 Data Preprocessing

We conduct several preprocessing steps. First, we need to retrieve the class labels "accepted" and "rejected" by choosing respective end activities. Then, we need to transform the input such as it is suitable for the employed models. For the XGBoost model, we have multiple events per case with various attributes that change during the process executions. However, the XGBoost model expects static (non-sequential input). We, therefore, preprocess the data to derive static properties (i.e., one n-dimensional vector of features per case) and convert all activities performed into categorical variables (encoding whether they occurred or not). All further categorical variables are one-hot-encoded (resulting in one additional feature per category level) to represent categorical variables using numerical values. Numerical variables are then standardized by removing the mean and scaling them to unit variance. Since we use BERT models for the textual data, we do not need extensive preprocessing steps. The model can process the textual data without significant assumptions and in considerable length. We, however, need to tokenize the dataset before feeding it into the BERT model with the model-specific tokenizer (in our case "BERT base model (uncased)").

3.4 Model Training and Explanation

For strategy 1, we focus on combining the class attribution probability of an XGBoost Model and a BERT model, which is fine-tuned on our dataset. We then decide per case which of the models' predictions results in a more significant absolute difference to the probability of 0.5 and, therefore, provide a clearer decision. Both models are fed into the SHAP explainer module and are individually explained. The SHAP framework is generally model-agnostic, but model-specific optimizations for faster calculation exist. The SHAP framework relies for BERT on the so-called PartitionExplainer and for XGBoost on Tree-Explainer.

For strategy 2, we first use the identical BERT setup described above. However, we then perform an explainability analysis using the SHAP framework to filter out the n most important words. We then feed these n features into an XGBoost model as the second stage to derive the final prediction. As mentioned above, BERT will be explained using the SHAP PartitionExplainer. As we use XGBoost in the second stage, we delete the stopwords before feeding these features into the XGBoost model. XGBoost disregards a word's left and right context and its sequential nature. The n most important features of the BERT explainability analysis after stopwords removal are represented using the well-known TF-IDF approach before using the XGBoost model. For the explainability analysis of strategy 2, we only consider the second-stage XGBoost model.

4   Results

Effect on Model Performance. The two strategies and their performance on the different augmented datasets are assessed using an F1-score and ROC AUC, which are common evaluation metrics for classification problems. We also introduce another baseline with "baseline unilateral" predicting all inputs with the majority class. Overall, we differentiate between strategies 1 and 2 on the augmented dataset and a baseline model on non-textual data only. The results in Fig. 5 show that already for purity of above 0.1, the proposed strategies lead to a net improvement of both ROC AUC and F1-score. The results suggest that the strategies provide a benefit even at low levels of textual data purity and improve the model performance. The combined incorporation of textual and non-textual information shows value in light of a low level of textual data purity as neither model alone can score these results. Using a pure textual model also creates similar results for high textual data purity (around 1.0), as shown by the pure BERT performance. Therefore, we can conclude that both strategies are valuable in that they provide higher predictive quality, especially for low levels of textual data purity, while the performance of the models converges for a very high purity on textual features. There is a slight difference discernible between strategies 1 and 2.

Effect on Rediscovery Rate. We calculate a metric of rediscovery to determine whether the artificial latent structures introduced during the dataset augmentation are uncovered and manifested in the explainability analysis. The rediscovery rate will be measured by the overlap between the most important textual features derived by the SHAP calculations and the input features used during the dataset augmentation via word2vec vector similarity. Word2vec represents words in a high-dimensional vector space [13]. We used the pre-trained word2vec vectors based on the Google News dataset². In our rediscovery calculation, we consider two words as rediscovered if the cosine similarity between the two words on the pre-trained word2vec vectors is above 0.3 and if the mean absolute feature importance via SHAP is above 0.005. Since both strategies show high rediscovery rates, one can conclude that the right latent structures seem to be found, and the strategies seem to work as intended. There is a difference between strategies 1 and 2, which indicates that strategy 1 rediscovers more of the latent features introduced during dataset augmentation. Strategy 2 incorporates a limited amount of features and thus leads to a lower yet still considerable rediscovery rate.

Effect on Quantitative Explainability Metrics. Stevens et al. propose an approach to quantitatively evaluate the explainability of ML models, particularly for the process domain. Their approach distinguishes interpretability (measured by parsimony), as well as faithfulness (measured by monotonicity) [18].

Parsimony. Parsimony as a property can describe the explainability models' complexity. Parsimony describes the number of features in the final model and can quantify the simplicity of a model. For post-hoc explainability analysis using

---

² https://code.google.com/archive/p/word2vec/.

feature importance, the non-zero feature weights are considered. The maximal value of the parsimony property is the number of features. A simple (or parsimonious) model is characterized by a small parsimony value [18]. To compare the parsimony, we take the parsimony for the baseline model, for strategy 1 (as a sum of both models' feature counts), and the second-stage model of strategy 2. We can see a significant difference between the baseline model and strategy 1 in Fig. 5. For strategy 2, the parsimony is only slightly higher than the baseline and converges against an upper boundary since we limit the number of textual features n in the second-stage model.

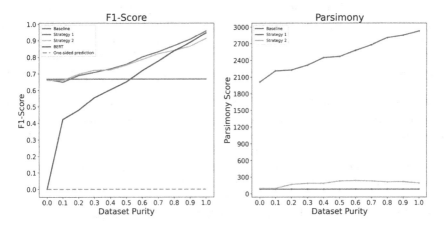

Fig. 5. F1-score and parsimony for augmented datasets with varying impurity

This implies that strategies 1 and 2 naturally consider substantially more features than the baseline. For strategy 1, even more features are incorporated in an explainability analysis with a higher purity of the augmented datasets and overall better model performance. As parsimony is a metric to determine how interpretable an explainability analysis is, this consequently means that models considering textual information (strategy 1 and strategy 2) are more challenging to interpret. We have to note here that the parsimony of strategy 2 is significantly below the parsimony of strategy 1. Therefore, the interpretability of strategy 2 is better as we limit the number of features to incorporate by the parameter n. In their elaboration on feature importance techniques specifically in the area of NLP, Danilevsky et al. argue in their work that "[t]ext-based features are inherently more interpretable by humans [...]" [5]. Following this line of reasoning, it is not entirely correct to assign non-textual and textual features the same negative impact on interpretability, which puts the results into relative terms.

Monotonicity. Monotonicity can be used as a metric to describe the faithfulness between the model and the explanation. Monotonicity describes the faithfulness between the feature importance resulting from the explainability analysis and the feature importance of the task model. For models that require post-hoc explainability, the monotonicity is denoted by the Spearman's correlation coefficient between the absolute values of the feature weights for the task model and the absolute values of the feature weights of the explainability model [18]. The range of the monotonicity lies between $[-1, 1]$ and describes the association of rank, where a perfectly faithful model would have a Monotonicity M of $+1$. In contrast, a less faithful model would score values closer to 0. A negative Spearman correlation coefficient implies a negative association of rank between the task model's feature importance and the explainability model's feature importance. For strategy 2 in the second stage and the baseline model, we use XGBoost as a model of choice, which provides inherent task model-specific feature importance. While there are multiple ways to assess XGBoost-specific feature importance, we will focus on the importance by the number of times a feature is used to split the data across all trees of the decision tree approach. We will not consider the monotonicity metric for strategy 1 because it is a BERT model for which task model-specific feature importance cannot be directly obtained.

We see that the monotonicity of the baseline model and the second-stage model in strategy 2 are almost similar. While there is only a small difference in monotonicity initially, it disappears with higher dataset purity. The results on monotonicity showed little to no difference between strategy 2 and the baseline. This indicates no notable difference in the faithfulness of the explainability analysis in comparison with the original prediction model. As elaborated before, we cannot calculate the monotonicity score for strategy 1 due to a lack of task model feature importance from the BERT model. Therefore, the statement relates to strategy 2 only.

Effect on Computation Time. For strategy 1, we add up both models' training time and the explanation time. For strategy 2, we add the training time of both stages together for training. At the same time, we only consider the explanation time of the second stage as we only perform an explanation computation via SHAP for this second stage.

The results show a significant difference between the baseline and strategies 1 and 2 for model training and explainability calculation. For the baseline, the training is performed quicker than the explanation, while this holds not true for strategies 1 and 2. The training and explanation of strategy 2 take only marginally longer than for strategy 1 but are considerably more expensive than for the baseline. There is also a noteworthy difference between training time and time for the SHAP calculations. The evaluations showed that the training times and explainability analyses required significantly more time for the proposed strategies than for the baseline. Our experiments suggest that for a high number of features and complex models, the computation for the explainability analysis far outweighs the training time. We can, however, not draw a conclusion regarding the ratio of training and explainability times, as this is highly dependent on the model choice and the dataset used for evaluation.

Prototype. To contemplate the practical implications of using textual data for explainable predictive monitoring of business processes, we developed a prototype illustrating how this might affect users. We differentiate between local explainability (for individual process instances) and global explainability (overview over all process instances). This screenshot shows a local analysis of strategy 1 divided into two separate models for the prediction as well as the explanation. A red color in the individual explainability plots indicates a positive change (towards a loan acceptance); blue color indicates a negative change in the expected model prediction (towards a loan rejection) (Fig. 6).

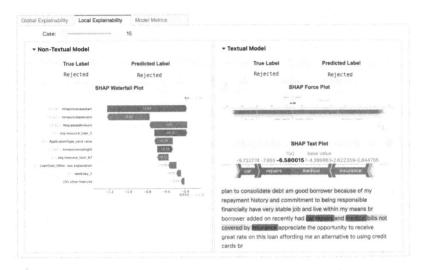

Fig. 6. Prototypical implementation of local explainability analysis (Strategy 1)

5   Related Work

Predictive process monitoring techniques have been developed for a wide range of purposes. The most prominent use cases include the prediction of the process outcome [19, 22] and the prediction of future process behavior, such as the next activity [9]. While most techniques build on categorical and numerical features to accomplish their prediction goal, some also take into account textual data. For instance, Pegoraro et al. use different strategies such as TF-IDF, Doc2Vec, or LDA to represent textual information and, in this way, integrate it into an LSTM architecture with further categorical and numerical data [15]. Teinemaa et al. perform predictive monitoring with structured and unstructured data by concatenating the textual features to the feature vector of the non-textual features. The text is represented, among others, using bag-of-n-grams, TF-IDF, and LDA [19]. A recent technique from Cabrera et al. [3] uses contextualized word embeddings to predict the next activity and the next timestamp of running cases.

Recognizing the need for explainability, several so-called explainable predictive process monitoring techniques have been developed. These techniques mostly rely on model-agnostic approaches such as SHAP [10,18] or LIME [14]. SHAP unifies existing model explanation techniques (which include six existing methods, amongst others, LIME [16]). SHAP is a unified measure to calculate post-hoc feature importance by using the Shapley values of the conditional expectation function of the original model [12]. All explainable predictive process monitoring techniques have in common that they rely on numerical and categorical features only and do not consider textual data. Hence, this paper empirically demonstrates the potential of explainable predictive process monitoring based on textual and non-textual data.

6   Conclusion and Future Work

This paper empirically explored the potential of combining textual and non-textual data in the context of explainable predictive process monitoring. To this end, we conducted extensive experiments on a synthetic dataset we created for this purpose. We found that using textual data alongside non-textual data requires more computation time but can lead to better predictions even when the quality of the textual data is poor. While the explainability metrics might decrease slightly depending on the chosen strategy, textual information is inherently more interpretable by humans, which allows for a more human-understandable explanation. Therefore, we conclude that combining textual and non-textual data in the context of explainable predictive process monitoring is a promising approach.

As for future work, we see two main directions. First, after an explainability analysis, it is unclear whether a variable is merely correlated with the outcome or causally related. Therefore, future work should combine the explainability analysis with a subsequent causality analysis. Second, it would be interesting to relate the results of an explainability analysis to real interventions.

References

1. Barredo Arrieta, A., et al.: Explainable artificial intelligence (XAI): Concepts, taxonomies, opportunities and challenges toward responsible AI. Inf. Fusion **58**, 82–115 (2020)
2. Blei, D.M., Ng, A.Y., Jordan, M.I.: Latent dirichlet allocation. J. Mach. Learn. Res. **3**, 993–1022 (2003)
3. Cabrera, L., Weinzierl, S., Zilker, S., Matzner, M.: Text-aware predictive process monitoring with contextualized word embeddings. In: Cabanillas, C., Garmann-Johnsen, N.F., Koschmider, A. (eds.) Business Process Management Workshops. BPM 2022, Lecture Notes in Business Information Processing, vol. 460, pp. 303–314. Springer, Cham (2023). https://doi.org/10.1007/978-3-031-25383-6_22
4. Chen, T., Guestrin, C.: Xgboost: a scalable tree boosting system. In: Proceedings of the 22nd ACM SIGKDD International Conference on Knowledge Discovery and Data Mining, KDD 2016, pp. 785–794 (2016)

5. Danilevsky, M., Qian, K., Aharonov, R., Katsis, Y., Kawas, B., Sen, P.: A survey of the state of explainable AI for natural language processing. In: Proceedings of the 1st Conference of the Asia-Pacific Chapter of the Association for Computational Linguistics and the 10th International Joint Conference on Natural Language Processing, pp. 447–459. AACL (2020)
6. Devlin, J., Chang, M.W., Lee, K., Toutanova, K.: BERT: Pre-training of deep bidirectional transformers for language understanding. In: Proceedings of the 2019 Conference of the North American Chapter of the Association for Computational Linguistics: Human Language Technologies, vol. 1, pp. 4171–4186 (2019)
7. Di Francescomarino, C., Ghidini, C., Maggi, F.M., Milani, F.: Predictive process monitoring methods: Which one suits me best? In: Business Process Management, pp. 462–479 (2018)
8. van Dongen, B.: Bpi challenge 2017 (2017). https://data.4tu.nl/articles/dataset/BPI_Challenge_2017/12696884/1
9. Evermann, J., Rehse, J.R., Fettke, P.: A deep learning approach for predicting process behaviour at runtime. In: Business Process Management Workshops, pp. 327–338 (2017)
10. Galanti, R., Coma-Puig, B., Leoni, M.d., Carmona, J., Navarin, N.: Explainable predictive process monitoring. In: 2020 2nd International Conference on Process Mining (ICPM), pp. 1–8 (2020)
11. George, N.: Lending club loan application data (2017). https://www.kaggle.com/wordsforthewise/lending-club. Accessed Dec 2021
12. Lundberg, S.M., Lee, S.I.: A unified approach to interpreting model predictions. In: Advances in Neural Information Processing Systems, vol. 30, pp. 4765–4774 (2017)
13. Mikolov, T., Chen, K., Corrado, G., Dean, J.: Efficient estimation of word representations in vector space. In: Proceedings of Workshop at ICLR 2013 (2013)
14. Ouyang, C., Sindhgatta, R., Moreira, C.: Explainable AI enabled inspection of business process prediction models. CoRR abs/2107.09767 (2021)
15. Pegoraro, M., Uysal, M.S., Georgi, D.B., van der Aalst, W.M.: Text-aware predictive monitoring of business processes. Bus. Inf. Syst. 1, 221–232 (2021)
16. Ribeiro, M.T., Singh, S., Guestrin, C.: "Why should I trust you?": explaining the predictions of any classifier. In: Proceedings of the 22nd ACM SIGKDD International Conference on Knowledge Discovery and Data Mining, San Francisco, CA, USA, 13–17 August 2016, pp. 1135–1144 (2016)
17. Rizzi, W., Di Francescomarino, C., Maggi, F.M.: Explainability in predictive process monitoring: when understanding helps improving. In: Fahland, D., Ghidini, C., Becker, J., Dumas, M. (eds.) BPM 2020. LNBIP, vol. 392, pp. 141–158. Springer, Cham (2020). https://doi.org/10.1007/978-3-030-58638-6_9
18. Stevens, A., De Smedt, J., Peeperkorn, J.: Quantifying explainability in outcome-oriented predictive process monitoring. In: Munoz-Gama, J., Lu, X. (eds.) ICPM 2021. LNBIP, vol. 433, pp. 194–206. Springer, Cham (2022). https://doi.org/10.1007/978-3-030-98581-3_15
19. Teinemaa, I., Dumas, M., Maggi, F.M., Di Francescomarino, C.: Predictive business process monitoring with structured and unstructured data. In: Business Process Management, pp. 401–417 (2016)
20. Teinemaa, I., Dumas, M., Rosa, M.L., Maggi, F.M.: Outcome-oriented predictive process monitoring: review and benchmark. ACM Trans. Knowl. Discov. Data (TKDD) 13(2), 1–57 (2019)

21. Verenich, I., Dumas, M., La Rosa, M., Maggi, F., Teinemaa, I.: Survey and cross-benchmark comparison of remaining time prediction methods in business process monitoring. ACM Trans. Intell. Syst. Technol. **10**, 1–34 (2019)
22. Weytjens, H., De Weerdt, J.: Process outcome prediction: CNN vs. LSTM (with attention). In: Del Río Ortega, A., Leopold, H., Santoro, F.M. (eds.) BPM 2020. LNBIP, vol. 397, pp. 321–333. Springer, Cham (2020). https://doi.org/10.1007/978-3-030-66498-5_24

Attribute-Based Conformance Diagnosis: Correlating Trace Attributes with Process Conformance

Michael Grohs$^{(\boxtimes)}$ (ID) and Jana-Rebecca Rehse (ID)

University of Mannheim, Mannheim, Germany
mgrohs@mail.uni-mannheim.de, rehse@uni-mannheim.de

Abstract. An important practical capability of conformance checking is that organizations can use it to alleviate potential deviations from the intended process behavior. However, existing techniques only identify these deviations, but do not provide insights on potential explanations, which could help to improve the process. In this paper, we present attribute-based conformance diagnosis (ABCD), a novel approach for correlating process conformance with trace attributes. ABCD builds on existing conformance checking techniques and uses machine learning techniques to find trace attribute values that potentially impact the process conformance. It creates a regression tree to identify those attribute combinations that correlate with higher or lower trace fitness. We evaluate the explanatory power, computational efficiency, and generated insights of ABCD based on publicly available event logs. The evaluation shows that ABCD can find correlations of trace attribute combinations with higher or lower fitness in a sufficiently efficient way, although computation time increases for larger log sizes.

Keywords: Process mining · Conformance checking · Correlations · Trace attributes · Root cause analysis

1 Introduction

The goal of conformance checking is to analyze the relation between the intended behavior of a process, captured in a process model, and the observed behavior of a process, captured in an event log [7]. It generates insights on where and how the observed behavior aligns with or deviates from the intended behavior. Organizations can use these insights for example to check whether their process execution is compliant with the originally designed process [22]. Over the last years, multiple conformance checking techniques have been developed, including rule checking, token-based replay, and alignments [7]. The techniques differ with regards to their algorithmic approach, computational complexity, and generated results, but they have one output in common: A measure of the conformance between log and model, called fitness, which quantifies the capability of a model to replay the behavior observed in the log [22].

© The Author(s) 2023
M. Montali et al. (Eds.): ICPM 2022 Workshops, LNBIP 468, pp. 203–215, 2023.
https://doi.org/10.1007/978-3-031-27815-0_15

One problem of existing conformance checking techniques is that they do not enable practitioners to reach their underlying goal, which is to improve the process [19]. As an example, consider a loan application process in a bank, where the application of a conformance checking algorithm yielded an overall fitness value of 0.8. From this number, a process analyst can conclude that some deviations between log and model occurred, but they do not know where, how, and—most importantly—why the process execution deviated and what the effects of the potential problem are. Therefore, explaining and understanding the underlying causes of conformance problems is an important part of leveraging the practical benefits of conformance checking [22]. Existing conformance checking techniques focus only on the identification of deviations and do not provide any potential reasons for their occurrence [5], although this would be a vital prerequisite for any deeper process analysis. For our exemplary loan application process, if the process analyst knows that loans with a higher amount more likely deviate from the intended process, they could specifically analyze those process instances to find and eventually address the root cause of those deviations.

In this paper, we present a novel approach for finding correlations between process conformance and trace attributes. This approach, called attribute-based conformance diagnosis (ABCD), builds on the results of existing conformance checking techniques and uses machine learning to find trace attribute values that potentially impact the conformance. Specifically, it creates a regression tree to identify those attribute combinations that correlate with higher or lower trace fitness. These correlations can be considered as potential explanations for conformance differences and therefore as a starting point for further analysis steps to find and address the causes of lower process conformance. ABCD is (1) inductive, i.e., it requires no additional domain or process knowledge, (2) data-driven, i.e., it requires only an event log and a process model as input, (3) universally applicable, i.e., it does not depend on process-specific characteristics, and (4) flexible, i.e., it can be configured to fit a specific case.

In the following, the ABCD approach is introduced in Sect. 2. Its explanatory power, computational efficiency, and potential practical insights are evaluated based on publicly available event logs in Sect. 3. We discuss related work in Sect. 4 and conclude with a discussion of limitations and future work in Sect. 5.

2   Approach

The goal of the ABCD approach is to find attribute value combinations in an event log that correlate with differences in conformance. Therefore, it analyzes trace attributes and correlates them with trace-level fitness, which is the most common way to measure conformance [22]. A schematic overview of ABCD can be found in Fig. 1. The approach requires two inputs, an event log and a corresponding process model, and consists of two major steps. In the first step, explained in Sect. 2.1, we enrich the event log with the trace-level fitness values with regard to the provided process model. This enriched log serves as input for the second step, called Inductive Overall Analysis (IOA) and explained in

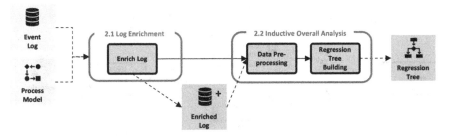

Fig. 1. Illustration of the Attribute-Based Conformance Diagnosis (ABCD) approach

Sect. 2.2. It determines the correlations between combinations of attribute values and process conformance. Therefore, it computes a regression tree. Regression trees are a data mining technique that relate a set of independent variables, in our case all trace attributes in an event log, to a real-valued dependent variable, in our case, i.e., average trace fitness in a log. To build the regression tree, the event log is iteratively split into sub-logs, based on trace attribute values. Each split defines a new node in the tree. These nodes are then used to predict the value of the dependent variable [10]. To find the best fitting tree, the algorithm minimizes the sum of errors in the prediction. An error is the difference between the predicted value in a leaf node and the actual value of the respective sub-log. The percentage of the true variation that can be explained by the predictions, i.e., 1 minus the sum of errors, is the coefficient of determination R^2, which can be used to determine the prediction quality of the regression tree [9].

2.1 Log Enrichment

Because the goal of ABCD is to correlate trace attributes with variations in conformance, it needs the trace-level fitness to perform any further analysis. Therefore, we compute the fitness of each trace with regard to the provided process model and add the value to the event log as a trace attribute. The user can choose between token-replay fitness and alignment-based fitness [7]. The latter is the default choice used in the remainder of this paper. This parametrization allows users to flexibly choose the best-suited technique, for example choosing token-based fitness if alignments require too much computation time.

After computing the trace fitness value, we also enrich each trace by its overall duration, defined as the time difference between start and end event in a timely ordered trace. This ensures that at least one trace attribute will always occur in the log. We decided on the trace duration as the default trace attribute, because it can be computed for every (time-stamped) event log and because the relation between process performance and process conformance is potentially relevant for all processes, independent of their context [24].

2.2 Inductive Overall Analysis

Following the log enrichment, Inductive Overall Analysis (IOA) determines correlations between combinations of attribute values and process conformance.

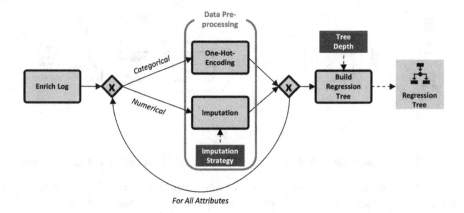

Fig. 2. Illustration of Inductive Overall Analysis (IOA)

Therefore, it first preprocesses the data and then constructs a regression tree that uses the trace attribute values as determinants for the fitness value. Figure 2 shows the schematic overview. IOA consists of two steps: preprocessing the data and building the regression tree.

Data Preprocessing. For the data pre-processing, we distinguish between categorical and numerical attributes. Due to requirements of the tree algorithm, pre-processing is necessary for both. First, because a regression tree can only handle numerical attributes, categorical variables need to be encoded to be used as a determinant. For this purpose, we use One-Hot-Encoding, which constructs one binary trace attribute per categorical attribute value. Second, the regression tree algorithm cannot handle missing data. If there are values missing for numerical attributes, we need to perform imputation, i.e., replace missing values with other values [31]. Assuming that raw data is the best representation of reality, no imputation will be the default. If it must be performed due to missing values, potential imputation strategies include replacing missing values with the mean, the median, the most frequent value, or a constant value. For IOA, users can select the imputation strategy as a parameter. Additional to no imputation, we allow for imputing with the most frequent value, a constant value of 0, the mean, and the median value. Imputation will only be necessary for numerical attributes since the encoding transforms the categorical attributes into binary attributes with no missing values. Missing values in categorical attributes will therefore lead to a 0 in all binary attributes.

Regression Tree Building. After the preprocessing, we build the regression tree. The goal is to find those combinations of attribute values that best predict variations in conformance. Therefore, the regression tree consists of nodes that split the event log based on one attribute value. A splitting node includes a condition for the attribute value, e.g., a duration smaller than 4 days. For all traces below the splitting node on the left side of the tree, the node condition is true. For all traces below on the right side, it is false. Leaf nodes do not state a condition, either because the tree has reached its maximum depth or because an additional split will not improve the result. Traversing the tree from root to leaves, each node divides the log according to its condition, iteratively dividing the log into one sub-log per leaf node. The sub-log of an internal node is the union of all sub-logs of its children. Each node reports on the average fitness for the sub-log created by all splits above it, which is used as a predictor for the fitness of the individual traces. The tree algorithm chooses attribute values and conditions by minimizing the total errors in the prediction, i.e., the sum of the differences between the true fitness value of each trace and the average fitness in the leaf node. The final tree consists of splitting nodes and leaf nodes. The leaf nodes indicate the overall prediction for the sub-logs created by the splitting nodes. The combination of conditions leading down to a leaf node indicates a combination of attribute values that well predicts the fitness of the given sub-log, i.e., it consistently determines the conformance level of these traces.

For building the tree, we use the sklearn-environment in Python[1]. As a parameter, we require the maximum tree depth, i.e., the number of node layers the algorithm may use to split the log. When choosing this depth, we need to balance the explanatory power of the tree with its visual clarity and the granularity of sub-logs. The returned regression tree includes those attribute value combinations that are correlated with higher or lower fitness and thus offer a potential explanation for differences in conformance.

3 Evaluation

We implemented the ABCD approach in Python.[2] Using this implementation, we conduct an evaluation to show that ABCD has explanatory power, is computationally efficient, and generates practical insights. For our evaluation, we used three publicly available data sets consisting of seven event logs (see Table 1):

MobIS-Challenge 2019 [26]. This event log from a travel management process contains trace attributes. It also comes with a matching process model that describes that process and can be used as a reference for conformance checking.

BPI Challenge (BPIC) 2020 [30]. This collection of five event logs, also from a travel management process, contains many trace attributes, which makes it well suitable to test ABCD's abilities to provide insights. Because there is no to-be model available for this process, we applied the PM4Py auto-filter on the event log to filter all common variants[3] and discovered a model using the Inductive Miner. This way, we check conformance against the most frequent behavior.

BPI Challenge (BPIC) 2017 [29]. This event log from a loan application process is comparably large, which makes it well suitable to test ABCD's computational feasibility. Because there also is no to-be model available for this process, we discovered one using the above-described method.

---

[1] https://scikit-learn.org/stable/modules/generated/sklearn.tree.DecisionTreeRegressor.html.

[2] https://gitlab.uni-mannheim.de/mgrohs/attribute-based-conformance-diagnosis/-/tree/main.

[3] https://pm4py.fit.fraunhofer.de/documentation.

Table 1. Public event logs used for evaluation

ID	Dataset	Name	Traces	Events	Trace attributes
(1)	MobIS	MobIS	6,555	83,256	Duration (Dur), Costs
(2)	BPIC 2020	Domestic Declarations	10,500	56,437	Dur, Amount (Amn), Budget Number (BudNo), Declaration Number (DeclNo)
(3)	BPIC 2020	International Declarations	6,449	72,151	Dur, Adjusted Amn, Amn, BudNo, DeclNo, Original Amn, Act. No., Org. Entity, Req. Bud
(4)	BPIC 2020	Request for Payment	6,886	36,796	Dur, Act., Cost Type, Org. Entity, Project, Req. Amon., Task, Rfp No.
(5)	BPIC 2020	Prepaid Travel Costs	2,099	18,246	Dur., Act., Cost Type, Org. Entity, Project No., Bud. No., Red. Budget, Project, Task
(6)	BPIC 2020	Travel Permit	7,065	86,581	Dur., Bud. No., Cost Type, Org. Entity, Overspent Amn, Project, Req. Amn
(7)	BPIC 2017	Loan Application	31,509	1,202,267	Dur, Application Type, Loan Goal, Requested Amn

3.1 Explanatory Power

To measure the explanatory power of ABCD, we use the coefficient of determination R^2, which shows the goodness of fit of the regression [8]. To determine the influence of our parameters, our evaluation setting varies the imputation strategy (none, mean, median, zero, constant), and the tree depth (from 3 to 7; a larger tree would not be visually clear anymore).

We first inspect the influence of the imputation strategy. This is shown in Table 2, where we list the R^2 for the four imputation strategies for the MobIS event log. No imputation is not possible for this event log due to missing attribute values. We do see not see any difference in R^2 for the different imputation strategies in the MobIS data. This is also the case for all other logs.[4] We can conclude that the imputation strategy has no effect on the explanatory power of ABCD. However, this might be different for highly variable real-life event logs, so the imputation option is necessary to remain universally applicable.

Table 3 shows the R^2 values for all event logs and tree depths. As expected, R^2 grows with tree depth, due to more allowed splits in the tree. This increase is log-dependent and ranges between 1% for log (2) and 13% for log (3). It is generally impossible to determine a universal threshold for a good R^2 value [25]. However, we see that ABCD is capable of explaining at least one fifth of the fitness variation in all logs and as much as 84% in one, meaning that it is capable of finding correlations of data attributes with (non-)conformance. All in all, our evaluation showed that for our inspected datasets, ABCD has moderate to high explanatory power and is not sensitive to imputation and tree depth.

---

[4] The full evaluation documentation is available in the GitLab repository.

Table 2. R^2 for the MobIS data set for working imputation strategies and tree depths 3 to 7

Log	Imp.	3	4	5	6	7
(1)	Mean	0.163	0.178	0.195	0.203	0.218
(1)	Median	0.163	0.178	0.195	0.203	0.218
(1)	Zero	0.163	0.178	0.195	0.203	0.218
(1)	Freq	0.163	0.178	0.195	0.203	0.218

Table 3. R^2 for tree depths 3 to 7

Log	Imp.	3	4	5	6	7
(1)	All	0.163	0.178	0.195	0.203	0.218
(2)	All	0.744	0.747	0.75	0.753	0.756
(3)	All	0.303	0.344	0.374	0.405	0.433
(4)	All	0.819	0.824	0.829	0.835	0.84
(5)	All	0.483	0.513	0.54	0.569	0.596
(6)	All	0.416	0.434	0.448	0.462	0.476
(7)	All	0.322	0.336	0.348	0.357	0.368

3.2 Computational Efficiency

For assessing the computational efficiency of ABCD, we measure the execution times, separated into the enrichment step in Table 4 and the analysis step in Table 5. Each reported value in those tables is an average of three separate executions, to account for outliers. For the analysis time, we only report the average execution time over all imputation strategies since there were no significant deviations between them.

Table 4. Enrichment times

Log	Traces	Events	Attr.	Time [s]
(1)	6,555	83,256	2	33.75
(2)	10,500	56,437	5	2.26
(3)	6,449	72,151	18	61.98
(4)	6,886	36,796	9	1.38
(5)	2,099	18,246	17	3.65
(6)	7,065	86,581	168	859.47
(7)	31,509	1,202,267	4	9,216.35

We see that the enrichment time increases with the number of traces and the number of events, because especially alignments become computationally expensive [7]. Additionally, the number of trace attributes negatively influences the enrichment time, which is visible for the Travel Permit log (6). At most, the enrichment takes 2.6 h for the largest log (7).

Like the enrichment time, the analysis time for IOA depends heavily on the number of traces and the number of trace attributes, again visible for logs (6) and (7). However, this increase is less significant compared to the increase in enrichment time and the maximum duration is below 25 min. 25 min. In case of more trace attributes, we consider more independent variables and in case of many traces we have a larger sample size, both increasing the explanatory power of ABCD. We conclude that

Table 5. Average computation time for IOA over all imputation strategies for tree depths 3 to 7 in s

Log	3	4	5	6	7
(1)	64.61	65.13	64.98	65.69	64.77
(2)	180.99	180.02	181.69	183.07	187.44
(3)	132.15	132.71	132.45	134.88	132.98
(4)	99.51	100.42	99.78	100.14	101.1
(5)	15.95	16.03	16.0	16.19	16.33
(6)	602.4	618.54	591.85	590.82	651.73
(7)	1,395.65	1,357.93	1,353.86	1,352.12	1,375.79

ABCD is computationally feasible even for larger logs, although the execution times are a potential drawback. Neither imputation strategy nor tree depth have a significant impact on the analysis time.

Overall, we see a negative influence of the log size on the computational efficiency. Still, execution takes less than 3 h for event logs with up to 1.2 million events. Considering the potential value of ABCD, the execution time does not limit its applicability. As alignment are the main cause for long executions, larger event logs could still be analyzed by means of a different fitness technique.

3.3 Practical Insights

The main benefit of ABCD is that it generates process insights without prior knowledge, which is supposed to provide value for practitioners. These insights are correlations between trace attributes and process conformance that serve as a starting point for further process analyses. To demonstrate some of these insights, we further examine the regression trees generated for the event logs. It is important to note that for all event logs except MobIS, the process model is generated based on variant filters. This means that conformance and fitness are based on the most common variants and not on a constructed process model. In the following, conformance of the BPI logs has to be interpreted as conformance to the most common variants. Detailed information about the practical insights provided by ABCD can be derived from the computed regression trees for all logs (available in the GitLab repository).

MobIS. An exemplary regression tree with depth 3 is provided in Fig. 3. It splits the log into six different sub-logs represented by the six leaf nodes. For example, the top node splits the log based on whether the trace has a duration above 0 (more than one event). The color indicates the fitness value: high fitness leads to darker color. We see that short duration above 0

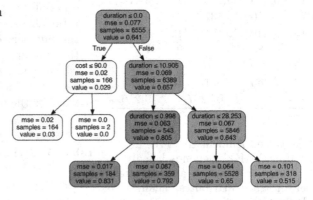

Fig. 3. Exemplary regression tree for the MobIS Log

correlates with better conformance. For traces with one event, lower costs correlate with slightly better fitness.

BPI Challenge 2020. Not knowing the trace ID, e.g., the declaration number, correlates with lower conformance in logs (2), (3), (4), and (5). For all five logs, the duration is an important feature in the trees, which shows the value of separately enriching this attribute. Longer traces conform better in log (2), but they conform worse in log (4). Another relevant trace attribute is the requested amount or budget, which also correlates with lower conformance in most cases.

BPI Challenge 2017. Longer traces conform better for log (7). Further, an unknown loan goal and a smaller requested amount correlate with lower fitness.

We conclude that ABCD can generate practical insights in form of correlations between trace attributes and trace fitness without relying on process or domain knowledge. These correlations can serve as starting points to identify causalities that explain conformance deviations. We show that it finds significant attribute values correlating with worse conformance, both for available to-be models and for mined models that represent the most common behavior. The identified correlations can be used to further examine the deviations that occur in the sub-logs created by the regression tree nodes. Comparing all sub-logs of MobIS data based on the leaf nodes in Fig. 3 could yield additional insights into conformance variation, including, e.g., the location and type of deviation that occurs in the individual sub-logs. For example, we see that for the leaf node with size 184, the deviations occur primarily in the reporting part of the travel management process.

4   Related Work

In this section, we elaborate on work related to the ABCD approach. Many other approaches combine data attributes and conformance checking. For example, data attributes are used while performing the conformance check to incorporate other perspectives into the optimal alignment of data-enriched process models and event logs [20–22]. Data attributes can also be used to define response moves (i.e., log moves that change data attributes that have been incorrectly changed by another log move in advance) [28] and to perform multi-perspective conformance checks on declarative models [6]. In all approaches, the data attributes refine the check itself but are not used to potentially explain conformance problems.

Data attributes can also be used to create sub-logs or sub-models in so called process cubes. Users can then analyze the differences between the sub-logs or sub-models and draw conclusions about what data attributes lead to the differences [1]. Main applications are process discovery [14,17] and performance analysis [2,4]. Applying process cubes for various purposes implicitly tries to use data attributes to explain differences in an event log or process model, often related to performance. This resembles attribute-based conformance diagnosis, but focuses on aspects other than conformance and metrics other than fitness.

The research stream that resembles ABCD the most closely is called root cause analysis (RCA). It aims to identify causal structures between different variables and show the influence these variables have on each other [23]. This can be achieved by using structural equation models based on data attributes [23], Granger-causal feature pairs, conventional correlations [3,18], or clustering techniques [12]. Also, to find reasons for deviations in processes, fuzzy mining and rule mining with data attributes can be applied without performing any conformance check [27]. Consequently, no deviations against a to-be model are investigated.

Another prominently used RCA technique are regression trees [10,16]. In process mining, regression trees have been applied to detect causes for performance issues [16], for example by analyzing data attributes not referring to the control-flow [10]. Also, tree structures can be applied to identify causes for control-flow deviations located through sub-group discovery [11]. However, all approaches require domain knowledge to identify deviations or validate root causes after the automated analysis. Further, current approaches do not use conformance as the dependent variable. The automation is limited and the approaches are very specific [10].

Correlation-based RCA is also supported by process mining tools like Appian Process Mining, ARIS PM, Celonis, Lana Labs and Mehrwerk Process Mining. Those tools among others have been identified as relevant in a recent study [15]. However, none of them include a to-be model in the analysis but try to find root causes for variations in the data instead variations in conformance.

ABCD further resembles approaches like [11,12] where correlations between data attributes and process flow metrics other than conformance are identified. However, no to-be models are included in the analysis and therefore no conformance checking can be performed.

5   Discussion and Conclusion

The goal of the ABCD approach is to identify combinations of trace attribute values that correlate with variations in process conformance. Therefore, we first enrich the event log with fitness values. After that, we investigate the correlation between process conformance and attribute combinations. Our evaluation shows that ABCD is able to generate practical insights with explanatory power in an acceptable computation time. ABCD is inductive because it does not rely on domain knowledge and data-driven because it only needs an event log and a corresponding process model. It is universally applicable because is only depends on generic event log attributes, such as timestamps, and flexible because users can parametrize it to fit their specific case.

ABCD is subject to multiple limitations, which should be addressed in future research. First and most importantly, ABCD identifies correlations between attribute values and process conformance. It is not capable to determine whether and how the identified values actually caused the process to deviate. Instead, they are meant as an orientation for practitioners that try to improve the conformance of their process. In future research, ABCD could be extended by causal analysis techniques that are capable of identifying causal relations between attribute values and process conformance. Currently, the causal identification is performed manually based on the found correlations (i.e., potential explanations).

Second, the computation times indicate that the enrichment might take long for larger event logs, mainly due to the duration of the alignments. To still make ABCD applicable to larger event logs, we could compute the trace fitness with other techniques such as token-based replay or heuristics [7]. This was not necessary for our evaluation, because the duration of under three hours at maximum was acceptable, but it might become necessary for larger data sets.

Third, we enriched traces by their duration only. This attribute was useful since the case study found it to be a potential explanatory factor in many regression trees. However, additional enrichment by other generic trace attributes might further increase the explanatory power. Possibilities are the weekday in which the trace started or the number of other active cases at the point of initiation. Such attributes could also relate to events, such as the occurrence of certain activities in a trace or the number of executions of the same activity. More sophisticated encoding approaches might be used [13].

Fourth, we limited our dependent variable to fitness. Therefore, we treat different causes for fitness differences similar. However, it might be better to include deviation information to find root causes of these fitness differences.

A limitation of our evaluation is that no to-be models were available for the BPI logs, meaning that our evaluation results have to be interpreted carefully. We tried to mitigate this limitation by applying ABCD in a case with to-be model. However, we acknowledge that the insights of ABCD heavily depend on the availability of these models. This could be addressed by data-driven approaches for deriving to-be models, reducing the necessary effort for the organizations.

Finally, ABCD only identifies that a certain attribute value or combination of attribute values is correlated with process conformance, but it does not explain how the conformance is influenced. As discussed in Sect. 3.3, the next step could be to incorporate a post-processing that investigates the alignments of the sublogs generated in the leaf nodes and analyzes where and how a deviation occurs.

References

1. van der Aalst, W.M.P.: Process cubes: slicing, dicing, rolling up and drilling down event data for process mining. In: Song, M., Wynn, M.T., Liu, J. (eds.) AP-BPM 2013. LNBIP, vol. 159, pp. 1–22. Springer, Cham (2013). https://doi.org/10.1007/978-3-319-02922-1_1

2. van der Aalst, W.M.P., Guo, S., Gorissen, P.: Comparative process mining in education: an approach based on process cubes. In: Ceravolo, P., Accorsi, R., Cudre-Mauroux, P. (eds.) SIMPDA 2013. LNBIP, vol. 203, pp. 110–134. Springer, Heidelberg (2015). https://doi.org/10.1007/978-3-662-46436-6_6

3. Adams, J.N., van Zelst, S.J., Quack, L., Hausmann, K., van der Aalst, W.M.P., Rose, T.: A framework for explainable concept drift detection in process mining. In: Polyvyanyy, A., Wynn, M.T., Van Looy, A., Reichert, M. (eds.) BPM 2021. LNCS, vol. 12875, pp. 400–416. Springer, Cham (2021). https://doi.org/10.1007/978-3-030-85469-0_25

4. Bolt, A., de Leoni, M., van der Aalst, W.M.P., Gorissen, P.: Business process reporting using process mining, analytic workflows and process cubes: a case study in education. In: Ceravolo, P., Rinderle-Ma, S. (eds.) SIMPDA 2015. LNBIP, vol. 244, pp. 28–53. Springer, Cham (2017). https://doi.org/10.1007/978-3-319-53435-0_2

5. Borrego, D., Barba, I.: Conformance checking and diagnosis for declarative business process models in data-aware scenarios. Expert Syst. Appl. 41, 5340–5352 (2014)

6. Burattin, A., Maggi, F., Sperduti, A.: Conformance checking based on multi-perspective declarative process models. Expert Syst. Appl. 65, 194–211 (2016)

7. Carmona, J., van Dongen, B., Solti, A., Weidlich, M.: Conformance Checking - Relating Processes and Models. Springer, Cham (2018)

8. Cheng, C.L., Shalabh, Garg, G.: Coefficient of determination for multiple measurement error models. J. Multivar. Anal. **126**, 137–152 (2014)
9. Chicco, D., Warrens, M., Jurman, G.: The coefficient of determination R-squared is more informative than SMAPE, MAE, MAPE, MSE and RMSE in regression analysis evaluation. PeerJ, Comput. Sci. **7**, e623 (2021)
10. De Leoni, M., van der Aalst, W., Dees, M.: A general process mining framework for correlating, predicting and clustering dynamic behavior based on event logs. Inf. Syst. **56**, 235–257 (2016)
11. Delias, P., Grigori, D., Mouhoub, M.L., Tsoukias, A.: Discovering characteristics that affect process control flow. In: Linden, I., Liu, S., Dargam, F., Hernández, J.E. (eds.) EWG-DSS -2014. LNBIP, vol. 221, pp. 51–63. Springer, Cham (2015). https://doi.org/10.1007/978-3-319-21536-5_5
12. Delias, P., Lagopoulos, A., Tsoumakas, G., Grigori, D.: Using multi-target feature evaluation to discover factors that affect business process behavior. Comput. Ind. **99**, 253–261 (2018)
13. Di Francescomarino, C., Ghidini, C.: Predictive process monitoring. In: van der Aalst, W.M.P., Carmona, J. (eds.) Process Mining Handbook. Lecture Notes in Business Information Processing, vol. 448, pp. 320–346. Springer, Cham (2022). https://doi.org/10.1007/978-3-031-08848-3_10
14. Fani Sani, M., van der Aalst, W., Bolt, A., García-Algarra, J.: Subgroup discovery in process mining. In: Abramowicz, W. (ed.) BIS 2017. LNBIP, vol. 288, pp. 237–252. Springer, Cham (2017). https://doi.org/10.1007/978-3-319-59336-4_17
15. FAU, Chair of Digital Industrial Service Systems: Process Mining Software Comparison (2020). https://www.processmining-software.com/tools/
16. Ferreira, D., Vasilyev, E.: Using logical decision trees to discover the cause of process delays from event logs. Comput. Ind. **70**, 194–207 (2015)
17. Gupta, M., Sureka, A.: Process cube for software defect resolution. In: APSEC 2014, pp. 239–246. IEEE (2014)
18. Hompes, B.F.A., Maaradji, A., La Rosa, M., Dumas, M., Buijs, J.C.A.M., van der Aalst, W.M.P.: Discovering causal factors explaining business process performance variation. In: Dubois, E., Pohl, K. (eds.) CAiSE 2017. LNCS, vol. 10253, pp. 177–192. Springer, Cham (2017). https://doi.org/10.1007/978-3-319-59536-8_12
19. Horita, H., Hirayama, H., Tahara, Y., Ohsuga, A.: Towards goal-oriented conformance checking. In: SEKE 2015, pp. 722–724 (2015)
20. Mannhardt, F., de Leoni, M., Reijers, H., van der Aalst, W.: Balanced multi-perspective checking of process conformance. Computing **98**, 407–437 (2016)
21. Mozafari Mehr, A.S., de Carvalho, R.M., van Dongen, B.: Detecting privacy, data and control-flow deviations in business processes. In: Nurcan, S., Korthaus, A. (eds.) CAiSE 2021. LNBIP, vol. 424, pp. 82–91. Springer, Cham (2021). https://doi.org/10.1007/978-3-030-79108-7_10
22. Munoz-Gama, J.: Conformance Checking and Diagnosis in Process Mining: Comparing Observed and Modeled Processes. Springer, Cham (2016)
23. Qafari, M.S., van der Aalst, W.M.P.: Case level counterfactual reasoning in process mining. In: Nurcan, S., Korthaus, A. (eds.) CAiSE 2021. LNBIP, vol. 424, pp. 55–63. Springer, Cham (2021). https://doi.org/10.1007/978-3-030-79108-7_7
24. Rozinat, A., van der Aalst, W.: Conformance checking of processes based on monitoring real behavior. Inf. Syst. **33**, 64–95 (2008)
25. Saunders, L., Russell, R., Crabb, D.: The coefficient of determination: what determines a useful R^2 statistic? Invest. Ophthalmol. Visual Sci. **53**, 6830–6832 (2012)
26. Scheid, M., Rehse, J.R., Houy, C., Fettke, P.: Data set for MOBIS challenge 2019 (2018)

27. Swinnen, J., Depaire, B., Jans, M.J., Vanhoof, K.: A process deviation analysis –
    a case study. In: Daniel, F., Barkaoui, K., Dustdar, S. (eds.) BPM 2011. LNBIP,
    vol. 99, pp. 87–98. Springer, Heidelberg (2012). https://doi.org/10.1007/978-3-
    642-28108-2_8
28. Tsoury, A., Soffer, P., Reinhartz-Berger, I.: How well did it recover? impact-aware
    conformance checking. Computing **103**, 3–27 (2021)
29. van Dongen, B.: BPI challenge 2017. https://data.4tu.nl/articles/dataset/BPI_
    Challenge_2017/12696884 (2017)
30. van Dongen, B.: BPI challenge 2020. https://data.4tu.nl/collections/_/5065541/
    1 (2020)
31. Zhang, Z.: Missing data imputation: Focusing on single imputation. Ann. Transl.
    Med. **4** (2016)

Detecting Surprising Situations in Event Data

Christian Kohlschmidt, Mahnaz Sadat Qafari$^{(\boxtimes)}$, and Wil M. P. van der Aalst

Process and Data Science Chair (PADS), RWTH Aachen University,
Aachen, Germany
christian.kohlschmidt@rwth-aachen.de,
{m.s.qafari,wvdaalst}@pads.rwth-aachen.de

Abstract. Process mining is a set of techniques that are used by organizations to understand and improve their operational processes. The first essential step in designing any process reengineering procedure is to find process improvement opportunities. In existing work, it is usually assumed that the set of problematic process instances in which an undesirable outcome occurs is known prior or is easily detectable. So the process enhancement procedure involves finding the root causes and the treatments for the problem in those process instances. For example, the set of problematic instances is considered as those with outlier values or with values smaller/bigger than a given threshold in one of the process features. However, on various occasions, using this approach, many process enhancement opportunities, not captured by these problematic process instances, are missed. To overcome this issue, we formulate finding the process enhancement areas as a context-sensitive anomaly/outlier detection problem. We define a process enhancement area as a set of situations (process instances or prefixes of process instances) where the process performance is surprising. We aim to characterize those situations where process performance is significantly different from what was expected considering its performance in similar situations. To evaluate the validity and relevance of the proposed approach, we have implemented and evaluated it on a real-life event log.

Keywords: Process mining · Process enhancement · Context-sensitive outlier detection · Surprising instances

1 Introduction

Considering the current highly competitive nature of the economy, it is vital for organizations to continuously enhance their processes in order to meet the best market standards and improve customer experience. Process enhancement involves many steps, including finding the process areas where improvements are possible, designing the process reengineering steps, and estimating the impact of changing each factor on the process performance. By conducting all these steps, organizations can benefit from applying process mining techniques. The first step

© The Author(s) 2023
M. Montali et al. (Eds.): ICPM 2022 Workshops, LNBIP 468, pp. 216–228, 2023.
https://doi.org/10.1007/978-3-031-27815-0_16

of process enhancement is detecting those process areas where an improvement is possible. Process mining includes several techniques for process monitoring and finding their friction points. However, these techniques have the hidden assumption that all the process instances (cases) are the same. So the set of problematic cases can be easily identified. For example, the problematic cases can be identified as the ones with an outlier value with respect to a process feature. Another common method is using a threshold for a specific process feature. However, considering the variety of the cases, it is possible that a solution solves the problem for one group of cases while aggravating the problem for another group. Moreover, using the current techniques, the performance of the process in some cases can be considered normal and acceptable compared to the overall behavior of the process, while it can be considered surprising (i.e. anomalous or undesirable) when just considering their similar cases. This phenomenon can lead to overlooking some of the process enhancement opportunities.

As another issue, there are several process instances where the process performs significantly better than other similar process instances. Analyzing the process behavior while performing these process instances can lead to invaluable clues on how to improve the process. Usually, this source of information is neglected by the current process mining techniques.

To overcome these issues, we formulate finding those areas where a process enhancement is possible as the problem of finding those groups of process situations where the process performance is significantly different from their similar situations. Here, we define a *process situation* (or simply a *situation*) as a process instance or a prefix of it. The proposed method includes four steps (1) enriching and extracting the data from the event log (2) finding a set of sets of similar situations (which we call a *vicinity cover* and each set of similar situations is a *vicinity*). Naturally, a measure is needed to measure the similarity between instances and identify vicinities. However, having access to such a measure is a strong assumption. Thus we use a machine learning technique to determine the vicinities in the absence of such a measure. (3) The next step involves finding the set of surprising situations in each vicinity (if any exist). (4) Finally, a list of detected sets of surprising situations is presented to the user ordered by their effect on the process and how surprising they are. These findings can be further analyzed to understand the reason for the different behavior of the process in these surprising situations and gain insights on how to improve the process. Figure 1 shows the general overview of the proposed method.

For example, consider that in a loan application process with 20 cases, we are interested in finding those cases where their throughput is surprising. In

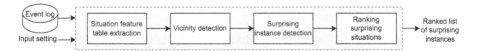

Fig. 1. The general overview of the proposed method.

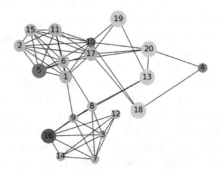

Fig. 2. A graph representing the similarity of situations in a loan application example. Each node represents a situation (a process instance). Two situations are similar if the Levenshtein distance of their activity sequences is at most one. The vicinity of a node is the set of process instances in the same community. Three vicinities have been detected in this example, which are colored red, blue, and green. Surprising situations are highlighted with a darker color. The throughput of each situation is proportional to the size of its corresponding node. (Color figure online)

this example, each process instance (case) is a situation. Also, we consider two situations similar if the Levenshtein distance of their activity sequence is at most one. Figure 2 shows the graph for the cases of this loan application, where each case corresponds to a node. Two cases are connected if they are similar. The size of each node is proportional to its throughput. The colors (blue, green, and red) indicate the vicinities found by the Louvain community detection algorithm [3]. The nodes highlighted with darker colors are the surprising cases where the throughput is significantly different from the other cases in the same vicinity. In this example, the throughput was worse than expected for cases 5 and 16 and better than expected for cases 4 and 10. The process owner can gain actionable insights by analyzing the behavior of the process in these cases, particularly in comparison with their vicinity, to enhance the performance of the process in other similar cases in the future. Note, if we just had considered the overall performance of this process, these four cases would not have been detected as their throughput are not far from the average throughput of all cases.

The rest of the paper is organized as follows. In Sect. 2, a brief overview of the related work is given. In Sect. 3, the proposed method is presented. The experimental results are discussed in Sect. 4. Finally, in Sect. 5, the conclusion is presented.

2   Related Work

Existing research on context-aware anomaly detection in process mining is closest to our work. Here we provide an overview of anomaly detection techniques.

Most existing methods investigate anomalies considering the control-flow perspective (e.g., [1,2,7,9,10,16]). These methods generate a reference model from the event log and apply conformance checking to detect anomalous behavior. A subgroup of these methods known as *deviance mining approaches* investigate performance anomalies [9]. In [16], the authors identify deviations and bottle-necks by replaying the event log on an enrich process model with performance information. In [7], the authors analyze the deviations between a process model and an event log to identify which deviations enforce positive performance. In [8], the anomalous cases in event logs are detected using window-based and Markovian-based techniques. The drawback of control-flow approaches is that they ignore a wide range of non-control-flow data, which can be used for more sophisticated context-sensitive anomaly detection methods.

The authors of [4] propose an anomaly detection approach that incorporates perspectives beyond the control-flow perspective, such as time and resource-related information. This approach marks events as anomalies based on a certain likelihood of occurrence, however, case anomalies are not considered.

Other approaches in this category only focus on specific use cases. The authors of [13] analyze suspicious payment transactions to identify money laun-dering within a money transfer service. They propose an approach to match the transactions with the expected behavior given by a process model to iden-tify many small transactions that end up on the same account. [14] identifies surprisingly short activity execution times in a process by automatically infer-ring a Bayesian model from the Petri net representation of the process model. The authors of [15] use fuzzy association rule learning to detect anomalies. As these approaches specialize in specific use cases, they do not apply to identify anomalies in a general process.

A third category is domain-based anomaly detection. For example, the authors of [11] propose an approach that supports the identification of unusual or unexpected transactions by encoding the cases and assigning an anomaly score to each case. They use the domain knowledge of domain experts to update the assigned anomaly scores. The approaches in this category require domain knowledge to label cases, which limits their applicability.

3   Method

Process mining techniques usually start by analyzing an event log. An event log is a collection of cases where each case is a sequence of events, in which each event refers to a case, an activity, and a point in time. More formally,

Definition 1 (Event, Case, Event log). *Let C be the universe of case identi-fiers, A be the universe of activities, T be the universe of timestamps. Moreover, let $D = \{D_1, \ldots, D_n\}$ be the universe of domain-dependent data attributes. We define the universe of events as $\mathcal{E} = C \times A \times T \times D_1 \times \cdots \times D_N$ and each element $e = (c, a, t, d_1, \ldots, d_n) \in \mathcal{E}$ an event. Let $\mathcal{E}^+$ be the universe of (non-empty) finite and chronologically ordered sequences of events. We define a case as a sequence of events $\gamma \in \mathcal{E}^+$ in which all events have the same case identifier; i.e. $\forall e_i, e_j \in \gamma \pi_c(e_i) = \pi_c(e_j)$ where $\pi_c(e)$ returns the case identifier of event $e \in \mathcal{E}$. We define an* event log, *L, as a set of cases in which each case has a unique* *case identifier; i.e.,* $\forall \gamma, \gamma' \in L(\exists e \in \gamma \exists e' \in \gamma \pi_c(e) = \pi_c(e')) \implies \gamma = \gamma'$. *We denote the universe of all event logs with* $\mathcal{L}$.

We assume that we know the process feature that captures the property of the process that the process owner is interested in its optimization. We call this feature *target feature* and denote it with *tf* where $tf \in \mathcal{TF} = \mathcal{A} \times \mathcal{D}$. Note that the target is composed of an attribute name and an activity name, which indicate the attribute value should be extracted from the events with that activity name. The attribute name can be any of the attributes captured by the event log or a derived one. Moreover, we assume that we know *descriptive features*, which are the set of process features that are relevant in measuring the similarity of the situations. In the following, we explain the surprising situation detection steps.

3.1 Situation Feature Table Extraction

To find the surprising situations, we have to extract the data in the form of tabular data from the event log. As the detected surprising situations are meant to be used for root cause analysis, it is important to respect the temporal precedence of cause and effect, indicating that the cause must occur before the effect. Therefore, we extract the data from that prefix of the case that has been recorded before the target feature. We call such a prefix a *situation*. More formally:

Definition 2 (Situation). *Let* $L \in \mathcal{L}$, $\gamma = \langle e_1, \ldots, e_n \rangle \in L$, $prfx(\langle e_1, \ldots, e_n \rangle) = \{\langle e_1, \ldots, e_i \rangle \mid 1 \leq i \leq n\}$, *a function that returns the set of non-empty prefixes of a given case, and* $tf \in \mathcal{TF} = \mathcal{A} \times \mathcal{D}$ *a target feature. We define the universe of all situations as* $\mathcal{S} = \bigcup_{L \in \mathcal{L}} S_L$ *where* $S_L = \{\sigma \mid \sigma \in prfx(\gamma) \wedge \gamma \in L\}$ *is the set of situations of event log* L. *We call each element* $\sigma \in \mathcal{S}$ *a situation. Moreover, we define sit* $\in (\mathcal{L} \times \mathcal{TF}) \times 2^{\mathcal{S}}$ *to be the a function that returns* $\{\sigma \in S_L \mid \pi_a(\sigma) = act\}$ *for a given* $L \in \mathcal{L}$ *and* $tf = (att, act)$, *where* $\pi_a(\sigma)$ *returns the activity name of the last event of* σ.

We call the data table created by extracting data from situations a *situation feature table*. Please note that each row of the situation feature table extracted from *sit*(*L*, *tf*) corresponds to a situation in it and this correspondence forms a bijection. To enrich the event log and extract the situation feature table, we use the method presented in [12].

3.2 Vicinity Detection

Informally, a vicinity is a set of similar situations and a vicinity cover of $S \subseteq \mathcal{S}$ is a set of vicinities of its situations such that their union covers S. Let $cov \in 2^{\mathcal{S}} \to 2^{2^{\mathcal{S}}}$ in which $\forall S \subseteq \mathcal{S} \forall S' \in cov(S)(S' \neq \emptyset \wedge (\forall \sigma, \sigma' \in S' sim(\sigma, \sigma') = 1))$ and $\forall S \subseteq \mathcal{S} \bigcup_{S' \in cov(S)} S' = S$. Here, $sim \in \mathcal{S} \times \mathcal{S} \to \{0, 1\}$ is an indicator function indicating if σ and σ' are similar, for $\sigma, \sigma' \in \mathcal{S}$.

Using a coverage function, we define a vicinity cover of a set of situations extracted from an event log with respect to a specific target feature as follows:

Definition 3 (Vicinity and Vicinity Cover). *Let $S = sit(L, tf)$ be the set of situations extracted from $L \in \mathcal{L}$ with respect to the target feature $tf \in \mathcal{TF}$ and $cov \in 2^{\mathcal{S}} \rightarrow 2^{2^{\mathcal{S}}}$ be a coverage function. We simply define a* vicinity cover *of S as $cov(S)$ and we call each member of $V \in cov(S)$ a* vicinity *of S. We denote the universe of all vicinities by $\mathcal{V}$.*

In the sequel, we explain the vicinity detection method separately for the case where we know the similarity measure and the case where such a similarity measure is not known.

Vicinity Detection with a Similarity Measure. Let $d \in \mathcal{S} \times \mathcal{S} \rightarrow \mathbb{R}$ be a distance measure. Then we can say a situation is similar to another situation if their distance is less than α. Now, we can define the similarity function as $sim_{d,\alpha} \in \mathcal{S} \times \mathcal{S} \rightarrow \{0, 1\}$ such that $sim_{d,\alpha}(\sigma_1, \sigma_1)$ returns 1 if $d(\sigma, \sigma') \leq \alpha$ and 0 otherwise, for all $\sigma, \sigma' \in \mathcal{S}$. In this case, we can determine the vicinity cover of the set of situations through the coverage function (Definition 3) in which $sim_{d,\alpha}(., .)$ is the similarity function. Another method is to create a graph $G = (S, E)$ in which each node corresponds to one of the situations extracted from the event log. There is an edge between two nodes if the distance of their corresponding situations is smaller than α. Using a *community detection* algorithm on this graph, we can determine the vicinities. Note that in this case two situations are similar if their corresponding nodes are in the same community and each detected community is a vicinity. A community detection function aims at finding (potentially overlapping) sets of nodes that optimize the modularity within the similarity graph. Modularity measures the relative density of edges inside the communities compared to edges outside the communities.

As another option we can use a clustering method to detect vicinities. We use k-means as the clustering model to explain the method; however, the general idea is similar to using other clustering models. To find the surprising situations using a clustering model, we first cluster the situations using k-means, with a predefined k, based on their descriptive features. In this method, two situations are similar if they belong to the same cluster and each cluster forms a vicinity. Please note that in this case the similarity measure is used to measure the distance between each situation and the centroids of clusters.

Vicinity Detection without a Similarity Measure. The availability of a distance function is a strong assumption. Considering the complexity of the real-life event data, even for specialists, it is a challenging task to determine such a distance function. Hence, we use machine learning techniques to detect surprising situations in the data. In this case, the process expert needs to know the set of process features relevant to measuring the similarity of the situations and not the exact distance measure. Here we briefly mention the vicinity detection method using a classification model.

We mainly use a decision tree as the classification model. We train a decision tree on the data trying to predict the target feature *tf* using descriptive features.

In this method, we consider two situations similar if they belong to the same node of the tree. Moreover, we consider the set of situations corresponding to each node of the decision tree (or each node in a subset of nodes of the decision tree, such as leaves) as a vicinity.

3.3   Surprising Situation Detection

We define the surprising situations in each vicinity as those situations in that vicinity that significantly differ from the other situations (in that vicinity). Suppose that $D \in \mathcal{V} \to \bigcup_{V \in \mathcal{V}} 2^V$ where $\forall V \in \mathcal{V} : D(V) \subseteq V$ is a function that, given a set of similar situations (a vicinity), returns its subset of surprising ones. We call such a function a *detector*. For example, a detector function can be a function that returns the subset of situations that exceed a user-defined threshold value for the target feature. Using this function, we define the set of surprising situations of a vicinity as follows:

Definition 4 (Surprising Situation Set). *Let $V \in \mathcal{V}$ be a vicinity and $D \in \mathcal{V} \to \bigcup_{V \in \mathcal{V}} 2^V$ where $\forall V \in \mathcal{V} : D(V) \subseteq V$ be a detector function. We define $D(V)$ as the set of surprising situations in V.*

We can find the set of all sets of surprising situations of the set of situations by applying the detector function on all the vicinities of its vicinity cover.

Definition 5 (Surprising Situation Sets). *Let $S = sit(L, tf)$ be the set of situations extracted from $L \in \mathcal{L}$ with respect to target feature $tf \in \mathcal{TF}$, $cov(S)$ a vicinity cover of S, and detection function $D \in \mathcal{V} \to \bigcup_{V \in \mathcal{V}} 2^V$. We define the surprising situation sets of S as $\{D(V) \mid V \in cov(S)\}$.*

3.4   Ordering Surprising Situations

We define two criteria to order the detected surprising situations: *surprisingness* and *effectiveness*. Suppose U is the set of surprising situations in a vicinity V. Surprisingness of U measures how rare it is to see such a situation in its vicinity, whereas effectiveness measures how beneficial it is to enhance the process based on the findings of root cause analysis of U. More precisely:

Definition 6. *Let $V \in \mathcal{V}$ be a vicinity and $U \subseteq V$ the set of surprising situations in V, and $\beta \in (0, 1]$ a threshold. We define the surprisingness of U as:*

$$surp(U) = \beta \mid avg(U) - avg(V \setminus U) \mid + (1 - \beta) \frac{\#(U)}{\#(V)}$$

and the effectiveness of U as:

$$eff(U) = \begin{cases} (avg(V \setminus U) - avg(U)) \times \#(V \setminus U) & avg(U) < avg(V \setminus U) \\ (avg(U) - avg(V \setminus U)) \times \#(U) & avg(U) > avg(V \setminus U) \end{cases}$$

where $\#(A)$ denotes the cardinality of A and $avg(A) = \frac{\sum_{s \in A} \pi_{tf}(s)}{\#(A)}$ for each $A \subseteq S$ is the average value of the target feature tf for the situations in A.

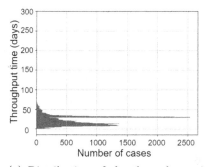

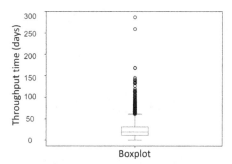

(a) Distribution of the throughput time for the BPI Challenge 2017 event log capturing the duration from the start to the end of each case.

(b) Detected outliers of throughput time of cases of BPI Challenge 2017 event log using boxplot. Cases durations above 61 days are considered anomalous.

Fig. 3. The throughput time for the BPI Challenge 2017 event log.

In the above definition, we assume that the lower values for *tf* are more desirable. If this assumption does not hold, the effectiveness can be similarly defined.

4   Experimental Results

To evaluate the proposed framework[1], we present the result of applying it on the event log for BPI Challenge 2017 [5]. This event log represents an application process for a personal loan or overdraft within a global financing organization taken from a Dutch financial institute. We consider throughput as the target feature. The majority of the cases in the process take between 5 and 40 days. The average duration for all cases in the event log is around 22 days. Figure 3a shows the distribution of the throughput time.

Boxplots are frequently used to identify performance anomalies [6]. Thus we use boxplots as the baseline and call this approach the *baseline*. The resulting boxplot is shown in Fig. 3b. Using this method, 255 cases with a throughput of more than 61 days have been considered anomalous. These are the detected anomalies without any context-awareness of the process.

To apply our approach, we used the following case-level attributes as descriptive features: *application type, loan goal, applicant's requested loan amount,* and the *number of offers* which is a derivative attribute indicating how many times the loan application institute offered a loan to the customer. Note that in this experiment, each case is a situation.

We apply surprising situation detection using a similarity measure, a classification method (using a decision tree), and also a clustering method (using *k*-means clustering). We call these three approaches *similarity based method,*

---

[1] The implemented tool is available at https://github.com/ckohlschm/detecting-surprising-instances.

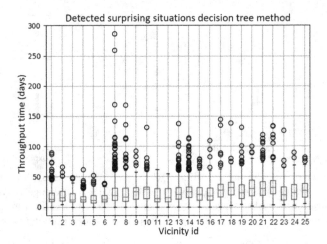

Fig. 4. Detected surprising situations in each vicinity defined by the decision tree method.

decision tree method, and *k-means clustering method* respectively. In all these methods, to maximize the applicability of the implemented tool and to minimize the required domain knowledge, we use the boxplot as the detector function (Definition 4) to find the surprising situations in each vicinity.

Decision Tree Method. For this experiment, we trained a decision (regression) tree with a maximum depth of 5 and a minimum number of instances per leaf of 100. We consider the vicinities described by the leaves of the tree. Figure 4 shows the detected surprising situations for the leaves in the decision tree where each leaf is labeled with a number. Some of the highlights of the comparison of the results of the decision tree method and the baseline are as follows:

– Application_1839367200 (Case duration 62 days) is barely considered an outlier in the total dataset, but in its vicinity (Vicinity 4: one offer, limit raise, loan goal car, requested amount > 11.150) it is far from the average which is 14 days.
– Vicinity 19, where the number of offers is more than 3 and the requested amount ≤ 13.162 includes seven surprising situations. These situations have not been considered outliers by the baseline method. One possible interpretation of this result is that high throughput is acceptable in such situations. The same applies to vicinity 20.
– Vicinity 5 (one offer, limit raise, Unknown loan goal, requested amount ≤ 3000) contains 3 surprising situations that are all overlooked by the baseline method. The vicinity contains 338 cases with an average throughput time of 13 days which makes cases with a duration of more than 40 days surprising. The same applies to vicinities 3 and 6.

Figure 5 shows the surprisingness (on the left) and effectiveness (on the right) of the sets of surprising situations detected by the decision tree method. The set of surprising situations in vicinity 17 has the highest surprisingness. This vicinity includes 126 situations, where 6 are surprising with an average throughput of 100 days, whereas the other situations in the vicinity have an average of 27 days. These are the cases with two offers that use their loan to pay their remaining home dept and the requested amount is at most 24.500. The set of surprising situations in vicinity 7 has the highest effectiveness. These situations correspond to the customers with one offer that apply for a new credit. Removing the problem that causes the delay in these surprising situations would reduce the average throughput time for similar cases by more than one day.

k-means Clustering Method. In this approach, we used k-means clustering to identify vicinities. For k we use the value 25, which is the number of the vicinities in the decision tree method and Euclidean distance as similarity measure. This method results in detecting a total of 280 surprising situations. The plot on the left side of Fig. 6 shows the surprising situations detected in each vicinity.

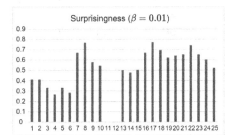
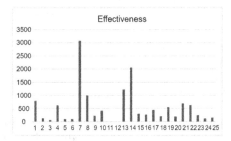

Fig. 5. Surprisingness and effectiveness of the surprising situations identified by the decision tree method.

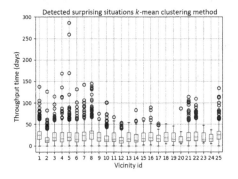
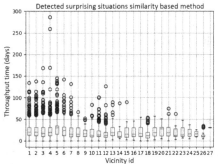

Fig. 6. Detected surprising situations by the k-means clustering and similarity based method.

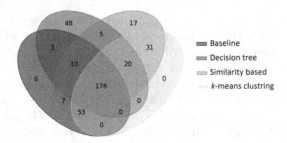

Fig. 7. Venn Diagram showing the intersection of detected surprising situations using the different methods.

Similarity Based Method. We run the similarity based approach where the distance measure is the Euclidean distance of normalized descriptive features (using min-max method). Then, we use 1.4, which results in 27 clusters (close to 25), as the threshold to generate a graph. To find the vicinities, we used the *Louvain community detection method* [3] on this graph. The plot on the right side of Fig. 6 shows the surprising situations detected in each vicinity.

It is worth noting that the set of surprising situations detected by different methods was not exactly the same. Figure 7 shows that all the methods agree on 176 detected surprising situations and for all other situations at least one method does not select it.

5   Conclusion

Finding the process enhancement areas is a fundamental prerequisite for any process enhancement procedure that highly affects its outcome. It is usually assumed that these process areas are known in advance or can be detected easily. However, utilizing simple methods have the danger of overlooking some of the opportunities for process enhancement or targeting the wrong ones. In this paper, we formulate the process of finding process enhancement areas as a method for finding surprising situations; i.e., detecting those situations where the process behavior is significantly different from similar situations.

We have implemented the proposed framework with different methods and evaluated it using real event logs. The experiment shows that the detected surprising (anomalous) situations are overlapping but not identical to the ones of the baseline, which is currently a common method for finding anomalies. It shows that to find the best result, it is best to use our framework complementary to the existing methods; i.e., using both context-sensitive and non-context-sensitive methods for finding the process enhancement areas.

Acknowledgment. We thank Alexander von Humboldt (AvH) Stiftung for supporting our research.

References

1. Bezerra, F., Wainer, J.: Fraud detection in process aware systems. Int. J. Bus. Process Integr. Manage. **5**(2), 121–129 (2011)
2. Bezerra, F.D.L., Wainer, J.: A dynamic threshold algorithm for anomaly detection in logs of process aware systems (2012)
3. Blondel, V.D., Guillaume, J.-L., Lambiotte, R., Lefebvre, E.: Fast unfolding of communities in large networks. J. Stat. Mech: Theory Exp. **2008**(10), P10008 (2008)
4. Böhmer, K., Rinderle-Ma, S.: Multi-perspective anomaly detection in business process execution events. In: Debruyne, C., et al. (eds.) OTM 2016. LNCS, vol. 10033, pp. 80–98. Springer, Cham (2016). https://doi.org/10.1007/978-3-319-48472-3_5
5. Carmona, J.J., de Leoni, M., Depaire, B., Jouck, T.: Process Discovery Contest 2017, vol. 5 (2021)
6. Conforti, R., La Rosa, M., ter Hofstede, A.H.M.: Filtering out infrequent behavior from business process event logs. IEEE Trans. Knowl. Data Eng. **29**(2), 300–314 (2016)
7. Dees, M., de Leoni, M., Mannhardt, F.: Enhancing process models to improve business performance: a methodology and case studies. In: Panetto, H., et al. (eds.) OTM 2017. LNCS, vol. 10573, pp. 232–251. Springer, Cham (2017). https://doi.org/10.1007/978-3-319-69462-7_15
8. Gupta, N., Anand, K., Sureka, A.: Pariket: mining business process logs for root cause analysis of anomalous incidents. In: Chu, W., Kikuchi, S., Bhalla, S. (eds.) DNIS 2015. LNCS, vol. 8999, pp. 244–263. Springer, Cham (2015). https://doi.org/10.1007/978-3-319-16313-0_19
9. Nguyen, H., Dumas, M., Rosa, M.L., Maggi, F.M., Suriadi, S.: Business process deviance mining: Review and evaluation. CoRR, abs/1608.08252 (2016)
10. Pauwels, S., Calders, T.: An anomaly detection technique for business processes based on extended dynamic Bayesian networks. In: Proceedings of the 34th ACM/SIGAPP Symposium on Applied Computing, pp. 494–501 (2019)
11. Post, R., et al.: Active anomaly detection for key item selection in process auditing. In: Munoz-Gama, J., Lu, X. (eds.) ICPM 2021. LNBIP, vol. 433, pp. 167–179. Springer, Cham (2022). https://doi.org/10.1007/978-3-030-98581-3_13
12. Qafari, M.S., van der Aalst, W.M.: Feature recommendation for structural equation model discovery in process mining. Prog. Artif. Intell., 1–25 (2022)
13. Rieke, R., Zhdanova, M., Repp, J., Giot, R., Gaber, C.: Fraud detection in mobile payments utilizing process behavior analysis. In: 2013 International Conference on Availability, Reliability and Security, pp. 662–669. IEEE (2013)
14. Rogge-Solti, A., Kasneci, G.: Temporal anomaly detection in business processes. In: Sadiq, S., Soffer, P., Völzer, H. (eds.) BPM 2014. LNCS, vol. 8659, pp. 234–249. Springer, Cham (2014). https://doi.org/10.1007/978-3-319-10172-9_15
15. Sarno, R., Sinaga, F., Sungkono, K.R.: Anomaly detection in business processes using process mining and fuzzy association rule learning. J. Big Data **7**(1), 1–19 (2020). https://doi.org/10.1186/s40537-019-0277-1
16. van der Aalst, W.M.P., Adriansyah, A., van Dongen, B.: Replaying history on process models for conformance checking and performance analysis. Wiley Interdisc. Rev.: Data Min. Knowl. Discovery **2**(2), 182–192 (2012)

LSTM-Based Anomaly Detection of Process Instances: Benchmark and Tweaks

Johannes Lahann[✉], Peter Pfeiffer, and Peter Fettke

German Research Center for Artificial Intelligence (DFKI) and Saarland University,
Saarbrücken, Germany
{johannes.lahann,peter.pfeiffer,peter.fettke}@dfki.de

Abstract. Anomaly detection can identify deviations in event logs and allows businesses to infer inconsistencies, bottlenecks, and optimization opportunities in their business processes. In recent years, various anomaly detection algorithms for business processes have been proposed based on either process discovery or machine learning algorithms. While there are apparent differences between machine learning and process discovery approaches, it is often unclear how they perform in comparison. Furthermore, deep learning research in other domains has shown that advancements did not solely come from improved model architecture but were often due to minor pre-processing and training procedure refinements. For this reason, this paper aims to set up a broad benchmark and establish a baseline for deep learning-based anomaly detection of process instances. To this end, we introduce a simple LSTM-based anomaly detector utilizing a collection of minor refinements and compare it with existing approaches. The results suggest that the proposed method can significantly outperform the existing approaches on a large number of event logs consistently.

Keywords: Business process management · Anomaly detection · Deep learning · LSTM

1 Introduction

Anomaly detection deals with the identification of rare articles, objects, or observations that differ significantly from the majority of the data and therefore raise suspicions [16]. In the context of business process analysis, businesses apply anomaly detection to automatically detect deviations in event logs which can be a sign of inconsistencies, bottlenecks, and optimization opportunities in their business processes [7]. A typical approach to detect anomalous behavior in business processes is to apply conformance checking [12], i.e., evaluating the real occurred behavior that is recorded in event logs against the business process model that business experts previously designed. However, to do this, such a process model is required beforehand. More recently, a variety of deep learning-based anomaly detection algorithms with different architectures have been developed that are

© The Author(s) 2023
M. Montali et al. (Eds.): ICPM 2022 Workshops, LNBIP 468, pp. 229–241, 2023.
https://doi.org/10.1007/978-3-031-27815-0_17

able to identify anomalous process behavior without requiring a process model or other prior knowledge about the underlying process. While there are apparent differences between the existing approaches, it is not clear how they perform in comparison. Furthermore, deep learning research in other domains has shown that advancements did not solely come from improved model architecture but are often due to minor training procedure refinements [6]. Thus, this paper aims to set up a broad benchmark between anomaly detection algorithms where we compare the performance of existing approaches with a simple LSTM-based anomaly detector that utilizes a number of minor refinements. The contribution of this paper is threefold:

- We examine a collection of different processing, model architecture, and anomaly score computation refinements that lead to significant model accuracy or run-time improvements.
- We show that the proposed methods lead to a significant performance improvement in comparison with state-of-the-art process mining-based and deep learning-based anomaly detection methods. To this end, we conduct experiments on the data sets from the Process Discovery Contests, the Business Process Intelligence Challenges, and additional synthetic event logs [7].
- We set up a comprehensive evaluation over a total of 328 different event logs, which can be utilized as a benchmark for further research.

The remaining sections of the paper unfold as follows: Sect. 2 introduces the reader to preliminary ideas of process mining and predictive process monitoring. Section 3 gives a brief overview of the approach before it discusses the applied refinements. Section 4 describes two experiments to evaluate the performance of the proposed approach. Section 5 shows the evaluation results covering an overall performance comparison with existing methods and a detailed analysis of the impact of different design decisions and refinements. Section 6 relates the developed approach to existing literature. Section 7 closes the paper with a summary of the main contributions and an outline of future work.

2　Preliminaries

This section introduces some preliminary concepts. In particular, we introduce the concepts of events, cases, and event logs and define next step prediction and (case-level) anomaly detection as we understand it during the scope of this paper.

Definition 1. *Event, Case, Event Log*
Let E be the universe of events. A case σ is a finite-length word of events, i.e.
$\sigma \in E^* \wedge |\sigma| = n$, $n \in \mathbb{N}$. An event log is a multi-set of cases, i.e. $L \in \mathbb{B}(E^*)$.

To describe a case σ, we also use the notation $\sigma := \langle e_1, \ldots, e_n \rangle$. There are further attributes next to the activity associated with events such as resource, timestamp, and others. These attributes can add additional information that can also be utilized for analysis and predictive tasks.

One process prediction task that has been researched intensively in recent years and also plays a major role in the proposed anomaly detection approach in this paper is next step prediction. Next step prediction aims to forecast the direct continuation of an ongoing process instance based on all available information regarding the process instance. We define next step prediction as follows:

Definition 2. *Next Step Prediction*
Given a prefix $p_t = \langle e_1, ..., e_t \rangle$ of a case $\sigma = \langle e_1, ..., e_n \rangle$ with $0 <= t < n$, $t, n \in \mathbb{N}$, we define Next Step Prediction as a relation $NSP \subseteq E^* \times E$ that predicts the next occurring event e_{t+1} based of the prefix p_t.

Next, we can define anomaly detection of process instances. There is a distinction between attribute and case-level anomaly detection in the literature. While the former detects irregular attribute values on event-level, such as false activities, resources, or timestamps, the latter aims to classify anomalous cases. For the scope of this paper, we are only concerned with case-level anomaly detection, which we conceptualize as follows:

Definition 3. *Case-level Anomaly Detection*
We define a case-level anomaly detector as a function f that receives a case σ and returns a label $\ell \in \{0, 1\}$, where 0 indicates a normal case and 1 indicates an anomalous case.

One may notice that we do not specify what makes a case normal or anomalous. We argue that depending on the context, the criteria for an anomaly may differ. Hence, a more vague definition is beneficial. In the first conducted experiment, we understand anomaly detection similarly to conformance checking, i.e., a case is normal if it fits a hidden process model; else, it is anomalous. In the second experiment, synthetic events and attributes are injected into the data sets based on a predefined rule-set. A case is considered anomalous if it contains at least one of the injected values.

3   Proposed Approach

3.1   Overview

The proposed method investigates prediction-based anomaly detection with a deep neural network as the predictive model. The approach can be divided into two stages - first, we train an LSTM-based model to learn the behavior of the process, while in the second stage, the trained model is used to assess whether a given trace is anomalous or not. In the first stage, we train the prediction model to solve the next step prediction task. The idea is to teach the model a hidden representation that contains the most relevant information to predict the possible next events. To assess whether a trace σ is anomalous or not, we use the trained model to predict all the steps of a given case. If the predicted behavior of the neural network and the real behavior differ significantly in at least one of the events, we consider this observation a strong indicator that the case is suspicious. Therefore, we mark the case as anomalous. We introduce DAPNN (Detection of Anomalous Processes through Neural Networks), which utilizes a collection of changes and refinements to previous work [8,9] that together led to significant performance improvements in the conducted experiments. We generated fixed sliding windows and switched to a LSTM-based network architecture. Furthermore, we used multiple training methods to improve the convergence of the neural networks. Last, we added normalization to the anomaly score computation, which creates a comparable anomaly score throughout different event logs.

3.2   Approach Characteristics and Refinements

Data Processing. DAPNN is trained on windows extracted from the cases σ of size w. Given a window of the $w - 1$ previous events, DAPNN's task is to predict the last event in the window. Thereby, we do not have to insert padding elements to counteract the different lengths of the prefixes. Furthermore, since the window size is usually much smaller than the maximum length of the prefixes, this results in a much faster training time. For a case $\sigma := \langle e_1, \ldots, e_n \rangle$ and a fixed window size w, we generate n-w windows $\langle e_t - w, e_t \rangle$, where $w < t \leq n$. In the conducted experiments, we used a fixed window size of 5. Next, we add special *Start* and *End* events to each case in the event log. Thereby, the next step prediction model can also learn to predict the beginning and the end of a case. This is especially effective since there are anomalous cases that only behave wrongly at the beginning or at the end.

Model Architecture and Training. We decided to use a simple LSTM-based architecture. Each case σ is split into separate sequences along the attributes, which are processed by individual LSTM blocks. Each block consists of an embedding layer, two LSTM-layer with hidden layer size 25, followed by a softmax layer. This allows obtaining a probability distribution $\vec{p}$ per attribute found in the event log, which serves as the basis to assess whether σ is anomalous or not.

We train each neural network for up to 25 epochs utilizing early stopping, the learning rate finder, and cyclic learning rates [13]. While early stopping primarily reduces training time, we see a significant improvement in the robustness of the results through the latter two methods throughout the conducted experiments.

Anomaly Score Computation. After training the prediction model, we can utilize it to detect anomalies. To do this, we compute all windows for a given case σ and feed them through the prediction model. For a case with n events and m attributes, we compute $m \times n$ probability distributions $\vec{p}$. In order to obtain the anomaly scores, we apply a scoring function Θ and store the anomaly scores per case in a matrix $M_{anomaly}$. We define Θ as follows:

$$\Theta(\vec{p}, y) = \frac{max(\vec{p}) - p_y}{max(\vec{p})}$$

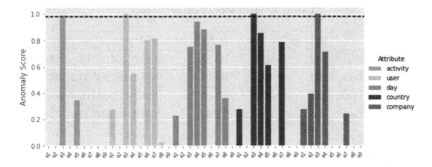

Fig. 1. Illustration of the anomaly scores of a case that resembles a skip sequence anomaly. For the 3rd predicted event, the threshold is exceeded for 4 out of 5 attributes.

y depicts the actual next occurred attribute in σ, and p_y represents the probability that the prediction model is assigned to the attribute y. The margin of $max(\vec{p})$ and p_y can be interpreted as a measure of certainty for an anomaly. If the margin is high, the prediction model is certain that another attribute should occur instead. Hence, this is a sign of an anomaly. By normalizing with $max(\vec{p})$, we make the anomaly score more robust so that it behaves similarly throughout all predictions. Additionally, it penalizes deviations stronger if it has low confidence regarding the occurred value. For example, if the predicted event has a probability of 0.75 and the occurred event has a probability of 0.25, the obtained anomaly score is $(0.75-0.25)/0.75 = 0.66$. However, if the predicted event has a probability of 0.5 and the occurred event has a probability of 0.0, the obtained anomaly score is $(0.5-0.0)/0.5 = 1.0$. The normalization pushes anomalies near 1.0 and enables easier differentiation between anomalies and normal events. Furthermore, it allows us to introduce a threshold that functions similarly to a significance measure, as the threshold is relatively stable over different event logs. Figure 1 shows the resulting anomaly scores for one particular case.

Anomaly Classification. Based on the anomaly scores, we can then determine if a case is anomalous, i.e., we define a function f that takes all anomaly scores M of a case and a threshold τ as input and outputs a label $l \in 0, 1$.

$$f(M_{anomaly}, \tau) = \begin{cases} 1, & \text{if } max(M_{anomaly}) > \tau \\ 0, & \text{otherwise} \end{cases}$$

The intuition behind the formula is that if a case contains at least one anomaly score greater or equal to the given threshold, it is flagged as an anomaly. In order to choose a suitable threshold, we compare different options:

- *Best Threshold*: we select the optimal threshold based on the achieved F1-score on the test set. I.e., we compute the F1-Score for all possible thresholds

Table 1. Data sets of experiment 1.

	# Logs	# Cases	# Activities	# Events	# Anomalies
PDC 2020 Train	192	1000	16–38	8867–70106	0/∼ 200
PDC 2020 Test	192	1000	16–38	8764–68706	412–515
PDC 2021 Train	480	1000	37–65	9867–32009	0/∼ 200
PDC 2021 Test	96	250	35–64	6612–11860	125

and choose the threshold with the highest F1-Score. Note that this heuristic requires labels and thus is not applicable in practice in an unsupervised scenario. However, it is still relevant as it allows us to measure the maximal achievable performance with the underlying prediction model.

– *Fixed Threshold:* we set a fixed threshold that we use throughout all experiments. We achieved reasonable results with a threshold of 0.98.
– *Anomaly Ratio:* we pick a threshold based on the total number or the ratio of predicted anomalies.
– *Elbow and Lowest Plateau Heuristic:* we utilize heuristics based on the anomaly ratio per potential threshold as introduced in [8].

4   Experimental Setup

4.1   Experiment 1

The first experiment compares the performance of the proposed anomaly detection approach with process discovery algorithms on the Process Discovery Contests 2020 and 2021 [14,15]. The process discovery contest (PDC) aims to assess tools and techniques that discover business process models from event logs. To this end, synthetic data sets are generated that comply with general concepts that influence process mining algorithms.

While the process discovery is designed to evaluate process discovery algorithms, it measures their performance indirectly through a classification task, identifying process cases that fit a hidden process model. Hence this task can also be accomplished through anomaly detection. Regarding the experimental setup, we follow the instructions from the process discovery contest. In particular, we consider the data sets from PDC 2020 and PDC 2021. Table 1 highlights the most important characteristics and statistics about the data sets. To achieve maximal comparability with the other algorithms that took part in the challenges, we also trained the next step prediction model on the training logs and measured the performance on the test sets.

4.2   Experiment 2

The second experiment provides a comparison with other machine learning-based anomaly detection approaches on the data sets generated by Nolle et al. [8]. The synthetic event logs are based on six process models with a different number of activities, model depths, and model widths, which are created randomly with the PLG2 framework [5]. Additionally, the authors utilized the event logs from the BPI Challenges 12, 13, 15, and 17. Subsequently, a variety of artificial anomalies was added to some of the cases of all event logs (Table 2):

- Skip: One or multiple events are skipped.
- Insert: Random events are inserted.
- Rework: Events are executed multiple times.
- Late: Events are shifted forward.
- Early: Events are shifted backward.
- Attribute: Other attribute values of some events are altered.

Table 2. Data sets of experiment 2.

	# Logs	# Cases	# Activities	# Events	# Attributes	# Anomalies
BPIC12	1	13087	73	289892	0	3927
BPIC13	3	819–7554	11–27	4068–81524	7	162–2257
BPIC15	5	832–1409	417–491	46110–62667	6	232–438
BPIC17	2	31509–42995	17–53	285211–1269176	2	9398–13193
Gigantic	4	5000	152–157	38774–42711	1–4	1499–1553
Huge	4	5000	109	46919–53627	1–4	1416–1479
Large	4	5000	85	61789–67524	1–4	1482–1529
Medium	4	5000	65	38990–41991	1–4	1459–1550
P2p	4	5000	27	48477–53193	1–4	1430–1563
Paper	1	5000	27	66814	1	1466
Small	4	5000	41	53437–56695	1–4	1481–1529
Wide	4	5000	58–69	39678–41910	1–4	1436–1513

4.3 Evaluation Metrics

In order to evaluate the performance of the approach, we use the F1 score, which is a common choice for evaluating anomaly detection. The F1 score is computed by the harmonic mean of precision and recall. The precision measures how precisely anomalies can be identified, i.e., how many of the predicted anomalies are actual anomalies. The recall measures how many anomalies are identified and how many anomalies are not recognized by the model:

$$F1\text{-}Score = \frac{2 * (precision * recall)}{(precision + recall)}$$

To comply with the specifications of the Process Discovery Contest and achieve comparability with the existing methods, we use an adapted version of the F1-Score in experiment 1, which is calculated by the balanced mean of the true positive rate tpr and the true negative rate tnr:

$$F\text{-}Score = \frac{2 * (tpr * tnr)}{(tpr + tnr)}$$

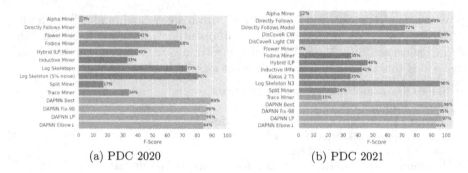

Fig. 2. Comparison by F-Score of the *DAPNN* approach with existing approaches extracted from the PDC website.

4.4   Reproducibility

All code used for this paper, including the implementation of *DAPNN* as well as the quantitative comparison with traditional and machine learning-based anomaly detection approaches, is available in our git repository[1].

5   Results

5.1   Overall Performance on the Process Discovery Contest

Figure 2 shows the performance of the *DAPNN* approach in comparison with existing process discovery algorithms as described in experiment 1. In PDC 2020, the *DAPNN* approach reaches an F-Score of 89% with the optimal heuristic, out-performing all other existing methods. Moreover, the *DAPNN* models with the other heuristics do not perform significantly worse. In PDC 2021, *DAPNN Best* and the *DAPNN LP* reach the highest F-Score with 98% and 97% respectively. The *DAPNN Fix-98* performs similarly to the DisCoveR CW, the DisCoveR Light CW, and the Log Skeleton N3 model. Since the latter models have not been applied to the PDC 2020, it would be interesting to see how they compare with the *DAPNN* approach. The results suggest that the *DAPNN* approach can effectively identify the non-fitting cases in the PDC contests and is able to reach state-of-the-art performances. The DAPNN approach can not be used straight-forwardly for process discovery as it does not directly output a process model. However, they seem to be superior in the detection of cases that do not fit the underlying process.

5.2   Overall Performance in Comparison with Other Anomaly Detection Approaches

Table 3 presents the results of experiment 2. It compares the F1-Score of 19 approaches on 40 event logs. Note that the event logs are grouped together as

---

[1] https://github.com/jolahann/dapnn.

Table 3. Comparison by F1-Score of the *DAPNN* approach with existing unsupervised anomaly detection approaches extracted from [8].

	BPIC12	BPIC13	BPIC15	BPIC17	Gigantic	Huge	Large	Medium	P2P	Paper	Small	Wide	Mean
Likelihood	0.0	0.0	0.0	0.0	0.0	0.0	0.0	0.0	0.0	0.0	0.0	0.0	0.0
OC-SVM	0.545	0.243	0.255	0.351	0.291	0.228	0.237	0.289	0.271	0.486	0.248	0.306	0.312
Naive	0.551	0.209	0.172	0.313	0.34	0.404	0.41	0.387	0.479	0.5	0.49	0.438	0.391
Naive+	0.551	0.209	0.173	0.276	0.383	0.454	0.49	0.439	0.48	0.5	0.488	0.469	0.409
Sampling	0.546	0.207	0.172	0.323	0.446	0.491	0.494	0.465	0.49	0.495	0.492	0.486	0.426
t-STIDE+	0.678	0.319	0.287	0.324	0.406	0.446	0.453	0.429	0.509	0.404	0.531	0.471	0.438
DAE	0.595	0.207	0.0	0.295	0.627	0.703	0.713	0.708	0.708	0.463	0.716	0.697	0.536
Likelihood+	0.625	0.445	0.329	0.399	0.665	0.676	0.622	0.654	0.611	0.656	0.688	0.637	0.584
BINetv2	0.607	0.397	0.375	0.43	0.68	0.704	0.71	0.719	0.768	0.757	0.775	0.733	0.638
BINetv1	0.621	0.398	0.346	0.469	0.711	0.713	0.713	0.734	0.768	0.739	0.772	0.761	0.645
BINetv3	0.664	0.446	0.362	0.489	0.662	0.693	0.692	0.709	0.769	0.791	0.762	0.738	0.648
$DAPNN_{FIX-98}$	0.636	0.425	0.459	0.565	0.735	0.776	0.744	0.789	0.842	0.898	0.847	0.805	0.71
$DAPNN_{AR-0.5}$	0.658	0.443	**0.484**	0.621	0.74	0.776	0.744	0.789	0.842	0.898	0.847	0.805	0.721
$DAPNN_{Elbow\downarrow}$	0.656	0.448	0.465	0.564	0.766	0.84	0.817	0.824	0.932	0.965	0.945	0.887	0.759
$DAPNN_{Elbow\uparrow}$	0.688	0.446	0.461	**0.689**	**0.829**	0.88	0.78	0.859	0.852	0.893	0.931	0.903	0.768
$DAPNN_{LP-Min}$	**0.72**	**0.473**	0.475	0.569	0.813	**0.939**	**0.927**	**0.899**	**0.973**	**0.996**	**0.973**	**0.955**	**0.809**
$DAPNN_{LP-Mean}$	**0.72**	**0.473**	0.475	0.569	0.813	**0.939**	**0.927**	**0.899**	**0.973**	**0.996**	**0.973**	**0.955**	**0.809**
$DAPNN_{LP-Max}$	**0.72**	**0.473**	0.475	0.57	0.813	**0.94**	**0.928**	**0.899**	**0.973**	**0.996**	**0.973**	**0.955**	**0.809**
$DAPNN_{Best}$	0.726	0.618	0.501	0.803	0.964	0.969	0.982	0.98	0.993	1.0	0.995	0.987	0.876

shown in Table 2 highlighting the mean F1-Score over the event logs of one data group. For example, the column *BPIC13* reports the mean F1-Score over all three event logs of the BPIC 2013. We reported the performance of the *DAPNN* approach with all heuristics. However, for the other approaches, only the performance with the *LP-Mean* heuristic is reported. The DAPNN approach reached top results on all examined event logs. In terms of the heuristics, the LP heuristics achieved better results than the elbow heuristics, followed by the anomaly ratio and the fixed threshold. Additionally, $DAPNN_{Best}$ reached a very high F1-Score for all synthetic event logs. This suggests that the prediction model is able to correctly separate anomalous and normal cases by assigning a higher anomaly score to anomalous events for most of the cases. However, the determination of the correct threshold is still a major challenge, as the $DAPNN_{LP-Max}$ with the second highest mean F1-Score performs significantly worse than the $DAPNN_{Best}$.

The results also show a clear performance gap between the synthetic event logs and the event logs of the BPI challenges. This can be explained by two reasons: On the one hand, the algorithms are only asked to find the artificial anomalies. However, it is unclear whether and how many unknown anomalies were already included in the original event logs that are not labeled as such. On the other hand, it might be the case that the synthetic event logs cover processes with simpler characteristics. In contrast, the processes of the BPI challenges are more difficult to comprehend for the approaches.

5.3   Detection of Anomaly Types

Given that we have different anomaly types, one question is how well the model can classify each anomaly type. Figure 3 compares the precision of the *DAPNN* with each heuristic for each anomaly type for the datasets from the second experiment. Aside from the best heuristic, there is no clear winner recognizable (Note that for multi-attribute event logs, we approximated the best heuristic with Naive Bayes optimization. Hence it is only a lower bound for the actual best score and can, in some cases, be lower than the scores of the other heuristics). The Elbow, Fix-98, and AR-0.5 heuristics tend to produce more false positives but have a slightly higher precision while detecting the anomalies. In contrast, the LP heuristics produce fewer false positives. Thus, the heuristics should be chosen based on the requirements of the business scenario.

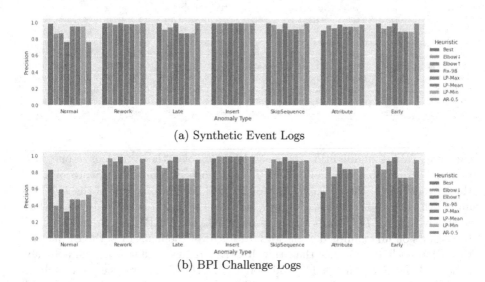

(a) Synthetic Event Logs

(b) BPI Challenge Logs

Fig. 3. Detection precision of the *DAPNN* approach for each anomaly type and heuristic

6   Related Work

Originally, anomaly detection on business process data was performed by evaluating process cases captured in an event log against a predefined process model [12]. However, this requires a reference model of the underlying process, which is not always available. To overcome this problem, Bezerra et al. define an anomalous case as an irregular execution that differs from a process model that was dynamically discovered by a process discovery algorithm [1]. The approach follows the hypothesis that anomalous cases are rare and differ significantly from normal cases. Therefore, the process discovery algorithm will focus on modeling the normal cases. Hence, the mined process model will require considerable modifications in order to fit anomalous cases leading to a high alignment score. According to this idea, the authors propose an anomaly detection approach that samples process cases from a discovered process model. If a case in the original event log does not correspond to one of the sampled cases, it is flagged as an anomaly. Building on this, Bezerra et al. introduce two parameters, fitness model degree and appropriateness of a process model, in order to formalize the degree of an anomaly [3]. Furthermore, they introduce two new variants of their anomaly detection approach, including a threshold and an iterative version [2]. Both of the approaches make use of the conformance fitness of each case according to the discovered model. Similarly, in the Process Discovery Contest, the detection of anomalous cases is used to measure the quality of the process discovery approaches [14,15]. Each process discovery approach is first trained on a training event log before assessing the F1-Score over a test log with normal and anomalous process cases, i.e., process cases that fit or do not fit a hidden process model.

More recently, a variety of model-less anomaly detection approaches have been developed that are able to detect anomalous process behavior without requiring an explicit process model. Böhmer et al. proposed a multivariate technique that builds up an extended likelihood graph on multiple event attributes in order to identify the anomalies [4]. Nolle et al. introduced three different deep learning-based anomaly detection approaches. In [7] they proposed a deep autoencoder to capture anomalous process cases. First, an autoencoder is trained by mapping each process case to itself. Afterward, the reconstruction error is calculated for each case. If the reconstruction error succeeds a predefined threshold, the case is flagged as an anomaly. Then, the same authors proposed BINET, which consists of a next step prediction model and a heuristic [8]. The heuristic determines if the deviation of the model predictions is a significant sign of a potential anomaly. Last, the same authors proposed DeepAlign [10], an extension of the previous approach that can also be used to correct the anomalous process behavior. The core components of the model are bidirectional LSTMs and beam search. Finally, Pauwels et al. developed an anomaly detection method based on Bayesian Networks [11].

7 Conclusion

This paper analyzed multivariate anomaly detection for detecting anomalous process instances (case-based anomaly detection) through LSTM neural networks. We showed that by various refinements in terms of data processing, neural network architecture, and anomaly score computation, we could improve the anomaly detection quality significantly. We evaluated the proposed approach against existing approaches on 328 different real-life and synthetic event logs. We were able to improve the mean F-Score on the PDC 2020 by 6% and the PDC 2021 by 2.3%. In comparison with the machine learning-based models, we achieved a performance gain of 26.1%. Additionally, the paper provides a benchmark for anomaly detection of process cases and can serve as a baseline for further research. In the future, we plan to investigate which design decisions lead to the highest performance improvements and which process features and anomalous behaviors are most difficult for neural networks to understand. Furthermore, we want to extend the anomaly score computation to support continuous attributes.

References

1. Bezerra, F., Wainer, J.: Anomaly detection algorithms in logs of process aware systems. In: Proceedings of the 2008 ACM Symposium on Applied Computing, pp. 951–952 (2008)
2. Bezerra, F., Wainer, J.: Algorithms for anomaly detection of traces in logs of process aware information systems. Inf. Syst. **38**(1), 33–44 (2013)
3. Bezerra, F., Wainer, J., van der Aalst, W.M.P.: Anomaly detection using process mining. In: Halpin, T., et al. (eds.) BPMDS/EMMSAD -2009. LNBIP, vol. 29, pp. 149–161. Springer, Heidelberg (2009). https://doi.org/10.1007/978-3-642-01862-6_13
4. Böhmer, K., Rinderle-Ma, S.: Multi-perspective anomaly detection in business process execution events. In: Debruyne, C., et al. (eds.) OTM 2016. LNCS, vol. 10033, pp. 80–98. Springer, Cham (2016). https://doi.org/10.1007/978-3-319-48472-3_5
5. Burattin, A.: PLG2: multiperspective process randomization with online and offline simulations. In: Azevedo, L., Cabanillas, C. (eds.) Proceedings of the BPM Demo Track 2016 Co-located with the 14th International Conference on Business Process Management (BPM 2016), Rio de Janeiro, Brazil, 21 September 2016. CEUR Workshop Proceedings, vol. 1789, pp. 1–6. CEUR-WS.org (2016)
6. He, T., Zhang, Z., Zhang, H., Zhang, Z., Xie, J., Li, M.: Bag of tricks for image classification with convolutional neural networks (2018). https://doi.org/10.48550/ARXIV.1812.01187. https://arxiv.org/abs/1812.01187
7. Nolle, T., Luettgen, S., Seeliger, A., Mühlhäuser, M.: Analyzing business process anomalies using autoencoders. Mach. Learn. **107**(11), 1875–1893 (2018). https://doi.org/10.1007/s10994-018-5702-8
8. Nolle, T., Luettgen, S., Seeliger, A., Mühlhäuser, M.: BINet: multi-perspective business process anomaly classification. Inf. Syst. **103**, 101458 (2022)
9. Nolle, T., Seeliger, A., Mühlhäuser, M.: BINet: multivariate business process anomaly detection using deep learning. In: Weske, M., Montali, M., Weber, I., vom Brocke, J. (eds.) BPM 2018. LNCS, vol. 11080, pp. 271–287. Springer, Cham (2018). https://doi.org/10.1007/978-3-319-98648-7_16
10. Nolle, T., Seeliger, A., Thoma, N., Mühlhäuser, M.: DeepAlign: alignment-based process anomaly correction using recurrent neural networks. In: Dustdar, S., Yu, E., Salinesi, C., Rieu, D., Pant, V. (eds.) CAiSE 2020. LNCS, vol. 12127, pp. 319–333. Springer, Cham (2020). https://doi.org/10.1007/978-3-030-49435-3_20
11. Pauwels, S., Calders, T.: An anomaly detection technique for business processes based on extended dynamic Bayesian networks. In: Proceedings of the 34th ACM/SIGAPP Symposium on Applied Computing, pp. 494–501 (2019)
12. Rozinat, A., van der Aalst, W.: Conformance checking of processes based on monitoring real behavior. Inf. Syst. **33**(1), 64–95 (2008)
13. Smith, L.N.: Cyclical learning rates for training neural networks (2017)
14. Verbeek, E.: Process discovery contest 2020 (2021)
15. Verbeek, E.: Process discovery contest 2021 (2021)
16. Zimek, A., Schubert, E.: Outlier detection. In: Liu, L., Ozsu, M. (eds.) Encyclopedia of Database Systems. Springer, Cham (2017). https://doi.org/10.1007/978-1-4899-7993-3_80719-1

Genetic Algorithms for AutoML
in Process Predictive Monitoring

Nahyun Kwon and Marco Comuzzi$^{(\boxtimes)}$

Ulsan National Institute of Science and Technology, Ulsan, Republic of Korea
{eekfskgus,mcomuzzi}@unist.ac.kr

Abstract. In recent years, AutoML has emerged as a promising technique for reducing computational and time cost by automating the development of machine learning models. Existing AutoML tools cannot be applied directly to process predictive monitoring (PPM), because they do not support several configuration parameters that are PPM-specific, such as trace bucketing or encoding. In other words, they are only specialized in finding the best configuration of machine learning model hyperparameters. In this paper, we present a simple yet extensible framework for AutoML in PPM. The framework uses genetic algorithms to explore a configuration space containing both PPM-specific parameters and the traditional machine learning model hyperparameters. We design four different types of experiments to verify the effectiveness of the proposed approach, comparing its performance in respect of random search of the configuration space, using two publicly available event logs. The results demonstrate that the proposed approach outperforms consistently the random search.

Keywords: AutoML · Genetic algorithm · Predictive process monitoring · Hyperparameter optimization

1 Introduction

Predictive process monitoring (PPM) is concerned with creating predictive models of aspects of interests of running process cases using the historical process execution data logged in so-called event logs [1]. Typical aspects predicted are the outcome of running cases or the next event to be executed in a running case.

PPM research has endured an exponential success in the last decade. However, the same cannot be said about the uptake of PPM solutions in practice. Existing commercial process mining tools, like Celonis or Apromore, have introduced simple PPM solutions only recently. We argue that the main reason for such a limited uptake is the gap between the typical developer of the PPM models (a process mining expert) and the typical user of these models (a process analyst). The latter have the knowledge to interpret the insights given by PPM models, but they often lack the technical skills of the former to develop the PPM models effectively. This gap can be seen as an instance of a more general gap between machine learning experts, who develop models, and business analysts,

M. Montali et al. (Eds.): ICPM 2022 Workshops, LNBIP 468, pp. 242–254, 2023.
https://doi.org/10.1007/978-3-031-27815-0_18

who are in charge of using the insights returned by these models to take business decisions.

AutoML [2] is one prominent solution to bridge this gap. It aims at creating automated ways to support multiple aspects of the traditional machine learning model development pipeline, like data preparation, feature extraction, model selection, or hyperparameter optimisation. Specifically, given a dataset and a machine learning problem, an AutoML framework aims at finding an optimal model for the user, hiding most of the inner details regarding the model development. AutoML solutions have proliferated in the last few years [3], even being touted to represent the "death of the data scientists".

In PPM, AutoML has received little attention. This is to some extent not surprising, since AutoML solutions for traditional machine learning problems cannot be directly instantiated into PPM problems. Besides the model hyperparameter optimisation, in fact, PPM requires to optimise other *parameters*, such as the type of trace encoding or bucketing used, which are PPM-specific and, therefore, cannot be directly understood by existing AutoML tools.

More broadly, the benchmark experiments for different PPM use cases [4–6] published in the literature provide only generic guidelines regarding the effectiveness of different ML techniques in specific PPM scenarios, but no automated solution. Nirdizati [7], i.e., a tool for automated development of PPM models, can develop different PPM models for a given PPM problem and show the results to the user. However, it has only limited facilities to optimise the models shown to the user. The only approach resembling AutoML is the one proposed by Di Francescomarino et al. [8] (also implemented within Nirdizati), in which genetic algorithms are adopted to optimise the parameters of outcome-based PPM models.

In this paper we propose a simple yet extensible AutoML framework for developing well-performing PPM models. The framework aims at optimising a set of PPM model parameters that comprise: the specific model used to create a predictive model (e.g., decision tree vs. random forest), the hyperparameters of the model, and other parameters specific to PPM, like the technique used to encode traces or the number of prefix buckets used to develop a model in the case of outcome prediction.

The presentation of the framework is split into two parts: (i) the solution space identification and (ii) a model optimisation method based on genetic algorithms (GA). In this paper, the proposed framework is instantiated in the case of outcome-based PPM. However, we argue that only little adaptation is required for its instantiation in other PPM use cases, like next-activity prediction, that yield a machine learning classification problem. The framework is evaluated on two publicly available real world event logs. We compare different experiment configurations in respect of a baseline that involves random search of the configuration parameter space.

The paper is organised as follows. Section 2 briefly discusses the related work. Section 3 presents the parameter optimisation space in the case of outcome-based PPM, while Sect. 4 presents the application of GA to solve the problem of finding a high performing model. The results of the evaluation are presented in Sect. 5, while conclusions are drawn in Sect. 6.

Table 1. PPM-specific model configuration space

Parameter	Range
drop_act	{2, 4, 6, 8}
bucketing	[1, 2 * mean trace length]
encoding	{'aggregate', 'index'}
model	{'DT', 'RF', 'XGB', 'LGBM'}

2   Related Work

AutoML automates the process of developing the *best* model, e.g., the most accurate, to address a given machine learning challenge, speeding up the model development phase and facilitating the application of ML techniques even by non-experts. Different AutoML frameworks, such as Auto-sklearn, the Tree-Based Pipeline Optimization Tool (TPOT), or H2O, provide different automated solutions for each step of the typical machine learning pipeline [2,3], such as data preparation or hyperparameter optimisation.

Predictive process monitoring [1,9] concerns various prediction tasks such as predicting the outcome of a process [4], the next event of a running case [6], or time-related measures [5]. Approaches in the literature often define process outcomes as the satisfaction of service level agreements or the satisfaction of temporal constraints defined on the order and the occurrence of tasks in a case. Extensive efforts have been devoted to enhancing the performance of predictive monitoring models. Recently, deep learning is increasingly applied to solve the problem of outcome prediction [10]. However, deep learning-based approaches require extensive specialist skills by model developers to set the model hyperparameters effectively.

As mentioned in the Introduction, AutoML has been generally neglected by the PPM literature, with the exception of [8]. In respect of the work of Di Francescomarino et al. [8], the framework proposed in this paper considers different encoding and bucketing methods, additional parameters, such as the dropping of infrequent activities, a broader set of models in the evaluation, including boosting ensemble models, and different experiment configurations instead of a single one in which all the parameters are optimised using the GA at once.

3   A Configuration Space for Predictive Monitoring

We consider the PPM use case of outcome-based predictive monitoring, where the aim is to predict a binary categorical outcome of running cases. An analysis of the literature prompted us to design a configuration space that includes four PPM-specific parameters, which are shown in Table 1 and discussed next.

Drop_act: This parameter captures the process of removing low-frequency activities from an event log. This can yield the benefit of reducing the computational

Table 2. Configuration space of hyperparameyters of classification models

Parameter		Range
DT	max_depth	(2, 20)
	min_samples_leaf	(5, 100)
	criterion	['gini', 'entropy']
RF	n_estimators	(10, 1000)
	max_depth	(2, 20)
	max_features	['auto', 'log2']
	bootstrap	[True, False]
	criterion	['gini', 'entropy']
XGB	max_depth	(2, 20)
	n_estimators	(10, 1000)
	learning_rate	[0.01, 0.05, 0.1]
LGBM	max_depth	(2, 20)
	num_leaves	(10, 500)
	min_child_samples	(2, 10)

cost when creating a predictive model and it has been demonstrated to improve the model performance in some cases [11]. We consider a discrete gap-based scale for this parameters, which includes dropping the 2, 4, 6, or 8 less frequent activities in an event log.

Bucketing: When pre-processing an event log for outcome-based prediction, the prefixes of each trace are extracted to construct a prefix log. In this paper, we consider prefix-length bucketing, which is concerned with grouping prefixes of the same length. A base strategy (zero-bucketing) groups all prefixes in a single bucket, thus training a single classifier. In prefix length bucketing, though, each bucket contains partial traces of a specific length, and one classifier is trained for each possible prefix length. Bucketing allows to group homogeneous prefixes, which is supposed to improve the performance of the trained models. For instance, if a lossless encoding that translates each event into a fixed of number features is adopted, then bucketing avoids the need to zero-pad prefixes of different length after encoding. Given an input event log, this parameter can assume values comprised between 1 (corresponding to zero-bucketing) up to two times the mean length of the traces in an event log.

Encoding: The prefixes extracted from an event log must be numerically encoded to be fed into the model. The problem of encoding prefixes is one of complex symbolic sequence encoding [12] and can be approached in multiple ways. In this paper, we consider *aggregation* and *index-based* encoding. Aggregation is a lossy encoding, which represents entire event sequence attributes into a single entity, for example, based on frequency. Index-based is a lossless encoding that maintains the order of events in a prefix. In index-based encoding, each event in a prefix is encoded into a fixed number of numerical features.

Model: This parameter concerns the choice of the classification model to use for developing the predictive model(s). Even though any classification model can be used, the literature highlights that tree-based classifiers show good performance

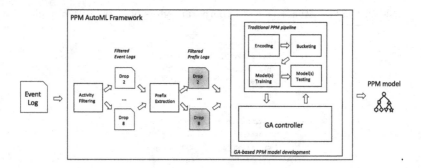

Fig. 1. GA-based framework for PPM model optimisation

in outcome-based PPM [4]. Thus, in this work we consider four kinds of tree-based models, including both individual and ensemble classifiers: Decision Tree (DT), Random Forest (RF), XGBoost (XGB), and LightGBM (LGBM).

Once a `model` is chosen, the hyperparameters of the model must be optimised. This is one of the typical functionalities of AutoML tools. In this work, we combine the optimisation of the model hyperparameters with the PPM-specific parameters mentioned above. Table 2 lists the domain of hyperparameters for each classifier that we consider in this work. Although several additional hyperparameters can be considered for each classifier, in this work we consider a restricted set of hyperparameters that are shown to have significant effect on the model performance in the literature [13–15]. For the hyperparemters not mentioned in Table 2, we use the default settings of the Python implementation (more details about this in Sect. 5).

After having introduced the PPM model configuration space above, we can now introduce the architecture of the proposed PPM AutoML framework, which is depicted in Fig. 1. We assume that the PPM use case has been defined, so the input of the framework is simply an event log. First, several pre-processed filtered event logs in which the low-frequency activities are dropped are generated, i.e., one for each possible value of `drop_act`. Then, for each filtered event log, the prefixes are extracted for each trace, which yields a set of filtered prefix logs. The filtered prefix logs are the input of the GA-based PPM model development module. This comprises the *GA controller*—implementing the logic of the GA-based optimisation presented in the next section—and a traditional PPM pipeline, which is called by the GA controller to generate new PPM models for given values of the configuration space parameters. The output of the framework is one PPM model, i.e., the highest-performing one identified by the GA-based optimisation.

4   GAs for Exploring the Configuration Space

GA was inspired from the Darwinian theory of evolution [16], according to which fitter individuals survive and their genes are passed to their offspring. In a GA, every individual solution, i.e., a PPM model in our case, corresponds to a chromosome and each parameter represents a gene of a chromosome, which assume a certain value in the configuration space. GA evaluates the fitness of each individual in the population using a fitness function. A selection process is used at each iteration to select the best chromosomes. These then mate to produce an offspring using the crossover operation. In addition, at each iteration several chromosomes are mutated, i.e., their value is randomly changed. Ideally, as generations go on, the fitness value of the offspring increases, until a sufficiently fit individual is identified. We describe next how the typical elements of a GA are customised in our framework.

Initial Population: The GA algorithm starts with creating an initial population. This population is generated by choosing the parameter values randomly within a domain in configuration space. In our framework, the size of the initial population is 20 individuals.

Evaluate Fitness: In this step, the GA computes the fitness value of each individual in the present population. Fitness is considered as an evaluation metric as well as objective function in GA. Individuals with high fitness value are likely to be selected, mutated and mated with another for crossover. In some simple GA implementations, fitness is defined as a single indicator, such as model accuracy. However, relying on only one metric can provide wrong insights. For example, when the distribution of classes is unbalanced, like in many PPM scenarios [4,6], the accuracy is not sufficient to evaluate the performance. It is then helpful to use multiple measures rather than only one. Thus, we designed the fitness $f(i)$ of an individual i, i.e., an outcome-based PPM model, to combine different measures as follows:

$$f(i) = \frac{sc(i) + re(i) + tr(i) + se(i)}{4}$$

where:

$$sc(i) = \frac{AUC(i) + acc(i)}{2},$$

$$re(i) = 1 - failure\ rate(i),$$

$$te(i) = \frac{\max(time) - time(i)}{\max(time) - \min(time)}$$

$$se(i) = \frac{sc(i) - \min(sc)}{\max(sc) - \min(sc)}$$

In the formulas above, the score $sc(i)$ combines the average Area Under the receiving operator Curve AUC and the average accuracy acc obtained by the model i. AUC is a more balanced performance measure that is often considered in PPM problems.

The reliability $re(i)$ is a measure that computes the overall reliability of the predictions made by an individual i over the test set. A classifier assigns to each observation in a dataset probabilities for each of the outcome labels. The label associated with the highest probability is chosen as the predicted one. When such a highest probability is less than a minimum threshold, we say that the prediction has *failed*, i.e. it is not reliable. In the GA, we compute the failure rate as 1 minus the fraction of observations (running cases) in a dataset for which the prediction failed. The minimum threshold value used in the experiments is 0.7, e.g., a prefix predicted with probability of 0.65 and 0.35 of having a positive or negative label, respectively, is considered a failed prediction.

The time efficiency $te(i)$ represents the relative amount of time required for an individual to be trained and tested (in respect of the maximum and minimum times observed in the current population). A main purpose of AutoML is in fact to reduce the time for identifying the best machine learning model. In this direction, the time efficiency represents how efficient the computation of a chromosome is compared to the other chromosomes in the same population. Similarly to the time efficiency, the score efficiency $se(i)$ represents the relative value of the score of the current individual i in respect of all the other individuals of the current population. This term is introduced to consider also the magnitude of the performance improvement when evaluating the fitness of a new individual i.

Selection: The main objective of the selection is to give a higher chance of being a parent to the fittest individuals in order to pass on better genes to the offspring. In other words, the higher the fitness of an individual, the higher the opportunity of selection. In this context, we adopted the *roulette wheel* strategy in our framework, in which the best individual has the largest chance to be selected, while the worst individual has the lowest chance.

Crossover and Mutation: Crossover is implemented by selecting a random point (or points) in a chromosome where the exchange of parents' genes happens. The crossover then brings up a new offspring based on the exchange point chosen with particular parts of the parents. Since we consider a limiter number of parameters defining a chromosome, we use the *one-point* crossover, in which only one crossover point along the chromosome is randomly selected.

The purpose of the mutation is to encourage diversity in the population, thus alleviating the local-optima problem in a GA implementation. When mutation is applied, a few genes in the chromosome are randomly changed to produce a new offspring. As a result, this creates new adaptive solutions to avoid local optima. We decided to change one gene for each mutation step.

The GA is thus characterised by the parameter crossover rate cr and the mutation rate mr. Both range between 0 and 1. The crossover rate indicates the chance that two chromosomes mate and exchange their genes, so that a new offspring is produced. If $cr = 1$ (100%), all the offspring are obtained applying the crossover. If $cr = 0$ then no mating at all occurs, i.e., a new generation is exactly the same as the previous one. The mutation rate determines how many chromosomes should be mutated in a generation. Setting $mr = 1$ (100%) results in mutating all the chromosomes in a population, while mutation never occurs when $mr = 0$. In the experiments, the values of these two parameters have been set experimentally through grid search (more details in the next section).

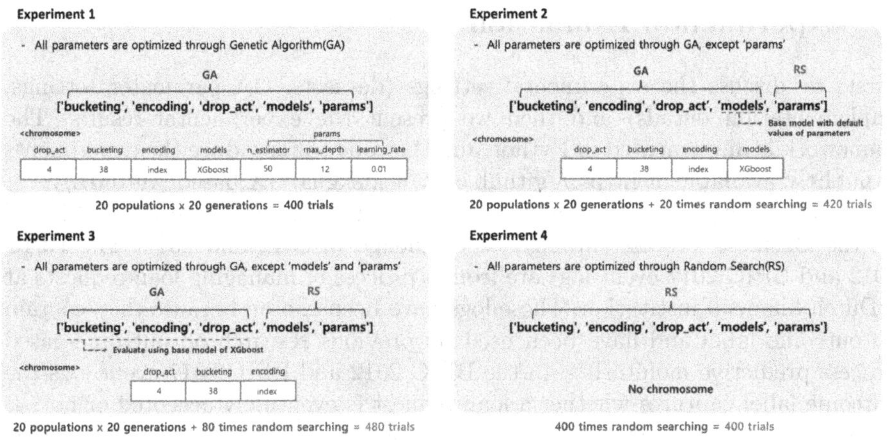

Fig. 2. Experiment configurations: illustration

New Population: A new population is generated by selection, crossover, and mutation. If the termination test (see next) is not passed, this population becomes the parent generation for the next population.

Termination Test: A GA algorithm must stop, returning the best solution found as a result. Therefore, a termination condition is tested for every generation. In the proposed framework, three conditions are tested and, if any of them are true, the algorithm stops: (i) the maximum number of iteration is reached, (ii) the number of times in which the average fitness of the new population is lower than the one of the previous population exceeds a certain limit (5 in the experiments), and (iii) the difference between the average fitness of the new population and the last one is less than 0.001. Note that (i) guarantees that the GA algorithms eventually stops.

4.1 Experiment Configurations

We designed four experiment configurations based on different ways of exploring the configuration space using GAs (see Fig. 2). In experiment 1, all the parameters in the configuration space are expressed by genes of the chromosomes and optimized using GA. In experiment 2, the hyperparameter values of the model are not part of the GA-based optimisation. First, the GA is run considering default parameter values for each model. Then, the hyperparameters of the model selected by the best individual using GA are optmised using random search. In experiment 3, only the PPM-specific parameters `bucketing`, `encoding` and `drop_act` are optimised using GA, considering XGB as the model with default hyperparmeter values. Then the model to be used and its hyperparameters are selected using random search. The fourth experiment is a totally random search (RS) baseline, in which all the values of all the parameters are optimised using random search. As can be seen in Fig. 2, all the experiments are configured to generate between 400 and 500 trials, i.e., models to train and test.

5   Experimental Evaluation

First, we discuss the experimental settings (datasets, GA parameter settings, implementation details) and then we present the experimental results. The framework is implemented in Python and the code to reproduce the experiments is publicly available at https://github.com/eekfskgus/GA_based_AutoML/.

We consider 2 event logs publicly available at https://data.4tu.nl/ published by the Business Process Intelligence Challenge in 2012 and 2017. The BPIC 2012 and BPIC 2017 event logs are from a process of managing loan requests at a Dutch financial institution. These logs have been chosen because they contain an outcome label and have been used by previous research on outcome-based process predictive monitoring. In the BPIC 2012 and BPIC 2017 event logs the outcome label captures whether a loan request is eventually accepted or not.

The design of GAs requires to set the values of several parameters. The value of the GA parameters can impact greatly on the solution found, even determining whether a solution is found at all by the algorithm [17].

Table 3. Grid search test for GA parameter setting

Parameter	Best score	Elapsed time(s)
cr = 0.9, mr = 0.1	0.76	4611
cr = 0.9, mr = 0.05	0.75	4538
cr = 0.9, mr = 0.01	**0.82**	**3848**
cr = 0.8, mr = 0.1	0.75	3947
cr = 0.8, mr = 0.05	0.71	4486
cr = 0.8, mr = 0.01	0.76	4233
cr = 0.7, mr = 0.1	0.77	4468
cr = 0.7, mr = 0.05	0.73	5424
cr = 0.7, mr = 0.01	0.7	4554

To find the best value of cr and mr, we conducted a grid search experiment using the BPIC 2012 dataset, in which $cr \in [0.9, 0.8, 0.7]$ and $mr \in [0.1, 0.05, 0.01]$. It is known that high crossover rate and low mutation rate effectively works in GA, since the low crossover rates lead to low rates of exploration, whereas high mutation rates increase the randomness of the search [18,19]. For every combination, we evaluated the best individual found and the elapsed time using the experiment 1 configuration. The results of this test are shown in Table 3 (the selected parameter values are in bold). For the other GA parameters, the initial population size is 20, with 5 individuals randomly generated for each of the 4 classification models considered. For the termination condition, the maximum number of iteration is 20.

For the training and testing of new individuals in a generation, the (training:test) ratio is set to (4:1). In addition, if the imbalance ratio of the minority

Table 4. Best solutions and corresponding parameter values

		Experiment 1			Experiment 2			Experiment 3			Experiment 4		
		Run 1	Run 2	Run 3	Run 1	Run 2	Run 3	Run 1	Run 2	Run 3	Run 1	Run 2	Run 3
BPIC2012	time(s)	93532	95454	83139	84823	113432	51252	157937	123628	82579	113952	119033	117269
	sc	0.83	0.74	0.96	0.94	0.78	0.89	0.78	0.92	0.99	0.84	0.82	0.84
	model	XGB	DT	RF	LGBM	RF		LGBM	LGBM	LGBM	XGB	RF	RF	RF
	drop_act	8	8	4	4	6	2	8	4	8	6	8	6
	bucketing	30	29	13	22	34	26	39	23	6	2	2	1
	encoding	index	index	index	index	index	index	index	index	aggregate	aggregate	index	index
BPIC2017	time(s)	77644	83140	101942	80839	54720	76564	102004	96954	109210	119351	93833	165861
	sc	0.83	0.96	0.96	0.94	0.84	0.73	0.76	0.99	0.96	0.75	0.74	0.78
	model	RF	RF	XGB	LGBM	XGB	RF	LGBM	XGB	LGBM	DT	RF	DT
	drop_act	6	4	6	8	8	8	4	4	4	6	8	8
	bucketing	25	13	6	7	28	34	37	18	9	1	1	3
	encoding	index	index	aggregate	index	index	index	index	index	index	index	index	index

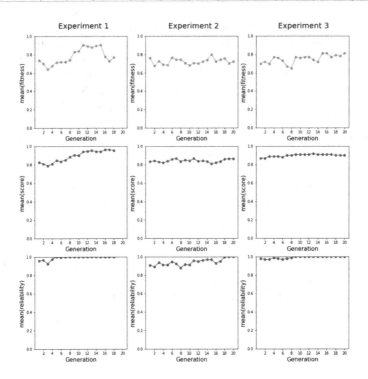

Fig. 3. Mean parameters values over generations in the GA-based experiments (BPIC 2017 event log)

class over the majority class is less than 0.33, then the dataset is automatically re-sampled using synthetic minority over-sampling, widely known as SMOTE. SMOTE sampling could lead to benefit the performance of classification in class imbalance problem, by improving the class boundary region especially with extremely imbalanced datasets.

Table 4 compares the best solution obtained by the four types of experiments. Given the randomness intrinsic to the experiments, for each type of experiment we show the results of three different runs. We compare the execution time, the accuracy-AUC-based score (sc), and the values of the parameters of the configuration space. The proposed GA-based framework (adopted in experiments 1, 2, and 3) generally outscore the RS (experiment 4), on both execution time and quality of the solution (score). Interestingly, the classifiers XGB and LGBM (especially the latter) are frequently selected in the experiments that use the proposed framework, whereas RF or DT are often selected by the RS experiment.

The RS baseline in experiment 4 selects the best individual from 400 samples obtained using parameter values randomly selected. These 400 individuals are independent of each other, i.e., their selection is not affected by the constraints on fitness, execution time and failure rate of the proposed GA-based framework. Therefore, a random search of the configuration space could work better for individual classifiers (like DT) or bagging-based classifiers (like RF), which do not try to improve iteratively the performance of the model. Another difference between XGB and LGBM when compared with DT and RF is that they use boosting. Boosting involves iterations, whereby the prediction results of a previous model affects the results of the next one. Based on the results shown in Table 4, the overlapping effect of boosting over generations improves the GA performance. In addition, LGBM is selected more frequently than XGB because of its superiority in terms of execution time. Being lightweight on execution time, LGBM is likely to lead to higher fitness of the solution found in a shorter time.

Regarding the other parameters, index encoding is more dominant in the solutions found than aggregation encoding. It appears also that dropping a higher number of infrequent activities leads to better results. Finally, Table 4 shows that the bucket size of the best chromosome tends to be higher when using the proposed framework when compared to the RS baseline.

To show the inner dynamic of the GA-based experiments, Fig. 3 shows the mean values across experiments 1, 2, and 3 of the three parameters fitness, score, and reliability over the generations for the BPIC 2017 dataset. We can see that the value of each parameter tend to converge to 1 as the number of generation increases, which shows the suitability of the GA-based approach as an optimisation strategy for identifying a PPM model.

6   Conclusions

This paper has presented an AutoML framework for identifying a high-performing PPM model. The framework relies on genetic algorithms for exploring a solution space that includes both traditional and PPM-specific model hyperparameters. In the future, we plan to extend the configuration space to more dimensions and use cases, e.g., next event prediction, and to compare the proposed GA-based approach with other bio-inspired heuristics, e.g. swarm or particle intelligence.

References

1. Di Francescomarino, C., Ghidini, C.: Predictive process monitoring. Process Min. Handb. LNBIP **448**, 320–346 (2022)
2. Yao, Q., et al.: Taking human out of learning applications: a survey on automated machine learning. arXiv preprint arXiv:1810.13306 (2018)
3. Karmaker, S.K., Hassan, M.M., Smith, M.J., Xu, L., Zhai, C., Veeramachaneni, K.: AutoML to date and beyond: challenges and opportunities. ACM Comput. Surv. (CSUR) **54**(8), 1–36 (2021)
4. Teinemaa, I., Dumas, M., Rosa, M.L., Maggi, F.M.: Outcome-oriented predictive process monitoring: review and benchmark. ACM Trans. Knowl. Discov. Data (TKDD) **13**(2), 1–57 (2019)
5. Verenich, I., Dumas, M., Rosa, M.L., Maggi, F.M., Teinemaa, I.: Survey and cross-benchmark comparison of remaining time prediction methods in business process monitoring. ACM Trans. Intell. Syst. Technol. (TIST) **10**(4), 1–34 (2019)
6. Tama, B.A., Comuzzi, M.: An empirical comparison of classification techniques for next event prediction using business process event logs. Expert Syst. Appl. **129**, 233–245 (2019)
7. Rizzi, W., Simonetto, L., Di Francescomarino, C., Ghidini, C., Kasekamp, T., Maggi, F.M.: Nirdizati 2.0: new features and redesigned backend. In: Proceedings of the Dissertation Award, Doctoral Consortium, and Demonstration Track at BPM 2019, vol. 2420, pp. 154–158 (2019)
8. Di Francescomarino, C., et al.: Genetic algorithms for hyperparameter optimization in predictive business process monitoring. Inf. Syst. **74**, 67–83 (2018)
9. Márquez-Chamorro, A.E., Resinas, M., Ruiz-Cortés, A.: Predictive monitoring of business processes: a survey. IEEE Trans. Serv. Comput. **11**(6), 962–977 (2017)
10. Rama-Maneiro, E., Vidal, J., Lama, M.: Deep learning for predictive business process monitoring: review and benchmark. IEEE Trans. Serv. Comput. (2021)
11. Tax, N., Sidorova, N., van der Aalst, W.M.: Discovering more precise process models from event logs by filtering out chaotic activities. J. Intell. Inf. Syst. **52**(1), 107–139 (2019)
12. Leontjeva, A., Conforti, R., Di Francescomarino, C., Dumas, M., Maggi, F.M.: Complex symbolic sequence encodings for predictive monitoring of business processes. In: Motahari-Nezhad, H.R., Recker, J., Weidlich, M. (eds.) BPM 2015. LNCS, vol. 9253, pp. 297–313. Springer, Cham (2015). https://doi.org/10.1007/978-3-319-23063-4_21
13. Bergstra, J., Komer, B., Eliasmith, C., Yamins, D., Cox, D.D.: Hyperopt: a python library for model selection and hyperparameter optimization. Comput. Sci. Discov. **8**(1), 014008 (2015)
14. Liang, W., Luo, S., Zhao, G., Wu, H.: Predicting hard rock pillar stability using GBDT, XGBoost, and LightGBM algorithms. Mathematics **8**(5), 765 (2020)
15. Kelkar, K.M., Bakal, J.: Hyper parameter tuning of random forest algorithm for affective learning system. In: 2020 Third International Conference on Smart Systems and Inventive Technology (ICSSIT), pp. 1192–1195. IEEE (2020)
16. Holland, J.H.: Genetic algorithms. Sci. Am. **267**(1), 66–73 (1992)
17. Mills, K.L., Filliben, J.J., Haines, A.: Determining relative importance and effective settings for genetic algorithm control parameters. Evol. Comput. **23**(2), 309–342 (2015)

18. Chiroma, H., Abdulkareem, S., Abubakar, A., Zeki, A., Gital, A.Y., Usman, M.J.: Correlation study of genetic algorithm operators: crossover and mutation probabilities. In: Proceedings of the International Symposium on Mathematical Sciences and Computing Research, pp. 6–7 (2013)
19. Hassanat, A., Almohammadi, K., Alkafaween, E., Abunawas, E., Hammouri, A., Prasath, V.S.: Choosing mutation and crossover ratios for genetic algorithms-a review with a new dynamic approach. Information **10**(12), 390 (2019)

Outcome-Oriented Predictive Process Monitoring on Positive and Unlabelled Event Logs

Jari Peeperkorn[1]([✉])[iD], Carlos Ortega Vázquez[1][iD], Alexander Stevens[1][iD], Johannes De Smedt[1][iD], Seppe vanden Broucke[1,2][iD], and Jochen De Weerdt[1][iD]

[1] Research Center for Information Systems Engineering (LIRIS), KU Leuven, Leuven, Belgium
{jari.peeperkorn,carloseduardo.ortegavazquez,alexander.stevens,
johannes.desmedt,seppe.vandenbroucke,jochen.deweerdt}@kuleuven.be
[2] Department of Business Informatics and Operations Management, Ghent University, Ghent, Belgium

Abstract. A lot of recent literature on outcome-oriented predictive process monitoring focuses on using models from machine and deep learning. In this literature, it is assumed the outcome labels of the historical cases are all known. However, in some cases, the labelling of cases is incomplete or inaccurate. For instance, you might only observe negative customer feedback, fraudulent cases might remain unnoticed. These cases are typically present in the so-called positive and unlabelled (PU) setting, where your data set consists of a couple of positively labelled examples and examples which do not have a positive label, but might still be examples of a positive outcome. In this work, we show, using a selection of event logs from the literature, the negative impact of mislabelling cases as negative, more specifically when using XGBoost and LSTM neural networks. Furthermore, we show promising results on real-life datasets mitigating this effect, by changing the loss function used by a set of models during training to those of unbiased Positive-Unlabelled (uPU) or non-negative Positive-Unlabelled (nnPU) learning.

Keywords: Process mining · Predictive process monitoring · OOPPM · XGBoost · LSTM · PU learning · Label uncertainty

1 Introduction

Outcome-Oriented Predictive Process Monitoring (OOPPM) refers to predicting the future state (labels) of ongoing processes, using the historical cases of business processes. Most recently, the literature in OOPPM has been focused on training machine and deep learning models on labelled historical data. However, to the best of our knowledge, no research has focused on training such models when the labels given to these historical cases are incomplete, uncertain, or even wrong. Accordingly, in this paper, a situation is investigated where part of the

M. Montali et al. (Eds.): ICPM 2022 Workshops, LNBIP 468, pp. 255–268, 2023.
https://doi.org/10.1007/978-3-031-27815-0_19

positive historical cases have been unnoticed and therefore mistakenly classified as negative in the data. A situation like this might be found when the positive label represents, e.g., detected outliers or fraud in a loan application, or customer (dis)satisfaction through a survey (which might not always be filled out) for a production process [10, 26]. Other examples can be found in medicine, e.g., when trying to predict the chances of complications which might go unnoticed, or when dealing with overall low-quality data and therefore uncertain labels [10, 14]. Other examples can be found in multi-organisational processes, where information flow can sometimes be limited. This setting can be understood as one-sided label noise, in which some seeming negatives are actually positive [1]. One-sided label noise is a common interpretation of positive and unlabelled (PU) data. In this setting, data consists of positive and unlabelled instances, in which an unlabelled example can be either positive or negative. Consequently, this field of machine learning research is called PU learning. We focus on methods based on the Expected Risk Minimization (ERM) in the literature of PU learning. Particularly, we use unbiased PU learning and non-negative PU learning [7,11] because of the state-of-the-art performance. These two methods have been successfully utilised in other domains such as imbalanced learning [21], and graph neural networks [27].

In our experimental setup, we flip different percentages of the positive labels in the training logs to a negative label, replicating a real-world situation with missing positive labels. By training models on these different training sets and evaluating their performance on the untouched test set, we can evaluate the impact of missing positive training labels on the models' actual performance. The models in question are gradient boosted trees (more specifically eXtreme Gradient Boosting, known as XGBoost or XGB) [3] and the Long Short-Term Memory neural networks (LSTM) [9]. Furthermore, we investigate the impact of replacing the binary cross-entropy loss functions with functions inspired by the Positive and Unlabelled (PU) learning literature. This can be summarised in the following hypotheses:

Hypothesis 1 (H1): *Incorrectly labelling deviant (positive) behaviour as normal (negative), can have an important impact on the (future) performance of a predictive model.*

Hypothesis 2 (H2): *Using loss functions from PU-learning, the problem above can be (partially) mitigated.*

To investigate these hypotheses, our setup has been applied to a selection of nine real-life process event logs from the literature. The rest of the paper is organised as follows. We start by discussing some relevant related work in Sect. 2. Second, Sect. 3 introduces essential background information, followed by an introduction to PU learning in Sect. 4. In Sect. 5, the experimental setup is described, before introducing the data and the hyperparameter search. This is succeeded by showing and discussing the results (Sect. 6). Finally, Sect. 7 provides a conclusion and some possible approaches for future research. The data, results, and code used and presented in this paper are available online[1].

---

[1] https://github.com/jaripeeperkorn/PU-OOPPM.

2   Related Work

Predictive Process Monitoring (PPM) is concerned with many tasks such as predicting the remaining time [25], next activity [22] or the outcome of the process [4,12,24]. The latter is also known as Outcome-Oriented Predictive Process Monitoring (OOPPM), a field of study that predicts the final state of an incoming, incomplete case. One of the pioneer studies in this field is [24], where they benchmark the state-of-the-art trace bucketing techniques and sequence encoding mechanisms used for different machine learning models. However, the use of classical machine learning models has been superseded by an avalanche of deep learning techniques. Here, the most frequent used predictive model in general predictive process monitoring literature has become LSTM neural networks, initiated by [22]. The introduction of this recurrent neural network has been motivated by the ability of this model to handle the dynamic behaviour of high-dimensional sequential data. In recent, many other sophisticated models have been benchmarked against this model in the field of predictive process monitoring, such as Convolutional Neural Networks (CNN) [16] or Generative Adversarial Networks (GAN) [23]. Some studies have already compared the predictive performance of different deep learning models [12,15,18].

Nonetheless, the predictions made by the majority of these works are based on data from past process instances, i.e. event logs, and therefore implicitly assume that the labelling made corresponds with the ground truth. Work on incremental predictive process monitoring [17,19] does provide a flexible alternative to deal with the rigidity of predictive models. Moreover, these incremental learning algorithms allow for the predictive model to deal with the variability and dynamic behaviour of business processes (i.e. different time periods have different characteristics [17]). Other recent work discusses a semi-supervised approach, also leveraging the power of deep neural networks, to handle scarcely labelled process logs in an OOPPM setting [8]. However, to the best of our knowledge, none of the related works has already used PU learning in the context of OOPPM, which incorporates that negatively labelled instances are possibly mislabelled.

3   Preliminaries

Executed *activities* in a process are recorded as an event in an Event Log L. Each *event* belongs to one *case*, indicated by its *CaseID* $c \in C$. An event e can also be written as a tuple $e = (c, a, t, d, s)$, with $a \in A$ the *activity* (i.e. *control-flow* attribute) and t the timestamp. Optionally, an event might also have event-related attributes (payload or *dynamic* attributes) $d = (d_1, d_2, \ldots, d_{m_d})$, which are event specific and might evolve during a case. Other attributes do not evolve during the execution of a single case and are called case or *static* attributes $s = (s_1, s_2, \ldots, s_{m_s})$. A sequence of events belonging to one case is called a trace. The outcome y of a trace is an attribute defined by the process owner. This attribute is often binary, indicating whether a certain criterion has been met [24]. We use the label *positive* when it is met, and call these cases *positive cases*. And *negative cases* otherwise. A prefix is part of a trace, consisting of the first l events (with l an integer smaller than the trace length). A prefix log L^* contains all possible prefixes which can be extracted from all traces in L.

XGBoost is an implementation of the gradient boosting ensemble method, which is constructed from multiple decision tree models. By adding additional trees to correct the prediction error from the prior iteration, an efficient yet powerful classifier can be trained [3]. Recurrent Neural Networks (RNNs) are neural networks specifically designed to work with sequential data by letting information flow between multiple time steps. LSTMs are a specific variant of RNN, specifically designed to handle long-term dependencies [9].

Both of these models rely on a proper choice of loss function for training. The loss function is used to score the model on its performance, based on the predicted probability $p \in [0, 1]$ and the actual label $y \in \{0, 1\}$. Formally, in the Empirical Risk Minimisation (ERM) framework, the loss function L is utilised within the risk function when scoring a classifier $g(x)$:

$$R(g(x)) = \alpha \mathbb{E}_{f_+}[L^+(g(x))] + (1 - \alpha)\mathbb{E}_{f_-}[L^-(g(x))], \tag{1}$$

where $L^+(g)$ and $L^-(g)$ are the losses for positive and negative examples; $\mathbb{E}_{f_+}$ and $\mathbb{E}_{f_-}$ are the expectation over the propensity density functions of the positive $f_+(x)$ and negative $f_-(x)$ instance space; and α is the positive class ratio or class prior as denoted in the literature. Usually for a binary classification problem, as is often the case in OOPPM, the binary cross entropy loss function is used. The binary cross-entropy can be calculated from a data set when $L^+(g(x_i)) = -log(p_i)$ and $L^-(g(x_i)) = -log(1 - p_i)$ in Eq. 1:

$$BCE = -\sum_{i=1}^{N} (y_i \log(p_i) + (1 - y_i) \log(1 - p_i)) \tag{2}$$

4 PU Learning

Despite the popularity of binary cross-entropy in the standard classification setup in which labels are accurate and complete, some real-world applications suffer from label uncertainty. In such scenarios, the binary cross-entropy is no longer valid for model learning. We focus on the PU setting in which the training data consists of only positive and unlabelled examples; the labelled instances are always positive, but some positives remain unlabelled. In PU learning, the label status $l \in \{0, 1\}$ determines if an example is either labelled or unlabeled. Formally, we assume that the positive and unlabelled instances are independent and identically distributed from the general distribution $f(x)$:

$$\mathcal{X} \sim f(x)$$
$$\sim \alpha f_+(x) + (1 - \alpha)f_-(x) \tag{3}$$
$$\sim \alpha c f_l(x) + (1 - \alpha c)f_u(x), \tag{4}$$

where $\mathcal{X}$ refers to the set of instances and the label frequency c is the probability of a positive example being labelled $P(l = 1 \mid y = 1)$. The general distribution can be formulated in terms of the positive distribution $f_+(x)$ and negative distribution $f_-(x)$ (see Eq. 3). In the PU setting, the general distribution consists of the labeled $f_l(x)$ and unlabeled distribution $f_u(x)$ as shown in Eq. 4. A proportion c of the positive instances of the data set is labelled, thus, a learner can only observe a fraction αc of instances with a positive label whereas the rest is unlabeled. Recent works have proposed methods based on the ERM framework, which are currently considered state-of-the-art [2,7,11]. These methods incorporate the information of the class prior (i.e., positive class ratio) to weight the PU data within the loss function. The weighting allows the empirical risk from the PU data to be the same in expectation as in the fully labelled data. From Eq. 1, we can transform the loss function into the PU setting as follows:

$$
\begin{aligned}
R_{upu}(g(x)) &= \alpha \mathbb{E}_{f_+}[L^+(g(x))] + (1-\alpha)\mathbb{E}_{f_-}[L^-(g(x))] \\
&= \alpha \mathbb{E}_{f_+}[L^+(g(x))] + \mathbb{E}_f[L^-(g(x))] - \alpha \mathbb{E}_{f_+}[L^-(g(x))] \\
&= \alpha c \mathbb{E}_{f_l}\left[\frac{1}{c}(L^+(g(x)) - L^-(g(x)))\right] + \mathbb{E}_f[L^-(g(x))] \\
&= \alpha c \mathbb{E}_{f_l}\left[\frac{1}{c}L^+(g(x)) + (1-\frac{1}{c})L^-(g(x))\right] + (1-\alpha c)\mathbb{E}_{f_u}[L^-(g(x))].
\end{aligned}
$$
$$(5)$$

In the first step of Eq. 5, we can substitute the term $(1-\alpha)\mathbb{E}_{f_-}[L^-(g(x))]$ with $\mathbb{E}_f[L^-(g(x))] - \alpha \mathbb{E}_{f_+}[L^-(g(x))]$ based on Eq. 3: the negative distribution f_- is the difference between the general distribution f and the positive distribution f_+. In the second step, we substitute $\mathbb{E}_f[L^-(g(x))]$ with $\alpha c \mathbb{E}_f[L^-(g(x))] + (1-\alpha c)\mathbb{E}_f[L^-(g(x))]$ based on Eq. 4. Now the unlabelled instances are considered negative with a weight of 1. Also, all labelled examples are added both as positive with weight $\frac{1}{c}$ and as negative with $1 - \frac{1}{c}$. The method is called unbiased PU (uPU) because the empirical risk for PU data (Eq. 5) is equal in expectation to the empirical risk when data is fully labelled (Eq. 1) [7]. The uPU can be used in modern techniques that require a convex loss function for training. However, the uPU method presents a weakness for flexible techniques that can easily overfit: the uPU risk estimator can provide negative empirical risks. This issue is problematic for powerful classifiers such as XGBoost [3] or deep learning models. Thus, the non-negative PU risk estimator is proposed that improves on uPU by adding a maximum operator [11]:

$$
R_{nnpu}(g(x)) = \alpha c \mathbb{E}_{f_l}\left[\frac{1}{c}L^+(g(x))\right] + \max\left(0, (1-\alpha c)\mathbb{E}_{f_u}[L^-(g(x))] + \alpha c \mathbb{E}_{f_l}\left[(1-\frac{1}{c})L^-(g(x))\right]\right). \quad (6)
$$

The maximum operator in Eq. 6 prevents the issue of negative empirical risks. We can derive an appropriate loss function for PU learning that can substitute the binary cross-entropy based on Eq. 6 and Eq. 5. Hence, the unbiased PU cross-entropy and non-negative PU cross-entropy can be estimated from a data set:

$$
uPU_{BCE} = -\sum_{i=1}^{N}\left(l_i\left[\frac{1}{c}\log(p_i) + (1-\frac{1}{c})\log(1-p_i)\right] + (1-l_i)\left[\log(1-p_i)\right]\right)
$$
$$(7)$$

$$
nnPU_{BCE} = -\sum_{i=1}^{N}\left(l_i\left[\frac{1}{c}\log(p_i)\right] + \max\left(0, (1-l_i)\left[\log(1-p_i)\right] + l_i(1-\frac{1}{c})\log(1-p_i)\right)\right) \quad (8)
$$

Unlike the binary cross-entropy, as shown in Eq. 2, the ground-truth label y is not available but the label status $l \in \{0, 1\}$. Notice that a labelled instance is always a positive example. We can, thus, use uPU_{BCE} and $nnPU_{BCE}$ as the loss function for a classification technique.

5   Experimental Setup

5.1   Setup

To address the hypotheses introduced earlier, two experimental setups were carefully constructed. Both share a similar setup, visualised in Fig. 1. An event log is taken and split into a training set and a test set. This is done 80–20% *out-of-time*, i.e. every case with time activity timestamps before a certain moment is added to the training set and later cases are added to the test set (in way that approximately 20% of the cases ends up in the test set). However, since we do not want to discard too much data, it was opted to do a split without discarding the whole cases in an overlapping period and only remove the specific event with overlap to the test log period, in correspondence to other works in literature [24]. Subsequently, we look at the different positively labelled traces in the training, and flip different percentages (25, 50 and 75%) of these labels to a negative label, hereby replicating situations where different positive cases in the training set would not have been classified as such. The negative label should therefore better be called *unlabelled*. We also keep one *Original* log, for which no labels have been flipped. For each of these training sets, the prefix log is obtained, which is then used to train different models. The models used are each time an XGBoost classifier and an LSTM neural network, albeit with varying loss functions. In **Experiment 1** we solely want to investigate the possible negative effect of mislabelling positive examples. For this purpose, we opt to use the standard binary cross entropy. After training, the classifier predicts the labels of all prefixes in the prefix log of the test log, and these labels are compared to the true labels. As a score, we use the area under the ROC curve (AUC), which can be used to express the probability a classifier will give a higher prediction to a positive example than to a negative example. This was chosen due to it being threshold-independent and unbiased with imbalanced data sets. Notice that we did not flip any labels in the test log, as we want to test the model's actual performance. The different models (trained on logs with different label flip percentages) are compared.

In **Experiment 2** we also train classifiers with the uPU and $nnPU$ loss functions introduced in Sect. 3. These classifiers are trained on the same training logs (only the one with label flips this time). By comparing the AUC on the test (untouched) examples, we can investigate the possible advantages of using PU learning loss functions over binary cross entropy. The XGBoost model is taken from [3] and the LSTM model is implemented by using the Python library Keras[2]. The uPU and $nnPU$ loss function implementations designed for this

---

[2] https://keras.io.

work are also working on top of these libraries. The PU loss functions demand the user to give a *class prior*. In this work, we have used the percentage of label flips as input, to derive an estimate for the class prior. This is not a fully realistic setting, as in real-life you might not know how many positive cases you will have missed. However, often an adequate guess can be made based on expert knowledge or previous samples. The class prior derived from the flip ratio does not lead to the exact class prior as well, as it is based on traces and not prefixes. Longer traces create more prefixes in the training log since every activity in a trace (minus the last) is used as the last activity in a prefix. In addition, the positive class ratio of the training log is different from that of the test set. With this not-exact estimate of the class prior, we, therefore, deem our setup suitable to investigate Hypothesis 2.

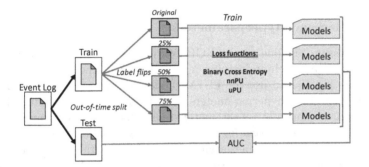

Fig. 1. Overview of the setup.

5.2 Event Logs

We have selected two sets of often used and publicly available event logs recorded from real-life processes. The outcomes are derived from a set of LTL rules similar as has been done in [4,13,20,24]. The first set of event logs, *BPIC2011* or *Hospital Log*, consists of four sublogs collected from the Gynaecology department of a Dutch Academic Hospital [6]. The different outcome LTL rules, and the accompanying trace cutting, are taken over from [24]. After collecting the patient's information, the patient's procedures and treatments are recorded. The *BPIC2015* event log consists of 5 different sublogs, each one having recorded a building permit application process in 5 different Dutch municipalities [5]. They share one LTL rule, checking whether a certain activity *send confirmation* receipt must always be followed by *retrieve missing data* [24]. The event logs' most important characteristics can be found in Table 1. Next to the number of traces in both train and test log, the minimum, maximum and median length of the traces can be found as well, together with the truncation length (prefixes longer than this length are not to be used). This can be due to computational considerations (cut off at 40 events) or earlier because the trace has reached all events determining its outcome. Also mentioned are the positive class ratio, $R(+)$ in both training and test set.

Table 1. An overview of the characteristics of the data sets used.

Dataset	Min Len	Med Len	Max Len	Trunc. Len	#Train	#Test	$R(+)$ Train	$R(+)$ Test
2011_1	1	25	1814	36	912	228	0.38	0.48
2011_2	1	54.5	1814	40	912	228	0.81	0.66
2011_3	1	21	1368	31	896	225	0.20	0.36
2011_4	1	44	1432	40	912	228	0.25	0.39
2015_1	2	42	101	40	555	140	0.22	0.26
2015_2	1	55	132	40	602	151	0.20	0.17
2015_3	3	42	124	40	1062	266	0.17	0.25
2015_4	1	42	82	40	460	116	0.17	0.13
2015_5	5	50	134	40	840	211	0.32	0.26

5.3   Encoding and Hyperparameters

The prepossessing pipeline of the XGBoost model is based on previous work discussing different machine learning approaches [24]. The adjustments to the preprocessing pipeline to use the LSTM model are taken from [20]. To ensure proper training, some hyperparameters have to be carefully selected. For this purpose, we have done a hyperparameters search for each of the variations (different label flip ratios) of each log, and this for each different model (using different loss functions). The hyperparameter selection is performed with the use of hyperopt. For the LSTM models these are the *size* of the LSTM hidden layers, the *batch size dropout rate*, *learning rate* and *optimizer* (*Adam, Nadam, SGD* or *RMSprop*) used during training. For the XGB models these are *subsample*, *maximum tree depth*, *colsample bytree*, *minimum child weight* and the *learning rate*. The XGB models also use the *aggregation* encoding setting to encode the features of a prefix, taken over from [24]. Although this sequence encoding mechanism ignores the order of the traces, the study of k [24] shows that it works best for our selected data sets (and similar pipeline). For the LSTM models, the features are encoded in an embedding layer. The rest of the model consists of two bidirectional recurrent layers, with a dense output layer.

6   Experimental Evaluation

6.1   Experiment 1

The AUC on the independent test set is assessed for each of the models trained on the training logs with different ratios of flipping the positive examples. The results can be found in Table 2 and, as expected, overall we can see a decreasing trend in AUC when adding more and more label flips to the training set. What stands out is the relative bad AUC of the LSTM model as compared to the XGB. The decrease in AUC when adding positive label flips to the training set, often also seems sharper and more volatile (not always decreasing when more label flips are added) for the LSTM classifiers. The LSTM classifier trained on the original '*bpic_2011_3*' training set seems to score a particularly low score, and

Table 2. AUC on an untouched test set for XGB and LSTM models, trained on training logs with different amounts of label flips.

Dataset	Method	Flip Ratio			
		0%	25%	50%	75%
bpic2011_1	LSTM	0.891	0.514	0.667	0.509
bpic2011_1	XGB	0.944	0.867	0.805	0.751
bpic2011_2	LSTM	0.882	0.520	0.783	0.494
bpic2011_2	XGB	0.972	0.962	0.905	0.785
bpic2011_3	LSTM	0.680	0.863	0.755	0.831
bpic2011_3	XGB	0.989	0.982	0.803	0.905
bpic2011_4	LSTM	0.873	0.680	0.680	0.736
bpic2011_4	XGB	0.865	0.855	0.813	0.720
bpic2015_1	LSTM	0.885	0.706	0.712	0.579
bpic2015_1	XGB	0.917	0.919	0.904	0.761
bpic2015_2	LSTM	0.937	0.854	0.803	0.807
bpic2015_2	XGB	0.947	0.952	0.914	0.909
bpic2015_3	LSTM	0.878	0.673	0.694	0.624
bpic2015_3	XGB	0.962	0.941	0.942	0.930
bpic2015_4	LSTM	0.858	0.784	0.715	0.465
bpic2015_4	XGB	0.917	0.898	0.837	0.847
bpic2015_5	LSTM	0.916	0.757	0.759	0.667
bpic2015_5	XGB	0.944	0.939	0.907	0.813

definitely stands out as an outlier. Another remarkable example can be found for data set 'bpic_2015_2', and 'bpic_2015_3', for which the relatively limited AUC decrease (for the XGB model) might be partially explained by this data set containing a lot of longer traces. The AUC results for the XGBoost model of [24] show that predictions for prefixes longer than length 15 are all almost 1. Intuitively, this boils down to the fact that the model is almost certain of the label prediction for prefixes with a minimal length of 15. In addition, the prefix log of the test set contains 63% prefixes of size larger or equal to 15, at which point the XGB model already has almost perfect predictions, such that the influence of the data flips in the training set has less influence on the overall AUC score. This is however only a partial explanation since it would not explain an actual increase of the XGB test performance when training on the training data with 25% of the positive labels flipped as compared to a model trained on the untouched training set. Possibly effects like the test set having a lower positive label ratio than the training set, or other data set-specific characteristics, might provide some extra explanation. Overall, we can confirm Hypothesis 1, however, the extent (and volatility) of the decrease can still be process dependent, or might even depend on which specific cases have a missing positive label.

6.2   Experiment 2

As mentioned earlier, in a second experiment we introduce the models using the *uPU* and *nnPU* loss functions, next to those using binary cross entropy (*CE*). We discard the original logs and only look at the logs for which positive labels have been flipped. The results of these experiments can be found in Table 3. Overall, an uplift can be seen in using the *nnPU* loss function over the *BCE*, for both LSTM and XGB. However, this is not always the case and the effectiveness of using PU learning seems to be log-dependent. Standing out again in the event log '*bpic_ 2015_ 2*', for which the *nnPU* function seems not to be effective (even

Table 3. AUC on an untouched test set for models trained with different loss functions on training logs with different amounts of label flips.

Dataset	Flip	LSTM			XGB		
		CE	nnPU	uPU	CE	nnPU	uPU
bpic2011_1	25%	0.514	**0.818**	**0.818**	0.867	**0.910**	0.897
bpic2011_1	50%	0.667	**0.736**	0.565	0.805	**0.889**	0.800
bpic2011_1	75%	0.509	0.505	**0.727**	0.751	**0.801**	0.684
bpic2011_2	25%	0.520	**0.752**	0.723	0.962	**0.963**	0.921
bpic2011_2	50%	0.783	**0.820**	0.662	0.905	0.922	**0.942**
bpic2011_2	75%	0.494	0.530	**0.612**	0.785	**0.827**	0.545
bpic2011_3	25%	**0.863**	0.838	0.750	0.982	0.975	**0.987**
bpic2011_3	50%	0.755	**0.773**	0.687	0.803	**0.925**	0.831
bpic2011_3	75%	**0.831**	0.779	0.707	0.905	**0.931**	0.911
bpic2011_4	25%	0.680	0.773	**0.775**	0.855	**0.868**	0.861
bpic2011_4	50%	0.680	**0.784**	0.734	**0.813**	0.812	0.718
bpic2011_4	75%	0.736	0.694	**0.840**	0.720	**0.797**	0.729
bpic2015_1	25%	0.706	0.804	**0.817**	**0.919**	0.916	0.917
bpic2015_1	50%	0.712	**0.803**	0.663	0.904	**0.918**	0.865
bpic2015_1	75%	0.579	0.609	**0.638**	0.761	0.631	**0.774**
bpic2015_2	25%	**0.854**	0.486	0.839	**0.952**	0.949	0.945
bpic2015_2	50%	0.803	0.594	**0.855**	**0.914**	0.902	0.867
bpic2015_2	75%	**0.807**	0.742	0.653	**0.909**	0.858	0.821
bpic2015_3	25%	0.673	**0.777**	0.592	0.941	**0.955**	0.947
bpic2015_3	50%	0.694	**0.715**	0.628	**0.942**	**0.942**	0.934
bpic2015_3	75%	0.624	**0.835**	0.583	**0.930**	0.904	**0.930**
bpic2015_4	25%	0.784	**0.821**	0.801	0.898	0.898	**0.923**
bpic2015_4	50%	**0.715**	0.615	0.678	0.837	**0.886**	0.844
bpic2015_4	75%	0.465	**0.664**	0.598	**0.847**	0.835	0.839
bpic2015_5	25%	**0.757**	0.710	0.684	**0.939**	0.937	0.924
bpic2015_5	50%	**0.759**	0.755	0.693	0.907	**0.921**	0.912
bpic2015_5	75%	0.667	**0.680**	0.576	0.813	**0.837**	0.777

very flawed in the LSTM's case). This event log also showed only slight decreases in AUC when adding the label flips. Overall, using the $nnPU$ loss function seems to lead to better scores than the uPU. Also in OOPPM the possibly negative risk values the uPU loss function can obtain, seem to have a negative impact on the learning. Depending on the process in question, using the $nnPU$ loss function seems to be able to increase the real performance of a classifier, so Hypothesis 2 can be (partially) confirmed. Further research will be needed to understand when and why PU learning seems (not) to work well in OOPPM.

7   Conclusion and Future Work

In this work, we have introduced OOPPM models to a setting where our training log consists of positive and unlabelled traces. This kind of situation might arise when the labelling of your positive cases is uncertain, e.g. when it is hard for the process owner to obtain all the information or be sure. A key example application is fraud detection, but also in other areas, obtaining accurate labels for all cases might be costly or even impossible, such as labels based on customer feedback or labels to be obtained from other parties collaborating in a multi-organisational business process. By training different LSTM and XGB models on different variations of an event log, each time with an increasing number of the positively labelled traces' label flipped to negative (and therefore changing the negative label to unlabelled), a drop in the classifiers' performance could be noticed, hereby confirming Hypothesis 1. Furthermore, we investigated the potential use of loss functions from the field of PU learning to mitigate this issue and found that generally, on our example event logs, a model trained with the $nnPU$ loss function would score higher in a situation where the training data had traces' positive labels flipped. This was generally true, but not for all event logs, so further investigations and fine-tuning might be interesting when applying this to data from other processes. This paper opens up a door for future research on OOPPM in positive and unlabelled settings.

In future work, a more extensive experiment with more event logs could be performed. Furthermore, creating multiple variations of the log for each random flip ratio, as well as flipping labels of examples closer or further from the decision boundary might have an impact. It would also be interesting to test this setup in data for which we know the labelling is uncertain by itself, in contrast to doing the ratio flips ourselves. One other limitation of this work is that our loss functions rely on knowing the *class prior*, and for this, we have used the flip ratio as an input. Because we purely wanted to investigate the potential use of the PU loss function (and because the class prior was still not the exact class prior of the training set), this was deemed acceptable. However, in future work, it might be interesting to investigate the impact of using different class prior values (or using class priors derived from different samples). A setting with 0% of the cases flipped has been excluded from experiment 2 since there would be little effect in changing the loss function (as the flip ratio was given). In future experiments on the sensitivity of having an (incorrect) class prior, this setting could be added, however. Other future work on dealing with unreliable negative labels could be found in investigating options besides altering the loss function. The process behaviour itself may also reveal valuable information concerning which negative labels can be considered more certain.

References

1. Bekker, J., Davis, J.: Learning from positive and unlabeled data: a survey. Mach. Learn. **109**(4), 719–760 (2020). https://doi.org/10.1007/s10994-020-05877-5
2. Bekker, J., Robberechts, P., Davis, J.: Beyond the selected completely at random assumption for learning from positive and unlabeled data. In: Brefeld, U., Fromont, E., Hotho, A., Knobbe, A., Maathuis, M., Robardet, C. (eds.) ECML PKDD 2019. LNCS (LNAI), vol. 11907, pp. 71–85. Springer, Cham (2020). https://doi.org/10. 1007/978-3-030-46147-8_5
3. Chen, T., Guestrin, C.: XGBoost: a scalable tree boosting system. In: Proceedings of the 22nd ACM SIGKDD International Conference on Knowledge Discovery and Data Mining, KDD 2016, pp. 785–794. Association for Computing Machinery, New York (2016). https://doi.org/10.1145/2939672.2939785
4. Di Francescomarino, C., Dumas, M., Maggi, F.M., Teinemaa, I.: Clustering-based predictive process monitoring. IEEE Trans. Serv. Comput. **12**(6), 896–909 (2019). https://doi.org/10.1109/TSC.2016.2645153
5. van Dongen, B.B.: BPI Challenge 2015 (2015). https://doi.org/10.4121/uuid: 31a308ef-c844-48da-948c-305d167a0ec1. https://data.4tu.nl/collections/BPI_ Challenge_2015/5065424/1
6. van Dongen, B.: Real-life event logs - Hospital log (2011). https://doi.org/10.4121/ uuid:d9769f3d-0ab0-4fb8-803b-0d1120ffcf54. https://data.4tu.nl/articles/dataset/ Real-life_event_logs_-_Hospital_log/12716513
7. Du Plessis, M., Niu, G., Sugiyama, M.: Convex formulation for learning from positive and unlabeled data. In: International Conference on Machine Learning, pp. 1386–1394. PMLR (2015)
8. Folino, F., Folino, G., Guarascio, M., Pontieri, L.: Semi-supervised discovery of DNN-based outcome predictors from scarcely-labeled process logs. Bus. Inf. Syst. Eng. (2022). https://doi.org/10.1007/s12599-022-00749-9
9. Hochreiter, S., Schmidhuber, J.: Long short-term memory. Neural Comput. **9**(8), 1735–1780 (1997)
10. Jaskie, K., Spanias, A.: Positive and unlabeled learning algorithms and applications: a survey. In: 2019 10th International Conference on Information, Intelligence, Systems and Applications (IISA), pp. 1–8 (2019). https://doi.org/10.1109/IISA. 2019.8900698
11. Kiryo, R., Niu, G., Du Plessis, M.C., Sugiyama, M.: Positive-unlabeled learning with non-negative risk estimator. In: Advances in Neural Information Processing Systems, vol. 30 (2017)
12. Kratsch, W., Manderscheid, J., Röglinger, M., Seyfried, J.: Machine learning in business process monitoring: a comparison of deep learning and classical approaches used for outcome prediction. Bus. Inf. Syst. Eng. **63**(3), 261–276 (2021)
13. Leontjeva, A., Conforti, R., Di Francescomarino, C., Dumas, M., Maggi, F.M.: Complex symbolic sequence encodings for predictive monitoring of business processes. In: Motahari-Nezhad, H.R., Recker, J., Weidlich, M. (eds.) BPM 2015. LNCS, vol. 9253, pp. 297–313. Springer, Cham (2015). https://doi.org/10.1007/ 978-3-319-23063-4_21

14. Martin, N.: Data quality in process mining. In: Fernandez-Llatas, C. (ed.) Interactive Process Mining in Healthcare. HI, pp. 53–79. Springer, Cham (2021). https://doi.org/10.1007/978-3-030-53993-1_5

15. Neu, D.A., Lahann, J., Fettke, P.: A systematic literature review on state-of-the-art deep learning methods for process prediction. Artif. Intell. Rev. **55**, 801–827 (2021). https://doi.org/10.1007/s10462-021-09960-8

16. Pasquadibisceglie, V., Appice, A., Castellano, G., Malerba, D.: Using convolutional neural networks for predictive process analytics. In: 2019 International Conference on Process Mining (ICPM), pp. 129–136. IEEE (2019)

17. Pauwels, S., Calders, T.: Incremental predictive process monitoring: the next activity case. In: Polyvyanyy, A., Wynn, M.T., Van Looy, A., Reichert, M. (eds.) BPM 2021. LNCS, vol. 12875, pp. 123–140. Springer, Cham (2021). https://doi.org/10.1007/978-3-030-85469-0_10

18. Rama-Maneiro, E., Vidal, J., Lama, M.: Deep learning for predictive business process monitoring: review and benchmark. IEEE Trans. Serv. Comput. (2021)

19. Rizzi, W., Di Francescomarino, C., Ghidini, C., Maggi, F.M.: How do I update my model? On the resilience of predictive process monitoring models to change. Knowl. Inf. Syst. **64**(5), 1385–1416 (2022)

20. Stevens, A., De Smedt, J., Peeperkorn, J.: Quantifying explainability in outcome-oriented predictive process monitoring. In: Munoz-Gama, J., Lu, X. (eds.) ICPM 2021. LNBIP, vol. 433, pp. 194–206. Springer, Cham (2022). https://doi.org/10.1007/978-3-030-98581-3_15

21. Su, G., Chen, W., Xu, M.: Positive-unlabeled learning from imbalanced data. In: IJCAI, pp. 2995–3001 (2021)

22. Tax, N., Verenich, I., La Rosa, M., Dumas, M.: Predictive business process monitoring with LSTM neural networks. In: Dubois, E., Pohl, K. (eds.) CAiSE 2017. LNCS, vol. 10253, pp. 477–492. Springer, Cham (2017). https://doi.org/10.1007/978-3-319-59536-8_30

23. Taymouri, F., Rosa, M.L., Erfani, S., Bozorgi, Z.D., Verenich, I.: Predictive business process monitoring via generative adversarial nets: the case of next event prediction. In: Fahland, D., Ghidini, C., Becker, J., Dumas, M. (eds.) BPM 2020. LNCS, vol. 12168, pp. 237–256. Springer, Cham (2020). https://doi.org/10.1007/978-3-030-58666-9_14

24. Teinemaa, I., Dumas, M., Rosa, M.L., Maggi, F.M.: Outcome-oriented predictive process monitoring: review and benchmark. ACM Trans. Knowl. Discov. Data **13**(2) (2019). https://doi.org/10.1145/3301300

25. Verenich, I., Dumas, M., Rosa, M.L., Maggi, F.M., Teinemaa, I.: Survey and cross-benchmark comparison of remaining time prediction methods in business process monitoring. ACM Trans. Intell. Syst. Technol. (TIST) **10**(4), 1–34 (2019)

26. Wang, H., Wang, S.: Mining incomplete survey data through classification. Knowl. Inf. Syst. **24**, 221–233 (2010). https://doi.org/10.1007/s10115-009-0245-8

27. Wu, M., Pan, S., Du, L., Tsang, I., Zhu, X., Du, B.: Long-short distance aggregation networks for positive unlabeled graph learning. In: Proceedings of the 28th ACM International Conference on Information and Knowledge Management, pp. 2157–2160 (2019)

Clustering Analysis and Frequent Pattern Mining for Process Profile Analysis: An Exploratory Study for Object-Centric Event Logs

Elio Ribeiro Faria Junior[1,2]([✉]) [iD], Thais Rodrigues Neubauer[1] [iD],
Marcelo Fantinato[1] [iD], and Sarajane Marques Peres[1] [iD]

[1] Universidade de São Paulo, São Paulo, SP 03828-000, Brazil
{elioribeirofaria,thais.neubauer,m.fantinato,sarajane}@usp.br
[2] Universidade do Contestado, Mafra, SC 89300-000, Brazil

Abstract. Object-centric event log is a format for properly organizing information from different views of a business process into an event log. The novelty in such a format is the association of events with objects, which allows different notions of cases to be analyzed. The addition of new features has brought an increase in complexity. Clustering analysis can ease this complexity by enabling the analysis to be guided by process behaviour profiles. However, identifying which features describe the singularity of each profile is a challenge. In this paper, we present an exploratory study in which we mine frequent patterns on top of clustering analysis as a mechanism for profile characterization. In our study, clustering analysis is applied in a trace clustering fashion over a vector representation for a flattened event log extracted from an object-centric event log, using a unique case notion. Then, frequent patterns are discovered in the event sublogs associated with clusters and organized according to that original object-centric event log. The results obtained in preliminary experiments show association rules reveal more evident behaviours in certain profiles. Despite the process underlying each cluster may contain the same elements (activities and transitions), the behaviour trends show the relationships between such elements are supposed to be different. The observations depicted in our analysis make room to search for subtler knowledge about the business process under scrutiny.

Keywords: Object-centric event log · Process mining · Trace clustering · Association rules

1 Introduction

Process mining aims to discover knowledge about how business processes actually occur [1]. This knowledge is primarily revealed by process model discovery and conformance checking techniques but can also come from modeling descriptive or predictive tasks. Once discovered, the knowledge is used for process improvement, through optimization of procedures in the organizations proposed either via human decisions or via automated prescriptive analysis.

M. Montali et al. (Eds.): ICPM 2022 Workshops, LNBIP 468, pp. 269–281, 2023.
https://doi.org/10.1007/978-3-031-27815-0_20

For about 20 years, the main input for process mining was event logs derived from a single business process notion, herein called traditional event logs. For instance, in an ITIL framework context, one would only consider events related to activities in the "incident" life cycle, leaving out the life cycle of a "problem" to which the incident relates. Recently, the Process and Data Science Group from RWTH Aachen University [8] proposed a new event log format for recording events related to the life cycle of over one process notion. The new format is called object-centric event log (OCEL). The use of this format is expanding rapidly due to scientific community efforts to adapt process mining techniques to work with it [2–4]. One challenge brought by this format is how to overcome the increase in complexity it causes. Spaghetti-style process models [1] are even more often obtained from OCEL-type event logs.

One way used in process mining with traditional event logs to deal with process model complexity is to cluster process instances. Through clustering analysis [6,14], the discovered process behaviour profiles provide knowledge about process particularities that simplifies subsequent applications of process mining techniques. For a proper profile analysis, the characterization of each profile is an important step that can be conducted by mining frequent patterns [10] existing in each profile or subset of profiles. In this paper, we describe an exploratory study consisted of applying clustering analysis followed by frequent pattern mining to facilitate the analysis of processes related to OCEL-type event logs. Even though the study was carried out on a synthetic and relatively simple event log, the results show the usefulness of the applied approach. The feasibility was also proved since the results brought knowledge for profile characterization in a semi-automated way – a business expert is required to extract semantic information from the frequently mined patterns. To the best of our knowledge, there is only one recent work [9] related to clustering analysis in OCEL-type event logs. In that work, the authors present a clustering strategy considering control-flow information and attributes values, while our approach focus on activities and transition occurrences. Besides, our approach goes beyond the discovery of clusters and presents a semi-automated way of characterizing them, while in [9] the authors present process models discovered upon clusters for visual analysis purposes. Both studies apply cluster analysis to flattened event logs, derived from different OCEL-type event logs, and present statistics that, although distinct, address the simplification provided by the resulting clusters.

This paper is organized as follows: Sect. 2 presents theoretical background on OCEL, clustering analysis and frequent pattern mining; Sect. 3 provides information on our exploratory study; Sect. 4 discusses the results related to cluster analysis, and the knowledge extracted from the mined frequent patterns; Sect. 5 resumes the contribution of our paper and highlights the research avenues raised from the exploratory study.

2   Theoretical Background

This section summarizes the theoretical concepts used in the exploratory study.

2.1 Object-Centric Event Logs

The process mining field aims to explore the knowledge latent to an event log generated from a business process execution. A traditional event log, as established by van der Aalst [1], contains data about events arising from the execution of activities of a specific *business case*. For example, an event log may concern the life cycle of purchase orders in an e-commerce system, while another event log concentrates data on the life cycle of deliveries of products purchased in this system. Therefore, each of these event logs assumes a *case notion*. However, the analysis provided by each of these event logs does not consider these life cycles are related, and a phenomenon observed in one life cycle may be because of facts occurred in the other life cycle. To overcome this limited and possibly incomplete analysis, the object-centric event logs were introduced [8]. In this new paradigm, multiple notions of cases are represented with information about the relationship between events and objects (e.g., orders, products, deliveries, etc.). According to van der Aalst [1] and van der Aalst and Berti [2], traditional event logs and object-centric event logs are defined as follows:

▷ *a traditional event log L is a set of cases, or process instances, $L \subseteq C$, being C a universe of cases with respect to a unique business case notion. Cases may be characterized by descriptive attributes, among which one is mandatory - the trace. A trace corresponds to a finite sequence of events $\sigma \in \mathcal{E}^*$, being $\mathcal{E}^*$ a non-empty universe of events. An event e is the occurrence of a process activity at a given time. Events may be characterized by attributes such as timestamp, activity label, resource, cost, etc. An event appears at most once in L.*

▷ *a object-centric event log L_{oc} is a set of events $e_{oc} \in \mathcal{E}_{oc}$ partially ordered in time, such that $e_{oc} = $ (ei, act, time, omap, vmap), and ei is an event identifier, act is an activity name, time is a timestamp, omap is a mapping indicating which object is included for each type of object in L_{oc} and vmap is a mapping indicating the values assumed by each attribute in L_{oc}. Although a L_{oc} is partially ordered, for practical effects, a time-based total order is applied[1].*

The diversity of information in the object-centric event log increases the complexity of the associated analyses, prompting the search for strategies to simplify the event log without losing relevant information. In [2], the authors present a suitable way of filtering the object-centric event log. In the proposed strategy, the authors suggest filtering out specific "activity - object type" combinations. Following this strategy, chosen objects and activities related to them are suppressed from the log without harmful effect to activities and relationships referring to other types of objects. Consequently, the event log can be reduced in relation to the number of objects it contains, or events related to infrequent activities can be deleted. Simplification by "activity - object type" combinations filtering is a convenient alternative to flattening the log or to separately analyzing each type of object. However, selecting the "activity - object type" combination to be filtered requires *a priori* knowledge of what is relevant for the intended analysis.

---

[1] There are definitions that assume the total order ($\leq$) for L_{oc} [4,9]. Such a definition states that L_{oc} is a tuple of events with total order.

2.2 Clustering Analysis

The task of clustering data is defined as a separation of data points into clusters according to a similarity metric. The goal is to allocate similar data points to the same cluster and dissimilar data points into different clusters. Although there are methods as density criterion or mutual information, distance measures based on the values of the features describing the data points are commonly used as similarity metrics [10]. The resolution of clustering tasks reveals descriptive information about the data set under analysis in an unsupervised form.

An assortment of clustering algorithms can be found in the literature. One category of fundamental clustering methods is the hierarchical methods, which partition the data into groups at different levels, as in a hierarchy. The provided hierarchical representation of the data points enables identifying that groups of a certain level can be further divided into respective subgroups. Hierarchical clustering methods are divided into agglomerative and divisive. We are interested in the first one, which is described as follows [10]:

▷ *the agglomerative clustering method starts at a level in which each data point forms a cluster and in each next level, the clusters are merged according to a similarity metric; by the end, it reaches a level in which there is only one cluster compound by all the data points. This method relies on measuring the distance being clusters to decide when to merge. The way of comparing the distance between clusters has to be defined, as a cluster is a set of objects. Possible ways are: single-linkage; complete-linkage; average-linkage; Ward's method.*

In process mining, we have observed applications of clustering analysis in the form of trace clustering [6,14]. Trace clustering strategies can be divided into three non-excluding categories [11]: *trace sequence similarity, model similarity* and *feature vector similarity*. We are interested in the latter strategy:

▷ *trace clustering based on feature vector similarity relies on mapping of traces to a vector space by extracting features from a specific profile (such as activity, transition, performance or resource profile [6]). Clustering algorithms are applied on such vector representation to analyze similarities and group data points.*

2.3 Frequent Pattern Mining

Patterns such as itemsets, subsequences, substructures and association or correlation rules that frequently appear in a data set are called *frequent patterns*. Frequent pattern mining is a data mining task whose aim is to mine relationships in a given data set [10]. Mining frequent itemsets enables the discovery of associations and correlations among data. In this paper, we are interested in mining itemsets and association rules:

▷ *an itemset refers to a set of items. An itemset that contains k items is a k-itemset. When an itemset is frequent in a given data set, it can be called frequent itemset. If we have a frequent 2-itemset as {milk, bread}, it means that such itemset is frequent in the corresponding data set.*

▷ *an* <u>*association rule*</u> *defines an if-then association between itemsets organized in the antecedent and the consequent of such rule. The rule* milk ⇒ bread *means that if a customer buys milk then they also buy bread, frequently.*

To identify which of the mined patterns are useful, the support is defined as an interestingness measure. The support informs the percentage of all the existing transactions in which the pattern occurred. For association rules, on top of the support measure, the confidence measure is defined as an interestingness measure to bring how certain is the rule. For instance, for the association rule *milk* ⇒ *bread*: a support of 10% means that this rule occurs in 10% of the transactions (e.g., all the sold baskets); and a confidence of 60% means that in 60% of the baskets in which there is milk, there is also bread. Typically, domain experts[2] define a minimum support threshold and a minimum confidence threshold to filter the useful rules [10]. The classic algorithm *Apriori* [5] is widely used for mining frequent patterns. This algorithm is based on the item's anti-monotonicity property. In the first phase of this algorithm, such a property allows an efficient implementation for the frequent itemsets search. Frequent itemsets will compose association rules mined in its second phase.

3   Exploratory Study

Figure 1 depicts the sequence of procedures performed in the exploratory study, the resources applied (material and human resources) and the artifacts created during the study. This exploratory study comprises two phases: in the former, clustering analysis is used to discover existing behaviour profiles in the business process under scrutiny; in the latter, discovered profiles are explored through frequent pattern analysis, and the itemsets and association rules identified as useful and meaningful are used to provide knowledge about the profiles.

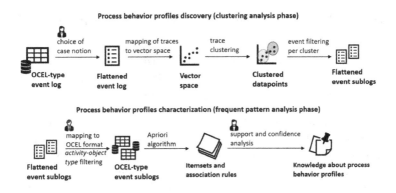

Fig. 1. Workflow followed in the exploratory study

---

[2] In this paper, the authors the authors played the role of domain experts.

3.1   Event Log

The input to our study is a synthetic object-centric event log referring to an "order management" process [8,9].[3,4] The process underlying the event log performs 11 activities on five types of objects (*orders, items, packages, customers,* and *products*). The execution registered in the event log comprises 22,367 events and 11,522 objects. Figure 2 represents an excerpt of this event log with all objects and attributes. We did not use the objects *product* and *customer*, and the attributes *price* and *weight*, since they do not represent an opportunity for control-flow perspective of analysis[5].

	attributes		objects				attributes		
Activity	**Timestamp**	**Order**	**Item**	**Package**	**Product**	**Customer**	**Weight**	**Price**	attribute names
place order	2019-05-20T09:07:47	{990001}	{880001, 880004, 880003, 880002}	{Ø}	{Echo Studio, Echo Show 8, Fire Stick 4K,	{Marco Pegoraro}	3.52	524.96	attribute values
place order	2019-05-20T10:35:21	{990002}	{880008, 880005, 880006, 880007}	{Ø}	{Kindle, iPad Air, iPad, MacBook Air}	{Gyunam Park}	2.656	3255.99	
pick item	2019-05-20T10:38:17	{990002}	{880006}	{Ø}	{Kindle}	{Gyunam Park}	0.483	79.99	
confirm order	2019-05-20T11:13:54	{990001}	{880001, 880004, 880003, 880002}	{Ø}	{Echo Studio, Echo Show 8, Fire Stick 4K,	{Marco Pegoraro}	3.52	524.96	
pick item	2019-05-20T11:20:13	{990001}	{880002}	{Ø}	{Fire Stick 4K}	{Marco Pegoraro}	0.28	89.99	

Fig. 2. "Order management" object-centric event log excerpt

Figure 3 shows the process model discovered from the filtered "order management" event log, represented by a direct flow graph. Activities and transitions are colored according to the object they refer to: green refers to object *order*; pink refers to object *item*; red refers to object *package*. Although a visual analysis of the process behaviour is possible in this case, it can be tiring and imprecise, especially when more complex processes are analyzed, justifying the application of strategies to simplify the knowledge discovery on the process under scrutiny.

3.2   Process Behaviour Profiles Discovery: Clustering Analysis Phase

The first phase of our study comprises the following procedures: choice of case notion; mapping traces to vector space; trace clustering; and event filtering per cluster. All procedures are described in this section.

Choice of Case Notion: The profile discovery proposed relies on a trace-based clustering analysis. Thus, we need to define a case notion (a *business case notion,* cf. Sect. 2.1) for establishing traces and create a flattened event log. We applied the case notion referring to the object type *order*. Since this object type is the only one related to all events in the event log, choosing such an object as case notion allowed that profile discovery considered information of all events.

---

[3] We used the JSON-OCEL serialized representation of the event log.

[4] http://ocel-standard.org/1.0/running-example.jsonocel.zip.

[5] Refer to [1] for information about control-flow perspective of analysis.

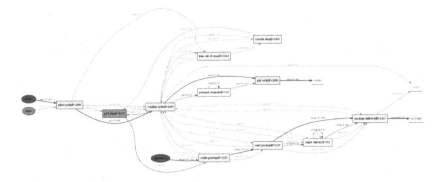

Fig. 3. Process model discovered from the filtered "order management" event log (process model discovered by using the package PM4Py for Python [7])

Mapping of Traces to Vector Space: We represented traces in a vector space using two sets of descriptive features: the occurrence of activities in a trace (activity-based representation); the occurrence of transitions in a trace (transition-based representation). The former does not consider the order in which activities occur, but provides a representation that incorporates similarity in the resulting data points (e.g., traces with the same activities but not the same execution order are mapped to the same data point). The latter represents the partial order in which activities occur, emphasizing a process-aware similarity analysis.

Trace Clustering: Trace clustering was applied using an agglomerative hierarchical clustering algorithm [13][6] with Ward as the linkage method, Euclidean distance as similarity metric and number of clusters set to six. The authors' experience in trace clustering showed the Ward's method allows finding clusters with slightly higher quality than using other linkage methods. The Euclidean distance was chosen as the first option for exploration in this study. We tested the number of clusters ranging from three to six. A profile associated with the "value chain" of the business process under scrutiny was found with five and six clusters considering the activity-occurrence representation; the number six was chosen to maximize the number of profiles for analysis. The same number was used with transition-occurrence representation for the sake of uniformity.

Event Filtering Per Cluster: Once the trace clusters are built, we separate the events associated with each cluster into independent files, the flattened sublogs.

3.3   Process Behaviour Profiles Characterization: Frequent Pattern Analysis Phase

The second phase of our study comprises the following procedures: mapping to OCEL format and *activity-object type* filtering; Apriori algorithm application; and support and confidence analysis. All procedures are described in this section.

---

[6] sklearn.cluster.AgglomerativeClustering: https://scikit-learn.org/.

Mapping to OCEL Format and Activity-Object Type Filtering: Flattened sublogs must be mapped back into OCEL-type event sublogs considering both the notion of case previously chosen and the *activity-object type* filter that relates activities to object types appropriately as suggested in [2]. The selection of *activity-object type* combinations to be used requires a business process-oriented decision making, usually carried out by a business expert.

Apriori Algorithm: For discovery of frequent patterns, the classic Apriori algorithm[7] was applied on each OCEL-type event sublog, considering the activities and transitions associated with each object type (*order, item, package*) separately. 18 sets of itemsets and association rules were created (i.e. one set per cluster per object). The input to the algorithm is a matrix of occurrences of activities (or transitions) in the object-type life cycle. The Apriori algorithm runs were performed with *minimum support* = 0.05 (for both itemsets and association rules) and *minimum confidence* = 0.9 (such values were set by experimentation).

Support and Confidence Analysis: The frequent patterns for each of the six clusters were compared following a one-versus-all strategy. This strategy enables selecting patterns which differs one cluster from the other clusters. Then, the selected frequent patterns were (manually) analyzed to extract expert knowledge about the discovered process behaviour profiles.

4   Analysis of Results

The first phase of our study aimed to reveal process behaviour profiles that provide simpler contexts for analysis and knowledge discovery than the context provided by the full event log. Table 2 and Table 3 show descriptive statistics for supporting analysis about simplicity of the context referring to each discovered profile (i.e. each cluster), considering activity-based and transition-based representation for traces. The descriptive statistics for the full event log were presented in [2] and are reproduced here for comparison purposes (see Table 1). Statistics refers to the *average* and *maximum number* of objects per event[8]. In these tables, "O", "I" and "P" stand for *orders, items* and *packages* respectively.

The comparison of statistics shows clustering generates more simplified contexts in two aspects: some clusters represent process profiles in which certain objects do not appear related to events of certain activities (e.g., there are no items associated with the activity "item out of stock" in the process profile of the clusters *a1, a4* and *a5*, showing these profiles do not suffer from the problem of an item not being found in stock while an order is processed); the occurrence of a maximum number of objects related to events of certain activity is lower in certain process profiles (e.g., fewer items enter the orders allocated in cluster *a1*

---

[7] Package Mlxtend: https://rasbt.github.io/mlxtend/.

[8] The statistic *minimum number* was suppressed from the Tables 1, 2 and 3 for simplicity. *Minimum* number = 1 if *maximum* number ≥ 1, and = 0 otherwise.

Table 1. Descriptive statistics about the full event log [2].

Activities	O	I	P	Activities	O	I	P
Place order	1.0, 1	4.0 15	0.0 0				
Confirm order	1.0, 1	4.0 15	0.0 0	Pay order	1.0 1	4.0 15	0.0 0
Item out of stock	1.0, 1	1.0 1	0.0 0	Create package	3.2 9	6.2 22	1.0 1
Reorder item	1.0, 1	1.0 1	0.0 0	Send package	3.2 9	6.2 22	1.0 1
Pick item	1.0, 1	1.0 1	0.0 0	Failed delivery	3.2 8	6.0 18	1.0 1
Payment reminder	1.0, 1	4.2 14	0.0 0	Package delivered	3.2 9	6.2 22	1.0 1

and $t4$ - citing only two clusters). However, in general, the averages of objects per event increase, as the number of events present in the clusters decreases.

In the second phase, we mined and analyzed the frequent patterns to reveal knowledge about the process profiles, alleviating the need to discover and inspect process models related to each sublog. We organized the analyses considering the two matrices of occurrences used as input for the Alpha algorithm.

Matrix of Activity Occurrences: We identified 13 association rules not common to all clusters. All rules involved 1-itemsets , achieved maximum confidence and the itemsets allocated to their consequents have maximum support. Thus, the rules analysis was reduced to the analysis of the support of itemsets allocated to their antecedents. The relevant knowledge that characterizes the profiles are:

- payment reminders occur on all process instances in the profiles $a0$ and $a1$;
- delivery failures occur in part of the process instances in profiles $a0$, $a1$, $a2$ and $a5$, with emphasis on profile $a5$ in which $\approx 60\%$ of the process instances present the occurrence of such a problem;
- out-of-stock items are observed in $\approx 30\%$ of process instances in profiles $a0$, $a2$ and $a3$.

The discovered frequent patterns concern the occurrence of activities that indicate some kind of problem in the order history. None of such patterns were highlighted for the profile $a4$. All association rules highlighted to profile $a4$ achieve maximum support and maximum confidence and do not involve activities related to failures or out-of-stock items. In view of these findings, we deduced the profile $a4$ concerns the process instances that follow the process's "value chain", or follow behaviours very close to it. To validate the deduction, we discovered the process model associated with this profile (Fig. 4).

Matrix of Transition Occurrences: We identified 26 association rules not common to all clusters. All rules involved 1-itemsets, 17 rules achieved the maximum confidence, the minimum confidence achieved was 0.91, and in two rules the consequent is not composed by an itemset with maximum support. The relevant knowledge that characterize the profiles are:

Table 2. Descriptive statistics about profiles discovered upon activity-based representation for traces. Statistics showing simplification are in bold.

Activities	O	I	P	O	I	P	O	I	P
	Cluster a0			Cluster a1			Cluster a2		
Place order	1.0, 1	4.7, 14	0.0, 0	1.0, 1	**3.3, 7**	0.0, 0	1.0, 1	4.9, 15	0.0, 0
Confirm order	1.0, 1	4.7, 14	0.0, 0	1.0, 1	**3.3, 7**	0.0, 0	1.0, 1	4.9, 15	0.0, 0
Item out of stock	1.0, 1	1.0, 1	0.0, 0	**0.0, 0**	**0.0, 0**	0.0, 0	1.0, 1	1.0, 1	0.0, 0
Reorder item	1.0, 1	1.0, 1	0.0, 0	**0.0, 0**	**0.0, 0**	0.0, 0	1.0, 1	1.0, 1	0.0, 0
Pick item	1.0, 1	1.0, 1	0.0, 0	1.0, 1	1.0, 1	0.0, 0	1.0, 1	1.0, 1	0.0, 0
Payment reminder	1.0, 1	4.8, 14	0.0, 0	1.0, 1	3.3, **7**	0.0, 0	**0.0, 0**	**0.0, 0**	0.0, 0
Pay order	1.0, 1	4.7, 14	0.0, 0	1.0, 1	3.3, **7**	0.0, 0	1.0, 1	4.9, 15	0.0, 0
Create package	3.9, 9	7.0, 22	1.0, 1	3.9, 9	7.3, 20	1.0, 1	3.7, 9	6.6, 22	1.0, 1
Send package	3.9, 9	7.0, 22	1.0, 1	3.9, 9	7.3, 20	1.0, 1	3.7, 9	6.6, 22	1.0, 1
Failed delivery	3.8, 8	6.7, 18	1.0, 1	3.8, 8	7.2, 18	1.0, 1	3.2, 8	6.1, 18	1.0, 1
Package delivered	3.9, 9	7.0, 22	1.0, 1	3.9, 9	7.3, 20	1.0, 1	3.7, 9	6.6, 22	1.0, 1
	Cluster a3			Cluster a4			Cluster a5		
Place order	1.0, 1	4.4, 14	0.0, 0	1.0, 1	3.2, 9	0.0, 0	1.0, 1	**3.5, 10**	0.0, 0
Confirm order	1.0, 1	4.4, 14	0.0, 0	1.0, 1	3.2, 9	0.0, 0	1.0, 1	**3.5, 10**	0.0, 0
Item out of stock	1.0, 1	1.0, 1	0.0, 0	**0.0, 0**	**0.0, 0**	0.0, 0	**0.0, 0**	**0.0, 0**	0.0, 0
Reorder item	1.0, 1	1.0, 1	0.0, 0	**0.0, 0**	**0.0, 0**	0.0, 0	**0.0, 0**	**0.0, 0**	0.0, 0
Pick item	1.0, 1	1.0, 1	0.0, 0	1.0, 1	1.0, 1	0.0, 0	1.0, 1	1.0, 1	0.0, 0
Payment reminder	**0.0, 0**	**0.0, 0**	0.0, 0	**0.0, 0**	**0.0, 0**	0.0, 0	**0.0, 0**	**0.0, 0**	0.0, 0
Pay order	1.0, 1	4.4, 14	0.0, 0	1.0, 1	**3.2, 9**	0.0, 0	1.0, 1	**3.5, 10**	0.0, 0
Create package	3.6, 9	6.6, 22	1.0, 1	3.8, 9	7.2, 22	1.0, 1	3.9, 9	7.2, 21	1.0, 1
Send package	3.6, 9	6.6, 22	1.0, 1	3.8, 9	7.2, 22	1.0, 1	3.9, 9	7.2, 21	1.0, 1
Failed delivery	**0.0, 0**	**0.0, 0**	0.0, 0	**0.0, 0**	**0.0, 0**	0.0, 0	3.8, 8	7.1, 18	1.0, 1
Package delivered	3.6, 9	6.6, 22	1.0, 1	3.8, 9	7.2, 22	1.0, 1	3.9, 9	7.2, **21**	1.0, 1

- payment of orders without sending a reminder is a majority behaviour (occurs in ≈80% to ≈98% of process instances) in five profiles (*t0*, *t1*, *t2*, *t4* and *t5*);
- reminders before the payment of an order is made occur in ≈99% of process instances allocated to the profile *t3*;
- repeated payment reminders occur only in profile *t3* and represent ≈21% of the processes instances allocated in this profile;
- in the profiles *t0*, *t2*, *t3* and *t5*, there are orders (≈30%, 15%, 6% and 8% respectively) in which the observation related to out-of-stock items occurs after the order is confirmed;
- although not really significant (rule with support from ≈0.0 to ≈13%), delivery failures are pointed at least twice in process instances of four profiles (*t1*, *t2*, *t4* and *t5*);
- packages successfully delivered on the first attempt occur in process instances allocated in all profiles (in 71/74/76/80/83/88% of process instances allocated respectively to profiles *t1*, *t2*, *t5*, *t4*, *t0*, and *t3*).

Table 3. Descriptive statistics about profiles discovered upon transition-based representation for traces. Statistics showing simplification are in bold.

Activities	O	I	P	O	I	P	O	I	P
	Cluster t0			Cluster t1			Cluster t2		
Place order	1.0, 1	4.0, **14**	0.0, 0	1.0, 1	**3.7, 11**	0.0, 0	1.0, 1	5.1, 15	0.0, 0
Confirm order	1.0, 1	4.0, **14**	0.0, 0	1.0, 1	**3.7, 11**	0.0, 0	1.0, 1	5.1, 15	0.0, 0
Item out of stock	1.0, 1	1.0, 1	0.0, 0	1.0, 1	1.0, 1	0.0, 0	1.0, 1	1.0, 1	0.0, 0
Reorder item	1.0, 1	1.0, 1	0.0, 0	1.0, 1	1.0, 1	0.0, 0	1.0, 1	1.0, 1	0.0, 0
Pick item	1.0, 1	1.0, 1	0.0, 0	1.0, 1	1.0, 1	0.0, 0	1.0, 1	1.0, 1	0.0, 0
Payment reminder	1.0, 1	4.2, **14**	0.0, 0	1.0, 1	**3.7, 10**	0.0, 0	1.0, 1	5.1, **13**	0.0, 0
Pay order	1.0, 1	4.0, **14**	0.0, 0	1.0, 1	**3.7, 11**	0.0, 0	1.0, 1	5.1, **15**	0.0, 0
Create package	3.8, 9	6.8, 22	1.0, 1	3.7, 9	7.0, 22	1.0, 1	3.6, 9	6.6, 22	1.0, 1
Send package	3.8, 9	6.8, 22	1.0, 1	3.7, 9	7.0, 22	1.0, 1	3.6, 9	6.6, 22	1.0, 1
Failed delivery	3.7, **7**	**5.6, 17**	1.0, 1	3.7, 8	6.8, **17**	1.0, 1	3.4, 8	6.3, 18	1.0, 1
Package delivered	3.8, 9	6.8, 22	1.0, 1	3.7, 9	7.0, 22	1.0, 1	3.6, 9	6.6, 22	1.0, 1
	Cluster t3			Cluster t4			Cluster t5		
Place order	1.0, 1	**3.7, 11**	0.0, 0	1.0, 1	**3.1, 10**	0.0, 0	1.0, 1	**3.9, 13**	0.0, 0
Confirm order	1.0, 1	**3.7, 11**	0.0, 0	1.0, 1	**3.1, 10**	0.0, 0	1.0, 1	**3.9, 13**	0.0, 0
Item out of stock	1.0, 1	1.0, 1	0.0, 0	1.0, 1	1.0, 1	0.0, 0	1.0, 1	1.0, 1	0.0, 0
Reorder item	1.0, 1	1.0, 1	0.0, 0	1.0, 1	1.0, 1	0.0, 0	1.0, 1	1.0, 1	0.0, 0
Pick item	1.0, 1	1.0, 1	0.0, 0	1.0, 1	1.0, 1	0.0, 0	1.0, 1	1.0, 1	0.0, 0
Payment reminder	1.0, 1	**3.8, 11**	0.0, 0	1.0, 1	**3.5, 5**	0.0, 0	1.0, 1	6.0, **6**	0.0, 0
Pay order	1.0, 1	**3.7, 11**	0.0, 0	1.0, 1	**3.1, 10**	0.0, 0	1.0, 1	3.9, 13	0.0, 0
Create package	3.8, **8**	6.9, **20**	1.0, 1	4.0, 9	7.3, 22	1.0, 1	4.3, **8**	7.7, **21**	1.0, 1
Send package	3.8, **8**	6.9, **20**	1.0, 1	4.0, 9	7.3, 22	1.0, 1	4.3, **8**	7.7, **21**	1.0, 1
Failed delivery	3.5, **6**	6.3, **13**	1.0, 1	3.6, 8	6.8, 18	1.0, 1	4.2, **7**	7.7, **16**	1.0, 1
Package delivered	3.8, **8**	6.9, **20**	1.0, 1	4.0, 9	7.3, 22	1.0, 1	4.3, **8**	7.7, **21**	1.0, 1

5   Final Remarks

In this paper, we introduce an approach to simplify the context of analysis related to OCEL-type event logs and present an exploratory experiment performed on a synthetic event log. The preliminary results show the usefulness and feasibility of our approach. The approach is useful because it allows extracting knowledge capable of highlighting, in each profile, characteristics that can direct subsequent in-depth analyses. It is feasible because, even in a low-complexity event log with little potential for profiling, it was possible to find and characterize a set of profiles. However, this is an exploratory study limited mainly by the choice of some parameters, such as the business case notion, the similarity metric or the number of clusters. In addition, the experiment considered a single event log, which undermines both statistical and analytical generalizations. The execution of this study opened up research opportunities: extension of the frequent pattern mining to discover association rules that characterize profiles considering the relationship among the life cycles of different objects types; using of attributes referring to the business context and available in the OCEL-type event logs to

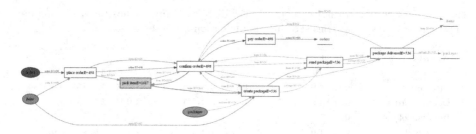

Fig. 4. Process model related to profile $a4$ involving the "value chain": place order, pick item, confirm order, pay order, create package, send package, package delivered.

enrich the relationships explored in the frequent pattern mining; adding frequent pattern mining outputs in tools for trace clustering visualization [12].

Acknowledgment. This study was partially supported by CAPES (Finance Code 001) and FAPESP (Process Number 2020/05248-4).

References

1. van der Aalst, W.M.P.: Process Mining - Data Science in Action. Springer, Heidelberg (2016). https://doi.org/10.1007/978-3-662-49851-4
2. van der Aalst, W.M.P., Berti, A.: Discovering object-centric petri nets. Fund. Inform. **175**(1–4), 1–40 (2020)
3. Aalst, W.M.P.: Object-centric process mining: dealing with divergence and convergence in event data. In: Ölveczky, P.C., Salaün, G. (eds.) SEFM 2019. LNCS, vol. 11724, pp. 3–25. Springer, Cham (2019). https://doi.org/10.1007/978-3-030-30446-1_1
4. Adams, J.N., Van Der Aalst, W.M.: Precision and fitness in object-centric process mining. In: Proceedings of the 3rd International Conference on Process Mining, pp. 128–135 (2021)
5. Agrawal, R., Srikant, R.: Fast algorithms for mining association rules in large databases. In: Proceedings of the 20th International Conference on Very Large Data Bases, pp. 487–499 (1994)
6. Appice, A., Malerba, D.: A co-training strategy for multiple view clustering in process mining. IEEE Trans. Serv. Comput. **9**, 832–845 (2016)
7. Berti, A., van Zelst, S.J., van der Aalst, W.M.: PM4Py web services: easy development, integration and deployment of process mining features in any application stack. In: International Conference on Business Process Managment (PhD/Demos) (2019)
8. Ghahfarokhi, A.F., Park, G., Berti, A., van der Aalst, W.M.P.: OCEL standard (2020). http://ocel-standard.org/
9. Ghahfarokhi, A.F., Akoochekian, F., Zandkarimi, F., van der Aalst, W.M.P.: Clustering object-centric event logs (2022). https://arxiv.org/abs/2207.12764
10. Han, J., Kamber, M., Pei, J.: Data Mining: Concepts and Techniques, 3rd edn. Morgan Kaufmann Publishers Inc., San Francisco (2011)
11. Lu, X.: Using behavioral context in process mining: exploration, preprocessing and analysis of event data. Ph.D. thesis, Eindhoven University of Technology (2018)

12. Neubauer, T.R., Sobrinho, G.P., Fantinato, M., Peres, S.M.: Visualization for enabling human-in-the-loop in trace clustering-based process mining tasks. In: 5th IEEE Workshop on Human-in-the-Loop Methods and Future of Work in BigData, pp. 3548–3556 (2021)
13. Pedregosa, F., et al.: Scikit-learn: machine learning in Python. J. Mach. Learn. Res. **12**, 2825–2830 (2011)
14. Song, M., Günther, C.W., van der Aalst, W.M.P.: Trace clustering in process mining. In: Ardagna, D., Mecella, M., Yang, J. (eds.) BPM 2008. LNBIP, vol. 17, pp. 109–120. Springer, Heidelberg (2009). https://doi.org/10.1007/978-3-642-00328-8_11

5th International Workshop on Process-Oriented Data Science for Healthcare (PODS4H'22)

Fifth International Workshop on Process-Oriented Data Science for Healthcare (PODS4H'22)

Data has become a highly valuable resource in today's world. The ultimate goal of data science techniques is not to collect more data, but to extract knowledge and valuable insights from existing data. To analyze and improve processes, event data is a key source of information. In recent years, a new discipline has emerged that combines traditional process analysis and data-centric analysis: Process-Oriented Data Science (PODS). The interdisciplinary nature of this new research area has resulted in its application to analyze processes in a wide range of different domains such as education, finance, and especially healthcare.

The International Workshop on Process-Oriented Data Science for Healthcare 2022 (PODS4H'22) provided a high-quality forum for interdisciplinary researchers and practitioners to exchange research findings and ideas on data-driven process analysis techniques and practices in healthcare. PODS4H research includes a variety of topics ranging from process mining techniques adapted for healthcare processes, to practical issues related to the implementation of PODS methodologies in healthcare organizations.

The fifth edition of the workshop was organized in conjunction with the International Conference on Process Mining in Bolzano (Italy). A novelty in this year's call for papers was that full papers could either be submitted as research papers or as case studies. While research papers had to focus on extending the state of the art of PODS4H research, case studies should focus on a practical application of PODS4H in a real-life context. In total, we received 19 full paper submissions, which were thoroughly reviewed by experts from our Program Committee such that each submission got three reviews. After the review process, 9 full papers were accepted. The distinction between research papers and case studies was also reflected in the accepted papers, which consisted of 5 research papers and 4 case studies. The research papers focused on a wide range of topics: integrating weighted violations in alignment-based conformance checking, discovering break behaviors, developing a taxonomy for synthetic data in healthcare, creating a semantic approach for multi-perspective event log generation, and establishing a method to generate event logs from MIMIC-IV. The case studies also considered a variety of healthcare-related problems and contexts: process modeling and conformance checking in a German hospital in a COVID-19 context, the early prediction of aftercare in a Dutch hospital, the prediction of care acuity in a Dutch hospital, and the investigation of the impact of COVID-19 on care pathways in a UK hospital. Besides the presentation of the full papers included in these proceedings, the workshop program also contained a poster session and a community discussion.

This edition of the workshop also included a Best Paper Award. The Best Paper Award of PODS4H'22 was given to Alistair Bullward, Abdulaziz Aljebreen, Alexander Coles, Ciarán McInerney, and Owen Johnson for their paper "Process Mining and Synthetic Health Data: Reflections and Lessons Learnt".

The PODS4H workshop is an initiative of the Process-Oriented Data Science for Healthcare Alliance (PODS4H Alliance) within the IEEE Task Force on Process Mining. The goal of the PODS4H Alliance is to promote awareness, research, development, and education regarding process-oriented data science in healthcare. For more information, we would like to refer the reader to our website www.pods4h.com.

The organizers would like to thank all the Program Committee members for their valuable work in reviewing the papers, as well as the ICPM 2022 workshop chairs and local organizers for supporting this successful event.

November 2022

Niels Martin
Carlos Fernandez-Llatas
Owen Johnson
Marcos Sepúlveda
Emmanuel Helm
Jorge Munoz-Gama

Organization

Workshop Chairs

Niels Martin — Hasselt University, Belgium
Carlos Fernandez-Llatas — Polytechnic University of Valencia, Spain
Owen Johnson — Leeds University, UK
Marcos Sepúlveda — Pontificia Universidad Católica de Chile, Chile
Emmanuel Helm — University of Applied Sciences Upper Austria, Austria
Jorge Munoz-Gama — Pontificia Universidad Católica de Chile, Chile

Program Committee

Davide Aloini — University of Pisa, Italy
Robert Andrews — Queensland University of Technology, Australia
Iris Beerepoot — Utrecht University, The Netherlands
Elisabetta Benevento — University of Pisa, Italy
Andrea Burattin — Technical University of Denmark, Denmark
Daniel Capurro — University of Melbourne, Australia
Marco Comuzzi — Ulsan National Institute of Science and Technology, South Korea
Benjamin Dalmas — Centre de Recherche Informatique de Montréal, Canada
Rene de la Fuente — Pontificia Universidad Católica de Chile, Chile
Claudio Di Ciccio — Sapienza University of Rome, Italy
Onur Dogan — Izmir Bakircay University, Turkey
Carlos Fernandez-Llatas — Polytechnic University of Valencia, Spain
Roberto Gatta — Università Cattolica S. Cuore, Italy
Emmanuel Helm — University of Applied Sciences Upper Austria, Austria
Owen Johnson — Leeds University, UK
Felix Mannhardt — Eindhoven University of Technology, The Netherlands
Ronny Mans — VitalHealth Software, The Netherlands
Mar Marcos — Universitat Jaume I, Spain

Weighted Violations in Alignment-Based Conformance Checking

Joscha Grüger[1,2]([envelope]) [ID], Tobias Geyer[2] [ID], Martin Kuhn[2] [ID],
Stephan A. Braun[3,4] [ID], and Ralph Bergmann[1,2] [ID]

[1] Business Information Systems II, University of Trier, Trier, Germany
grueger@uni-trier.de
[2] German Research Center for Artificial Intelligence (DFKI), Branch Trier,
Trier, Germany
[3] Department of Dermatology, University Hospital Münster, Münster, Germany
[4] Department of Dermatology, Heinrich Heine University, Düsseldorf, Germany

Abstract. Conformance checking is a process mining technique that
allows verifying the conformance of process instances to a given model.
Many conformance checking algorithms provide quantitative information
about the conformance of a process instance through metrics such as fitness. Fitness measures to what degree the model allows the behavior
observed in the event log. Conventional fitness does not consider the
individual severity of deviations. In cases where there are rules that are
more important to comply with than others, fitness consequently does
not take all factors into account. In the field of medicine, for example,
there are guideline recommendations for clinical treatment that have
information about their importance and soundness, making it essential
to distinguish between them. Therefore, we introduce an alignment-based
conformance checking approach that considers the importance of individual specifications and weights violations. The approach is evaluated
with real patient data and evidence-based guideline recommendations.
Using this approach, it was possible to integrate guideline recommendation metadata into the conformance checking process and to weight
violations individually.

Keywords: Process mining · Conformance checking · Alignments ·
Fitness · Weighted violations · Guideline compliance

1 Introduction

Process mining is an emerging research field and fills the gap between data
mining and business process management [3]. One technique of process mining
is conformance checking, whose approaches focus on measuring the conformance
of a process instance to a process model. The results of the measurement can

The research is funded by the German Federal Ministry of Education and Research
(BMBF) in the project DaTreFo under the funding code 16KIS1644.

M. Montali et al. (Eds.): ICPM 2022 Workshops, LNBIP 468, pp. 289–301, 2023.
https://doi.org/10.1007/978-3-031-27815-0_21

usually be output in the form of alignments [2], i.e., corrective adjustments for process instances, or metrics. A common metric is fitness, which measures to what degree the model allows the behavior observed in the event log that contains all process instances.

However, conventional fitness values each deviation, i.e., a rule violation against the specified behavior, equally. This becomes problematic in terms of assessment for use cases in which there are rules that are more important than others and, consequently, a violation of them is also worse. For instance, in the domain of medicine, there are clinical guidelines. Clinical guidelines are systematically developed statements that reflect the current state of medical knowledge to support physicians and patients in the decision-making process for appropriate medical care in specific clinical situations [11]. These statements have metadata (e.g., level of evidence or consensus strength) that provide information about their importance and soundness. Therefore, it is important to distinguish between the degree of deviation and to weight rule violations differently in order to obtain more accurate and meaningful results. In a scoping review, Oliart et al. [13] systematically assessed the criteria used to measure adherence to clinical guidelines and examined the suitability of process mining techniques. So far, there is no approach that allows different weighting of guideline statements [13]. Therefore, in this paper, we present a first approach for weighted violations in alignment-based conformance checking that incorporates the assessment of individual specifications in the calculation of fitness.

The approach is a promising solution to address medicine-specific characteristics and challenges for process mining presented in Munoz-Gama et al. [12]. Regarding the characteristics, we deal with the use of guidelines (D3) in the process mining context. In particular, concrete characteristics of guidelines are integrated to generate more valuable results. Furthermore, we built on characteristic D5, the consideration of data at multiple abstraction levels, by also integrating medical metadata. In addition, our research involves healthcare professionals (D6) who have made a valuable contribution to its realization. Regarding challenges, we address dealing with reality (C4) as we test and evaluate our approach with real patient data. Furthermore, the development of this approach should foster the use of process mining by healthcare professionals (C5), as it leads to helpful and valuable results.

The remainder of the paper is organized as follows. Section 2 provides background information on the components of our approach. Section 3 describes the methodological approach for the alignment-based conformance checking with weighted violations. Section 4 presents the evaluation process. In Sect. 5, the findings are discussed, and Sect. 6 concludes the paper.

2   Fundamentals

2.1   Event Logs

Process mining is based on event logs. Event logs can be viewed as multi-sets of cases. Each case consists of a sequence of events, i.e., the trace. Events are execution instances of activities. Here, the execution of an activity can be represented by multiple events. This can occur, for example, when multiple lifecycle stages of execution are logged [15]. In addition to the control flow perspective, event logs can also use attributes to represent other perspectives, such as the data perspective or the resource perspective. The following defines event logs, traces, events, attributes, and functions on them as a basis for the methodology.

Definition 1 *(Universes). For this paper, we define the following universes:*

- $\mathcal{V}$ *is the universe of all possible variable identifiers*
- $\mathcal{C}$ *is the universe of all possible case identifiers*
- $\mathcal{E}$ *is the universe of all possible event identifiers*
- $\mathcal{A}$ *is the universe of all possible activity identifiers*
- $\mathcal{AN}$ *is the universe of all possible attribute identifiers.*

Definition 2 *(Attributes, Classifier). Attributes can be used to characterize events and cases, e.g., an event can be assigned to a resource or have a timestamp. For any event $e \in \mathcal{E}$, any case $c \in \mathcal{C}$ and name $n \in \mathcal{AN}$, $\#_n(e)$ is the value of attribute n for event e and $\#_n(c)$ is the value of attribute n for case c. $\#_n(e) = \perp$ if event e has no attribute n and $\#_n(c) = \perp$ if case c has no attribute n. We assume the classifier $\underline{e} = \#_{activity}(e)$ as the default classifier.*

Definition 3 *(Trace, Case). Each case $c \in \mathcal{C}$ has a mandatory attribute trace, with $\hat{c} = \#_{trace}(c) \in \mathcal{E}^* \backslash \{\langle\rangle\}$. A trace is a finite sequence of events $\sigma \in \Sigma^*$ where each event occurs only once, i.e. $1 \leq i < j \leq |\sigma| : \sigma(i) \neq \sigma(j)$. By $\sigma \oplus e = \sigma$ we denote the addition of an e event to a trace σ.*

Definition 4 *(Event log). An event log is a set of cases $\mathcal{L} \subseteq \mathcal{C}$, in the form that each event is contained only once in the event log. If an event log contains timestamps these should be ordered in each trace. $\hat{\mathcal{L}} = \{e | c \in \mathcal{L} \wedge e \in \hat{c}\}$ is the set of all events appearing in the log $\mathcal{L}$.*

2.2 Alignments

To check the conformance of an event log $\mathcal{L}$ to a process model M, approaches to search for alignments are common for different process modeling languages [5]. An alignment shows how a log or trace can be replayed in a process model.

Definition 5 (Alignment, moves). *Let $\gg$ be the indicator for no move and $\mathcal{E}_\gg = \mathcal{E} \cup \{\gg\}$ the input alphabet including the no move. Then $\mathcal{E}_A = (\mathcal{E}_\gg \times \mathcal{E}_\gg) \backslash \{(\gg, \gg)\}$ is the set of legal moves. Let (s', s'') be a pair of values with $(s', s'') \in \mathcal{E}_A$, then holds:*

- *is a log move if $s' \in \mathcal{E}$ and $s'' = \gg$*
- *is a model move if $s'' \in \mathcal{E}$ and $s' = \gg$*
- *is a synchronous move if $(s', s'') \in (\mathcal{E} \times \mathcal{E}) \wedge s' = s''$*

An alignment of two traces $\sigma', \sigma'' \in \mathcal{E}^*$ is a sequence $\gamma \in \mathcal{E}_A^*$.

In other approaches, the alignment definition may differ from the above. However, the described approach can be adapted for all cost-based alignments.

2.3   MLMs and Arden Syntax

Medical Logic Modules are designed to represent medical knowledge in self-contained units that are both human-readable and computer-interpretable. Moreover, they should be transferable between several clinics [4,10]. The Arden syntax for MLMs allows the development of MLMs. It is a rule-based, declarative, HL7 standardized approach to open implementation of MLMs [14]. This was developed specifically to formalize and exchange medical knowledge. In the following, we interpret the term MLM as MLM in the Arden syntax. MLMs are text files divided into discrete slots (see Fig. 1). These slots then contain data, describe database queries or rules [10]. The basic orientation of MLMs are to formalize medical knowledge and to formulate rules, which are usually of the form "If patient has fever ≥ 40, then make a request for examination Z". This logic is formulated in the so-called logic slot and allows complex queries [4]. Among the operators are also operators with procedural reference like `before`, `after`, `within same day` or `n days before/after`. However, these do not directly compare events, only timestamps.

This approach was repurposed in the paper [8] to check the conformance of treatment sequences. For this purpose, part of the guideline for the treatment of malignant melanoma already used in [9] was transformed into MLMs using the CGK4PM framework [7]. The framework is inspired by the guideline creation process and enables the systematic transformation of guideline knowledge in an iterative procedure involving domain experts. Instead of MLMs being used to establish if-then rules, they were used in the approach to verify whether the particular guideline statement was followed. In case of non-compliance, manually modeled alignment steps were returned, which were then implemented by the client. This approach is used below to evaluate the approach in this paper.

2.4   MLM-Based Conformance Checking

To describe our approach, we introduce a simplified formalization of MLMs and the MLM-based conformance checking approach proposed by Grüger et al. [8].

Definition 6 (MLM and Slot). *We define an MLM m as a quadruple consisting of four categories with* $m = (maintenance, library, maintenance, resources)$. *Each category c consists of predefined slots. Let S be the set of all slots, then* $S_c \subset S$ *is the set of all slots defined for category c. Each slot consists of one to many values. So* $m[s]$ *returns the values of slot s for MLM m.*

Each MLM defines in the evoke slot at which evocation event it is evaluated. Here, the term evocation event extends the event concept to include the event classifier and data-level writing events. At the data level, events can be defined by the attribute name or the name in combination with the attribute value.

Definition 7 (evoke, evocation event). *Let* $e \in \mathcal{E}$ *be an event and m be an MLM.* E_e *defines the set of all evocation events evoked for event e:*

$$E_e = \{\underline{e}\} \cup \{e_n | n \in \mathcal{AN} \text{ if } e_n \neq \perp\} \cup \{(e_n, \#e_n) | n \in \mathcal{AN} \text{ if } e_n \neq \perp\}$$

Then there exists a function $evoke_m : \mathcal{E} \cup \mathcal{AN} \cup (\mathcal{AN} \times \mathcal{V}) \rightarrow \{0,1\}$ with:

$$evoke_m(E_e) = \begin{cases} 1 & \text{if } \#(m[evoke] \cap (x)) > 0 \\ 0 & else \end{cases}$$

Let $M \subseteq MLM$ be a declarative model consisting of many MLMs, and σ be a trace. Then holds:

$$M_\sigma = \{m \in M | \exists e \in (E) : evoke_m(E_e) = 1\}$$

is the shorthand for all evoked MLMs from M for σ.

The logic slot defines the actual conformance check based on the trace data from the data slot. The actual logic of the conformance checking and the alignment is adapted from [8] and described as a black box due to lack of space.

Definition 8 (Logic, Return). *Let A be the universe of alignment steps, K the universe of keys used in the slots and V the universe of values. Let m be an MLM, then there exists a logical function $l : MLM \rightarrow \{0,1\} \times A^* \times (K, V)^*$. The boolean value specifies whether the MLM was validated to be conform (1) or not (0). The alignment steps describe the steps for aligning a given trace.*

Definition 9 (Fitness). *Let MLM be the universe of all MLMs, $M \subseteq MLM$ be the declarative model, and σ be a trace. The function $eval : M \times \Sigma \rightarrow \{0,1\}$ evaluates whether a trace conforms to an MLM or not or was not evoked. The fitness is defined as:*

$$fitness(\sigma, M) = \frac{\sum_{i=1}^{n} eval(\sigma, M_i')}{|M_\sigma'|}$$

An outlined example of an alignment computed with an MLM is shown in Fig. 1. Here, event C is supposed to occur after event B. Since event B occurs in the trace, the MLM is evoked. The logic slot concludes to `false` since event C does not occur after event B. Hence, the defined alignment operation in the `else` block is executed and event C is inserted after event B. The timestamps of the events are used to find the correct position for the insertion.

3   Methodology

In order to incorporate the degree of a deviation into fitness to consider the importance of the violated part of the model, we introduce an approach to weight the cost of a deviation based on the given metadata. Consequently, we introduce a cost function $\mathcal{K} : \mathcal{E}_A \rightarrow \mathbb{R}_0^+$. Here, any cost function can be used that best represents the costs of the particular process and the domain-specific context.

For computing, the fitness of a trace $\sigma \in \mathcal{L} \subseteq \mathcal{E}^*$ to a process model M based on the cost function, a complete alignment with minimum cost γ^{opt} is sought. Moreover, the reference alignment $\gamma_{\sigma_\mathcal{L}}^{ref}$ is searched. Thereby, the type of process

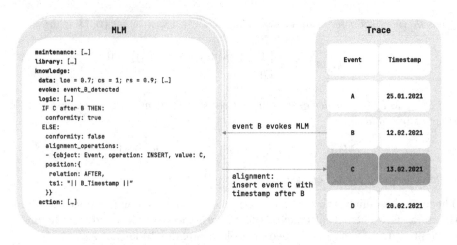

Fig. 1. Example showing a trace violating the MLM, which states that event B must be followed by C. The alignment step modeled manually in the MLM indicate that C is to be inserted after B.

modeling and the algorithm for calculating the alignment can be individually selected. Typically, the reference alignment with the highest cost is an alignment in which only moves exist in model and log:

$$\gamma_{\sigma_{\mathcal{L}}}^{ref} = \frac{\mathbf{L}\left|a_1^{\mathcal{L}}\right|...\left|a_n^{\mathcal{L}}\right|\gg\left|\gg\right|\gg}{\mathbf{M}\left|\gg\right|\gg\left|\gg\right|a_1^{M}\left|...\right|a_n^{M}}$$

While an alignment is a sequence γ of pairs $(s', s'') \in (\mathcal{E}_{\gg} \times \mathcal{E}_{\gg})\backslash\{(\gg, \gg)\}$, the cost of γ is the sum of the costs of each pair of alignments:

$$\mathcal{K}(\gamma) = \sum_{(s',s'')\in\gamma} \mathcal{K}((s', s''))$$

This is where the approach comes in. Each pair of an alignment (s', s'') with $s' \neq s''$ represents a deviation detected by the conformance checking algorithm using the model M. Therefore, there is a condition c in the model that caused this violation. We use condition as a term for modeling elements from imperative and declarative approaches (e.g., guards or rules).

Definition 10 (Condition, Condition weight). *Let M be a model and C be the set of all conditions. Then $C_M \subseteq C$ is the set of all conditions of M. Following functions are defined over C:*

- *$w : C \rightarrow \mathbb{R}_0^+$, the weighting for condition $c \in C_M$. As shorthand we use $w_c = w(c)$.*
- *$m_M : (\mathcal{E}_{\gg} \times \mathcal{E}_{\gg})\backslash\{(\gg, \gg)\} \rightarrow C$, a mapping of an alignment pair on the condition, causing the violation.*

Mapping the alignment pairs (s', s'') of an alignment γ to a condition c allows using w_c to assign a weight from $\mathbb{R}_0^+$ to each deviation in γ based on c.

Definition 11 (violation-weighted cost function). *Let* $\mathcal{E}_A = (\mathcal{E}_{\gg} \times \mathcal{E}_{\gg})\backslash\{(\gg, \gg)\}$, *then* $\mathcal{K}_{\mathcal{W}} : \mathcal{E}_A \rightarrow \mathbb{R}_0^+$ *is the violation-weighted cost function. If* $(s', s'') \in \mathcal{E}_A$, *then*

$$\mathcal{K}_{\mathcal{W}}((s', s'')) = w_{m((s', s''))} * \mathcal{K}(s', s'')$$

calculates the weighted cost for the alignment pair (s', s'').

Definition 12 (violation-weighted fitness function). *Let* $\sigma_L \in \mathcal{E}^*$ *be a log trace and* M *a model. Let* $\gamma_{\sigma_L}^{opt} \in \mathcal{E}_A^*$ *be an optimal alignment of* σ_L *and model* M *and* $\gamma_{\sigma_L}^{ref}$ *the reference alignment. The fitness level is defined as follows:*

$$\mathcal{F}_{\mathcal{W}}(\sigma_L, M) = 1 - \frac{\mathcal{K}_{\mathcal{W}}(\gamma_{\sigma_L}^{opt})}{\mathcal{K}_{\mathcal{W}}(\gamma_{\sigma_L}^{ref})}$$

Therefore, for each deviation in the optimal alignment $\gamma_{\sigma_L}^{opt}$ and in the reference alignment $\gamma_{\sigma_L}^{ref}$, the deviation weighted cost is calculated. This enables algorithm and process modeling language independent for all alignment-based conformance checking approaches to reflect the importance of violated rules in the fitness level.

4   Evaluation

For the evaluation, we used the data and model base from Grüger et al. [8]. In this paper, the authors present an MLM-based approach to conformance checking for clinical guidelines. Clinical guidelines are intended to support evidence-based treatment of patients. As a summary of systematically developed recommendations based on extensive literature studies, they are intended to optimize treatment of patients based on evidence [6]. In the original approach [8], part of the guideline for the treatment of malignant melanoma [1] (diagnosis and therapy in primary care and locoregional metastasis) was modeled as a declarative rule-based MLM model. We use this and the dataset consisting of five real patients from the University Hospital Münster to evaluate the approach described. This ensures immediate comparability with the conformance checking results from the original MLM-based conformance checking approach.

In addition, medical guidelines inherently contain information on the timeliness, importance, and foundation of each guideline recommendation, which could not be addressed in previous conformance checking approaches. Therefore, we adapt the approach to compute the violation-weighted fitness such that the weights are dynamically derived from the properties of the guideline statements represented by the MLMs. For calculation, we use the attributes *level of evidence, date of last review, consensus strength,* and *recommendation strength.*

- **level of evidence (loe):** evidence grading is according to Oxford (2009 version) and is divided into 10 grades (1a, 1b, 1c, 2a, 2b, 2c, 3a, 3b, 4, 5), with 1a (systematic review with homogeneity of randomized-controlled trials) highest loe and 5 (expert opinion without critical analysis or based on physiologic or experimental research or "basic principles") lowest loe.
- **consensus strength (cs):** indicates the strength of consensus in the expert panel on the respective statement in percent.
- **recommendation strength (rs):** for all recommendations, the strength of the recommendation is expressed as A (strong recommendation), B (recommendation), and C (recommendation open).
- **date of last review (dolr):** indicates the year of the last review of the statement. Considering constant progress, the topicality of recommendations is to be taken into account in the evaluation.

In order to incorporate the weighting attributes $WA = \{loe, cs, rs, dolr\}$ as weights into the fitness calculation, the individual classification values are mapped as values between 0 and 1, using the mapping function m. Let C be the set of MLMs. Let $m : C \times WA \to [0,1]$ be the mapping function for the weighting attributes for a concrete condition $c \in C$. For each of the weighting attributes, m is defined as follows.

For the 10-step gradation of the level of evidence (loe), the values are descending equally distributed over the range from 0 to 1. The strength of recommendation (rs) can be expressed by three different categorical values. Accordingly, the weighting is given in thirds of steps.

loe	1a	1b	1c	2a	2b	2c	3a	3b	4	5	**rs**	A	B	C
m(c,loe)	1	0.9	0.8	0.7	0.6	0.5	0.4	0.3	0.2	0.1	**m(c,rs)**	1	0.66	0.33

Since consensus strength (cs) is expressed in relative values from 0 to 100 percent, the mapping values are divided by 100. The date of the last review is divided into time intervals. Recommendations that have been reviewed since 2019 receive the highest recommendation. Review years below that receive a weight of 0.8. This expresses the strength of differentiating fine-grained between the informative value of the individual attributes. For example, the last review year was rated as less relevant by the domain experts.

$$m(c, cs) = \frac{c_{cs}}{100} \qquad\qquad m(c, dolr) = \begin{cases} 1 & \text{if } c_{dolr} \geq 2018 \\ 0.8 & \text{else} \end{cases}$$

Furthermore, it is necessary to differentiate between standard and critical MLMs. In a critical MLM, *loe*, *cs*, *rs* and *dolr* are all equal to 1. This means that this MLM is up-to-date and is seen as critical by medical experts. Thus, it is necessary to increase the weight of these MLMs. This is guaranteed by using the function below. In the case the MLM is critical, the defined if-condition holds and the value of 2 is assigned as weight. If the MLM is not critical, the else-condition is applied and the weight for a given MLM c is calculated as the sum of the mapped values $v \in WA$ divided by the number of weighting attributes.

$$w(c) = \begin{cases} 2 & \text{if } \sum_{a \in WA} m(c,a) = |WA| \\ \frac{\sum_{a \in WA} m(c,a)}{|WA|} & \text{else} \end{cases}$$

Grüger et al.'s approach [8] returns a semantically optimal alignment. This is manually pre-modeled for each of the MLMs and addresses violations of the MLMs in such a way that they are correctly resolved from a medical perspective, i.e., no overwriting of values in the data perspective, no changing of the guideline model, no most favorable path (e.g., by deleting nodes). This optimal alignment is then incorporated into the calculation of fitness in the denominator. Since the approach is built based on a set of rules in the form of MLMs, but not all of them are evoked for each trace, the reference alignment is computed based only on the set of evoked MLMs M_σ for the trace σ (see Definition 7).

Therefore, we adapt the fitness function established in Definition 9 and modify it as follows. For trace σ and the MLM-based model M, γ_σ^{opt} is the optimal alignment. Then γ_σ^{ref} is the reference alignment violating every MLM in M_σ.

$$\mathcal{F}_\mathcal{W}(\sigma_L, M) = 1 - \frac{\mathcal{K}_\mathcal{W}(\gamma_{\sigma_L}^{opt})}{\mathcal{K}_\mathcal{W}(\gamma_{\sigma_L}^{ref})} \qquad \mathcal{K}_\mathcal{W}((s', s'')) = (w_{c((s',s''))})^2 * \mathcal{K}(s', s'')$$

Since the guideline, according to its intention, mainly gives recommendations that have a higher degree of recommendation, a higher level of evidence, and a good consensus, the cost function was adjusted so that deviations from the optimum were weighted more heavily, this was ensured by squaring the weight term $w_{c((s',s''))}$. The computed fitness values for the five patients with the original approach [8] and the adapted weighted approach are shown in Table 1.

Table 1. Resulting fitness values compared with the non-weighting approach (log fitness and treatment trace for patients P21333-P87523).

	Violation weighted	Non-weighted
Log fitness	0.8642	0.8306
Fitness P87523	0.8787	0.8636
Fitness P56156	0.9258	0.8281
Fitness P21333	0.7840	0.8125
Fitness P23144	0.7769	0.8947
Fitness P23342	0.4444	0.3337

The results show that the fitness values of the entire logs differ only slightly. This is due to the fact that most of the guideline recommendations have a high degree of recommendation. Moreover, not only the optimal alignments are weighted, but also the reference alignments. Thus, the fitness is averaged here as well. This is clearly visible in patient P23342. Here, two guideline recommendations were violated and three were evoked. Each of the recommendations has the highest level of evidence, the highest consensus strength, recommendation strength and the year 2018, as the year of the last review and thus is critical. This results in a weight of 2 for each recommendation, resulting in a fitness of 0.4444 for the weighted and 0.3337 for the unweighted approach. For patient P87523 (see Fig. 2), three MLMs are evoked and one (guideline recommendation 4.22) is critical. Since each weighting attribute has the highest weight, the deviation from recommendation 4.22 has a weight of 2.

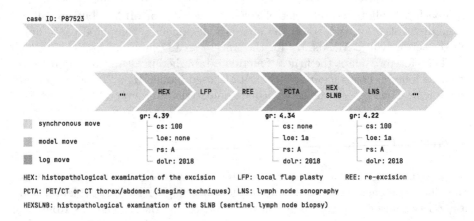

Fig. 2. Aligned trace of the patient case P87523. Containing three moves in the aligned trace: two model moves and one log move. For each alignment step, the guideline recommendation (gr) is shown, which is incorporated in the respective MLM. Below that, the weighting attribute information for deriving the weights is shown.

The high fitness values close to the unweighted values show that the treatment traces in particular violate important statements. There are nearly no recommendation violations weighted as less important. In total, the traces violated 21 statements, of which 11 rules have a weight of 1 (as in a crisp approach) and 4 are critical with a weight of 2. In six violations, all for patient P56156 (11 violations in total), the weights are less than 1, with an average weight of 0.6.

5   Discussion

As demonstrated in Sect. 4, the weighted fitness measure provides little difference from the crisp approach when (1) there are few or no strongly weighted deviations (2) there are few deviations in general, and they are not sufficient to make a difference (3) in our approach, few MLMs are activated for treatment. Addressing this issue would require further investigation of the effect of the weights. An extended weighting scale could generate larger differences between individual results and better differentiate deviations in terms of their importance.

Furthermore, it must be considered that the creation and assignment of the weights and their levels is done manually. This implies a certain amount of effort, which usually requires the contribution of one or more domain experts for the corresponding case. In our evaluation, we were able to derive the weights from the medical classifications. However, if weights are to be implemented when there is no default of importance, then they must be created based on the available data as well as a consensus of the respective domain experts. In addition, the assignment of numerical values to level of evidence and recommendation strength must be regarded critically, because it cannot be said with certainty that, e.g., the distance between *loe* 1a and 1b is the same as between 4 and 5.

The presented approach extends alignment-based conformance checking with weights to differentiate the severity of deviations. However, the data perspective is not currently considered, as it brings its own challenges, such as the semantically correct severity of a deviation from a given stage value.

When considering the results and the data set used, it should be noted that in an extended evaluation, the weighted fitness values may show greater differences from the unweighted fitness values. Since only a guideline section was modeled, only a delimited area of the entire treatment is tested for compliance. Accordingly, if a full treatment were reviewed, it is also very likely that more guideline violations of varying relevance would be identified, and the result would deviate much more significantly from the unweighted fitness score. Moreover, this work has shown that it is not straightforward to incorporate the importance of activities in the fitness value. On the one hand, the generated results could not show large differences in some cases and on the other hand, it is questionable to what extent fitness is the appropriate place to integrate the importance aspect. For medical process mining in particular, consideration should be given to introducing a new metric specifically designed for this purpose. In general, empirical research is needed on the association of greater guideline deviation and worse clinical outcomes addressed by clinical trials.

6   Conclusion

The presented approach for weighting violations of specific conditions allows the inclusion of attributes such as importance or soundness of modeled behavior. In the presented use case, this enables a more accurate knowledge representation in the process models and a higher expressiveness of the fitness value.

A limitation of the current approach is that it only considers the importance. However, the results show that the degree of deviation from the model is also important for calculating meaningful fitness values. This also applies to most cases of larger deviations in the time perspective since they should be weighted more heavily than small deviations. Accordingly, the replacement of one activity with another similar activity would also be less severe. An approach to include the degree of deviation for the data perspective could be the adaptation of the fuzzy set approach according to Zhang et al. [16]. Another factor could be the degree to which the conditions are met. Thus, it is interesting to know how close the trace could be to a threshold so that the respective condition still takes effect. Another challenge is the mapping of optional rules in the fitness value, which turned out to be very domain dependent. In future work, we intend to extend the approach to include the degree of deviation. In addition, the approach will be implemented and evaluated for several process modeling languages.

References

1. Leitlinienprogramm Onkologie (Deutsche Krebsgesellschaft, Deutsche Krebshilfe, AWMF): Diagnostik, Therapie und Nachsorge des Melanoms, Langversion 3.3. AWMF Registernummer: 032/024OL (2020). http://leitlinienprogramm-onkologie.de/leitlinien/melanom/. Accessed 20 Sept 2022
2. van der Aalst, W., Adriansyah, A., van Dongen, B.: Replaying history on process models for conformance checking and performance analysis. Wiley Interdisc. Rev.: Data Min. Knowl. Discov. **2**(2), 182–192 (2012)
3. van der Aalst, W.M.P.: Process Mining: Data Science in Action, 2nd edn. Springer, Heidelberg (2016). https://doi.org/10.1007/978-3-662-49851-4
4. Arkad, K., Gill, H., Ludwigs, U., Shahsavar, N., Gao, X.M., Wigertz, O.: Medical logic module (MLM) representation of knowledge in a ventilator treatment advisory system. Int. J. Clin. Monit. Comput. **8**(1), 43–48 (1991)
5. Dunzer, S., Stierle, M., Matzner, M., Baier, S.: Conformance checking: a state-of-the-art literature review. In: Betz, S. (ed.) Proceedings of the 11th International Conference on Subject-Oriented Business Process Management, pp. 1–10. Association for Computing Machinery, New York (2019)
6. Graham, R., Mancher, M., Miller Wolman, D., Greenfield, S., Steinberg, E. (eds.): Clinical Practice Guidelines We Can Trust. National Academies Press (2011)
7. Grüger, J., Geyer, T., Bergmann, R., Braun, S.A.: CGK4PM: towards a methodology for the systematic generation of clinical guideline process models and the utilization of conformance checking. BioMedInformatics **2**(3), 359–374 (2022)
8. Grüger, J., Geyer, T., Kuhn, M., Bergmann, R., Braun, S.A.: Declarative guideline conformance checking of clinical treatments. In: Business Process Management Workshops (2022). https://arxiv.org/abs/2209.09535
9. Grüger, J., Geyer, T., Kuhn, M., Braun, S.A., Bergmann, R.: Verifying guideline compliance in clinical treatment using multi-perspective conformance checking: a case study. In: Munoz-Gama, J., Lu, X. (eds.) ICPM 2021. LNBIP, vol. 433, pp. 301–313. Springer, Cham (2022). https://doi.org/10.1007/978-3-030-98581-3_22
10. Hripcsak, G.: Writing Arden syntax medical logic modules. Comput. Biol. Med. **24**(5), 331–363 (1994)
11. Lohr, K.N., Field, M.J.: Clinical Practice Guidelines: Directions for a New Program. Publication IOM, vol. 90–08. National Academy Press, Washington (1990)
12. Munoz-Gama, J., et al.: Process mining for healthcare: characteristics and challenges. J. Biomed. Inform. **127**, 103994 (2022)
13. Oliart, E., Rojas, E., Capurro, D.: Are we ready for conformance checking in healthcare? Measuring adherence to clinical guidelines: a scoping systematic literature review. J. Biomed. Inform. **130**, 104076 (2022)
14. Samwald, M., Fehre, K., de Bruin, J., Adlassnig, K.P.: The Arden syntax standard for clinical decision support: experiences and directions. J. Biomed. Inform. **45**(4), 711–718 (2012)

15. van Zelst, S.J., Mannhardt, F., de Leoni, M., Koschmider, A.: Event abstraction in process mining: literature review and taxonomy. Granular Comput. **6**(3), 719–736 (2020)
16. Zhang, S., Genga, L., Yan, H., Lu, X., Duan, H., Kaymak, U.: Towards multi-perspective conformance checking with fuzzy sets (2020). https://arxiv.org/abs/2001.10730

Event Log Generation in MIMIC-IV
Research Paper

Jonas Cremerius[1(✉)], Luise Pufahl[2], Finn Klessascheck[1], and Mathias Weske[1]

[1] Hasso Plattner Institute, University of Potsdam, Potsdam, Germany
{Jonas.Cremerius,Mathias.Weske}@hpi.de, Finn.Klessascheck@student.hpi.de
[2] Software and Business Engineering, Technische Universitaet Berlin,
Berlin, Germany
Luise.Pufahl@tu-berlin.de

Abstract. Public event logs are valuable for process mining research to evaluate process mining artifacts and identify new and promising research directions. Initiatives like the BPI Challenges have provided a series of real-world event logs, including healthcare processes, and have significantly stimulated process mining research. However, the healthcare related logs provide only excerpts of patient visits in hospitals. The Medical Information Mart for Intensive Care (MIMIC)-IV database is a public available relational database that includes data on patient treatment in a tertiary academic medical center in Boston, USA. It provides complex care processes in a hospital from end-to-end. To facilitate the use of MIMIC-IV in process mining and to increase the reproducibility of research with MIMIC, this paper provides a framework consisting of a method, an event hierarchy, and a log extraction tool for extracting useful event logs from the MIMIC-IV database. We demonstrate the framework on a heart failure treatment process, show how logs on different abstraction levels can be generated, and provide configuration files to generate event logs of previous process mining works with MIMIC.

Keywords: Event log generation · Process mining · Healthcare · MIMIC

1 Introduction

Process mining methods and techniques are experiencing a tremendous uptake in a broad range of organizations. These techniques help to make the real-world execution of business processes more transparent and support an evidenced-based process analysis and redesign [23]. Therefore, process mining receives increased attention in the healthcare domain, where traditionally manifold data is logged due to quality control and billing purposes [8,22].

Public available event logs, in which the process data is stored as an ordered list, are essential for developing new process mining techniques and methods and evaluating their impact and limitations. In recent years, different initiatives,

© The Author(s) 2023
M. Montali et al. (Eds.): ICPM 2022 Workshops, LNBIP 468, pp. 302–314, 2023.
https://doi.org/10.1007/978-3-031-27815-0_22

such as the BPI Challenges running since 2011, e.g., [7], or the conformance checking challenge [20], and additional research including [17] have provided publicly accessible event logs.

Public data sets are relevant to stimulate research in healthcare as well. For example, MIMIC (Medical Information Mart for Intensive Care) is a large, de-identified relational database including patients that received critical care in the Beth Israel Deaconess Medical Center [13] in Boston, USA. Whereas MIMIC-III contains data about activities in the intensive care unit (ICU) between 2001–2012, MIMIC-IV provides data on the complete hospital stay between 2008–2019, including procedures performed, medications given, laboratory values taken, triage information, and more. It provides the opportunity to develop and evaluate process mining techniques on patient care processes, such as in [2,15]. However, the uptake of this rich and data-intensive database is limited in the process mining community so far.

The relational database's complexity, the data's richness, and the need to flatten the data in a meaningful way in an event log has hampered the uptake of MIMIC-IV by the process mining community. Additionally, access to MIMIC-IV requires a data use agreement, including a training provided by the Collaborative Institutional Training Initiative (CITI) about collecting, using and disclosing health information. However, the process to gain access is clearly defined and usually does not take more than a few days.

This paper aims at simplifying the event log extraction from the MIMIC-IV database and its reusability. In particular, it provides a framework including an extraction method, an event hierarchy for MIMIC-IV, and a Python log extraction tool to ease the log extraction from MIMIC-IV. The remainder of this paper is organized as follows. In the next section, background on MIMIC is given in Sect. 2, and related work is discussed in Sect. 3. The event extraction framework for MIMIC-IV is presented in Sect. 4, followed by an evaluation in Sect. 5. The paper concludes in Sect. 6.

2   MIMIC-IV Database

MIMIC-IV is a publicly available dataset provided by the Laboratory for Computational Physiology (LCP) at the Massachusetts Institute of Technology (MIT). It comprises de-identified health data associated with thousands of hospital admissions. The project was launched in the early 2000s with MIMIC-I. It is still ongoing with the recent release of MIMIC-IV, including data from 2008–2019.

The data is derived from a hospital-wide Electronic Health Record (EHR) and an Intensive Care Unit (ICU) specific system, such as MetaVison [13]. So far, MIMIC-IV contains data from a single hospital. The ultimate goal is to incorporate data from multiple institutions capable of supporting research on cohorts of critically ill patients worldwide. To ensure the data represents a real-world healthcare dataset, data cleaning steps were not performed [13].

The MIMIC-IV relational database consists of 35 tables separated into four modules consisting of emergency department (ed), hospital (hosp), intensive care

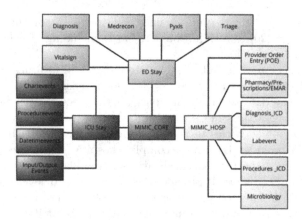

Fig. 1. MIMIC-IV 1.0 simplified data model. The colours represent the respective modules: Green: Core, Yellow: Hosp, Blue: ICU, Orange: ED (Color figure online)

unit (`icu`), and `core`. Figure 1 illustrates a simplified data model of the database with its modules. In `core`, demographic information, such as age and marital status, transfers between departments, and admission information including their admission location is stored. The `hosp` module provides all data acquired from the hospital-wide electronic health record, including laboratory measurements, microbiology, medication administration, billed diagnoses/procedures, and orders made by providers. The `ed` module adds information about patients' first contact with the hospital in the emergency department, including data about triage, suspected diagnosis, and measurements made. Lastly, the `icu` module contains precise information obtained from an ICU visit, including machine recordings and procedures performed. This schema is conforming with MIMIC-IV 1.0. In June 2022, MIMIC-IV 2.0 was released, which transferred the tables from `core` to `hosp`, which is a minor change, as it modifies the high-level schema and not the relations between the tables. However, the documentation is still structured as shown in Fig. 1. The provided method including the log extraction tool is conform with both versions.

To ensure patient confidentiality, all dates in MIMIC-IV have been shifted randomly. Thus, process mining techniques, such as bottleneck analysis, are not possible to apply. However, dates are internally consistent with respect to each patient, so the actual time between events is preserved.

3 Related Work

In this section, we want to review research works on event log extraction, and on applying process mining to data from MIMIC.

Event Log Extraction. An event log serves as the basis for process mining techniques. However, the preparation of an event log is often not trivial as business processes might be executed with the help of multiple IT systems and the

Table 1. Research works on applying process mining to MIMIC-III

Ref.	Year	Goal	Patient cohort	Notion	Events
[2]	2017	Reduce variation in pathways	Congestive heart failure patients	Hospital adm.	Admission, lab, prescription, ICU
[15]	2018	Assess the data quality	Cancer patients	Hospital adm.	Admission
[14]	2018	Analyse cancer pathways	Cancer patients	Hospital adm.	Admission and icustays
[16]	2020	Detect disease trajectories	≤ 16 years, btw. 2001-2012, ≤ 2 stays	Subject	Admission and diagnosis
[18]	2020	Compare ICU treatment	Cancer patients	Hospital adm.	ICU procedures

data is often stored not in the structure of an event log, but often in relational databases [6]. For the interested reader, Diba et al. [6] provide a structured literature review on techniques for event data extraction, correlation, and abstraction to prepare an event log. Remy et al. [22] present challenges in the event log abstraction from a data warehouse of a large U.S. health system. Jans and Soffers describe in [11] relevant decisions that need to be made to create an event log from a relational database: related (1) to the process as a whole, such as *"which process should be selected and its exact scope?"*, (2) to the selection of the process instance, such as *"what is the notion of an instance"* and to the event level, such as *"what type of events and attributes to include"*. In a later research work, the authors [12] provide a nine-step procedure to create an event log from a relational database, starting with stating a goal over identifying key tables and relationships until defining the case notion, and selecting event types and their attributes. This procedure will serve as a basis to create a method for extracting event logs from MIMIC-IV.

In the last years, event log extraction approaches and tools were developed to support practitioners in extracting event logs from their databases, such as *onprom* [4] using ontologies for the extraction, *eddytools* [9] for a case notion recommondation, and *RDB2Log* [3] for a quality-informed log extraction. Still, we observed that these tools could not be easily applied for MIMIC-IV. Reasons include the need to merge tables for obtaining complete information about events. Additionally, a patient cohort definition is necessary to deal with the complexity of healthcare processes. Thus, they are not used in this work.

Process Mining with MIMIC. This part presents research papers that used process mining to analyze the MIMIC database. The identified research works used the MIMIC-III database because MIMIC-IV has been published recently. We analyzed their goals, their used patient cohort, their used case notion, and selected event types for the event log preparation, summarized in Table 1.

Alharbi et al. [2], and Kurniati et al. [15] target methodological goals for the analysis of the healthcare data, such as reducing the variation in clinical pathway data and assessing the data quality. The other three research works follow medical analysis goals, such as analyzing cancer pathways, comparing the treatment of different cancer types at the ICU, and detecting disease trajectories. It can be observed that, on the one hand, patient cohorts with a specific diagnosis were selected, such as cancer and congestive heart failure patients. However, on the other hand, a broader patient cohort was also selected in a specific age range and a certain length of stay. As a notion of the process instance, two applied solutions can be observed: The subject (i.e., the patient with their *subject_id*) or the hospital stay (i.e., *hadm_id*) is selected. Whereas the subject covers all events that happen to a specific patient, including possibly several hospital admissions, the hospital admission comprises only events related to one admission. If a patient had several admissions for a specific diagnosis, it is represented as different traces for this patient. Finally, the research works applying process mining to the MIMIC data using different event data are presented. The high-level `admission` events of the `core` including information on the time of admission, discharge, etc. were used [2,14–16]. Kurniati et al. [14] select additionally high-level information on the ICU stay, such as `ICU intime`, whereas Marazza et al. [18] chose detail procedure events of the ICU stay. As Kusuma et al. [16] aim at detecting disease trajectories, they select additionally to the admission events also the diagnosis as an event. The diagnosis has no own timestamp, and the authors decided to use the time of admission. Alharbi et al. [2] select for their analysis a broad range of events, also lab, prescriptions, and ICU events.

It can be observed, that current research works on MIMIC use case-dependent SQL scripts that cannot be easily adapted for other use cases. This makes it difficult to reproduce the event log extraction and hinders researchers inexperienced with MIMIC to use this data source. In this research work, we want to provide an event log extraction tool to ease the access to MIMIC for the process mining community.

4   Event Log Extraction Framework for MIMIC-IV

This section presents the event log extraction framework for MIMIC-IV. It results from an analysis of related work and the MIMIC database and its documentation. Based on the event log preparation procedure by [12], we propose a method to derive event logs from MIMIC-IV including an event hierarchy in Sect. 4.1. In Sect. 4.2, the Python tool for event log extraction from MIMIC-IV is introduced.

4.1   Method and Event Hierarchy

The method to extract event logs from MIMIC-IV consists of six steps from goal definition and patient cohort definition, over selecting the case notion and attributes until the selection of event types and their enrichment, as shown in Fig. 2a. For each step, we describe the goal and activities, its mapping to the event preparation procedure by [12], and possibilities for configurations.

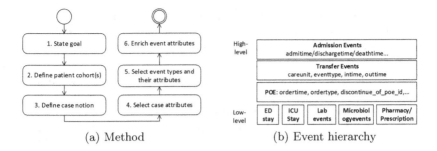

(a) Method   (b) Event hierarchy

Fig. 2. Method for event log extraction from MIMIC-IV and its event hierarchy.

1) State goal. As described by [12] in step P1, for a useful event log preparation, the goal of the process mining project needs to be defined. The need for
the goal definition also applies to the event log extraction from the MIMIC-IV
database. Possible medical analysis goals are the process variant exploration of
clinical pathways, disease trajectory modeling, conformance analysis to clinical
guidelines, etc. [21]. It can also be a methodological goal, such as analyzing the
data quality.

2) Define patient cohort(s). As suggested by [12] in step P2, the boundaries of
a process have to be defined. In healthcare, the scope of a process is usually
defined by selecting a particular patient cohort, e.g., congestive heart failure
patients [2] or cancer patients [15]. Patient cohorts are often selected via the
diagnosis of the **hosp** stay with the help of the International Statistical Classification of Diseases and Related Health Problems (ICD) codes[1]–a global system to
label medical diagnosis consistently. Another possibility are Diagnostic Related
Groups (DRGs), a code system that is used for determining the costs or the
reimbursement rate of a case. It is based on diagnoses, procedures, age, sex, discharge status, and the presence of complications or co-morbidities. Additionally,
an age range or the length of stay could be used to focus on specific patient
cohorts.

3) Define case notion. As given by [12] in step P5, an attribute has to be
selected that determines the process instance (i.e., the case id of an event log).
By analyzing the MIMIC-IV database and the related work, we identified two
possible notions of cases, the subject identifier (the patient with its *subject_id*) or
the hospital administration identifier (*hadm_id*). With *subject_id* the complete
patient history, including several admissions, can be analyzed. With *hadm_id*,
each patient admission is represented as an individual trace in the event log.
Further, each hospital admission consists of stays in different departments, such
as the ICU or ED stay, on which the focus could also be during the analysis.
The instance granularity needs to be selected (step P6 [12]) and its parent and
child activities. This is well-supported in MIMIC-IV: The main identifier, the

---

[1] https://www.icd10data.com/ICD10CM/Codes.

subject_id and *hadm_id*, is available in all tables as a foreign key. Only *hadm_id* is not available in the ed module, but the *stay_id* stored in ed tables can be mapped to an *hadm_id*.

4) Select case attributes. After the patient cohorts and the case notion have been selected, in the next step, additional attributes of cases, the traces in an event log, need to be selected as also suggested by [12] in step P8. Case attributes can be used to filter and cluster in the process mining project. Here available patient data, such as their *gender* or *age*, diagnosis data, such as the *ICD_code*, or admission data, such as *discharge_location* or *insurance* could be selected based on the selected case notion.

5) Select event types and their attributes. When the instances and their attributes are selected, the event types as also suggested by [12] in step P7 and event attributes in step P9 can be selected. Therefore, key tables (step P3 [12]) and their relationships (step P4) need to be identified. By analyzing MIMIC-IV and related work, we developed a hierarchy including possibly relevant event types for MIMIC-IV, as shown in Fig. 2b. The top shows the most high-level events, whereas the bottom shows low-level events. In the following, we present the different types of events in more detail, starting from the top:

Admission events, such as *admittime*, *dischargetime* etc., can be all together found in the admissions table of the core module. They provide high-level information about the patients' stays (e.g., when was the admission to the hospital or the discharge). Almost all related works have used this event type, either alone or with other event types, such as ICU stay information. If the admission events are requested, then all the "time"-events are provided including *admittime/dischargetime/deathtime* etc.

On the next level, the **transfer events** of the transfers table, also in the core, provide insights about which departments/care units a patient has visited during the hospital stay. These events can be used to analyze the path of a patient through the hospital. Each table entry represents one transfer event for which the *intime* or *outtime* can be selected to be used as a timestamp. The other attributes of this table are provided as event attributes.

The next level of detail is the **provider order entry (POE) events** that provide insights into ordered treatments and procedures for a patient. The POE table is part of the hosp module. These events do not represent the activities that have been finally executed, but they represent what has been planned and ordered for a patient. Additionally, the attributes *discontinue_of_poe_id* and *discontinued_by_poe* provide insights whether the order was cancelled. Each entry of the POE table represents one order for a patient of a specific hospital admission, and as timestamp, the *ordertime* can be used. The additional attributes of the POE table are added as event attributes. Some POE events, such as lab or medication events, can also be enriched with details about the activity execution from other tables. For instance, details on laboratory or microbiology examinations can be found in the labevents or microbiologyevents tables. The `pharmacy`, the `prescriptions` and the `EMAR` table provide details on the medications that a patient has received[2].

Finally, also low-level details on specific aspects of the hospital stay of a patient can be deduced from specific tables, such as events of the ED stay, ICU stay or the `labevents`. We allow deriving event data from any combination of low-level tables. For instance, medications prescribed (`prescription`) can be analysed in combination with procedures performed (`procedures_icd`).

6) Enrich event attributes. Optionally, events can be enriched by additional event attributes from any other table in MIMIC-IV if events have multiple timestamps. For example, the `transfers` table includes the times when patients entered and left the respective hospital department, or the `pharmacy` table includes the times when a medication was started and ended to be given. As shown in [5], events from the `transfers` table can be enhanced by aggregated laboratory values, such that for each department visit, the average laboratory value is known and can be analyzed. We allow adding aggregated information from any table in MIMIC-IV, so that not only laboratory values but also medication or procedure information can be added.

4.2   Event Log Extraction Tool

The event log extraction tool that forms an integral part of the framework presented in this paper has been implemented using Python 3.8 and is available as an open-source tool on GitHub[3]. It implements the method for event log extraction from MIMIC-IV (cf. Fig. 2a, Sect. 4.1). For this, access to and credentials for a MIMIC-IV instance running on PostgreSQL are required. The tool provides two ways of extracting logs: Either a user is guided interactively through the method, being prompted for input along with the six steps, starting at the second, as stating the goal is not supported by us.

Or, a user can provide a configuration file[4], which contains definitions and selections for one or more of the separate steps, as well as additional parameter configurations, such as the required database credentials. Then, the user is only asked to provide input for those steps that have not been configured using the configuration file. Thus, while logs that have been extracted out of MIMIC-IV cannot be shared due to the data use agreement, a configuration file defining the application of the extraction method on the MIMIC-IV database can be shared instead. We provide configuration files for the event logs presented in Sect. 5.

Besides that, it is possible to extract event logs either as a log file conforming to the XES standard (cf. [1]), or as a .csv file, depending on the desired format

---

[2] The reason for having three tables is that medications are prescribed first and then given to a patient. The prescription is stored in `pharmacy` with detailed information in `prescription`. Administration details can be found in `EMAR`, where nurses scan a barcode at the patient's bedside at the moment when the medication is given. The tables are connected through a common identifier *pharmacy_id*.

[3] https://github.com/bptlab/mimic-log-extraction.

[4] Example configuration files and an explanation of what they can configure can be found in the tool's GitHub repository.

and the tooling that is to be applied afterwards on the event log. For more in-depth information on how to install, configure, and run the tool, we refer the reader to the corresponding GitHub repository.

5   Evaluation

In the following, we evaluate the presented MIMIC log extraction framework in a twofold manner. First, we show how far we could replicate the event logs generated by other research works on process mining with MIMIC. Second, we apply the method to an example use case and demonstrate findings and research challenges.

Replicating Event Logs of Research Works in MIMIC. We were able to provide configuration files for almost all the related work presented in Sect. 3. One exception is [16], as they manually attached a timestamp to the diagnoses_icd table. It should be noted, that we could not generate the final event logs for all works, as some applied post-processing, such as event abstraction. However, we could replicate the cohort, case notion, case attribute, event, and event attribute selection of them, which is the goal of this tool so far. The configuration files can be found in the GitHub repository.

Demonstration on Heart Failure Treatment. We demonstrate the event log extraction method for MIMIC-IV and present one level of the event hierarchy in detail for the heart failure treatment case[5].

The **goal (1)** of this demonstration is to discover the hospital treatment process of patients having heart failure and to identify, if common treatment practices are applied. The **cohort (2)** consists of heart failure patients. Heart failure is the leading cause of hospitalizations in the U.S. and represents one of the biggest cohorts in MIMIC-IV besides newborns, with 7,232 admissions [10]. It was chosen based on ICD codes and DRG codes[6] related to heart failure. We have selected the hospital admission as the **case notion (3)**, because we want to focus on the steps taken specifically for patients with heart failure instead of analyzing the complete patient history. The chosen **case attributes (4)** are related to the hospital admission, such as *admittime*, *admission_location* and the list of diagnosis (from the diagnosis_icd table).

Regarding the chosen **event type (5)**, we will only present the POE level due to space limitations. The POE level provides a good overview of main activities of treating heart failure patients. The results for the other hierarchy levels can be found in the following report[7].

---

[5] The detailed event log descriptions with their configuration files can be found in a GitHub repository: https://github.com/bptlab/mimic-log-extraction/tree/main/ sample_config_files.

[6] The selected ICD and DRG codes can be found in the configuration files.

[7] https://github.com/bptlab/mimic-log-extraction/blob/main/EventLogGeneration Report.pdf.

The process model in Fig. 3 shows the sequence and frequency of heart failure related treatments and procedures ordered for the patients. We filtered manually for events that are typical activities performed for patients with heart failure [19]. We displayed frequency and case coverage in brackets for each activity. This process represents typical characteristics of healthcare processes, including highly repetitive tasks and flexible order of activities. It can be observed that monitoring is highly relevant for heart failure patients, especially telemetry is common for patients suffering from cardiac conditions, as well as X-rays or CT scans for the diagnosis. Additionally, activities for managing heart failure can be observed, such as oxygen therapy, renal replacement therapy in the form of hemodialysis, or palliative care [19].

Repetitive events, such as Vitals/Monitoring make it almost impossible to observe a process order, especially in directly follows graphs, as these events have a high amount of ingoing and outgoing arcs. Identifying these automatically and dealing with them can be an interesting way of making process models more readable. Additionally, one could think about methods and visualizations to analyse discontinued orders (*discontinue_of_poe_id* and *discontinued_by_poe*). As the POE level contains a high amount of different events, one could also think about methods supporting process analysts and domain experts to find events of interest.

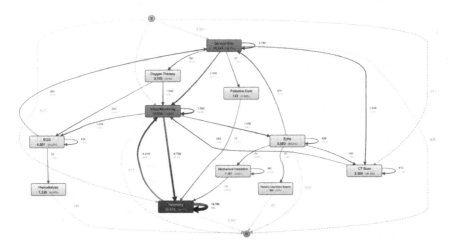

Fig. 3. POE events, showing treatments and procedures ordered at the hospital. Activity filter: Manually selected events given in a guideline [19] (10% of all with 100% case coverage), Paths filter: 45%

We see, that the POE level comes with interesting challenges for process mining in healthcare. Also, the other identified event abstraction levels demonstrated relevant research challenges, which are discussed in the above-mentioned report. As there is a need for healthcare tailored frameworks in process mining, MIMIC could provide a necessary data source to research innovative solutions working on real-world data [21].

6   Conclusion

This paper presented a method, an event hierarchy, and a tool to extract event logs from MIMIC-IV, an anonymized database on hospitals stays, in a structured manner. The rich database of interacting healthcare processes including a high amount of additional event data offers process mining research for healthcare a relevant source of event logs for developing and evaluating new process mining artifacts. We demonstrated for a heart failure use case how event logs can be created and presented challenges coming along with healthcare processes.

The presented MIMIC-IV log extraction tool focuses on event log extraction only, and does not provide functionality for further processing, which could be extended in the future. Additionally, the tool extracts currently one event of a medical activity with a selected timestamp and stores the other timestamps as event attributes. The XES standard allows having multiple events of an activity representing its lifecycle changes. In future, our framework could be extended, such that multiple events of a medical activity, such as the ordering, its start and end can be captured as individual events. In the use case demonstration, we have, on the lower abstraction level, manually filtered for relevant events after the event log extraction. This could be improved in the future by supporting the event selection based on user preferences.

Event logs from this database cannot be directly shared because of a data use agreement. With our tool, configuration files for the event log extraction can be easily shared supporting reproducibility and extensibility of research. As a result of this work, the configuration files of process mining research works on MIMIC-III/IV have been provided.

References

1. IEEE standard for extensible event stream (XES) for achieving interoperability in event logs and event streams. IEEE STD 1849-2016, pp. 1–50 (2016)
2. Alharbi, A., Bulpitt, A., Johnson, O.: Improving pattern detection in healthcare process mining using an interval-based event selection method. In: Carmona, J., Engels, G., Kumar, A. (eds.) BPM 2017. LNBIP, vol. 297, pp. 88–105. Springer, Cham (2017). https://doi.org/10.1007/978-3-319-65015-9_6
3. Andrews, R., van Dun, C.G., Wynn, M.T., Kratsch, W., Röglinger, M., ter Hofstede, A.H.: Quality-informed semi-automated event log generation for process mining. Decis. Support Syst. **132**, 113265 (2020)
4. Calvanese, D., Kalayci, T.E., Montali, M., Santoso, A.: The onprom toolchain for extracting business process logs using ontology-based data access. In: Proceedings of the BPM Demo Track and BPM Dissertation Award, co-located with BPM 2017, vol. 1920. CEUR-WS.org (2017)
5. Cremerius, J., Weske, M.: Supporting domain data selection in data-enhanced process models. In: Wirtschaftsinformatik 2022 Proc. 3 (2022)
6. Diba, K., Batoulis, K., Weidlich, M., Weske, M.: Extraction, correlation, and abstraction of event data for process mining. Wiley Interdiscip. Rev. Data Mining Knowl. Discov. **10**(3), e1346 (2020)

7. van Dongen, B.: BPI challenge 2020 (2020). https://data.4tu.nl/collections/BPI_Challenge_2020/5065541/1
8. Erdogan, T.G., Tarhan, A.: Systematic mapping of process mining studies in healthcare. IEEE Access **6**, 24543–24567 (2018)
9. Gonzalez Lopez de Murillas, E.: Process mining on databases: extracting event data from real-life data sources. Ph.D. thesis, Mathematics and Computer Science (2019). proefschrift
10. Jackson, S.L., Tong, X., King, R.J., Loustalot, F., Hong, Y., Ritchey, M.D.: National burden of heart failure events in the United States, 2006 to 2014. Circ. Heart Fail **11**(12), e004873 (2018)
11. Jans, M., Soffer, P.: From relational database to event log: decisions with quality impact. In: Teniente, E., Weidlich, M. (eds.) BPM 2017. LNBIP, vol. 308, pp. 588–599. Springer, Cham (2018). https://doi.org/10.1007/978-3-319-74030-0_46
12. Jans, M., Soffer, P., Jouck, T.: Building a valuable event log for process mining: an experimental exploration of a guided process. Enterp. Inf. Syst. **13**(5), 601–630 (2019)
13. Johnson, A., Bulgarelli, L., Pollard, T., Horng, S., Celi, L.A., Mark, R.: MIMIC-IV (2020). https://physionet.org/content/mimiciv/1.0/
14. Kurniati, A.P., Hall, G., Hogg, D., Johnson, O.: Process mining in oncology using the mimic-iii dataset. In: Journal of Physics: Conference Series, vol. 971, p. 012008. IOP Publishing (2018)
15. Kurniati, A.P., Rojas, E., Hogg, D., Hall, G., Johnson, O.A.: The assessment of data quality issues for process mining in healthcare using medical information mart for intensive care iii, a freely available e-health record database. Health Inform. J. **25**(4), 1878–1893 (2019)
16. Kusuma, G., Kurniati, A., McInerney, C.D., Hall, M., Gale, C.P., Johnson, O.: Process mining of disease trajectories in MIMIC-III: a case study. In: Leemans, S., Leopold, H. (eds.) ICPM 2020. LNBIP, vol. 406, pp. 305–316. Springer, Cham (2021). https://doi.org/10.1007/978-3-030-72693-5_23
17. Mannhardt, F.: Sepsis cases - event log (2016). https://data.4tu.nl/articles/dataset/Sepsis_Cases_-_Event_Log/12707639/1
18. Marazza, F., et al.: Automatic process comparison for subpopulations: application in cancer care. Int. J. Environ. Res. Public Health **17**(16), 5707 (2020)
19. McDonagh, T.A., et al.: 2021 ESC guidelines for the diagnosis and treatment of acute and chronic heart failure. Eur. Heart J. **42**(36), 3599–3726 (2021)
20. Munoz-Gama, J., de la Fuente, R.R., Sepúlveda, M.M., Fuentes, R.R.: Conformance checking challenge 2019 (CCC19) (2019). https://data.4tu.nl/articles/dataset/Conformance_Checking_Challenge_2019_CCC19_/12714932/1
21. Munoz-Gama, J., et al.: Process mining for healthcare: characteristics and challenges. J. Biomed. Inform. **127**, 103994 (2022)
22. Remy, S., Pufahl, L., Sachs, J.P., Böttinger, E., Weske, M.: Event log generation in a health system: a case study. In: Fahland, D., Ghidini, C., Becker, J., Dumas, M. (eds.) BPM 2020. LNCS, vol. 12168, pp. 505–522. Springer, Cham (2020). https://doi.org/10.1007/978-3-030-58666-9_29
23. van der Aalst, W.: Data Science in Action. In: van der Aalst, W. (ed.) Process Mining, pp. 3–23. Springer, Heidelberg (2016). https://doi.org/10.1007/978-3-662-49851-4_1

Process Modeling and Conformance Checking in Healthcare: A COVID-19 Case Study

Elisabetta Benevento[1,2]([⊠]) [iD], Marco Pegoraro[1]([⊠]) [iD], Mattia Antoniazzi[2] [iD], Harry H. Beyel[1] [iD], Viki Peeva[1] [iD], Paul Balfanz[3] [iD], Wil M. P. van der Aalst[1] [iD], Lukas Martin[4] [iD], and Gernot Marx[4]

[1] Chair of Process and Data Science (PADS), Department of Computer Science, RWTH Aachen University, Aachen, Germany
{benevento,pegoraro,beyel,peeva,vwdaalst}@pads.rwth-aachen.de
[2] Department of Energy, Systems, Territory and Construction Engineering, University of Pisa, Pisa, Italy
[3] Department of Cardiology, Angiology and Intensive Care Medicine, RWTH University Hospital, Aachen, Germany
pbalfanz@ukaachen.de
[4] Department of Intensive Care and Intermediate Care, RWTH Aachen University Hospital, Aachen, Germany
{lmartin,gmarx}@ukaachen.de

Abstract. The discipline of process mining has a solid track record of successful applications to the healthcare domain. Within such research space, we conducted a case study related to the Intensive Care Unit (ICU) ward of the Uniklinik Aachen hospital in Germany. The aim of this work is twofold: developing a normative model representing the clinical guidelines for the treatment of COVID-19 patients, and analyzing the adherence of the observed behavior (recorded in the information system of the hospital) to such guidelines. We show that, through conformance checking techniques, it is possible to analyze the care process for COVID-19 patients, highlighting the main deviations from the clinical guidelines. The results provide physicians with useful indications for improving the process and ensuring service quality and patient satisfaction. We share the resulting model as an open-source BPMN file.

Keywords: Process mining · Healthcare · COVID-19 · STAKOB guidelines · Business Process Management · Conformance checking

We acknowledge the ICU4COVID project (funded by European Union's Horizon 2020 under grant agreement n. 101016000) and the COVAS project.

M. Montali et al. (Eds.): ICPM 2022 Workshops, LNBIP 468, pp. 315–327, 2023.
https://doi.org/10.1007/978-3-031-27815-0_23

1   Introduction

At the turn of the decade, the logistics of operations in hospitals and healthcare centers have been severely disrupted worldwide by the COVID-19 pandemic. Its impact has been profound and damaging in all aspects of life, but in no context it has been more damaging than in healthcare: the safety and well-being of physicians and medical personnel, the supply chain of drugs and equipment, and the capacity of hospitals were all challenged by the pandemic.

One of the most critical points for healthcare systems involved in the treatment process is the management of COVID-19 patients needing acute and respiratory care. Therefore, healthcare organizations are increasingly pushed to improve the efficiency of care processes and the resource management for such category of patients. One way to attain such improvement is to leverage historical data from information systems of hospitals. These data can be then cleaned and analyzed, to individuate non-compliant behavior and inefficiencies in the care process.

The aim of our work is to analyze the care process for the COVID-19 patients treated at the Intensive Care Unit (ICU) ward of the Uniklinik Aachen hospital in Germany, in order to identify divergences or anomalies within the process. To do so, our work intends to develop an executable process model representing the clinical guidelines for the treatment of COVID-19 patients and evaluate the adherence of the observed behavior (recorded by the information system of the hospital) to such guidelines.

The STAKOB guidelines[1] ("Ständigen Arbeitskreis der Kompetenz- und Behandlungszentren für Krankheiten durch hochpathogene Erreger", "Permanent working group of competence and treatment centers for diseases caused by highly pathogenic agents") are widely accepted and recognized protocols for the treatment of COVID-19, compiled and verified by a large consensus of medical scientists, physicians, and research institutions. They provide a comprehensive overview of recommendations on the management of hospitalized COVID-19 patients. The process model was obtained starting from such guidelines, and was validated by the physicians working in the intensive and intermediate care unit of the Uniklinik. We openly share the resulting BPMN model, as well as the related documentation. The conformance with the guidelines was assessed by using process mining techniques. The results provide hospital managers with information about the main deviations and/or anomalies in the process and their possible causes. In addition, they suggest improvements to make the process more compliant, cost-effective, and performant.

The remainder of the paper is structured as follows. Section 2 explores related work and sets the context of our research. Section 3 lays out the methodology we employed in our case study. Section 4 illustrates the results of our case study. Finally, Sect. 5 concludes the paper.

---

[1] https://www.rki.de/DE/Content/Kommissionen/Stakob/Stakob_node.html.

2   Related Work

The global effort to fight the pandemic has stimulated the adoption of new technologies in healthcare practice [7]. An area where this effect has been radical is the digitization of healthcare processes, both medical and administrative. Data recording and availability have improved during the years of the pandemic. Stakeholders realized that data are a valuable information source to support the management and improvement of healthcare processes [9]. In addition, the reliance of medical personnel on digital support systems is now much more significant. Fields of science that have recently shown to be particularly promising when applied to healthcare operations are the process sciences, and specifically Business Process Management (BPM) and process mining [9]. This is mainly due to the characteristics of healthcare process, which are complex and flexible and involve a multidisciplinary team [9,13]. Particularly, process mining has emerged as a suitable approach to analyze, discover, improve, and manage real-life and complex processes, by extracting knowledge from event logs [1]. Currently, process scientists have gathered event data on the process of treatment for COVID-19 and leveraged process mining techniques to obtain insights on various aspects of the healthcare process [3,12,15] or on how other business processes have been impacted by the disruption caused by COVID-19 [17].

Among process mining techniques, conformance checking aims to measure the adherence of a (discovered or known) process with a given set of data, or vice-versa [6]. Conformance checking helps medics to understand major deviations from clinical guidelines, as well as to identify areas for improvement in practices and protocols [9]. Some studies have applied these techniques in different healthcare contexts, such as oncology [14]. However, no studies have addressed the compliance analysis on the care process of COVID-19 patients in a real-life scenario. To do so, it is essential to have a normative model, reflecting clinical guidelines and protocols, that can be interpreted by machines. Currently, executable process models representing the guidelines for the treatment of COVID-19 patients are still absent and needed, given the uncertainty and variability of the disease.

3   Methodology

The methodology conducted in this study consists of the following three main steps, also shown in Fig. 1:

- Development of a normative model based on the STAKOB guidelines. A normative model is a process model that reflects and implements rules, guidelines, and policies of the process, mandated by process owners or other supervisory bodies. This phase involves (i) the analysis of the STAKOB documentation and interview with ICU physicians, (ii) the development of the model from the guidelines, and (iii) the validation of the model with ICU physicians.

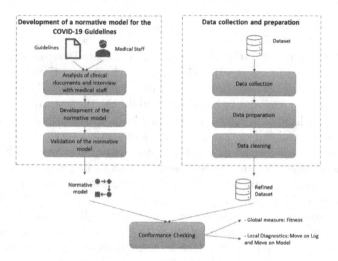

Fig. 1. Case study methodology. Our work measures the deviation between the expected and real behavior of the COVID-19 treatment process, respectively represented by the STAKOB guidelines, and by the COVAS dataset.

– Data collection and preparation, which involves the extraction and preprocessing of event data, gathered from the information system of the hospital.
  The event log is refined by removing duplicate and irrelevant data, handling
  missing data, and detecting outliers to ensure data reliability.
– Conformance checking, which involves the use of conformance checking techniques to compare the normative model with the event logs for the three
  COVID-19 waves and determine whether the behavior observed in practice
  conforms to the documented process.

3.1 Development of a Normative Model Based on the STAKOB Guidelines

The STAKOB guidelines provide information on the disease and its related symptoms, and describe the diagnostic and treatment activities to be performed on COVID-19 patients and the therapies to be administered. The treatment of COVID-19 patients requires a multi-disciplinary approach: in addition to intensive care physicians and nurses, specialists in infectious diseases and infection control must also be part of the team [8]. The guidelines guide the operations of the medical team involved in the inpatient care of COVID-19 patients, but are also intended to provide information for individuals and/or organizations directly involved in this topic.

To make the guidelines interpretable by machines—and thus suitable for conformance checking—we developed a normative process model of the STAKOB guidelines in the BPMN language using the Signavio tool[2]. The choice of the

---

[2] https://www.signavio.com/.

BPMN standard is due to its ability to be executable but, at the same time, easy to understand by physicians and practitioners. The BPMN model of the STAKOB guidelines was validated by using a qualitative approach. Specifically, the model was presented and discussed with three physicians working in the intensive and intermediate care unit of the Uniklinik during three meetings. During the meetings, several refinements were applied to the model, until it was approved by all.

3.2 Data Collection and Preparation

We collected and pre-processed data of COVID-19 patients monitored in the context of the COVID-19 Aachen Study (COVAS). The log contains event information regarding COVID-19 patients treated by the Uniklinik between January 2020 and June 2021. Events (patient admittance, symptoms, treatments, drug administration) are labeled with the date, creating timestamps with a coarseness at the day level. While here we exclusively focus on process mining, the COVAS dataset has also been analyzed in the context of explainable AI [16].

Data were gathered from the information system of the hospital. The initial database consisted of 269 cases, 33 activity labels, 210 variants, and 3542 events. Before the analysis, we refined the raw event log, to guarantee its quality. Data cleaning and preparation were executed with Python and included: (i) outliers and incomplete cases removal based on the number of hospitalization days, (ii) less significant activities abstraction, and (iii) filtering of infrequent variants. As an example, we removed the cases with a duration of more than 70 days: this value was validated with the doctors, according to whom durations longer than 70 days may be due to registration delays. In the end, the refined event log consisted of 187 patient cases, 32 activities, 135 variants, and 2397 events.

To evaluate the adherence of the COVAS dataset to the normative model during the three COVID-19 waves, we split the dataset into three sub-event logs. As illustrated in the next sections, this is done with the goal of examining how treatment operations for COVID-19 change between infection waves with respect to the adherence to the STAKOB guidelines. As shown by the dotted chart of the event log in Fig. 2, the three waves can be clearly identified. Such a choice of wave separation was also supported by the literature [5].

The event log of the first wave contains 106 cases and 1410 events. The average duration of the process is 25.38 days. The log of the second wave contains 59 cases and 892 events, with an average duration of 22.42 days. The log of the third wave contains 22 cases and 282 events, with an average duration of 16.38 days.

3.3 Conformance Checking

For each sub-event log, we applied conformance checking techniques to identify deviations within the process. Specifically, we utilized the plug-in "Replay a Log on Petri Net for Conformance Analysis" as implemented on ProM, with

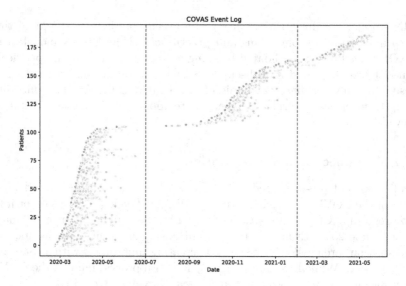

Fig. 2. Dotted chart of the COVAS event log. The cases are sorted by the first recorded event, which is highlighted in orange. Every blue dot corresponds to a recorded event. The vertical dashed lines separate the first, second, and third COVID-19 waves, based on the knowledge of physicians. (Color figure online)

standard setting parameters. The choice is due to the fact that alignment-based techniques can exactly pinpoint where deviations are observed [1, 2].

The alignment-based technique allowed to estimate a global conformance measure, which quantifies the overall conformance of the model and event log, and local diagnostics, which identify points where the model and event log do not agree. In the first case, we calculated fitness, which measures "the proportion of behavior in the event log possible according to the model" [1]. In the second case, we estimated for each activity within the model the following [4]:

- the number of "moves on log": Occurrences of an activity in the trace cannot be mapped to any enabled activity in the process model.
- the number of "moves on model": Occurrences of an enabled activity in the process model cannot be mapped to any event in the trace sequence.
- the number of "synchronous moves": Occurrences of an activity belonging to a trace can be mapped to occurrences of an enabled activity in the process model.

4   Results

In this section, we presented the results from the development of the normative model and the conformance checking analysis.

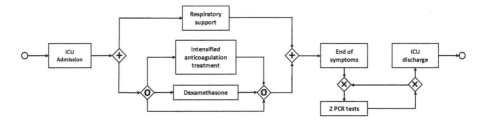

Fig. 3. A section of the STAKOB COVID-19 model, depicting some activities related to the ICU operations for COVID-19 patients.

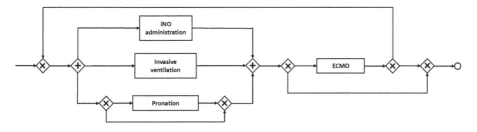

Fig. 4. A section of the STAKOB COVID-19 model, depicting some activities related to the respiration support operations for COVID-19 patients.

4.1 Normative Model

The developed normative model consists of 3 sub-processes, 23 activities and approximately 36 gateways (XOR, AND and OR). Figure 3 shows a section of the model.

The model clearly underlines the fact that the treatment of hospitalized patients with COVID-19 is complex and is characterized by several pursuable pathways (see the presence of XOR and OR gateways). It also requires the collaboration of different departments and specialists. More in detail, the care treatment includes an antibiotic/drug therapy phase and, if necessary, an oxygenation phase. At this point, if the patient's health condition deteriorates, the transfer to the ICU is planned (partially shown in Fig. 3). In the ICU, the patient may undergo mechanical ventilation, ECMO (ExtraCorporeal Membrane Oxygenation) or pronation in addition to the medical therapy. A section of the sub-process showing the respiratory support for the patient can be seen in Fig. 4. Recovery and subsequent discharge are confirmed by two negative COVID-19 tests.

The full model is openly available on GitHub[3]. It is rendered in the XML export format of the BPMN standard[4]. The folder also contains a PDF depicting

---

[3] https://github.com/marcopegoraro/pm-healthcare/tree/main/stakob.

[4] https://www.bpmn.org/.

Table 1. Results of conformance checking alignments with the STAKOB model for the patient sub-log corresponding to the first COVID-19 wave. For each activity in the log, we show the count of moves on log, moves on model, and synchronous moves.

Activity	Move on log	Syncro move	Move on model	Activity	Move on log	Syncro move	Move on model
Symptobegin	0	106	0	Ventilation Start	33	9	2
Hospitalization	1	105	1	Ventilation End	35	8	6
UKA Admission	12	96	10	NMB Start	4	11	0
Abx Start	2	58	0	NMB End	4	11	0
Abx End	2	58	0	CVVH Start	16	11	0
Start Oxygen	22	85	0	CVVH End	16	11	0
Remdesivir Start	0	3	0	Prone Start	25	10	0
Remdesivir End	0	3	0	Prone End	25	10	0
Admission ICU	35	20	0	ECMO Start	10	0	0
HiFlo Start	0	1	19	ECMO End	10	0	0
Hiflo End	0	1	19	End of Fever	22	53	53
NIV Start	6	5	9	Discharge ICU	48	6	14
NIV End	10	5	9	Last Oxygen Day	39	53	53
iNO Start	13	10	1	Discharge dead	0	33	0
iNO End	13	10	1	Discharge alive	0	73	0

the entire model, a license declaration, and an addendum describing the model schematic in more detail.

4.2 Conformance Checking Results

COVID-19 First Wave Results. For the first wave, the fitness between the model and the data is 0.69; some trace variants are not reproduced by the model. This may be due to the variability of the process (health conditions vary from patient to patient). In addition, the coarseness of the timestamps in the dataset has an impact: events are recorded at the date level, so the order in which they are recorded may vary in some instances. Table 1 shows the results of the conformance checking for the first wave. Specifically, for each activity, it shows the misalignments between the normative model and the event log.

Several misalignments can be observed. In particular:

- The *HiFlo Start* and *HiFlo End* activities (corresponding to high flow oxygenation) present 19 moves on model and one synchronous move. This means that, although it is required by the guidelines, this activity is only performed in one case. This indicates that, given the patient's condition, the physicians may have seen fit to skip this treatment.
- There are several tasks that have both moves on model and moves on log. This means that these tasks often deviate from the normative model (in some cases they are present in the model but not in reality, in others vice-versa). This may be due to the variability of patients' conditions and the lack of

Table 2. Results of conformance checking alignments with the STAKOB model for the patient sub-log corresponding to the second COVID-19 wave. For each activity in the log, we show the count of moves on log, moves on model, and synchronous moves.

Activity	Move on log	Syncro move	Move on model	Activity	Move on log	Syncro move	Move on model
Symptobegin	0	59	0	Dexamethasone End	24	14	1
Hospitalization	0	59	0	Ventilation Start	11	8	1
UKA Admission	8	50	9	Ventilation End	11	8	1
Abx Start	0	29	0	NMB Start	2	9	0
Abx End	0	29	0	NMB End	2	9	0
Start Oxygen	5	54	0	CVVH Start	7	8	1
Remdesivir Start	8	12	0	CVVH End	7	8	1
Remdesivir End	8	12	0	Prone Start	8	8	0
Admission ICU	8	15	1	Prone End	8	8	0
HiFlo Start	0	2	14	ECMO Start	7	0	0
Hiflo End	0	2	14	ECMO End	7	0	0
NIV Start	6	8	5	End of Fever	27	13	43
NIV End	8	5	8	Discharge ICU	20	2	14
iNO Start	2	9	0	Last Oxygen Day	19	36	23
iNO End	2	9	0	Discharge dead	0	17	0
Dexamethasone Start	23	15	0	Discharge alive	0	42	0

familiarity with COVID-19 and its standardized treatment, since this data was recorded in the early days of the pandemic. For example, the guidelines suggest that the *Discharge ICU* should occur after ventilation and pronation, while in reality, in some cases, it occurs before. Thus, many activities occur while the patient is hospitalized, but not still formally admitted to the ICU.

– Some activities present only moves on log and synchronous moves, i.e., they are present in reality but at times not in the normative model. This means that they are performed at different times than the guidelines suggest. For example, *Admission ICU* may be anticipated because of a particularly critical course not foreseen by the physicians or be delayed because no space in ICU is available at that time; or *Prone End* (the interruption of the treatment of pronation) may be brought forward because of the negative effects on the patient, e.g., the appearance of pressure sores. Alternatively, pronation may be delayed because the patient has not achieved optimal arterial blood oxygenation.

COVID-19 Second Wave Results. For the log of the second wave, the fitness with the STAKOB model is 0.66. Table 2 shows the results of conformance checking for the second wave.

In the second wave, *Hospitalization* is only performed after the onset of symptoms, as suggested by the guidelines. However, deviations are also encountered. As in the first wave, the most affected activities are *End Of Fever, Admission ICU* and *Discharge ICU*, and *Last Oxygen Day*, which have both moves on

Table 3. Results of conformance checking alignments with the STAKOB model for the patient sub-log corresponding to the third COVID-19 wave. For each activity in the log, we show the count of moves on log, moves on model, and synchronous moves.

Activity	Move on log	Syncro move	Move on model	Activity	Move on log	Syncro move	Move on model
Symptobegin	0	22	0	Dexamethasone End	8	4	0
Hospitalization	2	19	3	Ventilation Start	1	9	1
UKA Admission	0	22	0	Ventilation End	1	9	1
Abx Start	0	8	0	NMB Start	0	1	0
Abx End	0	8	0	NMB End	0	1	0
Start Oxygen	0	38	0	CVVH Start	2	1	0
Remdesivir Start	0	1	0	CVVH End	2	1	0
Remdesivir End	0	1	0	Prone Start	1	1	0
Admission ICU	1	2	1	Prone End	1	1	0
HiFlo Start	0	2	1	ECMO Start	0	0	0
Hiflo End	0	2	1	ECMO End	0	0	0
NIV Start	4	1	0	End of Fever	11	6	16
NIV End	5	0	1	Discharge ICU	3	2	1
iNO Start	1	1	0	Last Oxygen Day	3	17	5
iNO End	1	1	0	Discharge dead	0	3	0
Dexamethasone Start	9	3	1	Discharge alive	0	19	0

log and moves on model. This may be related to the mutability of the disease becoming difficult to manage with common protocols and the variability of the patients' conditions. Compared to the first wave, the use of drugs has changed. In particular, a new drug is being administered, i.e., Dexamethasone, and the use of Remdesivir is increased. The administration of both drugs has moves on log mismatches, indicating that the physicians needed to administer such treatments more frequently than recommended. The former is also used in patients who do not require intensive care, contrary to what the guidelines suggest. The second, which is preferred for non-critical hospitalized patients, is also used in intensive care. In addition, high flow oxygenation is rarely performed here, despite being included in the guidelines.

COVID-19 Third Wave Results. The fitness between the log and the model is 0.69 for the third COVID-19 wave. Table 3 shows the results of conformance checking for the third wave.

The physicians' experience and familiarity with the disease appear to have increased. However, many of the misaligned activities have similar behavior to those performed during past waves. Note that the ECMO treatment has zero values in all columns. This is because it is not performed in the third wave (unlike the first two). Since ECMO is the most invasive oxygenation treatment, this may be due to the fact that the severity of the patients' condition has decreased.

To summarize, alignments-based techniques make it possible to detect and analyze process deviations, providing useful insights for physicians. Furthermore, in the three waves, most activities remained misaligned, while some moved closer to the guidelines' suggestion. This shows that the process is highly variable and specific care pathways are required for each patient, which do not always coincide with those stated in the guidelines.

5   Conclusion

Our work aimed to analyze the care process for COVID-19 patients, bringing to light deviations from the clinical guidelines. Specifically, the work proposed a normative model bases on the STAKOB guidelines, which can be interpreted by software tools (e.g., process mining software). The BPMN model is openly accessible to any analyst, and can also be loaded into any commercial software supporting the BPMN standard, like Celonis and Signavio. This addresses the need for computer-interpretable and usable guidelines in healthcare, particularly for the treatment of COVID-19 patients [10]. In addition, the work provided physicians with guidance on the management of COVID-19 patients, highlighting deviations and critical points in the three infection waves.

The contributions of our work are:

- One of the first attempts to apply a process mining-based methodology for the analysis of process deviations in a real, complex, and uncertain healthcare context, like the recent and ongoing COVID-19 pandemic.
- The development of a normative model that can advise physicians in the treatment of COVID-19 patients by providing specific guidelines and procedures to follow. This is helpful in dealing with the uncertainty and complexity of healthcare operations brought about by the pandemic. In addition, the model can be used as input for the development of a decision support system, which alerts in real-time in case of violations of the guidelines.
- The extraction of valuable insights for physicians regarding the main deviations and the related causes in the COVID-19 patient care process. This knowledge is crucial for improving the process and ensuring service quality and patient satisfaction, e.g., better management of drug administration (when to administer and how often), more targeted execution of certain treatments—e.g., pronation—(who to treat and when to do it), and execution of treatments suggested by guidelines but never performed in reality that can enhance the care pathway and reduce hospitalization time (such as high flow oxygenation).

The work presents some open questions and directions for future research. The limited size, especially for the third wave, and the coarseness of the timestamps in the dataset may impact the results. To address this issue, a possible option is to weigh the results of analyses using the probability of specific orderings of events in traces [11]. Furthermore, the physician's consensus on both the validity of the STAKOB model and the interpretation of the conformance checking results can definitely be enlarged, by soliciting the expert opinion of a larger group of medics. As future developments, we plan to: (i) extend the research and collect new data from other German hospitals, in order to generalize the results and identify best practices in the treatment of COVID-19 patients; (ii) improve the validation of results; (iii) actively involve physicians in the analysis of deviations, using qualitative approaches such as interviews and field observations; (iv) conduct a more extensive comparative analysis based on process mining, including a structural model comparison, concept drift, and performance analysis.

References

1. van der Aalst, W.M.P.: Process Mining: Data Science in Action. Springer, Heidelberg (2016)
2. Adriansyah, A., van Dongen, B.F., van der Aalst, W.M.P.: Towards robust conformance checking. In: zur Muehlen, M., Su, J. (eds.) BPM 2010. LNBIP, vol. 66, pp. 122–133. Springer, Heidelberg (2011). https://doi.org/10.1007/978-3-642-20511-8_11
3. Augusto, A., Deitz, T., Faux, N., Manski-Nankervis, J.A., Capurro, D.: Process mining-driven analysis of COVID-19's impact on vaccination patterns. J. Biomed. Inform. **130**, 104081 (2022)
4. Dixit, P.M., Caballero, H.S.G., Corvo, A., Hompes, B.F.A., Buijs, J.C.A.M., van der Aalst, W.M.P.: Enabling interactive process analysis with process mining and visual analytics. In: HEALTHINF, pp. 573–584 (2017)
5. Dongelmans, D.A., et al.: Characteristics and outcome of Covid-19 patients admitted to the ICU: a nationwide cohort study on the comparison between the first and the consecutive upsurges of the second wave of the COVID-19 pandemic in the Netherlands. Ann. Intensive Care **12**(1), 1–10 (2022)
6. Gatta, R., et al.: Clinical guidelines: a crossroad of many research areas. challenges and opportunities in process mining for healthcare. In: Di Francescomarino, C., Dijkman, R., Zdun, U. (eds.) BPM 2019. LNBIP, vol. 362, pp. 545–556. Springer, Cham (2019). https://doi.org/10.1007/978-3-030-37453-2_44
7. Golinelli, D., Boetto, E., Carullo, G., Nuzzolese, A.G., Landini, M.P., Fantini, M.P., et al.: Adoption of digital technologies in health care during the COVID-19 pandemic: systematic review of early scientific literature. J. Med. Internet Res. **22**(11), e22280 (2020)
8. Malin, J.J., et al.: Key summary of German national treatment guidance for hospitalized COVID-19 patients. Infection **50**(1), 93–106 (2022)
9. Munoz-Gama, J., et al.: Process mining for healthcare: characteristics and challenges. J. Biomed. Inform. **127**, 103994 (2022)
10. Oliart, E., Rojas, E., Capurro, D.: Are we ready for conformance checking in healthcare? Measuring adherence to clinical guidelines: a scoping systematic literature review. J. Biomed. Informatics 104076 (2022)
11. Pegoraro, M., Bakullari, B., Uysal, M.S., van der Aalst, W.M.P.: Probability estimation of uncertain process trace realizations. In: Munoz-Gama, J., Lu, X. (eds.) ICPM 2021. LNBIP, vol. 433, pp. 21–33. Springer, Cham (2022). https://doi.org/10.1007/978-3-030-98581-3_2
12. Pegoraro, M., Narayana, M.B.S., Benevento, E., van der Aalst, W.M.P., Martin, L., Marx, G.: Analyzing medical data with process mining: a COVID-19 case study. In: Abramowicz, W., Auer, S., Stróżyna, M. (eds.) BIS 2021. LNBIP, vol. 444, pp. 39–44. Springer, Cham (2022). https://doi.org/10.1007/978-3-031-04216-4_4

13. Rebuge, Á., Ferreira, D.R.: Business process analysis in healthcare environments: a methodology based on process mining. Inf. Syst. **37**(2), 99–116 (2012)
14. Rojas, E., Munoz-Gama, J., Sepúlveda, M., Capurro, D.: Process mining in healthcare: a literature review. J. Biomed. Inform. **61**, 224–236 (2016)
15. dos Santos Leandro, G., et al.: Process mining leveraging the analysis of patient journey and outcomes: stroke assistance during the Covid-19 pandemic. Knowl. Manag. E-Learning Int. J. **13**(4), 421–437 (2021)
16. Velioglu, R., Göpfert, J.P., Artelt, A., Hammer, B.: Explainable artificial intelligence for improved modeling of processes. In: Yin, H., Camacho, D., Tino, P. (eds.) IDEAL 2022. LNCS, vol. 13756, pp. 313–325. Springer, Cham (2022). https://doi.org/10.1007/978-3-031-21753-1_31
17. Zabka, W., Blank, P., Accorsi, R.: Has the pandemic impacted my workforce's productivity? Applying effort mining to identify productivity shifts during COVID-19 lockdown. In: Proceedings of the Industry Forum at BPM 2021 co-located with 19th International Conference on Business Process Management (BPM 2021). CEUR Workshop Proceedings, vol. 3112, pp. 3–13. CEUR-WS.org (2021)

SAMPLE: A Semantic Approach for Multi-perspective Event Log Generation

Joscha Grüger[1,2](✉) ⓘ, Tobias Geyer[2] ⓘ, David Jilg[2] ⓘ,
and Ralph Bergmann[1,2] ⓘ

[1] Business Information Systems II, University of Trier, Trier, Germany
grueger@uni-trier.de
[2] German Research Center for Artificial Intelligence (DFKI), Trier, Germany

Abstract. Data and process mining techniques can be applied in many areas to gain valuable insights. For many reasons, accessibility to real-world business and medical data is severely limited. However, research, but especially the development of new methods, depends on a sufficient basis of realistic data. Due to the lack of data, this progress is hindered. This applies in particular to domains that use personal data, such as healthcare. With adequate quality, synthetic data can be a solution to this problem. In the procedural field, some approaches have already been presented that generate synthetic data based on a process model. However, only a few have included the data perspective so far. Data semantics, which is crucial for the quality of the generated data, has not yet been considered. Therefore, in this paper we present the multi-perspective event log generation approach SAMPLE that considers the data perspective and, in particular, its semantics. The evaluation of the approach is based on a process model for the treatment of malignant melanoma. As a result, we were able to integrate the semantic of data into the log generation process and identify new challenges.

Keywords: Process mining · Event log generation · Synthetic data · Data petri nets

1 Introduction

In many data-rich domains, the application of data analysis methods of data and process mining opens up great potentials. For example, with the right analytical approaches, operational processes can be designed more effective and efficient, new insights can be gained, and predictions can be made. However, there is a lack of data, especially in the context of research, as access is often difficult. This is particularly the case in areas where the data contains personal information (e.g., in medicine) or business secrets (e.g., in industry and business). This fact hinders progress in the development of new approaches and solutions.

One way to address this problem is to work on high-quality synthetic data. For instance, procedural data can be generated based on process models using

© The Author(s) 2023
M. Montali et al. (Eds.): ICPM 2022 Workshops, LNBIP 468, pp. 328–340, 2023.
https://doi.org/10.1007/978-3-031-27815-0_24

techniques such as token-based simulation, finite state automata simulation, abduction, constraint satisfactory problem, or Boolean satisfiability problem. However, all approaches either focus only on the control-flow perspective or, if they are able to generate variable values for the data perspective, they do so based solely on the defined conditions of the process model. In this case, the values are generated without considering the semantics and the focus of the data generation is only on the fulfillment of the conditions. This leads to unrealistic values for the variables and consequently to synthetic data with low quality.

Therefore, we present the SAMPLE approach, a multi-perspective event log generator that considers the data perspective and its semantics in particular. In the approach, variables are described by a meta-model and a triple of semantic information (values, dependencies, distributions). Using this, combined with a play-out algorithm to generate the control-flow perspective, leads to the creation of synthetic, correct data with semantically meaningful variable values. By generating synthetic data, this approach presents a method for preserving patient privacy and security that addresses challenge C7 of the characteristics and challenges for process mining by Munoz-Gama et al. [13].

The remainder of the paper is organized as follows. Section 2 provides information on related work and Sect. 3 on the components of our approach. Section 4 describes the methodological approach for the multi-perspective synthetic event log generator. In Sect. 5 the implementation is presented, Sect. 6 presents the evaluation process, and Sect. 7 concludes the paper.

2 Related Work

In token-based simulation, tokens are propagated through a process model and executed transitions are recorded to generate event logs. When using Petri nets, the propagation is achieved by firing enabled transitions until all transitions are disabled or a final state is reached. Different strategies can be used to determine which transition to fire, such as random selection. The order of the transitions fired is recorded to generate the traces. The transitions are then referenced with activities to obtain a valid trace, which can be added to the event log. The process is repeated until the desired number of traces is reached.

Token-based event log generation has evolved from work in modeling simulation, such as reference nets [8] or Colored Petri nets (CPNs) [6]. In [8], Kummer et al. developed the application RENEW which is a Java-based high-level Petri net simulator. It provides a flexible modeling approach based on reference nets as well as the feature to dynamically create an arbitrary number of net instances during a simulation. Alves de Medeiros and Günther [11] state the need for correct logs (i.e., without noise and incompleteness) for the development and tuning of process mining algorithms, since imperfections in the log hinder these activities. Their approach is an extension of Colored Petri nets to generate XML event logs with the simulation feature of the CPN Tools [16]. Nakatumba et al. [14] present an approach that incorporates workload-dependent processing speeds in a simulation model and how it can be learned from event logs. Moreover, they show how event logs with workload-dependent behavior can be generated by simulation using CPN Tools [14].

Many approaches address the lack of data for appropriate (process)mining algorithm testing and evaluation [1,11,12,15,17]. The approach of Shugurov and Mitsyuk [17] allows the generation of event logs and sets of event logs to support large scale automated testing. Furthermore, noise can be added to event logs to simulate more realistic data. Vanden Broucke et al. [1] present a ProM [3] plugin enabling the rapid generation of event logs based on a user-supplied Petri net. The approach offers features such as the configuration of simulation options, activities, activity and trace timings. Mitsyuk et al. [12] present an approach to generate event logs from BPMN models to provide a synthetic data base for testing BPMN process mining approaches. They propose a formal token-based executable BPMN semantic that considers BPMN 2.0 with its expressive constructs [12]. The approach simulates hierarchical process models, models with data flows and pools, and models interacting through message flows [12]. Pertsukhov and Mitsyuk [15] present an approach that generates event logs for Petri nets with inhibitor and reset arcs. These arc types improve the expressiveness of nets and are useful when ordinary place/transition-nets are not sufficient [15].

One rather unique use of token-based simulation is proposed by Kataeva and Kalenkova [7]. Their approach generates graph-based process models by applying graph grammar production rules for model generation. A production rule replaces one part of a graph by another [7]. The approach uses a simulation consisting of applying production rules that propagate tokens through the graph to generate event logs. Another approach is presented by Esgin and Karagoz [4], addressing the problem of unlabeled event logs, i.e., the lack of mapping of case identifiers to process instances in real event logs. Instead of fixing the log, the approach simulates a synthetic log from scratch using the process profile defining the activity vocabulary and the Petri net in tabular form as input [4]. In [2], the generation of random processes is extended by the complete support for multi-perspective models and logs, i.e., the integration of time and data. Furthermore, online settings, i.e., the generation of multi-perspective event streams and concept drifts, are supported [2].

Although important problems are addressed, a drawback of most related work in this field is the limitation to the pure control-flow. Besides exceptions such as [2], the data perspective is not considered. Overall, the semantics of data and its impact on the reality of event logs is not explicitly in addressed.

3   Fundamentals

In the following, we introduce the notions required for our approach.

3.1   Basic Notations

Definition 1 (universes, general function). *We define the following universes and functions to be used:*

- *C is the universe of all possible case identifiers*

- $\mathcal{E}$ is the universe of all possible event identifiers
- $\mathcal{A}$ is the universe of all possible activity identifiers
- $\mathcal{AN}$ is the universe of all possible attribute identifiers
- $dom(f)$ denotes the domain of some function f.

Definition 2 (attributes, classifier [18]). *Attributes can be used to characterize events and cases, e.g. an event can be assigned to a resource or have a timestamp. For any event $e \in \mathcal{E}$, any case $c \in \mathcal{C}$ and name $n \in \mathcal{AN}$, $\#_n(e)$ is the value of attribute n for event e and $\#_n(c)$ is the value of attribute n for case c. $\#_n(e) = \bot$ if event e has no attribute n and $\#_n(c) = \bot$ if case c has no attribute n. We assume the classifier $\underline{e} = \#_{activity}(e)$ as the default classifier.*

Definition 3 (trace, case [18]). *Each case $c \in \mathcal{C}$ has a mandatory attribute trace, with $\hat{c} = \#_{trace}(c) \in \mathcal{E}^* \setminus \{\langle\rangle\}$. A trace is a finite sequence of events $\sigma \in \mathcal{E}^*$ where each event occurs only once, i.e. $1 \leq i < j \leq |\sigma| : \sigma(i) \neq \sigma(j)$. By $\sigma \oplus e = \sigma$ we denote the addition of an e event to a trace σ.*

Definition 4 (event log [18]). *An event log is a set of cases $\mathcal{L} \subseteq \mathcal{C}$, in the form that each event is contained only once in the event log. If an event log contains timestamps, these should be ordered in each trace.*

Definition 5 (multiset [18]). *Let X be its set. A multiset is a tuple $M = (X, m)$ with $m : X \to \mathbb{N}$. We use $x \in M$ to express that x is contained in the multiset M, therefore $x \in X$ and $m(x) \geq 1$. We denote by $\mathcal{B}(X)$ the set of all multisets over X.*

3.2 Petri Nets, Marked Petri Net

Petri nets are process models that describe the control-flow perspective of a process while ignoring all other perspectives [10].

Definition 6 (Petri net [18]). *A Petri net is a triple $N = (P, T, F)$ where P is a finite set of places, T is a finite set of transitions, and $F \subseteq (P \times T) \cup (T \times P)$ is a set of flow relations that describe a bipartite graph between places and transitions. ${}^\bullet t$ denotes the input places of a transition t.*

3.3 Data Petri Nets

A data Petri net is a Petri net extended by the data perspective.

Definition 7 (data Petri net [9]). *A data Petri net (DPN) $N = (P, T, F, V, U, R, W, G)$ consists of:*

- *a Petri net (P, T, F);*
- *a set V of variables;*
- *a function U that defines the values admissible for each variable $v \in V$, i.e. if $U(v) = D_v$, D_v is the domain of variable v;*

- a read function $R \in T \to 2^V$ labeling each transition with the set of variables that it must read;
- a write function $W \in T \to 2^V$ labeling each transition with the set of variables that it must write;
- a guard function $G \in T \to G_V$ associating a guard with each transition.

For the naming of transitions, we introduce labeled data Petri nets. Invisible transition are enabled and fired, but do not refer to a process activity.

Definition 8 (labeled data Petri net [10]). Let $N = (P, T, F, V, U, R, W, G)$ be a Data Petri net. Then the triple $LN = (N, \lambda, \nu)$ is a labeled Petri net, with:

- $\lambda : T \to (\mathcal{E} \cup \{\tau\})$ is an activity labeling function, mapping transitions on an activity label and invisible transitions on τ.
- $\nu : V \to \mathcal{AN}$ a labeling function, mapping variables to attribute names.

Similar to Petri nets, data Petri nets always have a certain state described by the current markings and variable values. This is defined as follows.

Definition 9 (state of a DPN [9]). Let $N = (P, T, F, V, U, R, W, G)$ be a Data Petri net with $D = \cup_{v \in V} U(v)$, then tuple (M, A) is the state of N with

- $M \in \mathbb{B}(P)$ is the marking of the Petri net (P, T, F)
- $A : V \to D \cup \{\bot\}$. For $v \in V$ it holds, if no value is given for v, $A(v) = \bot$

With (M_0, A_0) the initial state and $M_0(p_0) = 1$, $\forall p \in P \setminus \{p_0\} : M_0(p) = 0$ and $\forall v \in V : A_0(v) = \bot$ and (M_F, A_F) the final marking.

Petri nets change their state by firing transitions. A valid firing of a transition is defined as follows.

Definition 10 (valid firing [10]). Let $N = (P, T, F, V, U, R, W, G)$ be a Data Petri net. A firing of a transition is a double (t, w) with $t \in T$ and variables that are written with the respective values. Let (M, A) be a state of N, then (t, w) is a valid transition firing, if

- $\forall p \in {}^\bullet t : M(p) \geq 1$, i.e. each place in t's preset contains at least one token.
- $dom(w) = W(t)$, the transition writes the prescribed variables
- $\forall v \in dom(w) : w(v) \in U(v)$, i.e. the assigned values for variables are valid
- Guard $G(t)$ evaluates true with A

4 Synthetic Multi-perspective Log Generation

To generate a realistic event log $\mathcal{L}$ for a given data Petri net N, SAMPLE divides the procedure into the control-flow perspective (Sect. 4.1) and data perspective (Sect. 4.2). While the generation of the control-flow perspective of the log is based on the token-based simulation approach, the generation of the data is built on a rule-based approach. Figure 1 depicts the log generation process. In the following, we first describe the generation of the control-flow perspective and extend the approach to the data perspective in the next step.

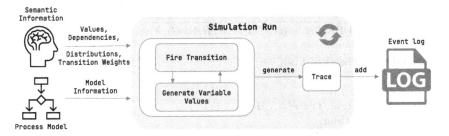

Fig. 1. The figure outlines the event log generation process of the approach. The model information and the semantic data serve as input for the simulation runs, in which traces (i.e., sequences of events with data) are generated and added to the log.

4.1   Generation of the Control-Flow Perspective

The control-flow perspective is realized through random trace generation, i.e., an approach that randomly traverses the Petri net to generate sequences of activities. Each single trace is generated by a simulation run. A simulation run starts with the initial marking of the model and starts firing random transitions until a deadlock or a final marking is reached.

Transitions can be weighted to generate particularly realistic logs. These weightings affect the probability of the transitions firing and could be learned, e.g., based on the distribution in real logs or manually defined by domain experts. For this purpose, we introduce a mapping of transitions to weights:

Definition 11 (transition weights). *Let* $N = (P, T, F, V, U, R, W, G)$ *be a data Petri net. Then* $\omega : T \rightarrow \mathbb{R}$ *is the mapping of transitions to weights. For all* $t \in T$, t_ω *is the short form for* $\omega(t)$.

Definition 12 (transition selection). *Let* $N = (P, T, F, V, U, R, W, G)$ *be a data Petri net and* (M, A) *the current state of the DPN. Then transition* t *is selected randomly by* $rt(N, (M, A))$ *by considering the weights* $\omega(t)$. R_ω *denotes*

$$\{t \in T | \forall p \in {}^\bullet t : M(p) \geq 1\} \xleftarrow{R_\omega} t$$

a weighted random selection. If no transition is enabled, $\perp$ *is returned.*

4.2   Generation of Data Perspective

The data perspective is addressed in data Petri nets by variables V and their values U. These are read and written by transitions and evaluated in guards. For the generation of realistic variable values for transitions, extensive knowledge about the variables is necessary. This can be partially learned from the process model or the event log, or must be specified by domain experts. Partially, this knowledge could be modeled in DPNs, but would grow the process models and reduce their maintainability. In the following, the knowledge and the procedure for the generation of realistic variable values are specified. To describe the variables, we introduce a variable meta-model.

Algorithm 1. Log Generation

Input labeled DPN $LN = ((P, T, F, V, U, R, W, G), \lambda, \nu)$, traces to generate $n \in \mathbb{N}$
Output Log $\mathcal{L}$

1: **procedure** GENERATE LOG(N,n)
2:     $\mathcal{L} \leftarrow \{\}$ ▷ empty log v
3:     **while** $|\mathcal{L}| < n$ **do**
4:         $\sigma = GenerateTrace(N, (M_0, A_9), \{\})$
5:         **if** $\sigma \neq \emptyset$ **then**
6:             $\mathcal{L} = \mathcal{L} \cup \{\sigma\}$
7: **procedure** GENERATE TRACE($LN, (M, A), \sigma$)
8:     $t \leftarrow rt(N, (M, A))$ ▷ random transition selection
9:     **if** $t = \perp$ **then**   ▷ Deadlock
10:        Return $\emptyset$
11:    **else**
12:        $(t, w) = GenerateVariable(t, N, (M, A))$ ▷ Generate Variables
13:        $e \leftarrow$ new event
14:        $\underline{e} \leftarrow \lambda(t)$ ▷ Set event name
15:        **for all** $v \in dom(w)$ **do**
16:            **if** $is\_tv(v)$ **then**
17:                $\#_{\nu(v)}(\sigma) \leftarrow w(v)$ ▷ add trace attributes (generated before)
18:            **else**
19:                $\#_{\nu(v)}(e) \leftarrow w(v)$ ▷ add event attributes (generated before)
20:        $\sigma \leftarrow \sigma \oplus e$ ▷ Add event to trace
21:        $(M, A) \rightarrow fireTransition(t, w)$ ▷ fire fransition and change Model State
22:        **if** $(M, A) = (M_F, A_F)$ **then**
23:            Return σ
24:        **else**
25:            Return Generate Trace($LN, (M, A), \sigma$)

Definition 13 (variable meta-model). *Let $N = (P, T, F, V, U, R, W, G)$ be a data Petri net, then the meta-model for a variable $v \in V$ is described by:*

- *$U(v)$ describing the domain of valid variable values.*
- *$is\_tv : V \rightarrow \{0, 1\}$ defining v is a trace variable (1) or an event variable (0)*
- *optional semantic information*

The semantic information allows the specification of values that the variable can take. The values can comprise the complete domain of the variable or only a section. In addition, frequency distributions can be specified via value weights.

Definition 14 (semantic information: values). *Let $N = (P, T, F, V, U, R, W, G)$ be a data Petri net with $v \in V$ and $D_v \subseteq U(v)$, the defined possible values for v. Then VW_v is a multiset with $VW_v = (D_v, m)$ with $m : D_v \rightarrow [0, 1]$, the weight function.*

Furthermore, the variables may be interdependent. This must be included to generate realistic values. Each dependency is described by a logical expression and a resulting constraint. If the logical expression is true, the constraint has implications on the possible values for a given variable.

Definition 15 (semantic information: dependencies). *Let $N = (P, T, F, V,$ $U, R, W, G)$ be a data Petri net with $v \in V$, $EXPR$ the Universe of all possible logical expressions (including disjunction and conjunction). Let $C =$ $(EXPR \times (O_C \times U))^*$ be the set of all possible dependencies, with $O_C = \{'==$ $', '! =', '<', '<=', '>', '>='\}$) the set of constraint operators. Then for all $v \in V$, the function $dep : V \rightarrow C$ defines the set of all dependencies holding for v. The following shorthands are defined for the dependency sets:*

- $dep_{int} : V \rightarrow (EXPR \times ((O_C \setminus \{'==', '! ='\}) \times U))^*$, *interval related dependencies*
- $dep_{eq} : V \rightarrow (EXPR \times (\{'=='\} \times U))^*$, *dependencies setting fixed values*
- $dep_{ne} : V \rightarrow (EXPR \times (\{'! ='\} \times U))^*$, *dependencies excluding values*
- *Let (M, A) be a DPN state and $c \in C$ a constraint, then $eval(c, (M, A))$ evaluates the logical expression building on the current DPN state. Let $C' \subseteq C$ be a set of dependency constraints, then $eval(C', (M, A))$ returns a set of all $c' \in C'$ with $eval(c', (M, A)) = 1$.*

This can be used, e.g., to specify dependencies excluding "prostate cancer" as a value for a variable for persons of female gender. It can also be used to define ranges of values or intervals by setting the logical expression to true.

$$\text{'gender == female'} \Rightarrow (!=, \text{'prostate cancer'})$$

$$\text{'true'} \Rightarrow (<, 5)$$

The third type of semantic information, distribution, refers to the weighting of the values. Instead of concrete weights, however, distribution functions can be specified here. While values are more suitable for discrete, categorical values, the possibility to define distribution functions is directed towards numerical values.

Definition 16 (semantic information: distribution). *Let $N = (P, T, F, V,$ $U, R, W, G)$ be a data Petri net, then for $v \in V$ a distribution function $distr_v :$ $\mathbb{R}^* \rightarrow \mathbb{R} \cup \{\bot\}$ provides values, considering the defined deviation (uniform, normal, ...). If $distr_v = \bot$, no distribution is defined for v.*

5   Implementation

For evaluation, SAMPLE was implemented using Python[1]. The tool allows the generation of multi-perspective event logs using semantic information about the variables. In addition to the random trace generation approach, the implementation allows to fully explore Petri nets for event log generation.

---

[1] https://github.com/DavidJilg/DALG, GNU GLP 3 license.

Algorithm 2. Generation of realistic variable values

Input Transition t, DPN N = (P, T, F, V, U, R, W, G), DPN State (M,A)
Output Firing (t,w)
1: **procedure** GENERATE VARIABLES(t,N,(M,A))
2:    **for all** $v \in W(t)$ **do**
3:       $PV \leftarrow U(v)$ ▷ Set of possible values for v
4:       **if** $|dep_{int}(v)| > 0$ **then**   ▷ intervall dependencies
5:          $PV \leftarrow \{value \; \forall value \in PV | value \; in \; dep_{int}(v)\}$
6:       **if** $|dep_{eq}(v)| > 0$ **then**   ▷ Dependencies setting fixed values
7:          $PV \leftarrow \{value | \forall (expr,(op,value)) \in eval(dep_{eq}(v),(M,A))\}$
           ▷ Dependencies excluding values
8:          $PV \leftarrow PV \setminus \{value | \forall (expr,(op,value)) \in eval(dep_{ne}(v),(M,A))\}$
           ▷ value restriction defined
9:       **if** $VW_v \neq \emptyset$ **then**
10:          set $w[v] = randByWeight(\{(val,wei) | (val,wei) \in VW_v : val \in PV\})$
11:       **else if** $distr_v \neq\perp$ **then**   ▷ distribution function defined
12:          set $w[v] = distr_v()|with \; distr_v() \in PV$
13:       **else**
14:          set $w[v] = randomValue(PV)$
15:    Return (t,w)

The implementation facilitates the configuration of semantic information about the variables (distribution, dependencies, etc.). Due to the large amount of semantic information that needs to be provided to generate realistic event logs, the tool offers a function that analyzes the model and tries to suggest semantic information based on the model. For example, guards are analyzed to identify data types, upper and lower bounds, or possible values. Furthermore, the described approach is extended by the time perspective and allows the generation of timestamps. For ease of use, the implementation provides a graphical user interface based on the QT framework, which allows the configuration of the simulation and semantic data and thus the event log generation (see Fig. 2).

6   Evaluation

The implementation described in Sect. 5 was used to evaluate the SAMPLE approach. First, the correctness of the approach was checked by the conformance of generated traces. For this purpose, process models were used including all combinations of semantic information types. All generated traces were conforming to the models and considered the given semantic information entirely. Subsequently, the realism of generated event logs was investigated, which is the main focus of the research. For preliminary investigations, the *activities of daily living of several individuals*[2] dataset was chosen to enable initial evaluations with respect to realism without expert knowledge. Afterwards, the approach was evaluated

---

[2] https://doi.org/10.4121/uuid:01eaba9f-d3ed-4e04-9945-b8b302764176.

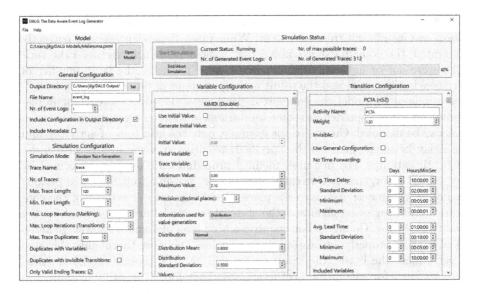

Fig. 2. Graphical user interface of the DALG-tool (Data Aware Event Log Generator)

by domain experts for skin cancer treatment. Therefore, a model was used that represents the diagnosis and treatment of malignant melanoma [5]. It consists of 51 places, 26 variables, 76 transitions, and 52 guards. Using the model, event logs were generated and a representative set of traces was used for evaluation. Therefore, a visual representation of the data was presented to the domain experts. The task of the evaluation was to investigate whether a physician with the same information would have chosen the same treatment options as in the synthetic traces. Additionally, it should be evaluated whether the generated variables are realistic for the given patient.

Compared to other existing approaches, the results show that the inclusion of semantic information enables the generation of data that is more meaningful and correct from a semantic point of view. This means that the sequence of activities shown in the trace makes sense in terms of the data available at a point in time. Consequently, the correct activities are performed based on the variable values. For example, an additional excision will only be performed on a patient if the variable indicating that there is still tumor residue in the skin is set to `true`. Additionally, the value ranges of the variables prevent the generation of unrealistic values. Moreover, specifying dependencies between variables leads to traces, where the variables' values in the trace also make sense when considered as a whole. For example, the variable representing the patient's cancer stage in the used model is dependent on several other variables, such as the presence of metastases or tumor thickness. The transition weights improved the realism of the event log data by influencing which transitions are triggered more frequently during random trace generation and thus which activities occur more frequently.

However, it was found that the semantic information provided for implementation was insufficient to some extent. While many dependencies were correctly integrated, the domain experts noted that some dependencies between the variables were not or not correctly integrated. This is due to the large number of variables in the model and the resulting large amount of time and expert knowledge required to model the complex dependencies. Besides, the current implementation of the approach has some limitations in terms of semantic information that can be modeled. Currently, for example, only the lead time of activities and the delay between them can be specified, resulting in some events with unrealistic timestamps. For instance, medical procedures are usually performed by day, except emergencies. Currently, it is not yet possible to define time periods during which an activity may take place. Besides functional extension, the configuration for log generation and the state of the model are also crucial for the quality of the log. Configuration requires a high level of domain knowledge and a lot of time to properly address all dependencies. The more thoroughly this step is performed, the better the resulting log will be. The process model is essential as a basis for generating synthetic data. Therefore, it must be examined in detail together with domain experts and checked whether all circumstances are represented correctly and all dependencies are taken into account.

In summary, generating synthetic event logs using the SAMPLE approach produces semantically more realistic data. Nevertheless, there are challenges in the definition of the dependencies, the integration of all necessary semantic data into the implementation, as well as in the effort of modeling the dependencies.

7   Conclusion

The presented SAMPLE approach of multi-perspective log generation sets itself apart from previous approaches by considering data semantics. The evaluation showed that the approach leads to medical event logs with higher quality, since the data perspective is implemented more realistically. Nevertheless, challenges were identified in the analysis of the results that need to be addressed.

In the future, we want to simplify the generation of logs and reduce the effort required. Therefore, we investigate possibilities to further automate the process and to optimize the configuration process. Furthermore, the semantic information identified as missing will be integrated into the approach. We also want to extend the approach to declarative process models. Future enhancements of the approach should enable the generation of more realistic logs. The evaluation of the domain experts is essential and guides the improvement of the approach.

References

1. vanden Broucke, S., Vanthienen, J., Baesens, B.: Straightforward petri net-based event log generation in prom. SSRN Electron. J. (2014)
2. Burattin, A.: PLG2: multiperspective processes randomization and simulation for online and offline settings. arXiv abs/1506.08415 (2015)

3. van Dongen, B.F., de Medeiros, A.K.A., Verbeek, H.M.W., Weijters, A.J.M.M., van der Aalst, W.M.P.: The prom framework: a new era in process mining tool support. In: Applications and Theory of Petri Nets 2005, pp. 444–454 (2005)

4. Esgin, E., Karagoz, P.: Process profiling based synthetic event log generation. In: International Conference on Knowledge Discovery and Information Retrieval, pp. 516–524 (2019)

5. Grüger, J., Geyer, T., Kuhn, M., Braun, S.A., Bergmann, R.: Verifying guideline compliance in clinical treatment using multi-perspective conformance checking: a case study. In: Munoz-Gama, J., Lu, X. (eds.) ICPM 2021. LNBIP, vol. 433, pp. 301–313. Springer, Cham (2022). https://doi.org/10.1007/978-3-030-98581-3_22

6. Jensen, K., Kristensen, L.M., Wells, L.: Coloured petri nets and CPN tools for modelling and validation of concurrent systems. Int. J. Softw. Tools Technol. Transfer 9(3), 213–254 (2007)

7. Kataeva, V., Kalenkova, A.: Applying graph grammars for the generation of process models and their logs. In: Proceedings of the Spring/Summer Young Researchers' Colloquium on Software Engineering proceeding (2014)

8. Kummer, O., et al.: An extensible editor and simulation engine for petri nets: RENEW. In: Cortadella, J., Reisig, W. (eds.) ICATPN 2004. LNCS, vol. 3099, pp. 484–493. Springer, Heidelberg (2004). https://doi.org/10.1007/978-3-540-27793-4_29

9. de Leoni, M., van der Aalst, W.M.P.: Data-aware process mining. In: Shin, S.Y., Maldonado, J.C. (eds.) Proceedings of the 28th Annual ACM Symposium on Applied Computing, p. 1454. ACM Digital Library, ACM, New York (2013)

10. Mannhardt, F.: Multi-perspective process mining. Ph.D. thesis, Mathematics and Computer Science (2018)

11. Medeiros, A., Günther, C.: Process mining: using CPN tools to create test logs for mining algorithms. In: Proceedings of the Sixth Workshop on the Practical Use of Coloured Petri Nets and CPN Tools (CPN 2005) (2004)

12. Mitsyuk, A.A., Shugurov, I.S., Kalenkova, A.A., van der Aalst, W.M.: Generating event logs for high-level process models. Simul. Model. Pract. Theory 74, 1–16 (2017)

13. Munoz-Gama, J., et al.: Process mining for healthcare: characteristics and challenges. J. Biomed. Inform. 127, 103994 (2022)

14. Nakatumba, J., Westergaard, M., van der Aalst, W.M.P.: Generating event logs with workload-dependent speeds from simulation models. In: Bajec, M., Eder, J. (eds.) CAiSE 2012. LNBIP, vol. 112, pp. 383–397. Springer, Heidelberg (2012). https://doi.org/10.1007/978-3-642-31069-0_31

15. Pertsukhov, P., Mitsyuk, A.: Simulating petri nets with inhibitor and reset arcs. Proc. ISP RAS 31, 151–162 (2019)

16. Ratzer, A.V., et al.: CPN tools for editing, simulating, and analysing coloured petri nets. In: van der Aalst, W.M.P., Best, E. (eds.) ICATPN 2003. LNCS, vol. 2679, pp. 450–462. Springer, Heidelberg (2003). https://doi.org/10.1007/3-540-44919-1_28

17. Shugurov, I., Mitsyuk, A.: Generation of a set of event logs with noise. Institute for System Programming of the Russian Academy of Sciences (2014)

18. Aalst, W.: Data science in action. In: van der Aalst, W. (ed.) Process Mining, pp. 3–23. Springer, Heidelberg (2016). https://doi.org/10.1007/978-3-662-49851-4_1

Research Paper: Process Mining and Synthetic Health Data: Reflections and Lessons Learnt

Alistair Bullward[1]([✉]), Abdulaziz Aljebreen[2] [iD], Alexander Coles[2],
Ciarán McInerney[2] [iD], and Owen Johnson[2] [iD]

[1] NHS England, Leeds, UK
alistair.bullward1@nhs.net
[2] University of Leeds, Leeds, UK
{ml17asa,scadc,c.mcinerney,o.a.johnson}@leeds.ac.uk

Abstract. Analysing the treatment pathways in real-world health data can provide valuable insight for clinicians and decision-makers. However, the procedures for acquiring real-world data for research can be restrictive, time-consuming and risks disclosing identifiable information. Synthetic data might enable representative analysis without direct access to sensitive data. In the first part of our paper, we propose an approach for grading synthetic data for process analysis based on its fidelity to relationships found in real-world data. In the second part, we apply our grading approach by assessing cancer patient pathways in a synthetic healthcare dataset (The Simulacrum provided by the English National Cancer Registration and Analysis Service) using process mining. Visualisations of the patient pathways within the synthetic data appear plausible, showing relationships between events confirmed in the underlying non-synthetic data. Data quality issues are also present within the synthetic data which reflect real-world problems and artefacts from the synthetic dataset's creation. Process mining of synthetic data in healthcare is an emerging field with novel challenges. We conclude that researchers should be aware of the risks when extrapolating results produced from research on synthetic data to real-world scenarios and assess findings with analysts who are able to view the underlying data.

Keywords: Process mining · Synthetic data · Simulacrum · Data grading · Taxonomy

1 Introduction

A care pathway is "a complex intervention for the mutual decision-making and organisation of care processes for a well-defined group of patients during a well-defined period" [1]. Care pathways describe ideal patient journeys and the extent to which individual patients follow this ideal can be explored through analysis of data extracted from healthcare information systems. Such data can include patient-level events like admissions, investigations, diagnoses, and treatments. Process-mining of healthcare data can help clinicians, hospitals and policy makers understand where care pathways are helping and hindering patient care [2]. However, healthcare data is sensitive and identifiable data,

© The Author(s) 2023
M. Montali et al. (Eds.): ICPM 2022 Workshops, LNBIP 468, pp. 341–353, 2023.
https://doi.org/10.1007/978-3-031-27815-0_25

which necessitates strong information governance to protect patients' privacy. This necessary governance can make it difficult to access healthcare data for beneficial analysis and research (especially for process discovery where a clear purpose is harder to pin down and hence link to a legal basis). One solution is to make highly-aggregated open datasets available. For example, NHS Digital publishes open data across 130+ publications spanning key care domains. However, such datasets are often not sufficiently detailed for patient-level process mining of care pathways. Consequently, there has been a growth in synthetic or simulated data that attempt to mirror aspects of the real, patient-level data without disclosing patient-identifiable information [3].

Generating synthetic data from real world data sets can be achieved via a number of methods. An example of synthetic healthcare dataset from the USA is Synthetic-Mass which is an unrestricted artificial publicly available healthcare dataset containing 1 million records generated using Synthea [4]. This dataset was generated using public healthcare statistics, clinical guidelines on care maps format and realistic properties inheritance methods. Another example from the UK is a project developed by NHSx AI Lab Skunkworks called Synthetic Data Generation [5]. In this project, a model previously developed by NHS called SynthVAE has been adopted to be used with publicly accessible healthcare dataset MIMIC-III in order to read the data (inputs), train the model then generate the synthetic data and check the data through a chained pipeline. A third example is synthetic datasets generated using Bayesian networks [6] have demonstrated good-to-high fidelity [7] and can be coupled with disclosure control measures [8] to provide complex, representative data without compromising patient privacy.

Regardless of generation method, rigorous evaluation of synthetic data is needed to assure and ensure representativeness, usefulness and minimal disclosivity. Approaches to evaluation include using generative adversarial networks that incorporate privacy checks within the data-generation process [9]; discrepancy, distance and distinguishability metrics applied to specific analysis goals [10]; meaningful identity disclosure risk [11]; multivariate inferential statistical tests of whether real and synthetic datasets are similar [12]; conditional attribute disclosure and membership disclosure [12]; and others [13]. What has not been suggested to date are approaches to evaluation that are specific to process mining. We hypothesise that process mining of health care pathways has a set of specific data requirements that may not be easily satisfied by current approaches to synthetic healthcare data creation. To explore this, we present a taxonomy for synthetic data in healthcare to help evaluate and grade synthetic datasets to identify those that would be useful for process mining. We apply our taxonomy to a case study of the Simulacrum cancer dataset, which is an openly available dataset of cancer treatment data based on the English National Cancer Registration and Analysis Service [14].

2   Method

Our methods are presented in four parts. In part 1, we propose a taxonomy of synthetic data for process mining in healthcare. In part 2, we define a set of tests to classify synthetic data against the taxonomy. In part 3, we describe the Simulacrum dataset that we use in our case study. Finally, in part 4, we evaluate the Simulacrum dataset using the tests from part 2, and classify the dataset according to our taxonomy from part 1.

2.1 Part 1: A Taxonomy for Synthetic Data in Healthcare

We present a 3-grade taxonomy to help classify the fidelity of a synthetic dataset. By fidelity, we refer to the extent to which synthetic data represents the real data it is attempting to replace. Random data presented in the format of the real data has low fidelity but might have functional value for testing analysis pipelines because it has the "right shape". If synthetic data also mirrors statistical relationships within variables, then it has greater fidelity and has some inferential value following analysis. Greater fidelity would be demonstrated by a synthetic dataset that mirrors the real data's statistical relationships between variables.

More formally, we define a minimum grade 1 synthetic dataset as one in which the format of the synthetic data matches that of the original dataset from which it was derived. The types of features represented in the original dataset must be faithfully represented. Examples for healthcare data include time-stamped events, patient identifiers, and treatment codes. Grade 1 synthetic datasets are not expected to retain any statistical or clinically-meaningful relationships within or between columns. From the perspective of process mining, we expect to be able to produce a process model but the sequences of events depicted in the model are not expected to be realistic, nor are the event and transition metadata (e.g. event counts or inter-event duration).

We define a grade 2 synthetic dataset as one in which the independent distributional properties of each synthetic variable are similar (statistically or clinically) from the same properties of each variable in the original dataset. Grade 2 datasets are not expected to retain any statistical or clinically-meaningful relationships between features. From the perspective of process mining, we expect to be able to produce a process model and for the event and transition metadata to be realistic, but we do not expect the sequences of events depicted in the model to be realistic.

We define a grade 3 synthetic dataset as one in which the multivariate distributional properties of all synthetic variables are similar (statistically or clinically) from the same properties of all variables in the original dataset. From the perspective of process mining, we expect to be able to produce a process model, for the event and transition metadata to be realistic, and for the sequences of events depicted in the model to be realistic. This paper focuses on assessing grade 3 for analytical process mining (Fig. 1 and Table 1).

Table 1. Summary of proposed taxonomy for synthetic healthcare data

Feature	Grade 1	Grade 2	Grade 3
Fidelity	Low	Medium	High
Data Format	Same	Same	Same
Independent Variable data	Random	Similar static/clinical meaningful distributions	Similar static/clinical meaningful distributions

(continued)

Table 1. (*continued*)

Feature	Grade 1	Grade 2	Grade 3
Relationships between variables	No	No	Similar static/clinical meaningful distributions
Produce process models	Yes	Yes	Yes
Event/transition metadata	Not realistic	Realistic	Realistic
Sequence of events	Not realistic	Not realistic	Realistic
Usage	Test analysis pipelines	Basic statistical analysis	Gain Insights through process discovery

A Proposed Model for Grading Synthetic Data in Health Care

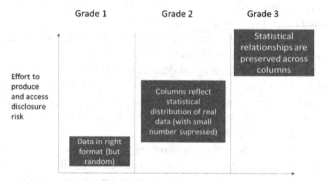

Fig. 1. A proposed model for grading synthetic data in healthcare

2.2 Part 2: Criteria for Grading Synthetic Data in Healthcare

In part 1, we presented a 3-grade taxonomy to help classify the fidelity of a synthetic dataset in healthcare. Below, we present a set of criteria that would identify the grade of a given synthetic healthcare dataset. Taken together, the taxonomy and the criteria provide a framework for evaluating the suitability of a synthetic dataset for process mining. We suggest some tests against these criteria but we encourage analysts to design, implement and share their own tests in keeping with the principles of the criteria, below.

Criterion 1: The variables within the real dataset are present within the synthetic dataset and are of the correct data type.

A sufficient test of this criterion is a basic one-to-one mapping of variable names and data types. If a process model can be derived from the synthetic dataset, then this criterion is also met.

Criterion 2: Each synthetic variable's typical value, range, and distribution are statistically- or clinically-meaningful similar to the relative variable in the real dataset.

If a statistical approach is preferred, then candidate tests of this criterion are null-hypothesis significance tests for similarity of, for example, each variable's mean or median. Importantly, each of these null-hypothesis tests would not be sufficient to meet this criterion if they are conducted in isolation. This is because these tests do not test all distributional parameters. Even tests of distributions like the Komolgorov-Smirnov test only test the minimum largest difference between two distributions rather than the entire distribution.

If a clinical approach is preferred, then clinical and administrative domain experts can audit distribution summary statistics. This is in keeping with the ethos of PM2 methodology where domain experts are involved in the process mining [15].

Criterion 3: The sequential, temporal, and correlational relationships between all variables are statistically- or clinically-meaningfully similar to those present in the real dataset.

Correlational relationships can be tested using a multivariate null-hypothesis statistical test for similarity but are subject to the same limitations as similar tests applied to Criterion 2. This criterion might also be satisfied if it is possible to progress with iterative, process-mining methodology involving the production, evaluation and review of event logs and process models. One could also meet this criterion by testing if a process model derived from the synthetic dataset passes tests of conformance with a process model derived from the real dataset.

2.3 Part 3: Case Study of the Simulacrum Cancer Dataset

The Simulacrum is a synthetic dataset derived from the data held securely by the National Cancer Registration and Analysis Service (NCRAS) within Public Health England [14]. NCRAS holds data on all cancer diagnoses in England and links them to other datasets collected by the English National Health Service. The Simulacrum uses a Bayesian network to provide synthetic data on patient demographics, diagnoses and treatments based on real patient data between 2013 and 2017. Table 2 shows a sample of the variables available in the Simulacrum that are relevant to process mining.

Table 2. Summary of activity data available in the simulacrum dataset for 2,200,626 patients.

Activity	Count of events across all cancers	Summary of information available for event
Diagnosis date	2,741,065	Site of neoplasm, Morphology, Stage, grade of tumour, age at diagnosis, Sex, cancer registry catchment area oestrogen receptor, EHRs status of the tumour, Clinical nurse specialist, Gleason Patterns, Date of first surgical event, Laterality Index of multiple deprivation
Decision to treat (Regimen)	749,721	Decision to treat date (Drug regimen)
First surgery	1,736,082	Date of first surgical event linked to this tumour recorded in the Cancer Registration treatment table
Start date on regimen	828,980	Patient's height (metres (m)), Patient's weight (kilograms (kg)), Drug treatment intent, Decision to treat date (Drug regimen), Start date (Drug regimen), Maximally granular mapped regimen, Clinical trial indicator, Chemo-radiation indicator, Regimen grouping (benchmark reports)
SACT cycle start	2,561,679	Pseudonymised cycle ID, Pseudonymised regimen ID, Cycle identifier, Start date (Cycle), Primary procedure (OPCS), Performance Status
Deaths	652,418	Date of Death

The Simulacrum dataset contains synthetic treatment events and associated variables for multiple cancers. We selected data from for malignant neoplasms of the brain (identified by the 3-character ICD10 code C71).

2.4 Part 4: Evaluation

We did not have access to the real world data on which the Simulacrum was based. We reviewed the Simulacrum for the presence of variables relevant to the brain cancer care pathway, and checked that the data types were appropriate, e.g. timestamp was a datetime data type. We assumed that the variables in the Simulacrum were also present in the real world. Regarding grade 2 fidelity, the producer of the Simulacrum synthetic dataset provided evidence that the distributions of each variable in the datasets were similar to those of the real dataset [16].

To test grade 3 fidelity, we sought to derive a process model of brain cancer from the Simulacrum synthetic data by applying process discovery to relevant variables. Patient ID was used as the case identifier, clinical events were used as the activity, and each event had an associated timestamp to produce an event log. PM4PY [17] packages were used to produce the process models and the PRoM was used to discover the processes [18]. Trace variants were extracted from the event log and reviewed by clinical experts for reasonableness.

To aid conformance checking, a normative model representing the expected pathway to be followed for brain cancer using available activities in Simulacrum was informed by brain tumour patient guides from the Brain Trust [19]. Conformance was quantified as the fitness of the synthetic event log when replayed on a petri net of the expected pathway [20]. This replay fitness provides a 0–1 measure of how many traces in the synthetic data's event log can be reproduced in a process model defined by the expected pathway, with penalties for skips and insertions.

The distributions of durations between diagnosis and first surgery was also reviewed in the synthetic and the real dataset with the assistance of the producers of the Simulacrum synthetic dataset. This permitted a simple evaluation of the reasonableness of the temporal relationship between variables.

3   Results

The fields required to inform the care pathway for brain cancers were all present and variables' data types were all correct. The discovered process model for brain cancer shows a substantial variety of sequences that differ from the care pathway derived from the Brain Trust (Fig. 2). Replay fitness of the synthetic event log on the expected pathway was 46%.

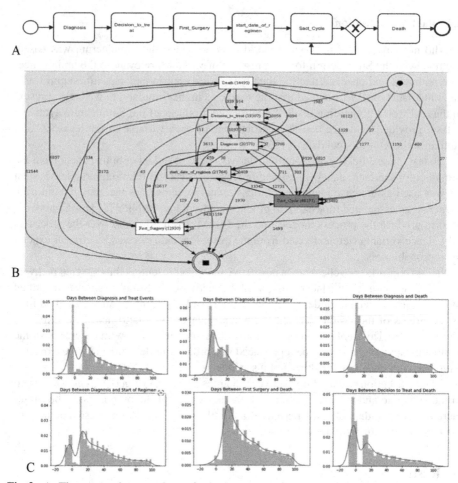

Fig. 2. A. The expected care pathway for brain cancer. B. Process discovery on Brain Cancer Pathways (ICD10 code C71). C. Histograms of durations between a sample of event pairs.

Of the 20,562 traces in the Simulacrum's brain cancer dataset, there were 4,080 trace variants (Fig. 3). Most variants were unique traces ($n_1 = 3,889$) and there were relatively few variants matching only two traces ($n_2 = 89$). The four-most-common variants represented 75.9% of traces (15,608/20,562). In 122 spurious traces, the "Death" event occurred before the "First_Surgery" event. Figure 4 presents the transition matrix between events with the care pathway being represented by the diagonal starting at the second cell from the top left, i.e. Start-Diagnosis date = 18,123.

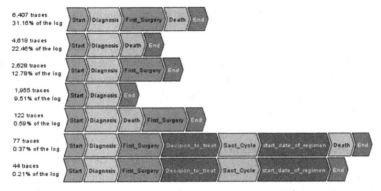

Fig. 3. The seven most common trace variants for brain cancer, accounting for over 77% of all trace variants.

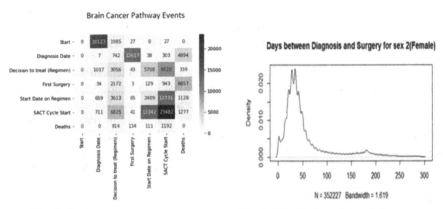

Fig. 4. Brain cancer event summary

Fig. 5. Distribution of days between diagnosis and first surgery for all cancers for Females

Figure 5 shows the distribution of computed duration between date of diagnosis and first surgery, in the female sub cohort. There is a typical value of approximately 35 days but a long skew duration in the low hundreds of days. There also appears to be a regular signal with a period of approximately 7–10 days.

4   Discussion

Care pathways are increasingly key in analysing health data. The aim of this paper was to present a taxonomy for synthetic data in healthcare to help evaluate and grade synthetic datasets to identify those that would be useful for process mining. We conducted an example evaluation on the Simulacrum dataset.

According to our tests, we conclude that the Simulacrum meets the grade 3 criterion of our taxonomy. Grade 1 was met by our finding that the fields required to inform the care pathway for brain cancer were all present and variables' data types were all correct.

Grade 2 was evidenced by the Simulacrum's producer's assuring that the distributions of each variable in the datasets were similar to those of the real dataset [16]. Grade 3 was evidenced by our ability to progress with an iterative, process-mining approach that involved the production of a process model and event log summary statistics that were reviewed with clinical experts and the producer of the synthetic dataset. In the remaining sections, we provide further details of the discussions with the producers of the Simulacrum synthetic dataset.

4.1 Meeting the Grade 3 Criterion

Our criterion for meeting grade 3 fidelity is if the sequential, temporal, and correlational relationships between all variables are statistically- or clinically-meaningfully similar to those present in the real dataset. We tested this criterion by progressing with an iterative, process-mining methodology and by testing if a process model derived from the synthetic dataset passes tests of conformance with a process model derived from the real dataset.

The Simulacrum synthetic dataset was able to produce a process model and trace variants that were similar to portions of the ideal care pathway.

The reasonableness of the synthetic dataset was also evidenced by our analysis of the distribution of days between diagnosis and first surgery, in female patients (Fig. 5). Figure 5 also shows what appears to be a regular signal with a period of approximately 7–10 days. Discussions with the producers of the Simulacrum synthetic dataset confirmed that this regular signal reflects the underlying non-synthetic data. Collaborative discussions suggested the signal reflects weekly patterns for booking surgery - for example non-urgent surgery tends to be booked on weekdays - but we have yet to test this hypothesis. Such analysis and representativeness would not be possible with synthetic datasets lower than grade 3.

Regarding a formal check of conformance, a replay fitness of 46% is considered low, suggesting that the expected care pathway does not represent the behaviour observed in the synthetic data's event log well [20]. It is not clear whether the poor replay fitness represents poor adherence to guideline care pathways or poor fidelity of the Simulacrum data set. Guideline care pathways represent ideal patient journeys but real-life cancer treatment is known to be complex [21]. For example, process models discovered for endometrial cancer show good replay fitness but require more-complex processes [22]. The replay fitness of our discovered process model for brain cancer was 66%, which, assuming the Simulacrum data is representative, suggests that the care pathways for brain cancer are more complex than what is presented in the idealised care pathways.

4.2 Data Quality

According to the ideal care pathway, we would expect all patients to experience all events that were selected from the Simulacrum synthetic dataset, and in the order specified by the ideal care pathway. On the contrary, Fig. 4 shows substantial deviation from the ideal care pathway. This is indicated partly by non-zero diagonal counts that indicate direct repeats of events (though repeated SACT cycles are not unexpected). Deviation from the ideal care pathway is also partly indicated by non-zero counts anywhere beyond the diagonal starting at the second cell from the top left. For example, there were 1,037 synthetic patient records that showed a patient receiving a decision to treat before a diagnosis date. These deviations could be accounted for if patients were diagnosed with multiple genetically-distinct cancers. For example, it is plausible that the 34 synthetic patients that underwent cancer-related surgery before diagnosis were undergoing diagnostic surgery, or were patients undergoing curative or debulking surgery and in whom an additional, genetically-unique cancer was discovered following analysis of the biopsy.

However, the observation that 1,192 synthetic patient records show a patient has died before their SACT cycle started cannot be explained by the real-life complexity of healthcare delivery. Alternative explanations for these cases include administrative errors or spurious simulation during the data generating process. Our collaborative discussions with the producers of the synthetic dataset revealed that this anomaly was a known feature of the generation of the synthetic data rather than being a feature of the real data.

4.3 Collaboration with Producers of the Synthetic Dataset

During the course of this work we have collaborated with the producers of the synthetic dataset under study. We felt that this was a crucial activity to aid in the efficient and effective use of the dataset. For example, without communication with producers of the synthetic datasets, it might not be possible to tell if a data quality issue is a result of the synthetic data generation or representative of the underlying data.

We have already presented two examples of the benefits of collaborating with the producers of synthetic datasets. The first was our analysis of the durations between date of diagnosis and first surgery (Fig. 5). It was only through discussion with the producers of the synthetic data that we were able to check that the distribution of computed durations was representative of real world data, and that we were able to collaboratively hypothesise an explanation for the regular 7–10 day signal. The second example was our ability to conclude that the anomalous transitions between death and SACT cycle were an artefact of the Simulacrum's data-generating process.

4.4 Recommendations

We make the following recommendations to producers of synthetic healthcare datasets that may be used by analysts (consumers) using process mining on the synthetic data:

1. Producers of synthetic health data should grade it and produce evidence using test cases that will help users determine whether the data is relevant to their study.

2. Consumers of synthetic data should expect to liaise with the producer. In particular, they should:

   a. Ask how the data were generated.
   b. Ask what tests of representativeness, usefulness and disclosivity were conducted.
   c. Apply our taxonomy to grade the dataset.
   d. Have a line of communication open to discuss data quality issues.

5 Conclusions

In conclusion, process mining of care pathways is an important approach for improving healthcare but accessing patient event based records is often burdensome. Synthetic data can potentially reduce this burden by making data more openly available to researchers, however the quality of the synthetic data for process mining needs to be assessed. We propose an evaluation framework and demonstrated this framework using the openly available Simulacrum Cancer data set and identified this data set can be thought of as grade 3 which makes it useful for process mining. Although researchers may be able to explore synthetic data and generate hypotheses, we argue that they will need to work with producers with access to the real data to confirm findings. This paper makes a number of recommendations for producers and consumers of synthetic data sets and highlights potential further work on the taxonomy to subdivide different types of grade 3 data.

References

1. Vanhaecht, K.: The impact of clinical pathways on the organisation of care processes. Doctoral dissertation (2007). Accessed 24 Aug 2022
2. Schrijvers, G., van Hoorn, A., Huiskes, N.: The care pathway concept: concepts and theories: an introduction. Int. J. Integrated Care 12(6) (2012). https://doi.org/10.5334/ijic.812
3. The NHS X Analytics Unit. https://nhsx.github.io/AnalyticsUnit/synthetic.html. Accessed 24 Aug 2022
4. Walonoski, J., et al.: Synthea: an approach, method, and software mechanism for generating synthetic patients and the synthetic electronic health care record. J. Am. Med. Inform. Assoc. "JAMIA" 25(3), 230–238 (2018)
5. AI Skunkworks projects. https://transform.england.nhs.uk/ai-lab/ai-lab-programmes/skunkworks/ai-skunkworks-projects. Accessed 24 Aug 2022
6. Kaur, D., et al.: Application of Bayesian networks to generate synthetic health data. J. Am. Med. Inform. Assoc. "JAMIA" 28(4), 801–811 (2021)
7. Shen, Y., et al.: CBN: constructing a clinical Bayesian network based on data from the electronic medical record. J. Biomed. Inform. 88, 1–10 (2018)
8. Sweeney, L.: Computational disclosure control: a primer on data privacy protection. Doctoral dissertation, Massachusetts Institute of Technology (2001). Accessed 24 Aug 2022
9. Yale, A., Dash, S., Dutta, R., Guyon, I., Pavao, A., Bennett, K.P.: Generation and evaluation of privacy preserving synthetic health data. Neurocomputing 416, 244–255 (2020)
10. El Emam, K., Mosquera, L., Fang, X., El-Hussuna, A.: Utility metrics for evaluating synthetic health data generation methods: validation study. JMIR Med. Inform. 10(4) (2022)
11. El Emam, K., Mosquera, L., Bass, J.: Evaluating identity disclosure risk in fully synthetic health data: model development and validation. J. Med. Internet Res. 22(11) (2020)

12. El Emam, K., Mosquera, L., Jonker, E., Sood, H.: Evaluating the utility of synthetic COVID-19 case data. JAMIA Open **4**(1) (2021)
13. El Emam, K.: Seven ways to evaluate the utility of synthetic data. IEEE Secur. Priv. **18**(4), 56–59 (2020)
14. Health Data Insight, The Simulacrum. https://healthdatainsight.org.uk/project/the-simulacrum. Accessed 24 Aug 2022
15. van Eck, M.L., Lu, X., Leemans, S.J.J., van der Aalst, W.M.P.: PM^2: a process mining project methodology. In: Zdravkovic, J., Kirikova, M., Johannesson, P. (eds.) CAiSE 2015. LNCS, vol. 9097, pp. 297–313. Springer, Cham (2015). https://doi.org/10.1007/978-3-319-19069-3_19
16. Health Data Insight, Testing the Simulacrum. https://healthdatainsight.org.uk/project/testing-the-simulacrum. Accessed 24 Aug 2022
17. Fraunhofer Institute for Applied Information Technology (FIT), PM4PY (2.2.24) [Software] (2022)
18. Van der Aalst, W.M., van Dongen, B.F., Günther, C.W., Rozinat, A., Verbeek, E., Weijters, T.: ProM: the process mining toolkit. BPM (Demos) **489**(31), 2 (2009)
19. Brain trust. https://brainstrust.org.uk. Accessed 24 Aug 2022
20. Buijs, J.C.A.M., van Dongen, B.F., van der Aalst, W.M.P.: On the role of fitness, precision, generalization and simplicity in process discovery. In: Meersman, R., et al. (eds.) OTM 2012. LNCS, vol. 7565, pp. 305–322. Springer, Heidelberg (2012). https://doi.org/10.1007/978-3-642-33606-5_19
21. Baker, K., et al.: Process mining routinely collected electronic health records to define real-life clinical pathways during chemotherapy. Int. J. Med. Inform. **103**, 32–41 (2017)
22. Kurniati, A.P., Rojas, E., Zucker, K., Hall, G., Hogg, D., Johnson, O.: Process mining to explore variations in endometrial cancer pathways from GP referral to first treatment. Stud. Health Technol. Inform. **281**, 769–773 (2021)

Discovering Break Behaviours in Process Mining: An Application to Discover Treatment Pathways in ICU of Patients with Acute Coronary Syndrome

Qifan Chen[1]($\boxtimes$) iD, Yang Lu[1] iD, Charmaine S. Tam[2] iD, and Simon K. Poon[1] iD

[1] School of Computer Science, The University of Sydney, Sydney, Australia
{qifan.chen,yang.lu,simon.poon}@sydney.edu.au
[2] Northern Clinical School, University of Sydney, Sydney, Australia
charmaine.tam@sydney.edu.au

Abstract. The inductive miner (IM) can guarantee to return structured process models, but the process behaviours that process trees can represent are limited. Loops in process trees can only be exited after the execution of the "body" part. However, in some cases, it is possible to break a loop structure in the "redo" part. This paper proposes an extension to the process tree notation and the IM to discover and represent break behaviours. We present a case study using a healthcare event log to explore Acute Coronary Syndrome (ACS) patients' treatment pathways, especially discharge behaviours from ICU, to demonstrate the usability of the proposed approach in real-life. We find that treatment pathways in ICU are routine behaviour, while discharges from ICU are break behaviours. The results show that we can successfully discover break behaviours and obtain the structured and understandable process model with satisfactory fitness, precision and simplicity.

Keywords: Process mining · Inductive miner · Process trees · Healthcare process discovery

1 Introduction

Process discovery algorithms are techniques that construct process models automatically from recorded data. Unlike many machine learning techniques, it has been discussed that process mining methods should return human-understandable results [3]. However, many existing process discovery algorithms return "spaghetti-like" process models which are hard to understand [3]. The inductive miner (IM) [17] is one of the most popular process discovery results that guarantees to return structured process models with high fitness. Although structured models are guaranteed to be discovered, as the direct output is a process tree [17], the possible represented behaviours are limited [20].

Q. Chen and Y. Lu—Contribute equally to the paper.

© The Author(s) 2023
M. Montali et al. (Eds.): ICPM 2022 Workshops, LNBIP 468, pp. 354–365, 2023.
https://doi.org/10.1007/978-3-031-27815-0_26

In process trees, a loop is composed of a "body" part and multiple "redo" parts. A loop should always start and end with the "body" part. For example, in $\circlearrowright(T_1, T_2)$, the loop should always start with T_1, then choose if it executes T_2 or exits the loop. However, in certain cases, it is possible to exit the loop from the "redo" part (e.g., exiting the loop during the execution of T_2). Such behaviours are called break behaviours which cannot be represented by the process trees or discovered by the IM.

Healthcare process discovery aims to get insights into how healthcare processes are executed and identify opportunities for improving services [23]. Tremendous efforts have been put into discovering various healthcare processes [9,21–23,26]. The Intensive Care Unit (ICU) is expensive, and its cost increases yearly. Carefully deciding on the discharging of patients from ICU is thus a critical issue to guarantee efficient treatments have occurred. Hence, the discovery of treatment processes in ICU can help domain experts better understand how patients are treated and improve the quality of medical services.

We present a motivation example (shown in Fig. 1) to demonstrate break behaviours in ICU treatment. The ICU treatment pathway is a routine loop behaviour that involves continued monitoring of vital measurements and repetitive orders several times a day (e.g., laboratory tests and medications) until discharge to normal wards. Patients are admitted to ICU and nurses start to monitor the vital measurements. Blood tests, followed by medications may be ordered for patients as requested by doctors. After staying in ICU for some time (i.e., executing the routine loop several times), patients can be discharged from ICU through three different ways. Typically, patients should be discharged if their vital measurements are normal, which is discharge pathway one in Fig. 1. Nevertheless, patients can be discharged after further ordering blood tests (discharge pathway two in Fig. 1) and medications (discharge pathway three in Fig. 1). Such discharge pathways are break behaviours (e.g., a break from the "redo" part of the routine treatment loop).

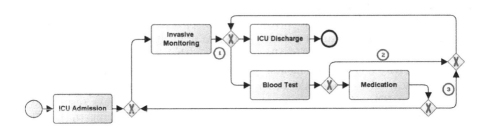

Fig. 1. A motivation example of a ICU treatment process

This paper proposes an extension to the process tree notation and the IM to discover and represent break behaviours. A case study is presented using a real-life healthcare event log to demonstrate the usability of the proposed approach. We aim to discover the treatment pathways in ICU of patients with Acute

Coronary Syndrome (ACS). Specifically, we plan to investigate the discharge behaviours from ICU, which can be regarded as break behaviours. The results show that we can obtain the structured and straightforward process model with satisfactory fitness, precision and simplicity.

The paper is structured as follows: Sect. 2 discusses the background. Section 3 explains the main approach. A real-life case study is presented in Sect. 4. Section 5 concludes the paper.

2   Background

2.1   Process Discovery Algorithms

The IMs [13–17] are a family of process discovery algorithms that apply the divide-and-conquer method to discover process trees. As process trees are discovered, the discovered process will always be structured and understandable. However, due to the limitation of process trees, certain behaviours are inherently harder to be represented and discovered. "Flower model" is often the result when the input log is complex and unable to be adequately represented by the process tree. Some extensions are proposed to discover more behaviours using the IM (e.g., recursive behaviours [12], switch behaviours [20], and cancellation behaviours [11]).

For those process discovery algorithms which can discover break behaviours in loops, like the alpha miner [1], the heuristics miner [25] and the split miner (SM) [4], structured process models cannot be guaranteed, instead "spaghetti like" process models are often returned [3].

2.2   Process Discovery in Healthcare

With the rapid development of process mining, healthcare process discovery has recently drawn even more attention [23]. [9,22] aim to analyse the trajectories of patients in hospitals, while [21,26] model the workflows in outpatient departments. Patient pathways in emergency departments are discovered in [2,8]. However, less attention is paid to the treatment process for patients in ICU, even though ICU is critical for patients with severe health conditions. Carefully deciding on the transfer out of patients in ICU is thus essential to ensure that patients receive efficient treatments. Apart from normal vital measurements, patients may need to undertake other examinations or treatments before discharging from ICU. Hence, we aim to discover treatment pathways (especially discharge behaviours for patients with ACS) in ICU. Additionally, due to the distinguishing characteristics of healthcare processes, the existing process discovery algorithms constantly fail to discover structured process models [23]. Therefore, unnecessary difficulties have been added to understanding the discovered process models for domain experts. Interactive process discovery is then proposed to address the issue [5,21]. Unfortunately, such domain knowledge is not always available under given conditions. Hence, we propose an approach to automatically discover structured and understandable process models, especially when complex behaviours (i.e., break behaviours) exist in healthcare event logs.

3   Methodology

3.1   The Break Process Tree

To represent break behaviours in process trees, we define the break process tree in this section to represent break behaviours. The break process tree is an extension based on the process tree model described in [16].

Definition 1 (Break Behaviour). *Assume there is a loop process tree* $T =\circlearrowleft$ *$(P_1, P_2, ..., P_n)$, where L is its corresponding event log. There is a break behaviour in T if there exists an activity $a_{end} \in End(L)$, $a_{end} \in P_i$, $1 < i \leqslant n$.*

Definition 2 (Break Process Tree). *Assume a finite alphabet A. A break process tree is a normal process tree with break leaf operators $a\otimes$, where $a \in A$. Combined with a loop operator $\circlearrowleft$, the break leaf node denotes the place where we execute activity a, and have an option to exit the loop. Assume there is a loop process tree $T =\circlearrowleft (P_1, P_2, ..., P_n)$ A break leaf node must be placed in the redo part of a loop process tree (i.e., $a\otimes \in P_i, 1 < i \leqslant n$).*

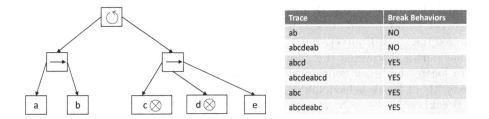

Fig. 2. An example break process tree and its corresponding traces

An example break process tree and its log are presented in Fig. 2. The process tree contains two break leaf operators $c\otimes$, $d\otimes$ that allow exiting the loop on the redo part of the loop process tree. If the process tree does not contain the break leaf operator, it will always start and end with "ab". The break loop operators allow the process tree to exit the loop after the execution of c and d.

3.2   Discovering Break Process Trees

Our method relies on the IM framework to discover process trees with break behaviours. The original loop cut is replaced with the following three steps:

Step 1: Finding Break Cut. In the first step, we aim to find a break loop cut. The break loop cut is similar to the original loop cut but allows the exit of loops from the "redo" part. The definition of the break loop cut is presented in Definition 3.

Definition 3 (Break Loop Cut). *Suppose G is a directly-follows graph of event log L_{break}. A break loop cut is a partially ordered cut $\sum_1, \sum_2, ..., \sum_n$ of G such that:*

1. *All start activities are in $\sum_1$: $Start(G) \subset \sum_1$*
2. *There must be at least one end activity in $\sum_1$: $\exists a \in \sum_1 : a \in End(G)$*
3. *There are only edges between $\sum_1$ and $\sum_n$: $\forall m \neq n \neq 1 \wedge a \in \sum_m \wedge b \in \sum_n : (a, b) \notin G$*
4. *If there are edges from $\sum_1$ to $\sum_n$, the sources of all such edges are end activities: $\exists (a, b) \in G \wedge a \in \sum_1 \wedge b \in \sum_n : a \in End(G)$*
5. *If there are edges from $\sum_n$ to $\sum_1$, the destinations of all such edges are start activities: $\exists (b, a) \in G \wedge b \in \sum_n \wedge a \in \sum_1 : a \in Start(G)$*
6. *If there is an edge from $\sum_1$ to $\sum_n$, there should be an edge from all end activities in $\sum_1$ to the same destination in $\sum_n$: $\forall a \in End(G) \wedge a \in \sum_1 \wedge b \in \sum_n : (\exists a' \in \sum_1 : (a', b) \in G) \iff (a, b) \in G$*
7. *If there is an edge from $\sum_n$ to $\sum_1$, there should be an edge from the same source to all start activities: $\forall a \in Start(G) \wedge b \in \sum_n : (\exists a' \in \sum_1 : (b, a') \in G) \iff (b, a) \in G$*

Step 2: Identifying Break Leaf Nodes. Once a break loop cut is identified, there can be two possibilities: 1) a loop process tree with break behaviours is discovered (i.e., $\exists a \in End(G) \wedge a \in \sum_i \wedge i \neq 1$); 2) a loop process tree without break behaviours is discovered (i.e., $\forall a \in End(G) \wedge a \in \sum_1$). We perform Algorithm 1 to locate the break behaviours. If an empty set is returned, a loop process tree without break behaviours is discovered. Otherwise, we mark the activities in BreakLeadNodes as break leaf nodes.

Algorithm 1: Identifying Break Leaf Nodes

Input: A break loop cut $\sum_1, \sum_2, ..., \sum_n$ of directly-follows graph G
1 BreakLeafNodes = {}
2 **for** *i in 2 ... n* **do**
3   **for** *a in $\sum_i$* **do**
4   **if** *$a \in End(G)$* **then**
5   BreakLeafNodes.add(a)
6   **end**
7   **end**
8 **end**
    Output: BreakLeafNodes

Step 3: Splitting Event Logs. The same loop cut split function for the original IM framework is applied to split the event log after a break loop cut. However, splitting the event logs directly after the break loop cut can bring extra behaviours into the discovered process model. For instance, in our example in Fig. 2, the activities are partitioned into two groups after the break loop cut: $\{a, b\}$ and $\{c, d, e\}$. The trace $< a, b, c, d >$ is then divided into $< a, b >$ and $< c, d >$, resulting in a process tree shown in Fig. 3, which allows traces such as $< a, b, c, d, a, b, c, d, a, b >$. To solve the problem, we remove all the traces with break behaviours before splitting the event logs (Algorithm 2).

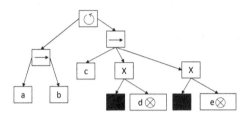

Fig. 3. Break process tree discovered from the log in Fig. 2 if traces with break behaviours are not removed before splitting the log

---

Algorithm 2: Removing Traces with Break Behaviours

    Input: A break loop cut $\sum_1, \sum_2, ..., \sum_n$ of directly-follows graph G, the event
           log L_{break} of G

1 **for** *Trace t in L_{break}* **do**
2   **if** $End(t) \in \sum_i \wedge i \neq 1$ **then**
3         $L_{break}.remove(t)$
4   **end**
5 **end**

A Running Example. Finally, a running example shown in Fig. 4 demonstrates the above three steps. The input is the log described in Fig. 2.

4 Case Study

We aim to discover the high-level treatment process in ICU for ACS patients. Specifically, domain experts are interested in how patients are discharged from the ICU. The goals of the case study are:

1. to discover the ACS patients' treatment pathways, especially discharge behaviours from ICU,
2. to quantitative and qualitative evaluate the proposed approach against existing process discovery methods with real-life break behaviours,
3. to gain insights into ICU discharge behaviours for ACS patient.

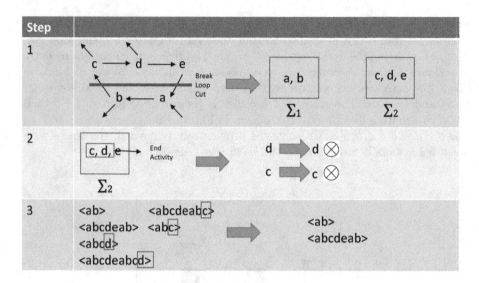

Fig. 4. A running example of our proposed approach based on the example in Fig. 2

4.1   Dataset and Event Log Generation

We utilise retrospective data from the EHR extracted between 2013 and 2018 from a single Cerner Millennium Electronic Medical Record domain in Sydney, Australia [7]. The Speed-Extract dataset comprises patients that presented with suspected ACS to facilities in Northern Sydney local health district (LHD) and Central Coast LHD [24]. Ethics and governance approval, including a waiver of informed patient consent, are provided by the Northern Sydney LHD Human Research Ethics Committee for the Speed-Extract dataset [7].

The Speed-Extract dataset consists of 18 tables; the following patient data is provided: Demographic and diagnosis information on patients, triage information after patients have arrived at hospitals, and transfer information between different ward levels. The orders placed during their stays, such as radiology, laboratory tests and procedures, are also provided.

We focus on a particular type of ACS, ST-elevation myocardial infarction (STEMI). STEMI patients are identified using the ICD-10 code (I21.3). We target at patients admitted to emergency wards and directly transferred to ICU. Patients who spent less than 24 h in hospitals are excluded. Furthermore, patients older than 85 or younger than 40 are excluded, as they have shown to be less informative in the treatment process development [7].

We treat each encounter as a case in the event log, as every encounter represents a unique hospital interaction. In total, 1,582 cases that have 666 variants are included. As behaviours in ICU can be relatively complex without proper abstractions, we categorise the behaviours into five activities: *Invasive Monitoring*, *Patient Care*, *Laboratory Test*, *Radiology* and *Procedure*. We follow [10] to extract frequent laboratory tests performed in ICU. *Radiology* represents the imaging operations in ICU [19], while *Procedure* involves the procedures performed on ICU patients (e.g., breathing assistance with ventilators). Overall, the event log contains events for 15 activities:

- two activities regarding the registration and triage in the emergency ward,
- three activities regarding patient conditions assessments in the triage,
- three activities regarding transfer to normal ward or ICU,
- five activities regarding treatments and measurements in ICU,
- two activities regarding discharge or death.

4.2   Results

Goal 1: ICU Treatment Process Discovery. The model discovered by our method is presented in Fig. 5 where the break process tree is translated into a BPMN model. The process starts with patient registration (*ER Registration*) and ends with different outcomes (*Discharge* or *Death*). One trajectory is that patients are directly admitted to ICU after registration. The remaining patients have been assessed before triage. We find that the treatment pathways in ICU are routine (i.e., a loop structure). The treatment pathway starts with invasive monitoring (i.e., "body" part in Fig. 5) for vital measurements [6]. The patients can be discharged from ICU at this point, given that they have received sufficient treatment and their monitoring results are normal. If not, nursing care (*Patient Care*) is conducted afterwards, involving care such as turning the patient in the bed. Patients can be asked to perform several treatments or measurements (i.e., "redo" part in Fig. 5) decided by the ICU team, depending on the monitoring results. Patients can also be discharged during the routine ICU treatment process, given that they have met the discharge criteria [18]. Such discharge behaviours (marked red in Fig. 5) can be considered break behaviours (i.e., a break from the "redo" part of the routine ICU treatment process). In fact, the orders placed in ICU are usually in bulk and made at the beginning of each day. We commonly observe that some orders are cancelled (e.g., discontinued or withdrawn) because patients have met the discharge criteria and been transferred out from ICU. After discharging from ICU, patients can be either discharged from the hospital or admitted to normal wards.

Goal 2: Validating with Existing Process Discovery Methods. To compare our method with existing process discovery algorithms, we apply our method, the inductive miner infrequent (IMF) [17], and the SM [4] on the extracted event log. We first apply conformance checking to the three process models. The results are presented in Table 1. Our method and the SM can achieve higher fitness and precision than the IMF. In addition, we adopt size and CFC (the number of branching caused by split gateways) to report the complexity of the process models. Although our model's size is slightly larger than the SM's, our method achieves a lower CFC.

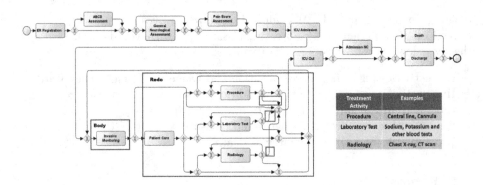

Fig. 5. The process model discovered by the proposed approach.

Table 1. Conformance checking results for the discovered process models.

Algorithms	Fitness	Precision	Size	CFC
Inductive Miner Infrequent (IMF)	0.98	0.60	49	46
Split Miner (SM)	0.98	0.80	**38**	41
Ours	**0.99**	**0.81**	41	**36**

Figure 6 shows the process model discovered by the SM. Although the process model can still describe the ICU treatment process according to the conformance checking results, it is hard to recognise the loop structure between *ICU Admission* and *ICU Out*. For instance, domain experts cannot tell which is the "redo" part. The discovered process model is unstructured and hard to understand compared to our model, because it barely produces valuable insights for domain experts. The process model discovered by the IMF is presented in Fig. 7. According to Table 1, the model has lower precision and higher complexity. Unlike our method, the discovered loop structure misses *Invasive Monitoring*, which is discovered as a parallel activity with the loop structure. Hence, the model cannot accurately represent the process since *Invasive Monitoring* cannot happen at an arbitrary time during the routine ICU treatment process. Besides, none of the break behaviours are discovered. To summarise, existing process discovery methods have difficulty discovering such break behaviours. The discovered models are unstructured, hard to understand and possess relatively low precision and high complexity.

Goal 3: Further Analysis of ICU Discharge Behaviours. More than 66.7% patients are discharged within 48 h, and no deaths are found among them. Most patients (64.4%) are normally discharged from ICU after invasive monitoring if their vital measurements are within the normal range. Some are further discharged from the hospital (i.e., transferred to other care facilities), and the remaining are admitted to normal wards in the hospital (i.e., *Admission NC*). Furthermore, three break discharge behaviours are discovered. 33.7% of patients

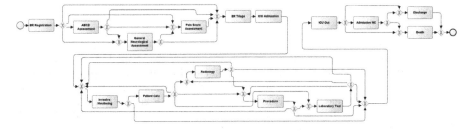

Fig. 6. The ICU pathways discovered by SM.

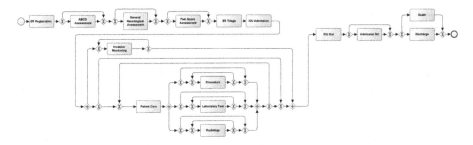

Fig. 7. The process model discovered by the IMF.

are discharged from ICU after performing further examinations ordered by doctors (i.e., laboratory tests and radiology), which is in line with the guideline [18]. Conversely, only 1.9% of patients are discharged after specific procedures are conducted. Further investigation indicates that the most are discharged because of death. Regarding discharge time, we find that 74.2% of patients are discharged in the morning, which indicates that although ICU usually have discharge rounds twice a day, the primary discharge decisions are made in the morning.

5 Discussion and Conclusion

This paper proposes a method to extend the IM framework to represent and discover break behaviours. The method is then applied to a healthcare event log to discover ICU discharge behaviours. Our method can discover more structured, understandable and accurate process models than existing process discovery algorithms.

It has to be noted that although our method can discover break behaviours in process trees, it may not always be possible to convert the break process trees into equivalent BPMNs/Petri nets. For example, in Fig. 5, there will be remaining tokens in the loop after break behaviours. Future work is needed to represent the break behaviours in other process modeling notations (e.g., using cancellation regions to represent break behaviours). Finally, our method can be potentially applied to other domains. Further evaluation is needed to demonstrate the performance of our method.

References

1. van der Aalst, W., Weijters, T., Maruster, L.: Workflow mining: discovering process models from event logs. IEEE Trans. Knowl. Data Eng. **16**(9), 1128–1142 (2004)
2. Abo-Hamad, W.: Patient pathways discovery and analysis using process mining techniques: an emergency department case study. In: Cappanera, P., Li, J., Matta, A., Sahin, E., Vandaele, N.J., Visintin, F. (eds.) ICHCSE 2017. SPMS, vol. 210, pp. 209–219. Springer, Cham (2017). https://doi.org/10.1007/978-3-319-66146-9_19
3. Augusto, A., et al.: Automated discovery of process models from event logs: review and benchmark. IEEE Trans. Knowl. Data Eng. **31**(4), 686–705 (2018)
4. Augusto, A., Conforti, R., Dumas, M., La Rosa, M., Polyvyanyy, A.: Split miner: automated discovery of accurate and simple business process models from event logs. Knowl. Inf. Syst. **59**(2), 251–284 (2019)
5. Benevento, E., Aloini, D., van der Aalst, W.M.: How can interactive process discovery address data quality issues in real business settings? evidence from a case study in healthcare. J. Biomed. Inf. **130**, 104083 (2022)
6. Berger, M.M., et al.: Monitoring nutrition in the ICU. Clin. Nutr. **38**(2), 584–593 (2019)
7. Chen, Q., Lu, Y., Tam, C., Poon, S.: Predictive process monitoring for early predictions of short-and long-term mortality for patients with acute coronary syndrome. In: Pacific Asia Conference on Information Systems (2022)
8. Delias, P., Manolitzas, P., Grigoroudis, E., Matsatsinis, N.: Applying process mining to the emergency department. In: Encyclopedia of Business Analytics and Optimization, pp. 168–178. IGI Global (2014)
9. Durojaiye, A.B., et al.: Mapping the flow of pediatric trauma patients using process mining. Appl. Clin. Inf. **9**(03), 654–666 (2018)
10. Ezzie, M.E., Aberegg, S.K., O'Brien, J.M., Jr.: Laboratory testing in the intensive care unit. Crit. Care Clin. **23**(3), 435–465 (2007)
11. Leemans, M., van der Aalst, W.M.P.: Modeling and discovering cancelation behavior. In: Panetto, H., et al. (eds.) OTM 2017. LNCS, vol. 10573, pp. 93–113. Springer, Cham (2017). https://doi.org/10.1007/978-3-319-69462-7_8
12. Leemans, M., van der Aalst, W.M.P., van den Brand, M.G.J.: Recursion aware modeling and discovery for hierarchical software event log analysis. In: 2018 IEEE 25th International Conference on Software Analysis, Evolution and Reengineering (SANER), pp. 185–196 (2018)
13. Leemans, S.J.J., Fahland, D., van der Aalst, W.M.P.: Discovering block-structured process models from incomplete event logs. In: Ciardo, G., Kindler, E. (eds.) PETRI NETS 2014. LNCS, vol. 8489, pp. 91–110. Springer, Cham (2014). https://doi.org/10.1007/978-3-319-07734-5_6
14. Leemans, S.J.J., Fahland, D., van der Aalst, W.M.P.: Using life cycle information in process discovery. In: Reichert, M., Reijers, H.A. (eds.) BPM 2015. LNBIP, vol. 256, pp. 204–217. Springer, Cham (2016). https://doi.org/10.1007/978-3-319-42887-1_17
15. Leemans, S.J.J., Fahland, D., van der Aalst, W.M.P.: Scalable process discovery and conformance checking. Softw. Syst. Model. **17**(2), 599–631 (2018)
16. Leemans, S.J.J., Fahland, D., van der Aalst, W.M.P.: Discovering block-structured process models from event logs - a constructive approach. In: Colom, J.-M., Desel, J. (eds.) PETRI NETS 2013. LNCS, vol. 7927, pp. 311–329. Springer, Heidelberg (2013). https://doi.org/10.1007/978-3-642-38697-8_17

17. Leemans, S.J.J., Fahland, D., van der Aalst, W.M.P.: Discovering block-structured process models from event logs containing infrequent behaviour. In: Lohmann, N., Song, M., Wohed, P. (eds.) BPM 2013. LNBIP, vol. 171, pp. 66–78. Springer, Cham (2014). https://doi.org/10.1007/978-3-319-06257-0_6
18. Lin, F., Chaboyer, W., Wallis, M.: A literature review of organisational, individual and teamwork factors contributing to the ICU discharge process. Aust. Crit. Care **22**(1), 29–43 (2009)
19. Lohan, R.: Imaging of ICU patients. In: Chawla, A. (ed.) Thoracic Imaging, pp. 173–194. Springer, Singapore (2019). https://doi.org/10.1007/978-981-13-2544-1_7
20. Lu, Y., Chen, Q., Poon, S.: A novel approach to discover switch behaviours in process mining. In: Leemans, S., Leopold, H. (eds.) ICPM 2020. LNBIP, vol. 406, pp. 57–68. Springer, Cham (2021). https://doi.org/10.1007/978-3-030-72693-5_5
21. Lull, J.J., et al.: Interactive process mining applied in a cardiology outpatient department. In: Munoz-Gama, J., Lu, X. (eds.) ICPM 2021. LNBIP, vol. 433, pp. 340–351. Springer, Cham (2022). https://doi.org/10.1007/978-3-030-98581-3_25
22. Mans, R., Schonenberg, M., Song, M., Van der Aalst, W., Bakker, P.: Process mining in health care. In: International Conference on Health Informatics (HEALTHINF 2008), pp. 118–125 (2008)
23. Munoz-Gama, J., et al.: Process mining for healthcare: characteristics and challenges. J. Biomed. Inf. **127**, 103994 (2022)
24. Tam, C.S., et al.: Combining structured and unstructured data in EMRs to create clinically-defined EMR-derived cohorts. BMC Med. Inf. Decis. Making **21**(1), 1–10 (2021)
25. Weijters, A., Ribeiro, J.: Flexible heuristics miner (FHM). In: 2011 IEEE Symposium on Computational Intelligence and Data Mining (CIDM), pp. 310–317 (2011)
26. Zhou, Z., Wang, Y., Li, L.: Process mining based modeling and analysis of workflows in clinical care-a case study in a Chicago outpatient clinic. In: Proceedings of the 11th IEEE International Conference on Networking, Sensing and Control, pp. 590–595. IEEE (2014)

Early Predicting the Need for Aftercare Based on Patients Events from the First Hours of Stay – A Case Study

Annika L. Dubbeldam$^{(\boxtimes)}$ ⓘ, István Ketykó ⓘ, Renata M. de Carvalho ⓘ, and Felix Mannhardt ⓘ

Department of Mathematics and Computer Science,
Eindhoven University of Technology, Eindhoven, The Netherlands
a.l.dubbeldam@student.tue.nl, {i.ketyko,r.carvalho,f.mannhardt}@tue.nl

Abstract. Patients, when in a hospital, will go through a personalized treatment scheduled for many different reasons and with various outcomes. Furthermore, some patients and/or treatments require aftercare. Identifying the need for aftercare is crucial for improving the process of the patient and hospital. A late identification results in a patient staying longer than needed, occupying a bed that otherwise could serve another patient. In this paper, we will investigate to what extent events from the first hours of stay can help in predicting the need for aftercare. For that, we explored a dataset from a Dutch hospital. We compared different methods, considering different prediction moments (depending of the amount of initial hours of stay), and we evaluate the gain in earlier predicting the need for aftercare.

Keywords: Early outcome prediction · Healthcare · Patient events · Aftercare demand

1 Introduction

Many people are admitted into a hospital every day, all of them different, taking their own personalized track, this makes for a lot of variability [10]. However, there is one thing all of these patients have in common during the hospitalization process, someone has to decide if the patient requires aftercare.

Currently, during the patient stay, a nurse might identify the need for aftercare and file an order. This means that some patients can be identified as soon as they enter the hospital, whereas others will only be identified near the end of their stay. As it takes time for the aftercare organizations to make room for a new patient, identifying patients that need this care very late means that they have to remain in hospital (even after their medical discharge date) in order to wait for the next available space. Patients that have to wait in the hospital no longer require any specialized treatment that can only be performed there. Furthermore, as they cannot be moved on, they will remain in their bed occupying a space that could be used by other patients that do require specialized treatment.

M. Montali et al. (Eds.): ICPM 2022 Workshops, LNBIP 468, pp. 366–377, 2023.
https://doi.org/10.1007/978-3-031-27815-0_27

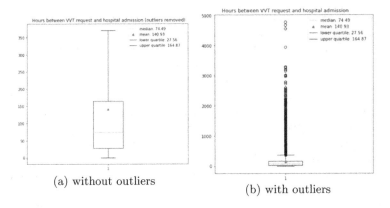

(a) without outliers

(b) with outliers

Fig. 1. Time for a patient to be identified as in need of aftercare

In order to establish the importance of this we must derive how long it currently takes the hospital to identify aftercare patients. Figure 1 depicts two box plots, showing how long (in hours) it took after admission for the patient to be marked for aftercare. Currently, on average after 140 h (or median of 74 h) a patient first gets noted. This leaves quite a lot of room for possible earlier detection, and consequently earlier arrangements with the aftercare organizations to make sure a place is available as soon as the patient gets discharged.

By noting these patients early on in their stay gives the hospital employees more time to inform the aftercare locations causing the patient's possible in-hospital wait time to be reduced. In this paper we aim to explore the possibility to identify those patients who need aftercare and to evaluate how early on during the process this can be done. For that we plan to make use of various decision tree related models which we will give different inputs (patient data with events from admission until a certain moment in time) to determine simultaneously if it is possible to predict aftercare and how soon in the process we can do this.

Within this paper we will first mention other similar studies in Sect. 2. After which in Sect. 3, the preliminaries will be explained as well as the importance of this study. Section 4 explains what the data looks like and how it was formatted accordingly. In Sect. 5 you can read about how we used the formatted data with the various models. Section 6 gives the results from the methods described in Sect. 5. Lastly Sect. 7 states the final conclusion.

2   Related Work

As can be read in the introduction, the main goal of this study is to determine if it is possible to detect early on which patients need aftercare and which do not. Not many other works can be found that deal with this specific topic of patient predictions. However, there are many that are related to developing a so called *early warning system* for hospital patients.

In [8], authors try to predict circulatory failure in the intensive care unit as early on as possible. Using three different machine learning techniques they tried to predict in a binary manner every 5 min after admission if a patient needed extra care or not. Similar to this, in [5] authors try to identify patients early on if they are at risk for Sepsis. Here they used gradient boosting at various timestamps within the first 24 h after admission to identify possible at risk patients. In [13], an architecture combining process mining and deep learning was proposed to improve the severity score measure for diabetes patients.

As the aforementioned works, our aim is also to make a reliable prediction as soon as possible. Contrary to [8], our research cannot focus on predictions every 5 min, as patients should be analyzed and confirmed by a hospital employee. In this context, we need to decide for a certain moment in time where the prediction can be done. Besides, while [5] compares different early moments to find the best time for an early prediction, they do not consider the events that happen during such period. Moreover, [13] combines both event and patient data, they also consider data only from the first hours, but their focus is to provide a severity score rather than a prediction with a high imbalanced positive class.

3   Background

3.1   Predictive Process Mining

Within process mining, predictions are usually made on incomplete traces regarding future events and/or outcome and related attributes [6]. A *trace* is a timely-ordered sequence of events related to the same context (in this research, such context is a patient admission). Commonly, the prediction is done (the *prediction moment*) based on all previous events known (denoted as *prefix*) and the prediction target is some event or outcome in the future. So, the prefix trace is used as input for the prediction model. Making predictions within process mining might be valuable for many organizations, as having an idea of the future might lead to early actions that can improve the remaining of the process.

3.2   Preliminaries

As the problem statement can be seen as a binary one (do/do not), it allows us to use decision trees, random forest, and XGBoost solutions within this study. A decision tree represents a series of sequential steps that can be taken in order to answer a question and provide probabilities, costs, or other consequences with it [9]. There is no way of knowing what the best tree depth is for a decision tree, which means that tests should be performed in order to reach a conclusion. One option is to use cross validation [11], which is a procedure that resamples the data it is been given to evaluate a machine learning model in many ways on a limited data set [7]. Random forest is a collection of decision trees producing a single aggregated result [9]. For random forests there is also the question of how many decision trees is best to use. Similarly to a single decision tree, this question cannot be answered very easily and requires for example cross validation as well over various combinations to find the best option [9]. Lastly, XGBoost, which is alike random forest but uses a different algorithm to build the needed trees. Random forest builds each tree independently whereas XGBoost builds them one at a time [9]. Also for XGBoost the problem of deciding on the amount of trees to use exists, and also here a possible solution is the usage of cross validation [9].

While a decision tree is a white box solution [3] and therefore preferred by the hospital due to it being explainable [10], random forest and XGBoost are also experimented with to allow for comparisons in the end. In order to be able to compare the results from the various models we keep track of the recall and precision scores [1]. With the hospital it was discussed that the recall scores weights more heavily than those of precision as it was deemed more important to be able to identify all of the aftercare patients (even though this might give many more false positives) than to miss them. Another way of comparing the models is by using a Receiver Operating Characteristic (ROC) curve or the Precision-Recall (PR) curve [4], which are also created. The preference in this paper goes to the usage of the PR curve, this due to the large class imbalance that we are dealing with. By computing the Area Under the Curve (AUC) for both ROC and PR allows for easy comparison between different models.

We will also make use of feature importance such that we can determine which datapoints we should keep and which can be removed. Feature importance is calculated as the decrease in node impurity weighted by the probability of reaching that node in a decision tree [12].

4   Data

4.1   Data Introduction and Processing

As a data set we received the patient records from 2018. We filtered this set to traces that are at least 24 h long but at most 2 months. Each patient used in this data set had given their permission to their data being used for analysis purposes. This resulted in a set containing 35380 unique hospital stays of which only 4627 required a type of aftercare, which is only 13% and could thus be classified as an infrequent behaviour [10].

For each hospital stay we collected the following patient information: aftercare required, aftercare type, age, gender, activities, timestamps, and additional information. Activities can be one of the following: hospital admission, hospital discharge, admit medication, poli appointment, start operation, end operation, start lab, and end lab. The additional information is related to the activity admit medication and specifies how it was admitted. Each stay was also assigned a random unique case id this to make sure patient information is anonymous [10].

We are currently not taking patient departments or any data regarding why they were admitted to the hospital into account. This is due to the fact that within this research we only considered the data of 2018. However, keeping in mind that a lot newer data exists and that this follow up data covers the Covid-19 years we had to create a dataset using features that stayed consistent throughout these years. After discussing with the hospital about what changed the most for patients during these years, and what would thus be an unreliable feature, we excluded the patient departments. The admission reason was excluded as this field is filled in manually within their systems, this creates a lot of possible different descriptions for the same issue.

In order to guarantee a certain quality event log, traces in which events happened before admission or after discharge were removed. Traces where end operation was before or at the same time as start operation or if either one of the two was missing (similar for start and end lab activities) were also removed.

4.2   Extending the Feature Set

We supplemented each trace with some manually created features of which the possible importance was questioned by the hospital. For each trace it was calculated how many times the same patient had been admitted previously, how many of those stays required aftercare, the average hospital duration of previous stays, the standard deviation of previous stays, the average duration in between admissions, and the standard deviation between admissions.

4.3   Formatting and Predicted Values

As decision trees do not take event logs as input data, we had to encode the datapoints in such a manner that all relevant points can be inputted at once. An initial dataset consisting of the manually created features combined with the patients age and gender was created. For a second dataset we had to make a distinction between *amount* and *occurrence*. With *amount* we count how often a certain activity took place (*how often did a patient receive medication? etc.*), whereas with *occurrence* we take note in a yes/no (1/0) manner if a certain activity took place at least once (*did the patient receive any medication? etc.*). This created two similar looking datasets, both containing the data from the first dataset one augmented with the *amount* and the other with the *occurrence* encoding. Later on, as will be described in Sect. 6, we also perform a count on specific medication and operation groups.

As prediction value, the dataset also contains a column indicating if that patient does need aftercare (denoted by 1) or not (denoted by 0).

5   Methods

The hospital records many different data points. It is of course not possible to just use everything and hope for the best. Therefore, we will approach the problem in the following manner. We start by using only data available at admission. This would give first insights for each patient at arrival moment if aftercare might be needed. Earlier than arrival time we cannot predict. This also provides us with a benchmark to which we can compare the models. Secondly, we will use a selection of features, after discussing with the hospital on possible relevancy, if based on the full trace data the same or an increase in prediction accuracy can be seen compared to the benchmark. Using feature importance we can eliminate features that are not as beneficial as expected and rerun the models.

While in this paper we do combine prediction making and process mining on incomplete traces, we do so in a different manner. We chose two different prediction moments to be evaluated: 24 and 48 h. As part of the research question is to determine how early we can predict for each patient, we will evaluate whether postponing the prediction moment contributes to an increase in prediction accuracy. For that, we will create two different models: one that considers only events happened within 24 h as a prefix trace, and 48 h for the other. They will be compared to the two benchmark models described.

The data used is split in two different ways. First in a 5-fold manner to perform cross validation for all three of the methods allowing us to find the best possible tree depth or number of trees used. Secondly, there is a 8:2 split for the final train/test set based on the results from the cross validation.

For the decision tree we will take cross validation over various tree depths (1 to 25), and for random forest and XGBoost we compare different amount of tree usages (1 to 50). For each step we calculate the accuracy and recall score, as can be seen in Fig. 2. The best possible tree depth/amount of trees is derived from where the recall score is highest along the plot. The recall score is taken here as we mentioned that this is the score the hospital is the most interested in.

6   Results

Admission Data Only. Starting with just the datapoints known upon arrival we get the recall plots over various depths/amount of trees using cross validation as can be seen in Fig. 2. From each plot we note the highest possible value with parameter and use those to create a final model. The final model results can be viewed in Table 1. Based on these results we can draw an intermediate conclusion that it is indeed possible to predict if a patient needs aftercare to a certain degree the moment they enter the hospital without knowing all too much about them. All three models appear very similar in overall results (F1).

Full Dataset. Next up was using the full dataset to determine feature importance. The full dataset was constructed in two manners (amount and occurrence). Similar to the previous section, here we also first tested using cross validation what the best depth/amount of trees is (Fig. 4). With this, we get the results in Table 1. Here we can clearly see an increase in scores for both the random forest and XGBoost compared to just the admission data. The decision tree results are similar with regards to just the recall score, however, the F1 scores did improve.

We did not find much difference in scoring between using either the amount or the occurrence datasets (hence we only show one of them). Given that the difference is minimal between the two means we can decide on one of them to use from this point forward. We decided on using the amount encoding.

Before we can do additional testing based on a shorter timeframe it is important to derive which of the features actually contributed to the results. Calcu-

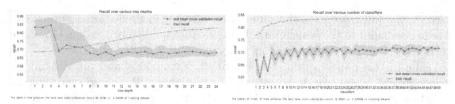

(a) Recall scores over various tree depths for a single decision tree

(b) Recall scores over various amount of trees for random forest

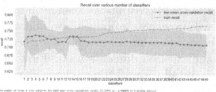

(c) Recall scores over various amount of trees for XGBoost

Fig. 2. Recall scores for various tree models using the admission data only dataset

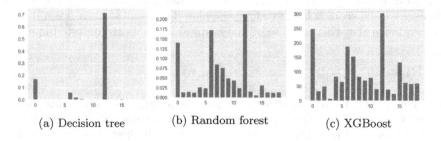

(a) Decision tree   (b) Random forest   (c) XGBoost

Fig. 3. Feature importance. 0 - age, 6 - medication, 12 - total time stay

lating the feature importance for each model we obtain the plots in Fig. 3. The three highest bars correspond to: the admission data, *total time stay*; the *age*; and the *medications*. From the first two features we cannot create a dataset based on time as they are constant values. Medication however is a value that might change throughout a patient stay. Therefore, we created a new dataset based on medications a patient received within 24 h. Within the hospital, more than 1000 different medications are used and creating a dataset that differentiates between them would result in very sparse dataset that takes a long time to train. Luckily, each medication comes with an ATC code [2]. An ATC code consists of 7 characters where the first four represent a medication group. There are only 268 medication groups. Grouping the medications quickly downsizes the dataset. Now, instead of counting each individual medication, we count how often a patient got admitted a medication from which medication group.

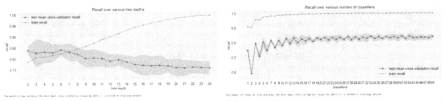

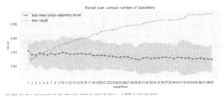

(a) Recall scores over various tree depths for a single decision tree
(b) Recall scores over various amount of trees for random forest

(c) Recall scores over various amount of trees for XGBoost

Fig. 4. Recall scores for various tree models using the full dataset with amount

Admission and First 24 h Medication Data. The combination of admission data and the first 24 h of medication group counts gives the third dataset. We again use cross validation to find the best parameters (Fig. 5) after which we obtain the final test scores (Table 1). Comparing these results to *admission data only* we can immediately tell that the recall score increased. Although the recall increased for all, the AUC PR for the decision tree was lower.

According to hospital domain experts, the way in which medication was admitted and the operation type might indicate a need for aftercare. Therefore a fourth and last test set was constructed based on the feature importance results and the domain knowledge of the hospital.

Admission, Medication, Admittance Way, and Operation Data (24 h & 48 h). The last dataset also took all the same steps as the previous datasets (Fig. 6, 7). For this dataset we did create an extra test for the first 48 h of events in order to see to what extent waiting for more information would provide better results, which can be found in Table 1. We can compare these results to the ones from the previous section. Here, one model had a slightly decrease in the recall score whereas others increased. Similarly for the AUC PR scores. Also, comparing the scores in Table 1, we do not see a major increase in using a dataset that considers 48 h.

There is one major downside with how the results are now portrayed. Our testset consists out of 1/5 from the total dataset, which was the entire year of 2018. However, this is not the amount of patients that the hospital will work with on a day to day basis. Therefore it is important to look at the effect that the final and best model would have each day for a certain timeframe (Fig. 8). Based on this figure we can see that on average the hospital will have to verify

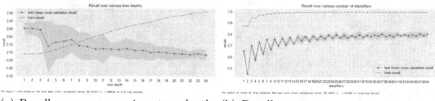

(a) Recall scores over various tree depths for a single decision tree

(b) Recall scores over various amount of trees for random forest

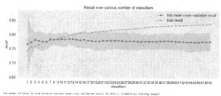

(c) Recall scores over various amount of trees for XGBoost

Fig. 5. Recall scores for various tree models using the admission with medication first 24 h dataset

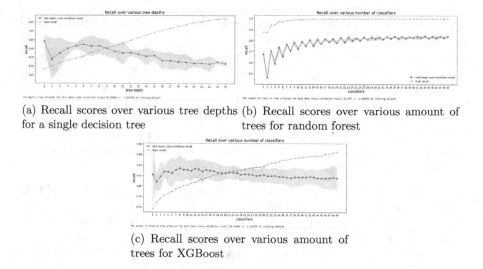

(a) Recall scores over various tree depths for a single decision tree

(b) Recall scores over various amount of trees for random forest

(c) Recall scores over various amount of trees for XGBoost

Fig. 6. Recall scores for various tree models using the admission with medication, admittance way and operation first 24 h dataset

between 40 and 60 patients per day of which 10 to 20 will indeed require aftercare. Generating these results daily only takes a matter of seconds and is thus very doable. After discussion with the hospital it was concluded that these numbers were reasonable which means we can draw a final conclusion.

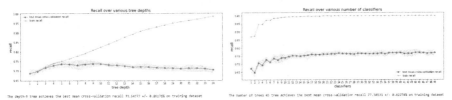

(a) Recall scores over various tree depths for a single decision tree

(b) Recall scores over various amount of trees for random forest

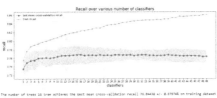

(c) Recall scores over various amount of trees for XGBoost

Fig. 7. Recall scores for various tree models using the admission with medication, admittance way and operation first 48 h dataset

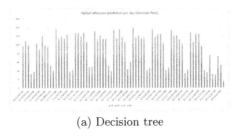

(a) Decision tree

Fig. 8. Model prediction per day based on the 24 h model of admission, medication, medication admittance way, and operations dataset

Table 1. All model scores for the various datasets

Dataset	Model	Accuracy	Recall	Precision	F1	AUC ROC	AUC PR	FP	TP
Admission data only	Decision Tree	0.60	0.82	0.23	0.35	0.70	0.52	2635	767
	Random Forest	0.68	0.66	0.24	0.35	0.67	0.45	1941	619
	XGBoost	0.64	0.74	0.23	0.35	0.68	0.49	2289	692
Full	Decision Tree	0.78	0.80	0.36	0.49	0.79	0.58	1351	750
	Random Forest	0.79	0.81	0.37	0.51	0.80	0.59	1319	760
	XGBoost	0.78	0.81	0.35	0.49	0.79	0.58	1379	754
Admission with Medication (24 h)	Decision Tree	0.57	0.83	0.21	0.34	0.68	0.52	2892	776
	Random Forest	0.71	0.80	0.29	0.42	0.75	0.54	1879	747
	XGBoost	0.71	0.78	0.28	0.42	0.74	0.53	1859	731

(continued)

Table 1. (*continued*)

Dataset	Model	Accuracy	Recall	Precision	F1	AUC ROC	AUC PR	FP	TP
Admission with Medication, Admittance way, Operation (24 h)	Decision Tree	0.66	0.80	0.24	0.37	0.72	0.52	2175	696
	Random Forest	0.70	0.81	0.27	0.40	0.75	0.54	1892	698
	XGBoost	0.72	0.75	0.27	0.40	0.73	0.51	1738	648
Admission with Medication, Admittance way, Operation (48 h)	Decision Tree	0.70	0.78	0.24	0.37	0.72	0.51	2100	677
	Random Forest	0.71	0.84	0.28	0.43	0.77	0.56	1847	732
	XGBoost	0.73	0.79	0.29	0.42	0.75	0.54	1719	686

7 Conclusions and Recommendations

Looking back at the research question stated in the introduction, we can definitely conclude that it is possible to predict which patients need aftercare and which do not to a certain degree.

We also wanted to analyze if patient could be identified earlier on in their trajectories compared to what is happening now. We had already derived that currently it takes about 74 h before a patient is marked for aftercare. Within this paper we provided models at three different timestamps that are of relevancy (0, 24, 48 h). How ever large the time benefit will be depends on what model the user chooses based on the first part of the research question.

Given that the hospital cares about the model being explainable only leaves one viable usable option for them, the decision tree. Comparing the third, fourth and fifth datasets from Table 1, we can say that there is no need to wait 48 h before making a prediction. The decision on which model to then use is more up to them. Both the 24 h results are very similar, one results in a slightly higher recall and the other in a slightly higher precision. Our recommendation would go to the model that uses admission, medication, medication admittance way, and operations given that the this one appears to be more of an increase compared to the first dataset.

If we were to give a final conclusion without being limited by the explainability rule, then we would recommend the random forest model at both the 24 h and the 48 h mark. This model has the highest AUC PR and overall higher F1 score.

In both conclusions we make use of the 24 h model, which compared to the current time median from Fig. 1, is a major speed up. Using these models to aid the nurses currently working on this to help identify patients as early as 24 h after admission, would give the employees who talk to the aftercare organization a lot more time to organise.

During the discissions with the hospital many more mentions were made about other datasets that they have in their possession. These can be used to possibly enhance the current models.

References

1. Singh, K.K., Elhoseny, M., Singh, A., Elngar, A.A.: Diagnosing of disease using machine learning. In: Machine Learning and the Internet of Medical Things in Healthcare, pp. 89–111. Academic Press (2021)

2. Medicijntab: Geneesmiddelen op ATC-code (4) (2022)
3. Carvalho, D.V., Pereira, E.M., Cardoso, J.S.: Machine learning interpretability: a survey on methods and metrics. Electronics **8**(8), 832 (2019)
4. Davis, J., Goadrich, M.: The relationship between precision-recall and ROC curves. In: Proceedings of the 23rd International Conference on Machine Learning - ICML 2006 (2006)
5. Delahanty, R.J., Alvarez, J., Flynn, L.M., Sherwin, R.L., Jones, S.S.: Development and evaluation of a machine learning model for the early identification of patients at risk for sepsis. Ann. Emerg. Med. **73**(4), 334–344 (2019)
6. Di Francescomarino, C., Ghidini, C.: Predictive process monitoring. In: van der Aalst, W.M.P., Carmona, J. (eds.) Process Mining Handbook. Lecture Notes in Business Information Processing, vol. 448, pp. 320–346. Springer International Publishing, Cham (2022). https://doi.org/10.1007/978-3-031-08848-3_10
7. Fushiki, T.: Estimation of prediction error by using k-fold cross-validation. Stat. Comput. **21**, 137–146 (2011)
8. Hyland, S.L., et al.: Early prediction of circulatory failure in the intensive care unit using machine learning. Nature Med. **26**(3), 364–373 (2020)
9. Larose, C.D., Larose, D.T.: Data Science Using Python and R. Wiley, Hoboken (2019)
10. Munoz-Gama, J., et al.: Process mining for healthcare: characteristics and challenges. J. Biomed. Inf. **127**, 103994 (2022)
11. Painsky, A., Rosset, S.: Cross-validated variable selection in tree-based methods improves predictive performance. IEEE Trans. Pattern Anal. Mach. Intell. **39**(11), 2142–2153 (2017)
12. Ronaghan, S.: The mathematics of decision trees, random forest and feature importance in scikit-learn and spark (2019). https://towardsdatascience.com/the-mathematics-of-decision-trees-random-forest-and-feature-importance-in-scikit-learn-and-spark-f2861df67e3
13. Theis, J., Galanter, W.L., Boyd, A.D., Darabi, H.: Improving the in-hospital mortality prediction of diabetes ICU patients using a process mining/deep learning architecture. IEEE J. Biomed. Health Inf. **26**(1), 388–399 (2022)

Predicting Patient Care Acuity: An LSTM Approach for Days-to-day Prediction

Jorg W. R. Bekelaar[1]([✉]) [ID], Jolanda J. Luime[2] [ID],
and Renata M. de Carvalho[1] [ID]

[1] Department of Mathematics and Computer Science, Eindhoven University of
Technology, Eindhoven, The Netherlands
`j.w.r.bekelaar@student.tue.nl`, `r.carvalho@ue.nl`
[2] Maxima Medical Center, Veldhoven, The Netherlands
`jolanda.luime@mmc.nl`

Abstract. In recent years, hospitals and other care providers in the
Netherlands are coping with a widespread nursing shortage and a directly
related increase in nursing workload. This nursing shortage combined
with the high nursing workload is associated with higher levels of burnout
and reduced job satisfaction among nurses. However, not only the nurses,
but also the patients are affected as an increasing nursing workload
adversely affects patient safety and satisfaction. Therefore, the aim of
this research is to predict the care acuity corresponding to an individual patient for the next admission day, by using the available structured
hospital data of the previous admission days. For this purpose, we make
use of an LSTM model that is able to predict the care acuity of the next
day, based on the hospital data of all previous days of an admission. In
this paper, we elaborate on the architecture of the LSTM model and we
show that the prediction accuracy of the LSTM model increases with the
increase of the available amount of historical event data. We also show
that the model is able to identify care acuity differences in terms of the
amount of support needed by the patient. Moreover, we discuss how the
predictions can be used to identify which patient care related characteristics and different types of nursing activities potentially contribute to
the care acuity of a patient.

Keywords: Nurse workload · LSTM model · Event data · Healthcare

1 Introduction

One hundred years ago, in 1922, the first paper on determination of appropriate
nurse staffing levels and bedside nursing time was published [7]. As of today,
both still are important topics that have only partially been solved over the
last 100 years. In the Netherlands, a number of big steps were made towards
the management of nurse staffing levels, including the international acceptance
of nurse-to-patient ratios, the introduction of policies and regulations regarding

© The Author(s) 2023
M. Montali et al. (Eds.): ICPM 2022 Workshops, LNBIP 468, pp. 378–390, 2023.
https://doi.org/10.1007/978-3-031-27815-0_28

shift duration and in general the labour conditions as prescribed in the collective labour agreement. Since this first publication, the effect and impact of bedside nursing time on the quality and the actual level of nursing care provided to the patient continued to become increasingly important for all healthcare actors.

In recent years, hospitals and other care providers are coping with a widespread nursing shortage and a directly related increase in nursing workload in the Netherlands. The nursing shortage results in a higher nursing workload, which is associated with higher levels of burnout and reduced job satisfaction among the nurses. Both could be predecessors for voluntarily stopping clinical nursing work by reschooling to a specialised nurse, nurse practitioner or even by leaving the nursing profession. However, not only the nurses, but also the patients are affected by the nursing shortage and the high workloads: an increasing nursing workload adversely affects patient safety and satisfaction. This emerges by the influence of the nurses on the care process including continuity of care, effective communication at discharge for the continuity of care at home or another care facility, patient centeredness and surveillance.

In order to solve such a complex problem, insights about care acuity - patient characteristics and the nursing care activities that can be expected for a patient - should be gathered. As a first step, we aim at predicting the care acuity expected for an individual patient. Such a prediction already provides a good overview of what nurses should expect for the next admission day and allows for improved decision making in terms of number of nursing staff per shift, which eventually leads to a more equal distribution of the care acuity among the nurses.

In this paper we make use of a Long Short-Term Memory (LSTM) neural network that is able to predict the care acuity per patient for the next admission day. The predictions are based on hospital data collected during the previous days of the corresponding admission, including the amount of care acuity on all previous admission days. Because the conditions of a patient might change due to deterioration or recovery, the LSTM model also considers the conditions of the patient at that particular day.

The remainder of the paper is organized as follows. Section 2 provides the concepts that are relevant for this research. Related research is discussed in Sect. 3. Section 4 describes the data used in this research, while the approach to data preprocessing and the prediction model are explained in Sect. 5. Then, Sect. 6 discusses the obtained results. Section 7 presents the final conclusions.

2   Background

2.1   Process Mining

Predictive process monitoring [1] is a segment of process mining interested in predicting the future of an ongoing process execution. For that, it relies on the *event log*, which is a structured dataset containing information about different executions of a process and can also be seen as a collection of traces. A *trace* is a non-empty sequence of events related to the same process execution, ordered by time. An *event* is then an atomic part of the process execution and is characterized by various properties, e.g., an event has a timestamp and it corresponds to an activity. Many approaches in predictive process monitoring leverage machine learning techniques, such as neural networks (cf. Sect. 3). For such approaches, the event log information should be encoded in terms of features. Usually, the event and its data *payload* are part of this feature set.

The predictive process is split into two phases: training and prediction. The *training* phase counts on the information of previously completed process executions to learn relations in the data. The *prediction* phase considers an ongoing process execution. This means that such a process execution is not completed yet. The known part of the trace is defined as the *prefix* and is used as the input for the prediction model. The future sequence of events that is supposed to take place after the prefix, is defined as the *suffix* and represents the prediction made by the model. Predictive process monitoring is also applied to predict the outcome of a process execution, or its completion time. For some organizations, it can be highly valuable to be able to predict in advance what is going to happen to a process execution. In this context, the organization can focus on *preventing* issues from happening, rather than *reacting* to them after their occurrence [10].

2.2   Long Short-Term Memory Neural Networks

The Long Short-Term Memory (LSTM) model is an advanced form of a Recurrent Neural Network (RNN) that allows information to persist [4]. LSTM models are explicitly designed to solve the problem of long-term dependencies by changing the structure of hidden neurons in a traditional RNN. A LSTM model can be used for predicting on the basis of time series data due to the characteristic of retaining the information for a long period of time. Hence, it is considered effective and general at capturing long term temporal dependencies [2].

In practice, the LSTM architecture consists of a set of recurrently connected sub-networks called memory blocks. An individual memory block contains a functional module that is known as the memory cell and a number of different gates. The memory cell is responsible for remembering the temporal state of the neural network over arbitrary time intervals, while the gates formed by multiplicative units regulate the flow of information associated with the memory cell. Together, the memory blocks form the key part of the LSTM that enhances its capability to model long term dependencies. A memory block contains both a hidden state and a cell state known as short term memory and long term memory respectively. The cell state encodes an aggregation of the data from all previous time steps that have been processed by the LSTM, while the hidden state is used to encode a characterisation of the input data of solely the previous time step.

A memory block contains three gates that together regulate the information flow: the *forget* gate, which decides what information should be removed from the previous cell state, the *input* gate, which quantifies the importance of the new information carried by the input and the *output* gate, which extracts the useful information from the current LSTM block by computing the new hidden state. LSTM models are appropriate to handle sequential data of different sizes and hence, process executions of different lengths. They are also able to consider additional information about the events, resources and any other data payload.

3   Related Work

Over the years, several attempts have been made to quantify and predict care acuity [3]. Some of the earliest methods that have been developed to quantify care acuity are the Therapeutic Intervention Scoring System (TISS), the TISS-28 method, the Nine Equivalents of Nursing Manpower (NEMS) and the Nursing Activities Score (NAS). All methods are based on an identical principle that distinguishes a number of activities that are scored on a 1–4 basis according to the intensity of involvement. Subsequently, the assigned scores are used to group patients into separate classes. The Project Research of Nursing (PRN) assigns a score to each nursing activity based on, among other factors, the corresponding duration, frequency and the number of nurses required to execute the activity, while the Time Oriented Scoring System (TOSS) is a time based system for quantifying care acuity that exactly times a number of preselected nursing tasks. Alternatively, the Rafaela method relates each activity to a domain with varying nursing intensities. The points assigned to the different domains are added up per patient and department to compute the actual workload per nurse.

As is mentioned in Sect. 2.2, a LSTM can be used for predicting on the basis of time series data. Today, applications and research of LSTM for time series prediction include usage in the healthcare sector to predict the day of discharge [9], hospital performance metrics [5] or to make clinical predictions [8].

Also in the context of process mining, the usage of LSTM is not new. LSTM models are notably suitable to deal with problems that involve sequences, such as event traces. Mostly, LSTMs are used in attempting to predict the next activity in a trace. Tax *et al.* [12] and Tello-Leal *et al.* [13] employ LSTM to predict the next event of a running case. Tax goes beyond, predicting its timestamp and showing how the method can be used to predict the full continuation of a case and its remaining time. Pham *et al.* [11] also uses LSTM models to predict the next activity in a trace and who would perform such an activity.

Building on the aforementioned works, we believe that simply representing the trace events with its data attributes is not enough for the problem of predicting care acuity. Firstly, we think it necessary to use all the historic hospital data of an admission, as it can show how fast the patient recovery process is. Therefore, we cannot use predefined prefix lengths. Secondly, there might be data to learn about this recovery process that are crucial for the model, but are not associated to any event directly. Such data mostly come from monitoring the patient's vital parameters.

To help in the decision making of the distribution of patients among nurses, we do not need to know the explicit sequence of events that will happen for a patient. However, it is necessary to know how much support is expected to be required from a nurse and if any critical task will take place. So, this work is different from previous research mainly on how we group and represent the workload of tasks. Besides this, we are interested in predicting a numeric value representing the care acuity on the next admission day. This objective is a regression task, rather than a classification task such as predicting the next event label.

4   Data Description

The data for this research have been obtained from the clinical departments of a hospital located in the Netherlands throughout 2018. The clinical departments consist of 8 different departments that are responsible for providing different levels of adult patient care services: cardiology, gastrointestinal surgery, general surgery, gynaecology, internal medicine, neurology, oncology, orthopaedics and pulmonary. The data from the intensive care unit (ICU) and the short stay unit (SSU) were not considered in this research. The resulting dataset distinguishes 62 features per record, including:

- five *patient features*: age, BMI, pre-hospitalisation physical mobility, sex, social economic status and the unique patient identifier;
- eight *admission features*, such as the admission department, inter-department transfers, reason and type of the admission and the specialism of the doctor;
- seven *time features*, such as the current date, day of the week, month, season, time and the current length of stay;
- eleven *medication features*, such as the daily number of inhaled, injected, intravenous, oncology, oral and pain medications and the daily number of either newly started or discontinued medications;
- four *examination features*: the daily number of bloodcount, imaging, laboratory and microbiology tests;
- eleven *vital parameter features*, including vital functions such as the daily maximum and minimum body temperature, early warning score, oxygen saturation level, pain score, respiratory rate and systolic blood pressure;
- six *nursing activity features*, such as the description, explanation and the type of the nursing activity and the maximum number of daily occurrences;
- three *nursing notes features*, such as the length (in terms of lines and words) and the daily amount of nursing notes;
- three *DBC features*, such as the amount of diagnosis treatment combinations in the three previous years per specialism;
- two *operation room (OR) features*: whether the patient underwent a procedure, or more than two procedures in the OR.
- two *discharge features*: whether the patient is going to be discharged in the next 24 or 48 h.

5   Methodology

Data was extracted using a software package on a copy of the electronic patient file system. This software (CTcue) allows for immediate pseudonymisation of the data using NLP and pseudo-IDs to de-identify all doctor and patient names in unstructured text. Data from the nurse activity plan was extracted by a dedicated SQL query. A common data model was created by representing each nursing care activity as a single record with the activity, the data source and the timestamp. Each of the records was assigned to a department, room and bed and an unique admission number. If multiple clinical departments were visited by the patient during a day, we assigned the final department to this day.

5.1 Workload Assignment

Based on the current daily nursing practice, 11 core activity categories were identified: *Activities of Daily Living (ADL), Bed rest, Communication, Drains, Excretion, Feeding tube, Infusions & Lines, Measurements & Observations, Reporting, Respiration* and *Woundcare*. Initially, a tree was built containing these categories and the individual nursing care activities, classified into each category. Points were assigned to each individual activity based on existing work by Jonker [6]. The research conducted by Jonker implemented a dedicated scoring system based on the Rafaela method [3] and assigns 0–3 points to each individual activity. This research implemented a similar scoring system with a similar scoring scale, but with a number of exceptions that received either 4 or 5 points, based on suggestions by the board of nurses. For each patient, all the activities in each category were summed to compute their daily care acuity. Care acuity is a latent variable that has no golden or reference standard, but of which the validity could be constructed via nurse opinion. Figure 1 provides an overview of the care acuity distribution in the training, validation and test datasets.

An exception was formed by the *ADL* and *Communication* categories that do not contain standalone activities. For the *ADL* category, we assigned a fixed baseline workload based on whether a patient was independent, partially independent or fully dependent on the nurse during *ADL* activities. These scenarios are used in daily nursing practice and were regarded as relevant by the nurses. Additional points were assigned for auxiliaries used for patient movement and transfer, equipment and medications, medical devices and the patient's mobility status, as they complicate the execution of the nursing care activities contained in the *ADL* category. The communication baseline workload consists of one scenario with four components that contribute to the care acuity: bedside rounds, communication with family members, medical handovers across shifts and time spent by nurses on registering medical notes and additional reporting. Special attention was paid to patients with a delirium. Delirium is a sudden change in the mental state of a patient. If patients are delusional or get a tendency to walk

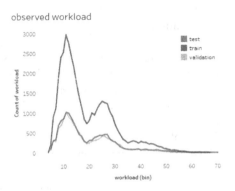

Fig. 1. The distribution of the care acuity.

away, nurses need to attend the patient more often. We used the results of the Delirium Observation Questionnaire for these patients to assign a workload to the delirium on a daily basis.

5.2   Prediction Preparation and Target

Finally, the time series data are compressed using a compression interval of exactly 1 admission day. As a results, each admission day is represented by a single record and the input for the LSTM model consists of a large input vector. Because of the different magnitude and unit of the different features, each feature is individually scaled and translated such that its values are in a range between 0 and 1. The scaler is fit on the training set and used to transform the data contained in both the validation and the test set. After the LSTM model has produced the predictions for the care acuity, it is necessary to reverse the scaling to retrieve the actual predictions of the care acuity.

The output of the LSTM model consists of the total care acuity of an individual patient for the next admission day. For the final day of an admission, there are no registered nursing activities on the next day. As a consequence, the value of target variable for each final day of an admission will be equal to 0. In order to predict the care acuity of the patient, the input variables are formed by the features that were contained in the original dataset and specified in Sect. 4, together with the additional features that were generated in the feature engineering steps during the data preprocessing. The LSTM model uses these features to predict the care acuity corresponding to an individual patient for the next admission day, based on the available date and time stamped hospital data of the current day. If the current length of stay is longer than 1 day, the prediction is made based on the available date and time stamped hospital data of the current day and the previous admission days.

5.3   LSTM Prediction Model

A LSTM neural network consists of different types of layers, including at least one LSTM layer. Figure 2 depicts the architecture of the LSTM neural network that was used in this research. The initial layer of the sequential model that represents the LSTM model is made up by a LSTM input layer. In order to pass the input data to the LSTM layer of the sequential model, the *input shape* parameter of the LSTM layer must be specified. The input to the LSTM layer must be three-dimensional and consists of samples, time steps and features. A sample is one sequence and represented by a unique admission in the dataset. A time step is one point of observation in the sample and represented by a single admission day, while each feature is one observation at a time step. Furthermore, the *units* parameter of the LSTM layer indicates the dimension of the hidden state and the number of parameters in the LSTM layer. Lastly, the *return_sequences* parameter of the LSTM layer ensures that the full output sequence is returned. By enabling the *return_sequences* parameter, one is allowed to access the output of the hidden state for each time step, leading to a prediction of the care acuity on the next

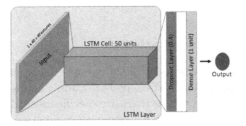

Fig. 2. The architecture of LSTM neural network

day for each admission day. This way, the LSTM layer eventually facilitates the prediction and subsequently the evaluation of the care acuity for each day contained in an admission, based on the previous admission days.

The LSTM layer is followed by a Dropout layer, which is a regularisation technique that randomly selects nodes to be dropped during each weight update cycle. To drop the inputs, the layer randomly sets input units to 0 with a frequency that is equal to the *dropout rate* parameter. To ensure that no values are dropped during inference, the Dropout layer only applies during training and not when the performance of the model is evaluated. It ensures that neurons do not end up relying too much on other neurons or on specific inputs, but that the model learns the meaningful interactions and patterns in the data. It produces a robust LSTM model, has the effect of reducing overfitting and eventually improving model performance, by ensuring that the weights are optimised for the general problem instead of for noise in the data.

Lastly, a dense output layer is added to the model. The dense layer is a regular densely-connected neural network layer that is used to consolidate output from the LSTM layer to the predicted values. Because the *return_sequences* parameter of the LSTM layer is enabled, the dense layer receives the hidden state output of the LSTM layer for each input time step. In order to ensure that the output of the LSTM model has the dimensionality of the desired target, so that the output of the dense layer consists of a prediction of the care acuity for each admission day contained in the test dataset, the value of the *unit* parameter for the dense layer is set to 1.

In order to determine the optimal values of the different hyperparameters, a random search followed by a grid search are executed. The random search randomly samples from a wide range of hyperparameter values to narrow down the search range for each hyperparameter, by performing k-fold cross validation. Subsequently, the grid search further refines the optimal values for the hyperparameters by evaluating the best hyperparameter values returned by the random search. The results of the grid search together with the specific characteristics of the hospital dataset indicate that the optimal model performance is achieved by training the model for 10 epochs, with a batch size of 4, using the *nadam* optimizer and the *mean absolute error* as the loss function.

6   Results

6.1   Data and Descriptive Statistics

In total, 16755 unique admissions of 12224 unique clinical patients of all ages in 2018 were available for analysis. We kept 15477 adult admissions corresponding to patients above 18 years of age, as there are specific medical procedures in place for patients under the age of 18 that come with specialized nursing care activities outside the scope of this research. Of those, we excluded 2782 admissions of women that were in labor, because the associated patient care at the Gynecology department differs significantly from the remaining clinical departments. In order to avoid incomplete admissions, we only included those that solely have admission days in 2018. This resulted in 12492 unique admissions corresponding to 9931 unique patients. The average length of stay was equal to 7 days (SD 10 days) with a median of 4 days (IQR 2–9 days). We subsequently split the dataset randomly in a 60% training set that included 7495 admissions, a 20% validation set ($n = 2498$) and a 20% test set ($n = 2499$). This resulted in an equal distribution of care acuity as is shown in Fig. 1, with a median equal to 16 (IQR 9-26) for the training dataset. The fact that the care acuity increases with the length of stay can be explained by the fact that sicker patients that require additional nursing care remain admitted to the hospital, while the relatively fitter patients that require less nursing care are discharged from the hospital.

6.2   Evaluation Metrics

To evaluate the performance of the model, a selection of different performance metrics are used. The three most well-known metrics that are used for evaluating and reporting the performance of a regression model are the Mean Absolute Error (MAE) – calculated as the average of the absolute error values –, the Mean Squared Error (MSE) – calculated as the mean of the squared differences between the predicted care acuity and the actual care acuity values – and the Root Mean Squared Error (RMSE) – calculated as the square root of the Mean Squared Error. Besides this, the R-squared score (R^2) indicates how well the model is able to predict the value of the target variable and is the percentage of the target variable variation that can be explained by the model. It is calculated by dividing the variance explained by the model by the total variance. Lastly, the symmetric Mean Absolute Percentage Error (sMAPE) returns the error of the model as a percentage, making it easy to compare and understand the model accuracy across different configurations, datasets and use cases.

6.3   Performance Measures

First of all, Fig. 3 shows the predicted care acuity for an exemplary patient contained in the test set. The lower part of the figure represents the actual daily workload for each activity category. The actual care acuity, which is the sum of

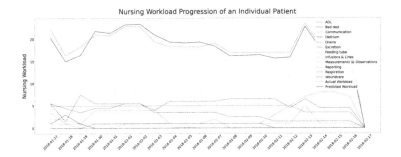

Fig. 3. Predicted Workload vs Actual Workload for an exemplary patient.

the different categories, and the predicted care acuity for each admission day are represented by the green and the red line in the top part of the figure respectively.

On top of this, Fig. 4 shows the average prediction error per consecutive admission day. Each bar represents the average prediction error for the admission day indicated by the value on the x-axis of the plot.

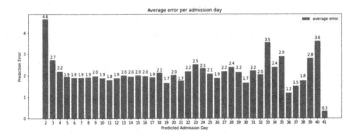

Fig. 4. Average prediction error per admission day.

It can be observed that the error decreases during the first five days of the admissions contained in the test set. After the fifth admission day, the prediction error stabilizes around a value of 2 and after the thirty-second admission day, the figure shows multiple outliers for which the value of the prediction error is 0.5 larger or smaller than the previously stable value of 2.0. This can be explained by the fact that it is harder for the model to learn about longer admissions, as they become more scarce. Longer admissions often consider patients that are exceptional, causing different and unexpected things to happen, such as infections or relapse. The highest errors are caused by an unexpected change of either the *ADL* or the *Communication* baseline scenario.

Furthermore, Table 1 displays the evaluation metrics for the predictions on the test set that indicate the performance of the LSTM model. The MAE indicates that the model performs well in general, as most of the errors are low. However, the high MSE value indicates that when the error is on the high side, it is far above the average. Finally, the R^2 score shows a high level of correlation.

Table 1. The evaluation metrics of the LSTM model on the test dataset.

Evaluation Metric	Value
MSE	19.376712799072266
RMSE	4.4018988609313965
MAE	2.230191946029663
R^2	0.8627777362127644
sMAPE	47.75%

7   Conclusions and Discussion

Nurses have a strong influence on the quality-of-care that patients receive in the hospital. To maintain high quality of care under the stress of the nurse staffing shortage, it has become critical to distribute workload evenly and to see what type of work maybe automated or done by others. This requires easy access to insights in the observed and expected care acuity of each patient in daily clinical nursing care. In this paper, we addressed this by digitally identifying and quantifying the care acuity corresponding to individual nursing activities and subsequently, predicting care acuity with a one-day time horizon to allow for an equal assignment of workload using an LSTM model. The architecture of the LSTM model proved itself suitable to facilitate this time series prediction for the hospital dataset. It displays the ability to adapt and make reliable predictions for the consecutive admission days.

The LSTM model was able to learn from the data and on group level resembles the observed data very well. If patients' care acuity fluctuates only slightly, the model is very well equipped to pick up small changes and predict the care acuity on the next day correctly. However, if there is a sudden deterioration of the patients' conditions, the model picks up the changes, but seemingly with one day delay. This suggests that the model drives to much on the previously observed care acuity and less on the change of the patient's condition. Future work needs to be done to weight the patients' characteristics and condition differently to stress the model to learn more from these features. Also, the initial care acuity that the model assigns to the first admission day seems rather arbitrary. This was to be expected as there is no data available to learn from. As a consequence, the model has no other means than to assign the average workload and optimize from there. One solution here could be to train another model to learn the care acuity for first day based on patient characteristics (e.g., reason for admission, vital functions) first and use these input values for the LSTM model to use. A similar approach was applied to predict the day of discharge by using the input of a GPboost model to determine the day of discharge.

More work is needed on the validity of the assignment of care acuity points to individual nursing care activities. The initial approach we took worked rather well. Consecutive rounds of discussion with nurses were performed to agree upon and optimize the current assignment of points. However, constructing validity against the nurses' opinions should be further researched to reflect daily nursing care well. Moreover, we need to put more weight on features related to patient characteristics, so that the ability of the model to make predictions for individual patients improves. In the end, this research contributed in digitally identifying and quantifying the care acuity corresponding to individual nursing activities and show that patients' care acuity can be predicted one-day ahead.

References

1. Di Francescomarino, C., Ghidini, C.: Predictive Process Monitoring. In: van der Aalst, W.M.P., Carmona, J. (eds.) Process Mining Handbook. Lecture Notes in Business Information Processing, vol. 448, pp. 320–346. Springer, Cham (2022). https://doi.org/10.1007/978-3-031-08848-3_10
2. Greff, K., Srivastava, R.K., Koutník, J., Steunebrink, B.R., Schmidhuber, J.: LSTM: a search space odyssey. IEEE Trans. Neural Netw. Learn. Syst. **28**(10), 2222–2232 (2017)
3. Griffiths, P., Saville, C., Ball, J., Jones, J., Pattison, N., Monks, T.: Nursing workload, nurse staffing methodologies and tools: a systematic scoping review and discussion. Int. J. Nurs. Stud. **103**, 103487 (2020)
4. Houdt, G.V., Mosquera, C., Nápoles, G.: A review on the long short-term memory model. Artif. Intell. Rev. 1–27 (2020)
5. Jia, Q., Zhu, Y., Xu, R., Zhang, Y., Zhao, Y.: Making the hospital smart: using a deep long short-term memory model to predict hospital performance metrics. Ind. Manag. Data Syst. (2022)
6. Jonker, J.: De validiteits- en betrouwbaarheidstest van het verpleegkundig zorgzwaartemodel (2019)
7. Lewinski-Corwin, E.H.: The hospital nursing situation. Am. J. Nurs. **22**(8), 603–606 (1922). http://www.jstor.org/stable/3406790
8. Lu, W., Ma, L., Chen, H., Jiang, X., Gong, M.: A clinical prediction model in health time series data based on long short-term memory network optimized by fruit fly optimization algorithm. IEEE Access **8**, 136014–136023 (2020)
9. Luo, L., Xu, X., Li, J., Shen, W.: Short-term forecasting of hospital discharge volume based on time series analysis. In: 2017 IEEE 19th International Conference on e-Health Networking, Applications and Services (Healthcom), pp. 1–6 (2017)
10. Ly, L.T., Maggi, F.M., Montali, M., Rinderle-Ma, S., van der Aalst, W.M.: Compliance monitoring in business processes: functionalities, application, and tool-support. Inf. Syst. **54**, 209–234 (2015)
11. Pham, D.L., Ahn, H., Kim, K.S., Kim, K.P.: Process-aware enterprise social network prediction and experiment using LSTM neural network models. IEEE Access **9**, 57922–57940 (2021)
12. Tax, N., Verenich, I., La Rosa, M., Dumas, M.: Predictive business process monitoring with LSTM neural networks. In: Dubois, E., Pohl, K. (eds.) CAiSE 2017. LNCS, vol. 10253, pp. 477–492. Springer, Cham (2017). https://doi.org/10.1007/978-3-319-59536-8_30
13. Tello-Leal, E., Roa, J., Rubiolo, M., Ramirez-Alcocer, U.M.: Predicting activities in business processes with LSTM recurrent neural networks. In: 2018 ITU Kaleidoscope: Machine Learning for a 5G Future (ITU K), pp. 1–7 (2018)

Measuring the Impact of COVID-19
on Hospital Care Pathways

Christin Puthur[1]([⊠]), Abdulaziz Aljebreen[1], Ciarán McInerney[2],
Teumzghi Mebrahtu[3], Tom Lawton[3], and Owen Johnson[1]

[1] University of Leeds, Leeds, UK
{sc21cp,ml17asa,o.a.johnson}@leeds.ac.uk
[2] University of Sheffield, Sheffield, UK
ciaran.mcinerney@sheffield.ac.uk
[3] Bradford Teaching Hospitals NHS Foundation Trust, Bradford, UK
{teumzghi.mebrahtu,tom.lawton}@bthft.nhs.uk

Abstract. Care pathways in hospitals around the world reported significant disruption during the recent COVID-19 pandemic but measuring
the actual impact is more problematic. Process mining can be useful
for hospital management to measure the conformance of real-life care
to what might be considered normal operations. In this study, we aim
to demonstrate that process mining can be used to investigate process
changes associated with complex disruptive events. We studied perturbations to accident and emergency (A&E) and maternity pathways in
a UK public hospital during the COVID-19 pandemic. Co-incidentally
the hospital had implemented a Command Centre approach for patient-
flow management affording an opportunity to study both the planned
improvement and the disruption due to the pandemic. Our study proposes and demonstrates a method for measuring and investigating the
impact of such planned and unplanned disruptions affecting hospital care
pathways. We found that during the pandemic, both A&E and maternity
pathways had measurable reductions in the mean length of stay and a
measurable drop in the percentage of pathways conforming to normative
models. There were no distinctive patterns of monthly mean values of
length of stay nor conformance throughout the phases of the installation
of the hospital's new Command Centre approach. Due to a deficit in
the available A&E data, the findings for A&E pathways could not be
interpreted.

Keywords: Process mining · Process changes · Conformance
checking · Normative model · Perturbations · Care pathways ·
Patient-flow · COVID-19 · Maternity · A&E

1 Introduction

Process mining techniques can be used to measure the level of compliance by
comparing event data to a de jure or normative model [19]. In the healthcare

© The Author(s) 2023
M. Montali et al. (Eds.): ICPM 2022 Workshops, LNBIP 468, pp. 391–403, 2023.
https://doi.org/10.1007/978-3-031-27815-0_29

domain, normative models can be extracted from clinical guidelines and proto-cols. Deviations from clinical guidelines occur frequently as healthcare processes are intrinsically highly variable - a challenge described in the process mining for healthcare (PM4H) manifesto [16]. In healthcare it is sometimes very impor-tant to deviate from guidelines for the safety of the patient. Other distinctive characteristics of healthcare processes include the need to consider contextual information during analysis and be aware of process changes brought about by advances in medicine and technology.

Changes in healthcare processes can also be caused by external factors that are unplanned, for example the COVID-19 pandemic, or planned, for exam-ple the implementation of a new hospital IT system. We propose a method to examine the impact of these planned and unplanned factors on patient care by analysing pathway changes using process mining techniques. We are building on an approach for checking conformance of event logs to discovered models to detect sudden process changes that was originally developed and validated against synthetic data [5]. The method proposed in this paper investigates pro-cess changes due to known perturbations to real-life care pathways using process mining techniques including checking conformance to normative models.

Distinctive characteristics of healthcare such as high variability and frequent process changes lead to certain key challenges in mining healthcare processes identified in the PM4H manifesto [16]. Challenge C2 in the manifesto describes the need for novel techniques for checking conformance of healthcare processes to available clinical guidelines. This is relevant to our study as we compare real-life care pathways in event logs with normative models by checking conformance. As highlighted in challenge C3 of the PM4H manifesto, changes in healthcare processes over time due to factors such as seasonal changes or the introduction of a new work system should also be considered. This challenge directly affects our study on the impacts of two major perturbations on care pathways.

We studied patient pathways at Bradford Royal Infirmary (BRI) which is a public hospital in Bradford, UK. During the period of our study there were two potential sources of perturbations. These were the COVID-19 pandemic and the near co-incident implementation of a new Command Centre approach to patient-flow management. A study protocol had been designed [11] to evaluate impacts of the newly implemented Command Centre system on patient safety and healthcare delivery. However, shortly after the Command Centre was intro-duced, COVID-19 disrupted the hospital activities along with the rest of world. Thus, we have a unique opportunity to study effects of two co-incident sources of perturbations on hospital processes, one of which was planned and the other was unplanned.

The Command Centre approach was based on a new IT system and a corre-sponding redesign of patient-flow management processes and implemented in a series of planned interventions. The Command Centre aims to improve health-care delivery by providing relevant information to assist staff in making real-time complex decisions [6]. Designated staff monitor continuously updated hospital information summarised on a wall of high-resolution screens through applications called 'tiles'. The 'tiles' present process status data from established hospital information systems used across the different units of the hospital. The Command Centre software uses rule-based algorithms to warn about impending bottlenecks and other patient safety risks to support optimised patient care and effective management of resources. The intention of the Command Centre approach is to provide centralised surveillance of hospital patient flow to a team of people empowered to manage that flow in the best interests of patients and the hospital, following approaches that are well established in other industries such as air traffic control centres at airports.

The COVID-19 pandemic has impacted healthcare around the world, notably with a great reduction in the use of healthcare services [15] as available resources were allocated to the high demand of care for COVID-19 patients. The reprioritisation of resources to meet the challenges of the pandemic affected normal care processes. For instance, in England, major disruptions to the pathway for colorectal cancer diagnosis led to a considerable reduction in detection of the disease in April 2020 [14]. In the city of Bradford, UK, surveys for studying the pandemic's impacts on families showed increases in mental health issues in adults as well as children [3]. Our hypothesis is that the impact of external disturbances on care processes can be detected and measured in event log data extracted from BRI's Electronic Health Records (EHR) data. In this paper, we propose a method for identifying and measuring impacts of disruptive events by building on previously established approaches of detecting process changes and apply this method on a real-life case study.

1.1 Related Work

This process mining work is part of a larger project based on the study protocol [11] to evaluate impacts of the Command Centre at BRI. Our focus is on a subsection of the study protocol aiming to analyse effects of the Command Centre on patient journeys using process-mining techniques. Investigation of patient flow is expected to contribute towards assessing the installation of the Command Centre under the hypothesis that productivity, associated processes and patient outcomes are influenced by patient flow. The study protocol also hypothesised that the recording of hospital data is influenced by the Command Centre's installation. Studies on quality of data, patient flow and patient outcomes throughout the phases of the Command Centre's installation are proposed in the protocol.

In related work, Mebrahtu et al. [13] investigated quality of data and patient flow to test the hypothesis that the Command Centre positively impacts recorded data and flow of patients through the hospital. They considered five time periods based on different interventions involved in the Command Centre's installation as shown in Fig. 1. They also explored A&E patient records for missing timestamps of certain events and the relative occurrence of the valid A&E pathway to assess the Command Centre's impact on data quality. To study the impact on patient flow, time intervals between selected timestamped events recorded for A&E patients were analysed. They observed no notable improvements to A&E

patient flow and quality of data suggesting the Command Centre had no measurable impact. A drawback of the investigation was that the COVID-19 pandemic that disrupted normal hospital function occurred nearly co-incidentally with the launch of the Command Centre. This suggests the need for further research to understand how command centres may influence data quality and patient journeys in hospital settings.

1.2   Study Design

In this paper, we aim to extend the previous work by including an investigation of the impacts on patient pathways using process mining. Process mining methods have been previously used in describing hospital journey of patients in different healthcare domains. For instance, process mining has been used to discover that few patients undergoing chemotherapy followed an ideal care pathway [1]. A study of A&E pathways using process mining attributed the reason for longer stays in the department to a loop in the pathway [17]. This paper proposes a method aiming to measure and investigate process changes associated with disruptive events which is demonstrated using a case study of in-hospital care pathways.

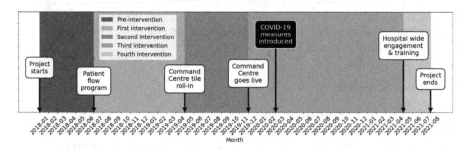

Fig. 1. Timeline of the study period indicating the interventions involved in installing the Command Centre.

Our study focuses on the perturbations to A&E and maternity pathways through BRI arising from COVID-19 and the co-incident implementation of a new patient-flow management system. We aim to add to the previous investigation of A&E pathways through the hospital described in the related work. The choice of maternity pathways is justified by the ease of identifying maternity patients in the data and of obtaining a predetermined normative model as maternity processes can be expected to be reasonably consistent in nature. Moreover, maternity patients were possibly the least affected by COVID-19 measures that prevented other patients from accessing timely medical treatment. Exploring impacts of two simultaneous perturbation sources on hospital pathways presents a unique opportunity to reflect on the challenges of PM4H. Through this case study, we demonstrate a method to measure the impact of perturbations on the quality of hospital service in the context of in-hospital care pathways.

2   Methods

2.1   PM^2 for Exploring Impacts on Care Pathways

We followed the PM^2 process mining methodology [4] as adapted by Kurniati et al. [10] to analyse process changes using a multi-level approach. The first two stages of PM^2 are focused on formulating basic research questions followed by two stages of analysis which delve deeper into the objectives while the last two stages focus on process improvements and real-world implementation. In our investigation we applied stages 1 to 4 of PM^2 but not stages 5 and 6 as process improvement and clinical intervention were out of the scope of this work. For the multi-level approach, we focused on model and trace-level process comparisons to explore impacts of potential perturbations on care pathways.

For Stage 1 (Planning), our research questions were drawn based on the process mining subsection of the study protocol [11] to evaluate impacts of the new Command Centre at BRI. Previous related studies of impacts on patient flow [13] and patient safety [12] were also included in framing the process mining objectives. Research questions were further adapted to studying A&E and maternity pathways during the time period covering the two perturbations. In Stage 2 (Extraction), selection of data attributes relevant to the patient pathways was guided by previous related work [13], advice from clinicians and our understanding of attribute labels with the help of public information resources. A clinician familiar with the study data was part of the project team, while other clinicians were engaged as interviewees as described in Stage 2 of the ClearPath method [9].

In the next stage, Stage 3 (Data Processing), we used patient admission as the case identifier to create event logs for in-hospital care pathways. The models that were discovered in Stage 4 (Mining and Analysis) identified the key activities for building normative models based on clinical advice. Our main analysis involved process comparisons over the period of interest by studying durations at the trace-level and conformance and precision between event logs and normative models at the model-level. The conformance is measured by checking the proportion of traces in the event log that fit the model. Precision is a measure obtained by comparing the set of traces that are allowed by the model with the set of traces in the event log fitting the model. Thus, precision is not a meaningful measure for unfit traces [2]. In this paper, the precision was calculated only for traces that were fitting the respective process model.

For obtaining normative models for A&E and maternity pathways, we followed a framework proposed by Grüger et al. [7] for the non-trivial transformation of clinical guidelines into computer-interpretable process models. The framework known as the Clinical Guideline Knowledge for Process Mining (CGK4PM) comprises five steps that include identification of required key inputs, conceptualisation through workshops with stakeholders, formalisation to obtain a semi-formal process representation of guidelines, implementation by translating into a selected process modelling language and finally the testing step for verifying and validating the implemented model.

For the first step of identification, clinical guidelines were selected based on discovered process models and discussions with clinicians. We skipped the conceptualisation step due to resource constraints and instead we consulted clinicians for the transformation of clinical guidelines into semi-formal process models. This was achieved by identifying relevant activities through process discovery and consulting clinicians on the expected order of events for patients who were progressing well. The process representation of clinical guidelines was then translated into Business Process Model and Notation (BPMN). The BPMN model was verified by conformance checking and reviewed by clinicians for validation.

2.2 Data

The data source for our case study was the EHR data from BRI. A data extract was provided for our study by the Connected Bradford [18] data linkage project. The Connected Bradford project brings together data covering a wide range of factors influencing population health for the Bradford region through data linkage. In particular we used the summary of activity produced as a part of integrating hospital data to Secondary User Services (SUS) which is created as a data feed to the national data warehouse for healthcare data in England, augmented by timings from a data feed used to drive the Command Centre tiles. The data extract included information on A&E patients, outpatients and inpatients along with diagnoses, procedures, surgeries, prescriptions and some patient demographics.

Our study uses the A&E and inpatient data during the period from January 2018 to August 2021. The A&E timing data that was used in this study came from the Command Centre system which recorded 100% of the data starting only from September 2020. However, it did also include a small amount of data (approximately 20% of attendances, which may not be a representative sample) from prior to this point. Thus, the findings from the A&E data in this study cannot be interpreted.

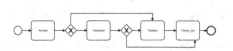

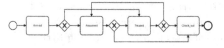

(a) BPMN diagram of the normative model for A&E attendance.

(b) BPMN diagram of a model for A&E attendance based on the discovered process map shown in Fig. 5.

Fig. 2. A&E models.

For analysing A&E pathways, we identified 193,772 A&E attendances that occurred during the period of study. For analysing maternity pathways, we selected admissions of patients who registered in one of the 'maternity wards' which included a birth centre for uncomplicated labour cases, a labour ward for patients needing specialist care during labour, two maternity operating theatres and two wards for patients needing care before or after birth, referred to in this paper as 'natal wards'. A total of 18,076 maternity admissions were identified for analysis of which 16,905 resulted in the delivery of a newborn baby with a recorded timestamp. Data on admissions, ward stays and delivery timestamps were distributed across three tables which were linked through admission and patient identifiers.

2.3   Tools

The summary of activity data from BRI was made accessible on the cloud by the Connected Bradford service via Google Cloud Platform (GCP). Accessing data was possible through the relational database management system BigQuery provided by GCP. Timestamped data was extracted to RStudio Server Pro storage using SQL-based queries for the analysis. Event logs and process maps in the form of directly-follows graphs were generated using the open-source process mining platform called bupaR [8] in the RStudio Server Pro environment. An open-source Python package known as PM4Py [2] was used for conformance checking against normative models.

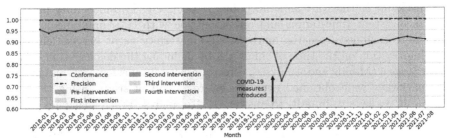

(a) Conformance and precision between monthly event logs and the normative A&E model.

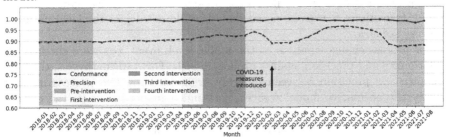

(b) Conformance and precision between monthly event logs and the A&E model based on the discovered process map.

Fig. 3. Metrics depicting process changes associated with A&E pathways.

Directly-follows graphs discovered from the event logs identified activities relevant for building normative models following the CGK4PM framework. BPMN diagrams of normative models reviewed by clinicians were drawn using an online tool (https://demo.BPMN.io) and uploaded to Jupyter notebook for conversion into Petri nets using the PM4Py package. The resulting Petri nets were used for checking conformance of event logs by token-based replay to obtain percentage of traces in the event log that fit the normative model.

3   Results

These are the research questions that were identified during Stage 1 (Planning) of the PM^2 methodology: *Q1. What are the discovered pathways for A&E attendance and maternity admissions in BRI? Q2. What are the normative models for A&E and maternity pathways in BRI? Q3. Can process changes due to potential perturbations be identified and measured in discovered pathways using normative models?* In Stage 2 (Extraction), we selected timestamps of arrival, assessment, treatment and check-out for A&E attendance. For maternity admissions, we selected the timestamps of admission, ward stays in any specialty, and discharge.

During Stage 3 (Data Processing), the event logs were filtered for the time period of interest. We filtered out A&E attendances that did not have arrival and check-out as the start and end points respectively. Two maternity patients with inconsistent timestamps and one admission with two simultaneous ward stays were excluded from the analysis. The maternity event log was enriched with information on the time of childbirth by including the delivery timestamp.

In Stage 4 (Mining and Analysis), directly-follows graphs for A&E and maternity pathways were obtained over the entire period of study, using the processmapR package in bupaR, to answer Q1. To analyse process changes at the trace-level, we examined the mean and median length of A&E attendances and maternity admissions. The CGK4PM framework was followed to obtain normative models for A&E (see Fig. 2a) and maternity pathways to answer Q2. Although the notation in the normative models suggests typical clinical rationale for transitions, it is to be noted that these do not depict the ideal pathway for every scenario.

For process change analysis at the model-level, event logs were checked for conformance and precision against process models. For A&E pathways, the conformance and precision between monthly event logs and two process models, namely the normative model (see Fig. 2a) and a model based on the discovered process map (see Fig. 2b), are shown in Figs. 3a and 3b. The conformance and precision between monthly event logs and the normative maternity model are shown in Fig. 4. For obtaining monthly values of conformance and precision, event logs for each month were selected by including cases that started within the month. It was found that for both A&E and maternity, the conformance between event logs and corresponding normative models reduced during the period after COVID-19 measures were introduced (April 2020 to August 2021) compared to pre-pandemic times (April 2018 to February 2020). No significant difference in the precision was observed in these two periods for both A&E and maternity pathways. To answer Q3, the trace-level analysis of durations showed that the lowest median length of stay over the period of study occurred in April 2020 for both A&E and maternity pathways. It was also observed that the mean length of stay reduced after national pandemic measures were introduced for both A&E and maternity compared to pre-pandemic times.

4   Discussion

In this case study we have added conformance checking against the normative model as an extension to the multi-level approach of Kurniati et al. [10] to address challenge C2 of PM4H [16]. Changes in healthcare processes over time could be analysed by this method but identifying the cause of process changes requires further research. For obtaining a clearer picture of the impacts of the two perturbations, other inherent influences such as seasonal factors need to be controlled for as described in challenge C3. Since one of the perturbations was planned, while the other was unplanned, there is scope for further research to try to differentiate the impacts of the two perturbations.

In this study, the most noticeable process change was the drop in conformance of A&E pathways to the normative model in April 2020 (see blue curve in Fig. 3a) following the introduction of nationwide pandemic measures in March 2020. For the normative A&E model, the precision is high throughout (see red curve in Fig. 3a). For the model based on the discovered process map, the conformance remains high throughout (see blue curve in Fig. 3b), while the precision is lower and changes significantly during the 'Third intervention' period (see red curve in Fig. 3b).

From conformance values with respect to the normative A&E model, we can see some disturbances in the pathways in April 2020. The precision values between monthly A&E event logs and the model based on the discovered process showed fluctuating behaviour during 'Third intervention' period. The extra path in the A&E model based on the discovered process map (see Fig. 2b), indicating an alternative way of working, captured deviations that were not detected by the normative model. Thus, the model based on the discovered process map contains a useful level of complexity which is the occurrence of the activity 'Assessed' after 'Treated'. This only shows what has been recorded by the IT system but not necessarily what happens in the A&E department and is thus not part of the normative model. On discussion with clinicians, assessment might be recorded after treatment due to a technical need to progress with the treatment. This suggests that it might be a regular feature of work in practice to record assessment after the event.

The drop in conformance in April 2020 and the changes in precision during the 'Third intervention' period could be detected using the identified metrics. Further research using the full A&E dataset and discussion with clinical experts is required to accurately identify causes of the process changes. If the detected perturbations can be attributed to external disturbances, the ability to capture them could be implemented in information systems to warn about disruptions to the normal workflow. The integration of process mining into process aware information systems would enable perturbations to be detected in real time allowing clinicians and hospital managers to identify and react to adverse events taking place in the hospital.

As described before, the reasonably consistent nature of maternity pathways can be seen in the more stable values of conformance and precision (see Fig. 4) over the period of study. The significant differences in the impact on A&E and maternity pathways under the influence of the same external perturbation sources might be attributed to the contrasting nature of the two pathways. A&E pathways are very dynamic whereas maternity pathways are often predetermined. Through this study we have demonstrated that process changes due to complex perturbations can be detected using process mining techniques. In future work, the frequency of traces following a selected sequence of activities over the time period of interest can be studied at the trace-level [10]. The care pathways can also be studied at the activity-level for further investigation of the process changes.

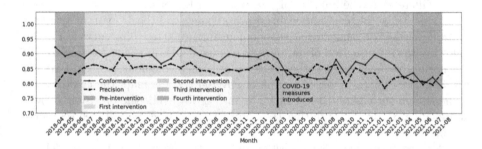

Fig. 4. Conformance and precision between monthly event logs and the normative maternity model.

Since only a subset of the data for A&E attendances was available until August 2020, we are not in a position to draw conclusions about the length of stay and the overall conformance and precision measures of the A&E pathway. We have demonstrated the proposed method but cannot state that all our results are representative since we do not know the bias. Further work would be necessary to rerun the analysis on the complete set of data. However, the full dataset was not available at the time of writing.

5   Conclusion

We used the proposed method to identify process changes at the trace and model levels. Causes of identified changes cannot be determined with confidence as the perturbations were nearly co-incident. In further research, the results may be compared with another hospital that did not implement a change in the management system during the same period.

Acknowledgements. This study is based on data from Connected Bradford (REC 18/YH/0200 & 22/EM/0127). The data is provided by the citizens of Bradford and district, and collected by the NHS and other organisations as part of their care and support. The interpretation and conclusions contained in this study are those of the authors alone. This project is funded by the National Institute for Health Research Health Service and Delivery Research Programme (NIHR129483).

We thank Dr Allan Pang and Dr Timothy Harrison for their invaluable input regarding the clinical aspects of this work. We thank the PPIE representatives for their contribution to the conception, development, ongoing implementation and future communication of this project. This research is supported by the National Institute for Health Research (NIHR) Yorkshire and Humber Patient Safety Translational Research Centre (NIHR Yorkshire and Humber PSTRC). The views expressed in this article are those of the authors and not necessarily those of the NHS, the NIHR, or the Department of Health and Social Care.

Ethics Approval. The study was approved by the University of Leeds Engineering and Physical Sciences Research Ethics Committee (#MEEC 20-016) and the NHS Health Research Authority (IRAS No.: 285933).

A   Appendix

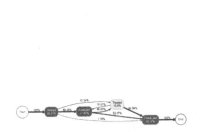

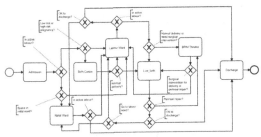

Fig. 5. Directly-follows graph for A&E attendances.

Fig. 6. BPMN diagram of the normative model for maternity pathways.

References

1. Baker, K., et al.: Process mining routinely collected electronic health records to define real-life clinical pathways during chemotherapy. Int. J. Med. Inform. **103**, 32–41 (2017)
2. Berti, A., Van Zelst, S.J., van der Aalst, W.: Process mining for python (PM4Py): bridging the gap between process-and data science. arXiv preprint arXiv:1905.06169 (2019)

3. Dickerson, J., et al.: The impact of the COVID-19 pandemic on families living in the ethnically diverse and deprived city of Bradford: findings from the longitudinal Born in Bradford COVID-19 research programme. In: COVID-19 Collaborations, pp. 73–87. Policy Press (2022)

4. van Eck, M.L., Lu, X., Leemans, S.J.J., van der Aalst, W.M.P.: PM^2: a process mining project methodology. In: Zdravkovic, J., Kirikova, M., Johannesson, P. (eds.) CAiSE 2015. LNCS, vol. 9097, pp. 297–313. Springer, Cham (2015). https://doi.org/10.1007/978-3-319-19069-3_19

5. Gallego-Fontenla, V., Vidal, J., Lama, M.: A conformance checking-based approach for sudden drift detection in business processes. IEEE Trans. Serv. Comput. (2021)

6. GE Healthcare: Bradford announces AI-Powered Hospital Command Center, first of its kind in Europe. https://www.ge.com/news/press-releases/bradford-announces-ai-powered-hospital-command-center-first-its-kind-europe. Accessed 21 Aug 2022

7. Grüger, J., Geyer, T., Bergmann, R., Braun, S.A.: CGK4PM: towards a methodology for the systematic generation of clinical guideline process models and the utilization of conformance checking. BioMedInformatics **2**(3), 359–374 (2022)

8. Janssenswillen, G., Depaire, B., Swennen, M., Jans, M., Vanhoof, K.: bupaR: enabling reproducible business process analysis. Knowl.-Based Syst. **163**, 927–930 (2019)

9. Johnson, O.A., Ba Dhafari, T., Kurniati, A., Fox, F., Rojas, E.: The ClearPath method for care pathway process mining and simulation. In: Daniel, F., Sheng, Q.Z., Motahari, H. (eds.) BPM 2018. LNBIP, vol. 342, pp. 239–250. Springer, Cham (2019). https://doi.org/10.1007/978-3-030-11641-5_19

10. Kurniati, A.P., McInerney, C., Zucker, K., Hall, G., Hogg, D., Johnson, O.: Using a multi-level process comparison for process change analysis in cancer pathways. Int. J. Environ. Res. Public Health **17**(19), 7210 (2020)

11. McInerney, C., et al.: Evaluating the safety and patient impacts of an artificial intelligence command centre in acute hospital care: a mixed-methods protocol. BMJ Open **12**(3), e054090 (2022)

12. Mebrahtu, T.F., et al.: The effect of a hospital command centre on patient safety: an interrupted time series study (in publication)

13. Mebrahtu, T.F., et al.: The Impact of a Hospital Command Centre on Patient Flow and Data Quality: findings from the UK NHS (in publication)

14. Morris, E.J., et al.: Impact of the COVID-19 pandemic on the detection and management of colorectal cancer in England: a population-based study. Lancet Gastroenterol. Hepatol. **6**(3), 199–208 (2021)

15. Moynihan, R., et al.: Impact of COVID-19 pandemic on utilisation of healthcare services: a systematic review. BMJ Open **11**(3), e045343 (2021)

16. Munoz-Gama, J., et al.: Process mining for healthcare: characteristics and challenges. J. Biomed. Inform. **127**, 103994 (2022)

17. Rojas, E., Cifuentes, A., Burattin, A., Munoz-Gama, J., Sepúlveda, M., Capurro, D.: Performance analysis of emergency room episodes through process mining. Int. J. Environ. Res. Public Health **16**(7), 1274 (2019)

18. Sohal, K., et al.: Connected Bradford: a whole system data linkage accelerator. Wellcome Open Res. **7**(26), 26 (2022)

19. Van Der Aalst, W.: Process Mining: Data Science in Action, vol. 2. Springer, Heidelberg (2016). https://doi.org/10.1007/978-3-662-49851-4

1st International Workshop on Data Quality and Transformation in Process Mining (DQT-PM'22)

The First International Workshop on Data Quality and Transformation in Process Mining (DQT-PM'22)

The First International Workshop on Data Quality and Transformation in Process Mining (DQT-PM'22) aimed to facilitate the exchange of research findings, ideas, and experiences on techniques and practices to data transformation and quality improvement at Stage 0 of a process mining project.

These days, the amount of available data has increased in organizations, so has its perceived value for stakeholders. A broad spectrum of process mining techniques (e.g., process discovery, conformance checking, and performance analysis) exists to derive actionable business insights from the recorded process data. As these process mining techniques rely on historical process data as 'the single source of truth', working with data that is of low and dubious quality poses significant hurdles to successfully translating data into actionable business insights.

It is also well-known that significant time and effort associated with process mining projects is being spent on data preparation tasks. A recent survey within the process mining community (XES) shows that more than 60% of the overall effort is spent on data preparation, where challenges such as complex data structures, incomplete, and inconstant data are being addressed. Current approaches to data preparation (e.g., data transformation, data quality auditing and remedies for repairs) are mostly ad-hoc and manual. Thus, there is a need for systematic and preferably automated approaches to event data transformation that will speed up the production of high-quality process data for decision-making purposes.

The first edition of DQT-PM workshop attracted six submissions. In a rigorous review process, each submission was reviewed by three PC members. Further discussions among the reviewers were conducted to resolve disagreements. In the end, three papers were accepted, all of which are included in the proceedings. The papers cover the topics of event log creation, transformation, and quality for process mining.

This year, the DQT-PM workshop had a joint program with the RPM workshop on the related topic of responsible process mining. During the final panel discussion of the workshop, the panel members and the authors discussed trustworthiness of process mining results in the presence of poor-quality data, complex processes, and biases.

The workshop chairs wish to thank all authors of the submitted papers for their efforts, participants of the workshop for sharing insights on data quality and transformation in process mining, the PC members for contributing their valuable time to review the submissions and finally the workshop organisers and the organisers of ICPM 2022, for bringing this workshop to life.

November 2022

Sareh Sadeghianasl
Jochen De Weerdt
Moe Thandar Wynn

Organization

Workshop Chairs

Sareh Sadeghianasl   Queensland University of Technology, Australia
Jochen De Weerdt   KU Leuven, Belgium
Moe Thandar Wynn   Queensland University of Technology, Australia

Program Committee

Robert Andrews   Queensland University of Technology, Australia
Behshid Behkamal   Ferdowsi University of Mashhad, Iran
Andrea Burattin   Technical University of Denmark, Denmark
Marco Comuzzi   Ulsan National Institute of Science and Technology, South Korea
Johannes De Smedt   KU Leuven, Belgium
Claudio Di Ciccio   Sapienza University of Rome, Italy
Kanika Goel   Queensland University of Technology, Australia
Sander J. J. Leemans   RWTH Aachen, Germany
Henrik Leopold   Kühne Logistics University, Germany
Xixi Lu   Utrecht University, The Netherlands
Felix Mannhardt   Eindhoven University of Technology, The Netherlands
Niels Martin   Hasselt University, Belgium
Pnina Soffer   University of Haifa, Israel
Eric Verbeek   Eindhoven University of Technology, The Netherlands
Arthur ter Hofstede   Queensland University of Technology, Australia
Han van der Aa   University of Mannheim, Germany

Deriving Event Logs from Legacy Software Systems

Marius Breitmayer[1]([⊠]) ⓘ, Lisa Arnold[1] ⓘ, Stephan La Rocca[2],
and Manfred Reichert[1] ⓘ

[1] Institute of Databases and Information Systems, Ulm University, Ulm, Germany
{marius.breitmayer,lisa.arnold,manfred.reichert}@uni-ulm.de
[2] PITSS GmbH Stuttgart, Stuttgart, Germany
slarocca@pitss.com

Abstract. The modernization of legacy software systems is one of the
key challenges in software industry, which requires comprehensive system analysis. In this context, process mining has proven to be useful for
understanding the (business) processes implemented by the legacy software system. However, process mining algorithms are highly dependent
on both the quality and existence of suitable event logs. In many scenarios, existing software systems (e.g., legacy applications) do not leverage
process engines capable of producing such high-quality event logs, which
hampers the application of process mining algorithms. Deriving suitable
event log data from legacy software systems, therefore, constitutes a relevant task that fosters data-driven analysis approaches, including process
mining, data-based process documentation, and process-centric software
migration. This paper presents an approach for deriving event logs from
legacy software systems by combining knowledge from source code and
corresponding database operations. The goal is to identify relevant business objects as well as to document user and software interactions with
them in an event log suitable for process mining.

Keywords: Event log generation · Legacy software system · Software
Modernization · Process mining

1 Introduction

Economically, one of the most important sectors in software industry concerns
the modernization of legacy software systems. These systems need to be replaced
by modern software systems showing better usability, higher performance, and
improved code quality. A successful modernization of a legacy software system
requires the analysis of the (business) processes implemented by the legacy software, the interactions users have with the system, and the access points to system
information (e.g., source code or databases).

Process mining offers a plethora of analysis approaches to gain a broad understanding of the processes implemented in software systems. Process discovery, for
example, enables the derivation of process models from event logs [1]. In turn,

© The Author(s) 2023
M. Montali et al. (Eds.): ICPM 2022 Workshops, LNBIP 468, pp. 409–421, 2023.
https://doi.org/10.1007/978-3-031-27815-0_30

conformance checking correlates modeled and recorded behavior of a business process, enabling the analysis of the observed process behavior in relation to a given process model [2]. Finally, process enhancement allows improving business processes based on the information recorded in event logs. In summary, most process mining approaches highly depend on the existence of process event logs as well as the quality of these logs.

In software modernization projects, legacy software systems need to be analyzed. In this context, the use of process mining approaches is very promising for analyzing the processes implemented in these systems. However, most existing legacy software systems neither have been designed based on pre-specified executable process models nor do they provide extensive process logging capabilities. As a consequence, the application of process mining to legacy software systems is hampered and alternatives for obtaining models of the implemented processes and, thus, for supporting the migration of the legacy software system to modern technology are needed. Alternatives include, for example, extensive interviews with key system users and process owners [3]. Both alternatives, however, are time-consuming and prone to incompleteness.

This paper presents an approach to generate event logs from running legacy software systems by combining knowledge from source code analysis, including database statements, to discover the relevant business objects of a process as well as to document user and software interactions in an event log suitable for process mining. We consider the following research questions:

RQ1: How can we generate event logs from running legacy software systems?
RQ2: How can we ensure that the performance of legacy software systems is not affected during event log generation?

The remainder of this paper is structured as follows: Sect. 2 introduces the concepts necessary for understanding this work. Section 3 discusses the requirements for generating event logs from running legacy software systems. Section 4 presents the legacy software system analysis required for generating event logs. Section 5 describes our approach and shows how one can extend a legacy software system to generate event logs. Section 6 evaluates our work using a requirements evaluation, a performance comparison, and a user survey. Section 7 discusses related work. Section 8 provides a short summary as well as an outlook.

2   Fundamentals

2.1   Legacy Software Systems

Legacy software systems are widespread in enterprises, but very costly to maintain due to bad documentation, outdated operating or development environments, or high complexity of the historically grown system code basis [4]. As a result, the replacement of such legacy software systems is often significantly delayed beyond the initial system lifespan. Legacy software systems consist of a plethora of artifacts and resources such as servers, (non-normalized) databases,

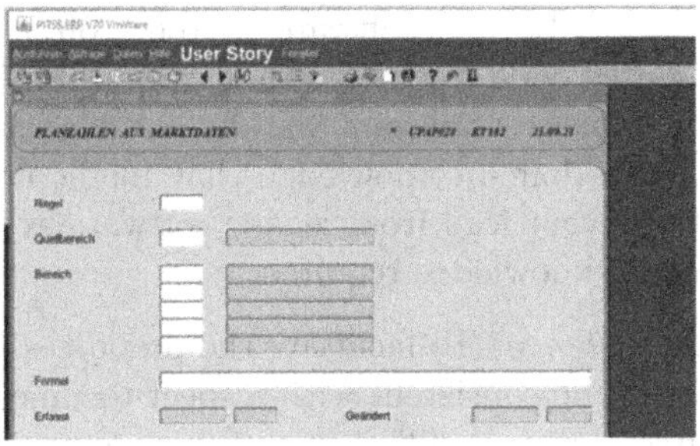

Fig. 1. Screenshot of a legacy software system

source code, or user forms, which all may be used during legacy software system analysis. Figure 1 depicts a screenshot of an Oracle legacy software system implemented in the 1990s. We will refer to this example in the following.

2.2 Event Logs

Event logs build the foundation for process mining algorithms and capture information on cases, events, and corresponding activities [5]. In general, event logs record events related to the execution of process instances. Mandatory attributes of a log entry include the case identifier, the timestamp, as well as the executed activity [5].

In the context of legacy software systems, which may support multiple process types (e.g., order-to-cash, purchase-to-pay, or checking an invoice), it might be unclear to which process type an activity belongs. Therefore, an additional attribute indicating the process type is required when deriving event logs from legacy software systems.

3 Requirements

In most cases, there exist no suitable event logs for process mining in legacy software systems. This section elicits fundamental requirements to be met when generating event logs from user and software interactions with legacy software systems. On one hand, we gathered the requirements from literature [5]. On the other, we conducted interviews with domain experts (e.g., software engineers, and process owners) to complement these requirements. Amongst others, we identified the following requirements:

Requirement 1: (*Relevance*) The event log should only contain process-relevant data that refers to those interactions with the legacy software system that correspond to a process (e.g., filling or completing a form). If an interaction triggers an automated procedure (e.g., invocation of an operation in the legacy software system), the resulting changes (e.g., to the database) should be recorded in the event log as well.

Requirement 2: (*Scope*) Legacy software systems often use a plethora of database tables and source code fragments that contain business-relevant data. Identifying and scoping process-relevant database tables and code fragments usually requires extensive domain knowledge that might not be available. An approach for generating event logs from legacy software systems should therefore minimize the domain knowledge required.

Requirement 3: (*Consistency*) To facilitate the preprocessing of the event log data, the event log should be consistent with respect to timestamps, data types, and additional resources, even if different software components of the legacy software system (e.g., database and user forms) are involved.

Requirement 4: (*Performance*) The event log generation from a running legacy system should not influence its performance, i.e., the user and software interactions should not be influenced (e.g., due to increased loading times).

4   Legacy Software System Analysis

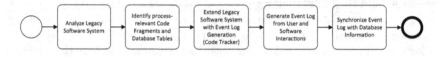

Fig. 2. Preparation steps of our approach

We derived the approach for generating event logs from running legacy software systems (cf. Fig. 2) by applying design science research [6].

In the first step, we analyze the legacy software system, including source code, database tables, and additional resources (e.g., configuration files, user forms displayed by the running legacy software system).

In the second step, we transform the source code of the legacy application to an abstract syntax tree in order to identify those code elements that trigger database operations (e.g., the selection, insertion, deletion or update of tuples in database tables). Using the database tables in combination with the information provided from the source code (e.g., the exact SQL statement), we address an important problem of legacy software systems, i.e., we are able to identify relations between tables that have not been explicitly specified using foreign-key constraints. In other words, we identify additional relations between database tables specified in the legacy application source code.

We can further build clusters of database tables that most likely belong to the same process based on these identified relations. In Fig. 3, for example, tables belonging to the cluster marked in green correspond to orders, whereas tables of the purple cluster correspond to articles. We identify the center of a cluster using a page rank algorithm [7]. Note that checking the identified clusters with

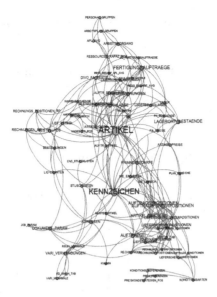

Fig. 3. Clusters derived from database and source code

a domain expert (if possible) might further improve the event log generation (cf. Requirements 1 and 2 in Sect. 3).

After having identified the clusters in the database tables, we can determine which source code fragments are relevant for the generation of the event log, i.e., which code fragments affect process-relevant database tables. This information can then be used to configure and install the code tracker into the legacy software system.

The code tracker is able to automatically inject code fragments into the source code, which, in turn, are then executed together with the legacy software system code enabling the generation of event logs at runtime. To ensure that the performance of the legacy software system is not negatively affected, the necessary data is passed using common log mechanisms (e.g., *java.util.logging* or *Oracle message-builtIns*) already available in the legacy software system. This yields the advantage that the existing infrastructure, in which the legacy software system operates, takes care of managing files, rotating data and, thus, providing methods for writing data to an event log in a performant manner. Consequently, the transfer of event log data becomes possible with minimal footprint. In a last step, we synchronize the event log with the information from the database (e.g., redo logs) enabling the generation of high-quality event logs.

5   Event Log Generation

In the context of a legacy software system, a business process can be derived from the sequences of interactions the users have with the legacy application. Each interaction of such a sequence is then subject-bound (i.e., the interactions of a sequence belong to the same transaction). In a legacy software system, such processes may be initiated and terminated using pre-defined actions, for example, menu items or key combinations. The addition of corresponding actions to an event log, together with the associated application object (e.g., a product identified by a unique product number, or an order identified by its order number) constitutes the basis for generating an event log. Subsequently, this event log may then serve as input for process mining algorithms.

5.1   Legacy Software System Extension

After showing how process-relevant source code fragments can be identified in the legacy software system (cf. Sect. 4), we discuss how to augment the legacy software system with event log generation capabilities by installing the *code tracker*. This installation utilizes our ability to parse the relevant source code fragments and to map them as an abstract syntax tree [8].

Leveraging this source code information, we can add the code tracker nodes at the relevant positions of the software code, i.e., "start", "end", "return", "exit", and "exception", surrounding a create-, read-, update- or delete-statement (CRUD-statement). Each code tracker statement then captures the context (i.e., the position of the relevant source code in the entire legacy software system), the timestamp, the identifier of the corresponding user session, and, optionally, additional parameters of the identified source code fragments.

Adding the code tracker to the legacy software system is implemented as a pre-deployment task. Thus, no developer interaction becomes necessary. In a deployment chain, relevant code is checked out, parsed, added to the tracker, saved, compiled, and then deployed to the running legacy software system. This integration ensures that any kind of source code change or release of new software versions can be captured, hence, preventing mismatches between the running code and the information captured in the generated event log. As an example, consider the code fragment depicted in Fig. 4a, which is responsible for handling a user interaction event. When applying the code tracking pre-deployment task to this code fragment, we obtain the code fragment depicted in Fig. 4b. In the latter, the event log generation is added to lines 2, 5, 7, and 9. Note that *ScreenName* and *EventName* constitute placeholders that are replaced by the actual values at runtime. An example of such actual values could be ORDERS.MAIN_CANVAS.BUTTON_SAVE.WHEN_BUTTON_PRESSED.

```
1   declare
2   |   var as number;
3   begin
4   |   do_something(var);
5   exception when others then
6   |   capture_error;
7   end:
```

(a) Source Code

```
1   declare
2       ":A" number;
3       var as number;
4   begin
5       Rec.LogStory(Rec.GetStory, '10.ScreenName.EventName','*start*',":A"):
6       do_something(var);
7       Rec.LogStory(Rec.GetStory, '10.ScreenName.EventName','*exit*',":A"):
8   exception when others then
9       Rec.LogStory(Rec.GetStory, '10.ScreenName.EventName','*exception*',":A"):
10      capture_error;
11  end;
```

(b)   Extended Source Code

Fig. 4. Example source code fragments

During event log analysis, such values provide important contextual information and enable a failure-free identification of documented user and software interactions. There exists a plethora of user interactions, e.g., pressing a button, entering a value into a form field, clicking on a check box, or navigating between elements. As long as the legacy software system implements these events as process-relevant in the source code, the code tracker is added.

Merging User Interactions with Database Events. In addition to the user interaction events gathered by the code tracker, we analyze all database updates (i.e., insert, update and delete) expressed in terms of Data Manipulation Language (DML) statements. For this analysis, we utilize the redo log capabilities provided by the legacy software system database. Redo logs are created by transactional databases, to enable recovery in case of failures (e.g., after crashes). The information contained in a redo log consists, for each recorded operation, of the name of the database table, the performed operation (i.e., insert, update, or delete), the timestamp, the session-id, and the original DML statement applied to the database [9].

From the source code extension (cf. Fig. 4b), for each event, we can also extract the timestamp, session-id, and the affected database table. Combining these three attributes enables the allocation between user or software interactions and the corresponding changes to the persistence layer of the legacy software system. Leveraging the information from redo logs, again ensures that no performance penalties emerge due to the event log generation.

Using the code tracker functions, the information captured in the event log is significantly increased compared to an event log solely generated from the database schema [10], as we can unambiguously link processes with both program code and related data. Therefore, time-consuming reverse engineering and root cause analysis are not needed as the connection between source code, data, and processes already exists.

Finally, one valuable effect for software modernization can be achieved: missing entries in the event log indicate that process parts implemented in the legacy software system have never been used. This information is vital for modernizing legacy software systems as the code fragments may correspond to technical debt and must therefore not be migrated [11].

5.2   Recording User Interactions

Once the code tracker is installed, we are able to document the interactions of users with the legacy application, including resulting software interactions. For recording user interactions, we support two variants [12]:

Silent Recording. Shall record the use of the legacy application, starting with the login a of user until closing the legacy application. We allow specifying which information shall be recorded and in which form. For example, personal data may only be logged in an anonymized way. By only recording selected user sessions (e.g., sessions of users from a certain department), we can further restrict the recording of user interactions to relevant user groups (e.g., users handling invoices) in a fine-grained fashion.

Dedicated Recording. Aims to record existing (i.e., already identified) processes implemented in the legacy software system. Users may define the start and end of the recording (e.g., through predefined key combinations), and provide additional information about the recorded process. This, in turn, allows for a precise delimitation of the interactions corresponding to a process.

6 Evaluation

The evaluation of our approach is threefold: First, we assess whether the identified requirements are met. Second, we analyze the performance of an Oracle legacy software system to which we applied our approach. Third, we applied process discovery algorithms to the derived event logs and evaluate the resulting process models with domain experts. In total, the legacy software system used to evaluate the approach comprises 589 database tables with 9977 columns. Additionally, 60712 database statements (including more than 8000 different statements) were implemented in a total of over 5 million lines of code. Furthermore, the legacy software system comprises 1285 forms and 6243 different screens. The event log was created using dedicated recording (cf. Sect. 5). In other words, the users in this event log were able to provide additional information of the recorded business process (e.g., name and description of the process). Additionally, we applied the approach using silent recording to the legacy software system of an insurance company[1].

6.1 Requirements Evaluation

To evaluate *Requirement 1 (Relevance)*, according to which the event log shall solely contain process-relevant information, we conduct an in-depth and automatic analysis of the legacy software system by identifying and clustering important tables and source code fragments (cf. Sect. 4). This enables us to distinguish between relevant and non-relevant information. As a result, we are able to configure the code tracker to ensure that only relevant data is collected.

Requirement 2 (Scope) deals with the scope of the legacy software system and aims to minimize the amount of domain knowledge needed for the analysis. By analyzing the source code, we are able to identify which code fragments refer to which database tables. Clustering the database tables (cf. Sect. 4) allows grouping the tables that belong to the same context. This enables a best guess approach that may be checked by domain experts to further improve the event log generation. Compared to alternative approaches (e.g., extensive interviews), our approach requires significantly less domain knowledge.

---

[1] Event logs provided: https://cloudstore.uni-ulm.de/s/7jYeRnXtcsk2Wfd.

Requirement 3 (Consistency) refers to consistency with respect to data types, timestamps, and resources. While we account for consistency regarding data types (e.g., timestamp formats and variables), due to the automated nature of our approach, the fulfillment of this requirement also depends on the consistency of the analyzed legacy software system as well as the underlying database.

According to *Requirement 4 (Performance)* the event log generation must not affect the performance of the legacy software system or user interactions with the legacy application. Typically, the generation of redo log files, archive log files based on the redo log files, as well as the log rotation capabilities are tuned to not influence the performance of the analyzed legacy software system. For further analysis, the generated event log is extracted asynchronously to ensure that the extraction neither impacts users nor the performance of the running legacy software system. Additionally, the logging of user interactions focuses on the relevant actions identified during legacy software analysis. Furthermore, the logging is running in a separate, isolated transaction to the user session. Finally, the collected event data is also persisted in a separate storage to not affect performance.

6.2   Performance Analysis

To further evaluate the performance effects of our approach on the considered legacy software system, we executed the same 3 processes multiple times ($N = 10$) with and without event log generation and measured the duration of the following performance metrics: navigation, loading time, and function call. Note that due to limitations of the legacy software system, timestamps could only be collected every 10 ms. In other words, differences of up to 20 ms might exist. Figures 6 - 7 depict the collected performance metrics. When navigating through the legacy software system the average duration decreased by 25 ms. The average loading times decreased by 30 ms after adding the event log generation. These differences are in range of the timestamp limitations of the legacy software system. Therefore, we can conclude that the event log generation does not significantly impact navigation and loading times. On average, the duration of function calls increased by 0.65 s (+18.2%) per function call. However, after closer inspection, this increase is mainly due to recursive function calls that generate event log entries with each iteration. We are able to only record one event log entry for recursive function calls, consequently reducing the increase to the level of non-recursive function calls. Concerning the latter, we observed an average increase of 14 ms (1.73%). Across all observed performance metrics, the differences do not impact typical user and software interactions (Figs. 5, 6 and 7).

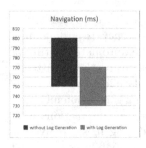
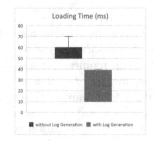
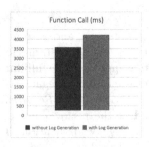

Fig. 5. Navigation   **Fig. 6.** Loading time   **Fig. 7.** Function calls

6.3 Initial Process Discovery

We applied several process discovery algorithms to the event logs generated with our approach using default algorithm configurations. Next, we showed the resulting process models to domain experts ($N = 13$) and asked them to evaluate to which degree they are able to recognize the legacy software system in each process model on a 5-Point Lickert scale from *not at all* to *completely*. Overall, the domain experts rated the process model generated by the Heuristic Miner (threshold $= 0.9$) best (Mean $= 4.45$, SD $= 0.63$). This indicates that process models discovered from the generated event log adequately represent the behavior of processes implemented by the legacy software system (Table 1).

Table 1. Domain expert recognition of discovered process models ($N = 13$)

	Inductive (Tree)	Inductive (BPMN)	DFG	Heuristic (thold $= 0.75$)	Heuristic (thold $= 0.9$)	Heuristic (thold $= 0.95$)
Mean (SD)	3.08 (1.07)	3.08 (0.73)	2.31 (1.2)	4.15 (0.77)	4.46 (0.63)	3.38 (1.27)

While the results could be improved using additional process discovery algorithms or fine-tuning parameters, they emphasize the high quality of generated event logs as no additional event log preparation was required.

7 Related Work

This paper is related to event log generation, robotic process automation, and legacy software system analysis.

Process mining algorithms require event logs and, therefore, the generation of event logs from various sources has gained great attention [13]. Databases are often used as the main resource for extracting event data from information systems [10,14]. A quality-aware and semi-automated approach to extract event logs from relational data is presented in [15]: users may select event log attributes from available data columns, assisted by data quality metrics. In the context of legacy software systems, however, relying solely on the information present in databases is not sufficient, as important process-relevant knowledge is often captured in the source code as well as the displayed user forms, but cannot be discovered from the database solely. For example, legacy databases are often not normalized and miss important information, e.g., foreign key constraints.

In the field of Robotic Process Automation (RPA) [16], user interface interactions and software robots are used to replicate human tasks. An approach for recording the interactions with user interfaces and the generation of user interface event logs is presented in [17]. A pipeline of processing steps enabling robotic process mining tools to generate RPA scripts from UI logs is presented in [18]. [19] presents an UI logger that generates an event log from multiple user interfaces. As opposed to [17–19], our approach accounts for the effects on the legacy software system (e.g., exact database statements), i.e., it does not only consider the user interface interactions in isolation.

In [20], a framework to recover workflows from an e-commerce scenario is presented, leveraging static analysis to identify business knowledge from source code. Similarly, [21] presents an approach for recovering business knowledge from legacy application databases by inspecting the data stored within the database. As our approach also aims to identify business knowledge from legacy software systems, it differs from [20,21]. Instead of extracting business knowledge from static analysis, we generate event logs that represent business knowledge using interactions with the legacy software systems.

[22] deals with the generation of event logs from legacy software systems by first extending the source code and then recording the event logs. In contrast, our approach requires less domain knowledge for generating the event logs as we derive relevant source code fragments from the clusters identified in the database (including foreign-key constraints specified in the source code) rather than domain experts or system analysts. Additionally, we support two event log generation variants (silent and dedicated) that enable further insights into specific processes implemented in the legacy software system.

8   Summary and Outlook

This paper presented an approach for generating event logs from running legacy software systems with minimal domain knowledge. We combine information from source code analysis and the database structure to identify tables and source code fragments relevant in the context of supported business processes.

Further, we identify which database tables and source code fragments may correspond to a specific process (e.g., handling an invoice) using a cluster analysis. We then automatically inject event log generation functions to the legacy software system to track user and software interactions with the legacy software system, while at the same time recording the resulting database transactions. Next, we document user interactions with the application and the resulting database changes from the running legacy application in a user-decided fashion. We then combine both logs to correlate user interactions with corresponding database changes to obtain event logs suitable for process mining.

We evaluated the approach based on the requirements identified with domain experts, a performance analysis of the legacy software system, and the application and evaluation of initial process discovery algorithms. The requirements are met, enabling the generation of comprehensive event logs from legacy software systems with the approach. A performance evaluation using an Oracle legacy software system has shown that our event log generation does not impact the performance of the legacy software system, and initial process models discovered were able to adequately represent the legacy software system for domain experts using the event logs generated with the approach.

In future work, we will apply the presented approach to additional legacy software systems. Additionally, we will increase the quality of the discovered process models for non-experts using more intuitive event log labels based on the legacy software system.

Acknowledgments. This work is part of the SoftProc project, funded by the KMU-innovativ Program of the Federal Ministry of Education and Research, Germany (F.No. 01IS20027A)

References

1. van der Aalst, W.M.P., et al.: Process mining manifesto. In: Daniel, F., Barkaoui, K., Dustdar, S. (eds.) BPM 2011. LNBIP, vol. 99, pp. 169–194. Springer, Heidelberg (2012). https://doi.org/10.1007/978-3-642-28108-2_19
2. Rozinat, A., van der Aalst, W.M.P.: Conformance checking of processes based on monitoring real behavior. Inf. Syst. **33**(1), 64–95 (2008)
3. Dumas, M., Rosa, M.L., Mendling, J., Reijers, H.A.: Fundamentals of Business Process Management, 2nd edn. Springer, Heidelberg (2018). https://doi.org/10.1007/978-3-642-33143-5
4. Feathers, M.: Working Effectively with Legacy Code. Addison-Wesley, Boston (2013)
5. van der Aalst, W.M.P.: Process Mining: Data Science in Action, 2nd edn. Springer, Heidelberg (2016). https://doi.org/10.1007/978-3-662-49851-4
6. Wieringa, R.J.: Design Science Methodology for Information Systems and Software Engineering. Springer, Heidelberg (2014). https://doi.org/10.1007/978-3-662-43839-8
7. Page, L., Brin, S., Motwani, R., Winograd, T.: The pagerank citation ranking: bringing order to the web. Stanford InfoLab, Technical Report 1999-66, previous number = SIDL-WP-1999-0120 (1999)
8. Fluri, B., Wursch, M., Pinzger, M., Gall, H.: Change distilling: tree differencing for fine-grained source code change extraction. IEEE Trans. Softw. Eng. **33**(11), 725–743 (2007)
9. de Murillas, E.G.L., van der Aalst, W.M.P., Reijers, H.A.: Process mining on databases: unearthing historical data from redo logs. In: Motahari-Nezhad, H.R., Recker, J., Weidlich, M. (eds.) BPM 2015. LNCS, vol. 9253, pp. 367–385. Springer, Cham (2015). https://doi.org/10.1007/978-3-319-23063-4_25
10. van der Aalst, W.M.P.: Extracting event data from databases to unleash process mining. In: vom Brocke, J., Schmiedel, T. (eds.) BPM - Driving Innovation in a Digital World. MP, pp. 105–128. Springer, Cham (2015). https://doi.org/10.1007/978-3-319-14430-6_8

11. Cunningham, W.: The wycash portfolio management system. SIGPLAN OOPS Mess. **4**(2), 29–30 (1992)
12. Breitmayer, M., Arnold, L., Reichert, M.: Towards retrograde process analysis in running legacy applications. In: Proceedings of the 14th ZEUS Workshop, vol. 3113, pp. 11–15. CEUR-WS.org (2022)
13. Dakic, D., Stefanovic, D., Lolic, T., Narandzic, D., Simeunovic, N.: Event log extraction for the purpose of process mining: a systematic literature review. In: Prostean, G., Lavios Villahoz, J.J., Brancu, L., Bakacsi, G. (eds.) SIM 2019. SPBE, pp. 299–312. Springer, Cham (2020). https://doi.org/10.1007/978-3-030-44711-3_22
14. Calvanese, D., Montali, M., Syamsiyah, A., van der Aalst, W.M.P.: Ontology-driven extraction of event logs from relational databases. In: Reichert, M., Reijers, H.A. (eds.) BPM 2015. LNBIP, vol. 256, pp. 140–153. Springer, Cham (2016). https://doi.org/10.1007/978-3-319-42887-1_12
15. Andrews, R., et al.: Quality-informed semi-automated event log generation for process mining. Decis. Supp. Syst. **132**, 113265 (2020)
16. Wewerka, J., Reichert, M.: Robotic process automation - a systematic mapping study and classification framework. Enterprise Information Systems (2022)
17. Choi, D., R'bigui, H., Cho, C.: Enabling the gab between RPA and process mining: User interface interactions recorder. IEEE Access **10**, 39604–39612 (2022)
18. Leno, V., Polyvyanyy, A., Dumas, M., La Rosa, M., Maggi, F.: Robotic process mining: vision and challenges. Bus. Inf. Syst. Eng. **63**, 06 (2021)
19. López-Carnicer, J.M., del Valle, C., Enríquez, J.G.: Towards an opensource logger for the analysis of RPA projects. In: Asatiani, A., et al. (eds.) BPM 2020. LNBIP, vol. 393, pp. 176–184. Springer, Cham (2020). https://doi.org/10.1007/978-3-030-58779-6_12
20. Zou, Y., Hung, M.: An approach for extracting workflows from e-commerce applications. In: 14th IEEE ICPC 2006, pp. 127–136 (2006)
21. Pérez-Castillo, R., Caivano, D., Piattini, M.: Ontology-based similarity applied to business process clustering. J. Softw. Evol. Process **26**(12), 1128–1149 (2014)
22. Pérez-Castillo, R., Weber, B., Pinggera, J., Zugal, S., de Guzmán, I.G.R., Piattini, M.: Generating event logs from non-process-aware systems enabling business process mining. Enterp. Inf. Syst. **5**(3), 301–335 (2011)

Defining Data Quality Issues in Process Mining with IoT Data

Yannis Bertrand[(✉)][iD], Rafaël Van Belle[iD], Jochen De Weerdt[iD],
and Estefanía Serral[iD]

Research Centre for Information Systems Engineering (LIRIS), KU Leuven,
Warmoesberg 26, 1000 Brussels, Belgium
{yannis.bertrand,rafael.vanbelle,jochen.deweerdt,
estefania.serralasensio}@kuleuven.be

Abstract. IoT devices supporting business processes (BPs) in sectors
like manufacturing, logistics or healthcare collect data on the execution
of the processes. In the last years, there has been a growing awareness of
the opportunity to use the data these devices generate for process mining
(PM) by deriving an event log from a sensor log via event abstraction
techniques. However, IoT data are often affected by data quality issues
(e.g., noise, outliers) which, if not addressed at the preprocessing stage,
will be amplified by event abstraction and result in quality issues in the
event log (e.g., incorrect events), greatly hampering PM results. In this
paper, we review the literature on PM with IoT data to find the most
frequent data quality issues mentioned in the literature. Based on this,
we then derive six patterns of poor sensor data quality that cause event
log quality issues and propose solutions to avoid or solve them.

Keywords: Data quality · Process mining · IoT data

1 Introduction

As IoT devices, i.e., sensors and actuators, are becoming increasingly more
important for supporting the execution of business processes (BPs), there is a
growing awareness of the opportunity to use the data collected by these devices
for process mining (PM). Such IoT data can serve as a source for the derivation
of an event log of the process around which IoT devices are placed, which can
then be used to apply PM techniques (e.g., discovery, conformance checking).

However, IoT data (in particular sensor data) are well-known to be of poor
general quality, i.e., suffering from noise, containing missing data, etc. There is a
risk that underlying sensor data quality issues lead to data quality issues in the
event log extracted from them, e.g., erroneous activity names, missing events,
imprecise event-case relationships, etc.

Previous research has identified various event log quality issues [3] and patterns leading to some of those issues [27]. This being said, no work to date has

This research was supported by the Flemish Fund for Scientific Research (FWO) with
grant number G0B6922N.

M. Montali et al. (Eds.): ICPM 2022 Workshops, LNBIP 468, pp. 422–434, 2023.
https://doi.org/10.1007/978-3-031-27815-0_31

studied how the intrinsic characteristics of sensor data lead to event log quality issues and which specific patterns characterise event log quality issues stemming from quality issues in the source sensor data. This is of interest for research as identifying and understanding these patterns makes it easier for other researchers and practitioners to improve their IoT data quality to prevent event log quality problems and ultimately improve PM results.

In this paper, we address this gap and investigate data quality issues in PM that make use of IoT data. To do so, we review papers from the literature on IoT PM that mention data quality issues, both in sensor data and in the event logs derived from the sensor data. Based on this, we identify patterns of event log quality issues caused by quality issues in the source IoT data.

The remainder of the paper is structured as follows. In Sect. 2, we first go over the literature on data quality in general, before mentioning data quality in PM and IoT and outlining PM using IoT data. Then, in Sect. 3, we introduce our research questions and detail the methodology we followed to review the literature on data quality in IoT PM and derive patterns from it. After this, in Sect. 4, we present the results of our literature review and the patterns found in the literature. The results and the patterns are discussed in Sect. 5. We conclude our paper with suggestions to improve the quality of sensor data in IoT PM and ideas for future work.

2   Background

2.1   Data Quality

Data quality is a vast research topic and many definitions of data quality exist. In general, data quality is seen as the extent to which data meet the requirements of their users [25,30]. Various dimensions have been defined to describe and quantify data quality, among which: accuracy, timeliness, precision, completeness, reliability, and error recovery [16]. Note that the importance of each of these dimensions depends on the use case and the type of data.

2.2   Data Quality in Process Mining

Process mining assumes as input an event log consisting of all the events that took place in the process that is being analysed within a certain time frame. In order to apply process mining, an event log should include at least the following data elements: a case ID, indicating to which instance of the process an event belongs; a timestamp; and the label of the activity performed [24].

Data quality issues in PM revolve around errors, inconsistencies and missing data in event logs. The authors of [3] propose to classify these issues along two axes: the type of issue (incorrect, irrelevant, imprecise or missing data) and the event log entity affected (case, event, event-case relationship, case attribute, position, activity name, timestamp, resource, and event attribute). Some issues affecting events, timestamps and activity names are argued to be more important and are therefore analysed in further detail.

In [27], the authors build upon this framework and identify 11 event log quality issues in the form of imperfection patterns. For each of these patterns, a usual cause is identified, an example is given, a link is made with a event log quality issue from [3], and advice to detect and solve the issue is provided.

However, both seminal works focus on data quality issues arising in traditional event logs, while process mining on IoT data is faced with event log quality issues stemming from intrinsic characteristics and limitations of IoT devices.

2.3   IoT Data Quality

IoT data quality is a broad topic ranging from detecting IoT data quality issues to improving data quality through cleaning methods [16,28]. IoT applications often rely on low-cost sensors with limited battery and processing power, frequently deployed in hostile environments [28]. This leads to sensor issues such as low sensing accuracy, calibration loss, sensor failures, improper device placement, range limit and data package loss. Such sensor faults, in turn, cause various types of errors in the generated data complicating further analysis.

The authors of [28] reviewed the sensor data quality literature and listed the following error types (in decreasing order of frequency): outliers; missing data; bias; drift; noise; constant value; uncertainty; stuck-at-zero. When left untreated these errors result in incorrect data, and subsequent analysis will yield unreliable results, ultimately leading to wrong decisions.

To prevent misguided decision making, it is important to assess the underlying data quality. To this end, the authors of [21] introduced measures for sensor data quality: completeness, timeliness, plausibility, artificiality and concordance.

2.4   Process Mining with IoT Data

IoT devices usually sense the environment and produce at runtime a sequence of measurements called a *sensor log*, usually in the form shown in Table 1.

Table 1. Example of a sensor log generated by in smart spaces.

Timestamp	Sensor	Value
...	...	...
2022-05-31 12:34:52	M3	ON
2022-05-31 12:34:58	M5	OFF
2022-05-31 12:35:04	M3	OFF
2022-05-31 12:35:22	T2	22
2022-05-31 12:38:17	M29	OFF
...	...	...

The vast majority of the process mining literature involving IoT data focuses on deriving an event log from a sensor log. Traditional process mining techniques can then be applied to this event log to, e.g., discover control-flow models of the processes. Typical steps include preprocessing the raw data (i.e., cleaning, formatting), event correlation to retrieve the cases each event belongs to and event abstraction to derive meaningful process events from sensor data (see, e.g., [5,15,18,26,29]).

These papers often report errors in the event logs derived from sensor data, which cause issues in the PM results (e.g., spaghetti models due to irrelevant events). In this paper, we argue that a large portion of the errors in the event log are due to data quality problems in the source sensor log, which are amplified by the event abstraction step and result in errors in the event log used for PM.

3   Methodology

In this section, we detail the methodology followed to review the literature on PM with IoT data and to derive patterns from the literature. It consists of three main steps: research question definition, literature selection and data extraction.

3.1   Research Questions

Three research questions (RQs) are addressed in this research:

- RQ-1: Which IoT data quality issues do IoT process mining papers face?
- RQ-2: Which event log quality issues do IoT process mining papers face?
- RQ-3: Which patterns can be found between IoT data and event log quality issues in IoT process mining?

3.2   Literature Selection

To answer these RQs, we scanned the literature on IoT PM that mentioned IoT data and event log quality issues. To do so, we devised a query consisting of three parts: process mining keywords, IoT data keywords and data quality keywords. After some refinements, the following query was finally selected:

("process mining" OR "process discovery" OR "process enhancement" OR "conformance checking") AND ("sensor data" OR "iot data" OR "internet of things data" OR "low-level log" OR "low-level data") AND ("data quality" OR "data challenges" OR "data issues" OR "data preparation" OR "data challenge" OR "data issue")

The query was executed on the Scopus and Limo online search engines, which access articles published by Springer, IEEE, Elsevier, Sage, ACM, MDPI, CEUR-WS and IOS Press. Because the literature tackling data quality in PM with IoT data is still very scarce, all fields were searched, yielding 177 results in total.

After removing duplicates and non-English results, papers were scanned based on title and abstract, before a full paper scan was performed. Papers were included based on their ability to answer the RQs, i.e., they had to apply PM with sensor data and mention data quality issues in sensor data or event logs derived from sensor data or both. Review papers that could answer RQs were usually very generic and for this reason were excluded and replaced with the original studies, which answered the RQs in more detail. At the end of the review process, 17 studies remained for analysis (see Fig. 1 for more detail).

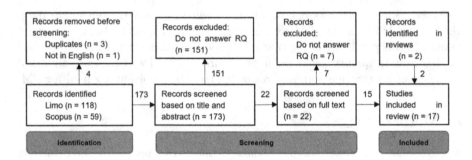

Fig. 1. Literature selection: included and excluded papers.

3.3 Data Extraction

The following information was extracted from the studies: The environment; The types of IoT data used and whether process data (i.e., a traditional event log) were also available; the IoT data and event log quality issues, following the classifications of [3,28], respectively; and the analytical goal of the study (i.e., the type of PM to apply).

Based on this, patterns linking IoT data quality issues with event log quality issues were derived. For each pattern, its origin (cause of IoT data quality issue), effects (resulting event log quality issues) and potential remedies are discussed.

4   Results

4.1   Mapping of Data Quality Issues in IoT PM

The results of the data extraction can be found in Table 2. As can be seen, most of the papers report on process mining conducted in an industrial or healthcare environment. The vast majority of the literature uses only sensor data, from which an event log is derived (occasionally, mined models are shown in the papers), as discussed in Sect. 2.4. In line with the two most frequent environments considered by the papers, two main types of sensor data emerge: individual location sensor (ILS) data in healthcare and time series (TS) and discrete sensor data in industrial scenarios. These different data types are often affected by different data quality issues, which are discussed in the next paragraph. Finally, a slight upward trend can be seen in the number of publications over time, with a peak in 2018.

Concerning data quality issues, the most frequent IoT data quality issues encountered (RQ1) are noise (7), outliers (4) and missing data (4). Next to this, many papers also mention volume (5) as a sensor data issue, which does not make the data erroneous, but can make the data considerably more difficult to analyse. Regarding event log quality issues (RQ2), the most frequent is incorrect event (7), followed by missing event (3), incorrect activity name (2) and incorrect

Table 2. Summary of the information extracted from the literature.

ID	Environment	Data type(s)	Data quality issue(s)		Goal	Year	Ref
			IoT data	Event log			
S1	Healthcare	Process data, TS sensor data	Outliers, noise	Incorrect events, irrelevant events	Process discovery	2012	[17]
S2	Healthcare	Individual location sensor (ILS) data	Outliers, noise	/	Process discovery	2013	[11]
S3	Logistics, healthcare	Process data, TS sensor data (simulated)	/	Missing event-case relationship, missing event attributes	Decision mining	2014	[9]
S4	Industry	TS sensor data	Volume, variety, velocity	/	Event log creation	2016	[20]
S5	Healthcare	ILS data	Inaccurate, granularity	Incorrect activity names, incorrect event-case relationship, missing events	Process redesign	2016	[31]
S6	Commerce	ILS data	/	Imprecise event-case relationship	Process discovery	2017	[14]
S7	Industry	GPS data	Missing data, volume	/	Predictive process monitoring	2018	[1]
S8	Industry	TS sensor data, discrete sensor data	Outliers, noise, duplicates	Incorrect event-case relationship	Event log creation	2018	[5]
S9	Industry	TS sensor data, discrete sensor data	Volume, granularity	/	Event log creation	2018	[6]
S10	Healthcare	ILS data	Volume	Incorrect events, incorrect timestamps	Queue mining	2018	[12]
S11	Healthcare	Hospital information system (HIS) and ILS data	Missing data, inaccurate data, granularity	Incorrect events	Event log repair	2018	[23]
S12	Home	ILS data	Noise	Incorrect events	Habit mining	2019	[8]
S13	Industry	TS sensor data, discrete sensor data	Outliers, noise	/	Event log creation	2020	[4]
S14	Industry	TS sensor data	Noise	Incorrect events, duplicate events	Anomaly detection	2020	[22]
S15	Various	Process data, sensor data	Noise, missing data, volume, granularity	/	Event log creation	2021	[2]
S16	Healthcare	ILS data	Noise , missing data	Missing events, incorrect events, duplicate events	Process discovery	2021	[10]
S17	Home	Video camera data	Noise	Incorrect events, missing events, incorrect activity names	Event log creation	2022	[19]

event-case relationship (2). Note that slashes in Table 2 indicate that the paper did not report data quality issues, which does not necessarily mean that no issue was encountered in the study.

4.2 Patterns Description

In this section, we present the patterns we have derived from the literature (RQ3). Note that papers that mention only either IoT data or event log quality issues cannot be used to derive patterns and, in addition to this, S11 cannot be used because the IoT data and event log quality issues described are unrelated (the event log is not derived from the IoT data). For each pattern, we discuss its origin, effects and potential remedies. Table 3 provides an overview.

Pattern 1: Incorrect Event-Case Relationship Due to Noisy Sensor Data. In many cases, when trying to derive an event log from sensor data, one of the main issues is that no case ID is present in the sensor log (e.g., in S8, S14, S17). To solve this problem, an event correlation step has to be performed, which will annotate events derived from the sensor log with the ID of the case they relate to. This correlation can be done either based on domain knowledge or using data-driven techniques. However, as noted in S8, this step is highly sensitive to the quality of the sensor data. In particular, noise and outliers can lead data-driven techniques to split cases mistakenly, resulting in labelling events with incorrect case IDs.

To avoid this issue, the use of sensor data cleaning methods is very important. The authors of S8 recommend in their follow-up paper S14 to use robust quadratic regression to clean and smoothen noisy sensor data.

Pattern 2: Erroneous Events Due to Inaccurate Location Sensor. ILS data is often used for PM, the assumption that different activities take place in different locations enabling a straightforward conversion of the sensor log into an event log (see, e.g., [13]). However, when different activities are executed in adjacent locations, there is a risk that several sensors will register the passage of a user (e.g., a patient, a resource) simultaneously. This generates erroneous events in the sensor log, which hinder the event abstraction step and result in incorrect events and activity names in the event log. This can have important consequences on PM: S16 reports that less than 0.5% errors in the event log already have a considerable impact on the quality of the process models mined.

This issue can best be treated by improving the sensor infrastructure. Using more accurate sensors or placing them further from each other can help avoid the issue completely. Otherwise, ex-post treatment can be applied by, e.g., deleting passages that last less than a given threshold (e.g., one minute in [7], cited by S12; 24 s in S5).

Pattern 3: Missing Events Due to Sampling Rate. Inadequate sampling rates can cause missing events in the event logs. It arises when the sampling rate of the sensors is too low, hence events that should be detected by these sensors are not. In S5, for instance, the sampling rate of the system is 12 s, which means that passages of less than 12 s through a given location might not be recorded (which is realistic when the location is, e.g., a corridor), resulting in missing events.

The authors of S16 also propose a post-hoc solution to impute missing events based on the characteristics of the physical process environment. For example: given rooms A, B and C, if C is only accessible via B, then a user must have been through B even if the sensor log only contains passages in A and C. Other possibilities involve improving sensor logging a priori by fine-tuning the sampling rate for each location (so there are neither missing events nor incorrect events), e.g., lowering the sampling rate of the sensor in the corridor while increasing the sampling rate of the sensor in the doctor's practice. A second possibility is to filter out passages that are too short (e.g., in S5, passages of less than 24 s are considered as noise and removed). This technique can be refined by using a low sampling rate in all locations and filtering out events that are obviously too short or too long, depending on the location.

Pattern 4: Missing Events Due to Sensor Range Limit. A similar pattern arises in the dimension of space rather than time. In this case, the range of sensors (e.g., location sensors) is too narrow and does not encompass the whole area where an activity could take place. This issue leads to missing events that happened beyond the sensor's reach. For instance, in S5, the range of location sensors is two meters, which means that any movement beyond this range will remain unnoticed, hence if an activity of the process is executed more than two meters from the sensor, it will not be detected.

The post-hoc solution suggested by S16 (see Pattern 3) can be applied to impute missing events that are caused by a lack in sensor range. In addition to this, improving the coverage of the physical process space by installing additional sensors can help prevent this issue from happening.

Pattern 5: Erroneous Events Due to Noisy Sensor Data. In this pattern, noise is present in the sensor data due to issues during logging or due to the presence of noise affecting the phenomenon measured by the sensors (e.g., in S17, video data contain sequences that are irrelevant for the process). This noise in the sensor data is picked up in the event abstraction phase and translates into noise in the event log in the form of incorrect events and events that carry incorrect activity name.

To solve this issue, S17 uses the inductive miner - infrequent (IMf) discovery algorithm, which has a parameter that can be adjusted to determine the level of infrequent behaviour to include in the model mined. The same approach is followed by S14, also using the noise threshold of the IMf algorithm to determine which events to leave out of the model.

Pattern 6: Incorrect Timestamps Due to Sensor Range Limit. This issue is related with P4, and arises when the arrival of a user in a room/at a location does not coincide with the beginning of the activity executed here. This causes the beginning of the activity to be recorded earlier than the actual beginning of the activity. E.g., in S10, it is assumed that the beginning of a consultation with a doctor is the moment when the patient is detected by the location sensor in the office of the doctor. However, as noted by the authors, it may be that the doctor is still busy in another room, or finishing taking notes for the previous patient. The same issue can also affect the end of the activity, when a user leaves the room with a certain delay after the end of the activity.

This issue can sometimes be solved by modifying the placement of the sensors, to make them detect users more precisely when events happen, or by adapting the range of the sensors to make them only detect users when the activity actually started or ended (and not after it started or before it ended either).

Table 3. Overview of identified patterns linking sensor faults and data quality issues to the associated errors in process mining.

	Sensor fault/characteristic	References
	$\implies$ Sensor data issue	
	$\implies$ Process mining errors	
P1	Unstable environment	S8,
	$\implies$ Noisy sensor data & outliers	S14,
	$\implies$ Incorrect case ID	S17
P2	Inaccurate sensor location	S16
	$\implies$ Duplicate or inconsistent sensor readings	
	$\implies$ Incorrect events, incorrect activity names	
P3	Inadequate sensor sampling rate	S5
	$\implies$ Events not captured in sensor log	
	$\implies$ Missing events	
P4	Sensor range limit	S5,
	$\implies$ Activities outside sensor range are missing	S16
	$\implies$ Missing events	
P5	Unstable environment	S1,
	$\implies$ Noisy sensor data	S12
	$\implies$ Incorrect events, incorrect activity names	S14, S17
P6	Sensor range limit	S10
	$\implies$ Activity start/end time is logged incorrectly	
	$\implies$ Incorrect timestamps	

5 Discussion

It is interesting to note that the most frequently IoT data quality issues are among the most cited error types in the IoT literature. However, the high number of papers mentioning noise as an issue and the absence of other, more refined, IoT data quality issues from [28] makes us suspect that some of the papers reviewed used noise and outliers as bucket terms for more specific sensor data quality issues (e.g., drift, bias). This may have also had an effect on the precision of the patterns we found.

Next to this, it is remarkable that the patterns identified usually result in issues with the most critical event log elements (i.e., event, case ID, activity name, timestamp). This is mainly due to the fact that PM using IoT data often focuses on extracting these required elements from the sensor log. Moreover, these elements being the most essential also makes it more likely that errors concerning them are searched for (and detected). This effect can also be observed in [27], where most patterns detected cause event log quality issues affecting events, activity names or timestamps.

The literature mentions two main strategies to improve sensor data quality: post-hoc data cleaning (e.g., removing outliers, smoothing; for a complete discussion of sensor data cleaning techniques, see [28]) and fostering good data logging practices (e.g., careful sensor data placement, constant environmental conditions). While the latter has the advantage of preventing the issue rather than solving it, it must be noted that completely preventing sensor data quality issues is impossible. E.g., sensor failure is typically hard to detect, let alone predict [16]. Moreover, some of the patterns are interrelated, and avoiding one of them sometimes comes at the cost of aggravating another one. For instance: ILS can only avoid blind spots (Pattern 4) at the cost of having zones where multiple location sensors overlap (Pattern 2). This means that some data cleaning will always have to be performed, e.g., to impute missing events due to blind spots in between location sensors.

Finally, it is worth noting that some papers use sensor data to repair traditional event logs collected by information systems. S11, for instance, uses ILS data to detect sequences of events that are not realistic given the path followed by patients in a hospital and correct them. S11 also argues that neither sensor data nor event logs collected by traditional sources are fully reliable, and that the main advantage of using two (or more) data sources is to be able to compare them to find anomalous data and hopefully correct them.

6   Conclusion

In this paper, we investigated data quality issues in PM using IoT data. After reviewing background literature and related works on sensor data quality and event log quality, we scanned the literature to find the most common sensor data quality issues (RQ1) and event log quality issues (RQ2) in IoT PM papers, following well-established data quality taxonomies [3,28]. Based on this, we identified six patterns of sensor data quality issues that cause event log quality issues and hinder IoT PM (RQ3), and mentioned possible remedies to the underlying IoT issues.

Following this, our advice for improving sensor data quality for PM is to first improve the logging practices, with 1) thoughtful sensor placement to avoid missing and duplicate events; 2) use devices to identify the users tracked by IoT devices to have case IDs at logging time; 3) careful choice of sensors to obtain data at the best granularity level (i.e., accuracy, frequency) to avoid huge volumes of data. Second, we encourage researchers to investigate more generic and more automated techniques (i.e., requiring little expert input) to detect and correct sensor data quality issues, as data cleaning approaches mentioned in the literature are often ad-hoc and highly tailored for data from specific sensors. Finally, we align ourselves with [23] in advising researchers and practitioners to try to combine different data sources whenever possible.

One key limitation of this study is the fact that we restricted ourselves to patterns that could be derived from the existing IoT PM literature. Accordingly, given the still fairly low maturity of this subdomain of PM, we cannot make founded claims on completeness of these patterns. In particular, with IoT PM focusing heavily on the derivation of events and subsequent control-flows from sensor data, there is a lack of research into using IoT data for non-control-flow related data, including event and case attributes, e.g., in function of decision mining, trace clustering, etc. Such uses of IoT data are very likely to produce additional data quality patterns. Another important area for future research concerns the streaming nature of typical IoT data, given the additional complexity this creates for data quality detection and rectification strategies. Finally, while well-known as a data quality issue in the field of IoT, the level of measurement precision of sensors is currently not yet taken into account within the IoT PM literature. Given the importance of delicately tuned thresholding approaches, e.g. for event abstraction, we consider research on the impact of sensor data precision on process mining results to be another promising area for future work.

References

1. Bandis, E., Petridis, M., Kapetanakis, S.: Business process workflow mining using machine learning techniques for the rail transport industry. In: Bramer, M., Petridis, M. (eds.) SGAI 2018. LNCS (LNAI), vol. 11311, pp. 446–451. Springer, Cham (2018). https://doi.org/10.1007/978-3-030-04191-5_37

2. Beverungen, D., et al.: Seven paradoxes of business process management in a hyper-connected world. BISE **63**(2), 145–156 (2021)

3. Bose, R.J.C., Mans, R.S., van der Aalst, W.M.: Wanna improve process mining results? In: 2013 IEEE CIDM, pp. 127–134. IEEE (2013)

4. Brzychczy, E., Gackowiec, P., Liebetrau, M.: Data analytic approaches for mining process improvement-machinery utilization use case. Resources **9**(2), 17 (2020)

5. Brzychczy, E., Trzcionkowska, A.: Creation of an event log from a low-level machinery monitoring system for process mining purposes. In: Yin, H., Camacho, D., Novais, P., Tallón-Ballesteros, A.J. (eds.) IDEAL 2018. LNCS, vol. 11315, pp. 54–63. Springer, Cham (2018). https://doi.org/10.1007/978-3-030-03496-2_7

6. Brzychczy, E., Trzcionkowska, A.: Process-oriented approach for analysis of sensor data from longwall monitoring system. In: Burduk, A., Chlebus, E., Nowakowski, T., Tubis, A. (eds.) ISPEM 2018. AISC, vol. 835, pp. 611–621. Springer, Cham (2019). https://doi.org/10.1007/978-3-319-97490-3_58

7. Dogan, O., Bayo-Monton, J.L., Fernandez-Llatas, C., Oztaysi, B.: Analyzing of gender behaviors from paths using process mining: a shopping mall application. Sensors **19**(3), 557 (2019)

8. Dogan, O., et al.: Individual behavior modeling with sensors using process mining. Electronics **8**(7), 766 (2019)

9. Dunkl, R., Rinderle-Ma, S., Grossmann, W., Anton Fröschl, K.: A method for analyzing time series data in process mining: application and extension of decision point analysis. In: Nurcan, S., Pimenidis, E. (eds.) CAiSE 2014. LNBIP, vol. 204, pp. 68–84. Springer, Cham (2015). https://doi.org/10.1007/978-3-319-19270-3_5

10. Fernandez-Llatas, C., Benedi, J.M., Gama, J.M., Sepulveda, M., Rojas, E., Vera, S., Traver, V.: Interactive process mining in surgery with real time location systems: interactive trace correction. In: Fernandez-Llatas, C. (ed.) Interactive Process Mining in Healthcare. HI, pp. 181–202. Springer, Cham (2021). https://doi.org/10.1007/978-3-030-53993-1_11

11. Fernández-Llatas, C., Benedi, J.M., García-Gómez, J.M., Traver, V.: Process mining for individualized behavior modeling using wireless tracking in nursing homes. Sensors 13(11), 15434–15451 (2013)

12. Gal, A., Senderovich, A., Weidlich, M.: Challenge paper: data quality issues in queue mining. JDIQ 9(4), 1–5 (2018)

13. Grefen, P., Brouns, N., Ludwig, H., Serral, E.: Co-location specification for iot-aware collaborative business processes. In: CAISE 2019, pp. 120–132. Springer, Heidelberg (2019). https://doi.org/10.1007/978-3-030-21297-1_11

14. Hwang, I., Jang, Y.J.: Process mining to discover shoppers' pathways at a fashion retail store using a wifi-base indoor positioning system. IEEE T-ASE 14(4), 1786–1792 (2017)

15. Janssen, D., Mannhardt, F., Koschmider, A., van Zelst, S.J.: Process model discovery from sensor event data. In: Leemans, S., Leopold, H. (eds.) ICPM 2020. LNBIP, vol. 406, pp. 69–81. Springer, Cham (2021). https://doi.org/10.1007/978-3-030-72693-5_6

16. Karkouch, A., Mousannif, H., Al Moatassime, H., Noel, T.: Data quality in internet of things: a state-of-the-art survey. JNCA 73, 57–81 (2016)

17. Kaymak, U., Mans, R., Van de Steeg, T., Dierks, M.: On process mining in health care. In: SMC 2012, pp. 1859–1864. IEEE (2012)

18. Koschmider, A., Janssen, D., Mannhardt, F.: Framework for process discovery from sensor data. In: EMISA, pp. 32–38 (2020)

19. Kratsch, W., König, F., Röglinger, M.: Shedding light on blind spots-developing a reference architecture to leverage video data for process mining. DSS 158, 113794 (2022)

20. Krumeich, J., Werth, D., Loos, P.: Prescriptive control of business processes. BISE 58(4), 261–280 (2016)

21. Kuemper, D., Iggena, T., Toenjes, R., Pulvermueller, E.: Valid. iot: a framework for sensor data quality analysis and interpolation. In: ACM MMSys 2018, pp. 294–303 (2018)

22. Maeyens, J., Vorstermans, A., Verbeke, M.: Process mining on machine event logs for profiling abnormal behaviour and root cause analysis. Ann. Telecommun. 75(9), 563–572 (2020)

23. Martin, N.: Using indoor location system data to enhance the quality of healthcare event logs: opportunities and challenges. In: Daniel, F., Sheng, Q.Z., Motahari, H. (eds.) BPM 2018. LNBIP, vol. 342, pp. 226–238. Springer, Cham (2019). https://doi.org/10.1007/978-3-030-11641-5_18

24. Reinkemeyer, L.: Process mining in a nutshell. In: Process Mining in Action, pp. 3–10. Springer, Cham (2020). https://doi.org/10.1007/978-3-030-40172-6_1

25. Scannapieco, M.: Data Quality: Concepts, Methodologies and Techniques. Data-Centric Systems and Applications. Springer, Heidelberg (2006). https://doi.org/10.1007/3-540-33173-5

26. Seiger, R., Zerbato, F., Burattin, A., Garcia-Banuelos, L., Weber, B.: Towards iot-driven process event log generation for conformance checking in smart factories. In: EDOCW, pp. 20–26. IEEE (2020)
27. Suriadi, S., Andrews, R., ter Hofstede, A.H., Wynn, M.T.: Event log imperfection patterns for process mining: towards a systematic approach to cleaning event logs. ISJ **64**, 132–150 (2017)
28. Teh, H.Y., Kempa-Liehr, A.W., Wang, K.I.K.: Sensor data quality: a systematic review. J. Big Data **7**(1), 1–49 (2020)
29. Valencia Parra, Á., Ramos Gutiérrez, B., Varela Vaca, Á.J., Gómez López, M.T., García Bernal, A.: Enabling process mining in aircraft manufactures: extracting event logs and discovering processes from complex data. In: BPM2019IF (2019)
30. Wang, R.Y., Strong, D.M.: Beyond accuracy: what data quality means to data consumers. JMIS **12**(4), 5–33 (1996)
31. Zhang, Y., Martikainen, O., Saikkonen, R., Soisalon-Soininen, E.: Extracting service process models from location data. In: Ceravolo, P., Guetl, C., Rinderle-Ma, S. (eds.) SIMPDA 2016. LNBIP, vol. 307, pp. 78–96. Springer, Cham (2018). https://doi.org/10.1007/978-3-319-74161-1_5

Creating Translucent Event Logs
to Improve Process Discovery

Harry H. Beyel$^{(\boxtimes)}$ and Wil M. P. van der Aalst

Process and Data Science, RWTH Aachen University, Aachen, Germany
{beyel,wvdaalst}@pads.rwth-aachen.de

Abstract. Event logs capture information about executed activities. However, they do not capture information about activities that could have been performed, i.e., activities that were enabled during a process. Event logs containing information on enabled activities are called translucent event logs. Although it is possible to extract translucent event logs from a running information system, such logs are rarely stored. To increase the availability of translucent event logs, we propose two techniques. The first technique records the system's states as snapshots. These snapshots are stored and linked to events. A user labels patterns that describe parts of the system's state. By matching patterns with snapshots, we can add information about enabled activities. We apply our technique in a small setting to demonstrate its applicability. The second technique uses a process model to add information concerning enabled activities to an existing traditional event log. Data containing enabled activities are valuable for process discovery. Using the information on enabled activities, we can discover more correct models.

Keywords: Translucent event logs · Robotic process mining · Task mining · Desktop activity mining

1 Introduction

In today's digital environment, a high amount of data is generated and stored. In organizations, a lot of these data are related to processes, for example, a production process or hiring new people. These data can be stored in *event logs*. By using process mining techniques, event logs can be turned into real value. Process mining techniques are categorized into three areas: process discovery, conformance checking, and process enhancement [1]. Process discovery techniques aim to construct a process model given an event log. Such a model aims to represent the underlying process comprehensively. Conformance checking describes and quantifies how well a model corresponds to an event log. Process enhancement aims to combine a process model and an event log to extend or improve the provided model. Traditionally, event logs only capture what happened — not what *could*

We thank the Alexander von Humboldt (AvH) Stiftung for supporting our research.

M. Montali et al. (Eds.): ICPM 2022 Workshops, LNBIP 468, pp. 435–447, 2023.
https://doi.org/10.1007/978-3-031-27815-0_32

have happened. Nevertheless, the information on *enabled activities* besides the executed action is valuable. Process discovery gets more straightforward if this information is accessible. There are information systems from which these data can be extracted. Examples of such systems are workflow-management systems and user interfaces. We call event logs which possess the information of enabled activities *translucent event logs* [2]. To illustrate the benefits of translucent event logs in process mining, consider the excerpt of an event log shown in Table 1 and the Petri nets shown in Fig. 1.

Table 1. Excerpt of an example translucent event log.

Case ID	Activity	Timestamp	Enabled activities
404	a	2022-10-23	a
404	b	2022-10-24	b, c
404	c	2022-10-25	c
404	e	2022-10-26	d, e
911	a	2022-10-27	a
911	c	2022-10-28	b, c
911	b	2022-10-29	b
911	d	2022-10-30	d, e
911	b	2022-10-31	b, c
911	c	2022-11-01	c
911	e	2022-11-02	d, e

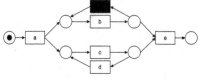

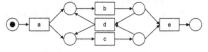

(a) Accepting labeled Petri net based on considering executed activities of the event log displayed in Table 1 and applying the inductive miner [9].

(b) Accepting labeled Petri net based on considering enabled and executed activities of the event log displayed in Table 1. We apply the baseline discovery algorithm presented in [2].

Fig. 1. Two different process models based on the event log displayed in Table 1.

Using only the information of executed activities, the process model depicted in Fig. 1a is discovered by using the inductive miner [9]. However, suppose we use the information of enabled activities and apply the baseline discovery algorithm presented in [2]. In that case, we receive the Petri net shown in Fig. 1b. As we observe, the latter Petri net suits the event log better than the former Petri net. As a result, this small example demonstrates the value of translucent event logs since process discovery can already benefit from the additional information. Dedicated process discovery techniques that use this information are described in [2].

However, translucent event logs are not widely available or used. To increase the availability of translucent event logs, we propose two techniques. The first technique uses snapshots describing a system's state linked to each event in an event log, labeled patterns, and pattern matching. The second technique generates translucent event logs given a process model and a traditional event log. Both approaches produce more informative event logs that allow for translucent-based discovery techniques.

The remainder is structured as follows. In Sect. 2, we present the preliminaries of our work. Related work is presented in Sect. 3. Subsequently, we present the formerly mentioned techniques in Sect. 4. Afterward, we demonstrate the applicability of our techniques in Sect. 5. Finally, we provide a conclusion of our work and provide an outlook in Sect. 6.

2   Preliminaries

Translucent event logs allow us to consider enabled activities. Multiple activities may be enabled for each event in a translucent event log, whereby the executed activity of each event is part of the enabled activities of an event. Therefore, we define translucent event logs as follows.

Definition 1 (Event Logs and Translucent Event Log). *Let C be the universe of case identifiers, A be the universe of activity names, and T be the universe of timestamps. An event log is a non-empty set of events $\mathcal{E}$ such that for any $e \in \mathcal{E}$: $\pi_{case}(e) \in C$, $\pi_{act}(e) \in A$, $\pi_{time}(e) \in T$. In addition, for any $e \in \mathcal{E}$, $\pi_{en}(e) \subseteq A$, $\pi_{act}(e) \in \pi_{en}(e)$, denotes the set of enabled activities when e occurred.*

We assume that the reader is familiar with alignments. If not, the work in [1] provides an overview. We denote an alignment given an arbitrary Petri net N and case σ as $\gamma^N(\sigma)$. In the remainder, we are only interested in the moves on the model. $\gamma^N(\sigma)(i)$ denotes the model move at position i. In addition, we assume that the reader is familiar with the construction and the meaning of a reachability graph; otherwise, [1] provides an introduction. We assume that at most one directed edge connects the states of a reachability graph if they are connected, i.e., no multiple arcs in one direction. Applying the function l on an edge returns the set of transition labels, i.e., activities, such that a firing of a transition leads from one marking to another. We denote the activity of τ-transitions with $\perp$.

3   Related Work

To our knowledge, no work has been conducted on creating translucent event logs. Moreover, there are seldom translucent event logs available [5]. However, there is work that connects translucent event logs with lucent process models. A process model is lucent if the states are characterized by their enabled transitions

[3]. In [2], it is shown that a translucent event log can be used to rediscover a lucent process model. In [4], lucency is further elaborated. In [13], lucent process models may be best suited for a prefix-based conformance checking technique.

Lucency can be a desired property for information systems with user interfaces. If lucency is a property, it implies that the system behaves consistently from a user's viewpoint. As a result, Robotic Process Mining (RPM) seems to be a field of interest for lucent process models and translucent event logs. RPM deals with the analysis of user interaction logs [8]. RPM and Robotic Process Automation (RPA) are closely related. The goal of RPA is to automate tasks that demand a high effort if automated traditionally, for example, tasks executed by users in a complex user interface environment [12]. RPM should provide help to create automation for RPA. Since a user interface has to be recorded for this analysis, capturing enabled activities besides the executed activities is convenient. An example of capturing this information is by taking screenshots. The screenshots taken during a task's execution are valuable for several reasons. First, we can use screenshots to document the execution of a task. Second, we can use screenshots to identify flaws in the interface design. Third, we can use screenshots to add information about enabled activities to the recorded log. There are already recording tools for user interaction logs available, for instance, the work presented in [11].

4   Creating Translucent Event Logs

Translucent event logs allow us to observe enabled activities besides the executed activities. However, the problem of creating translucent event logs has not been tackled. We provide two techniques to create translucent event logs, as depicted in Fig. 2. As one can observe, the two approaches do not share any similarities. The first technique relies on pattern matching and snapshots. An event log and a snapshot database linked to the event log are needed. We can check if a labeled pattern appears in a snapshot. If so, we add the associated label as an enabled activity to the event linked to the snapshot. The second technique adds the enabled activities to an existing event log using a process model. Given an event log and a process model, alignments are computed. Given these alignments and a reachability graph based on the process model, we compute the enabled activities.

In the remainder of this section, we explain our techniques in more detail. First, we present the approach of adding enabled activities using pattern matching and snapshots. Second, we describe our alignment-based technique.

4.1   Snapshots and Pattern Matching

Figure 3 illustrates an abstract illustration of our approach. As depicted, our approach uses an event log with information about snapshots, a snapshot event log. Moreover, our approach relies on patterns associated with a label. Combining

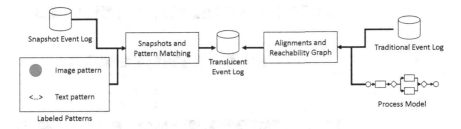

Fig. 2. Overview of our two approaches to generate translucent event logs. The first technique relies on a snapshot event log, a combination of an event log and snapshots, describing a system's state and linked to events, and labeled patterns. Each pattern is labeled with an activity. If a pattern appears in a snapshot, its label is added as an enabled activity. The second technique relies on process models and traditional event logs. Using this information to generate alignments and a reachability graph, we can create a translucent event log.

a snapshot event log with labeled patterns results in a translucent event log. In the following, we describe our approach in more detail.

During the execution of a process, snapshots of a system can be taken. These snapshots reveal the different states a system has.

Definition 2 (Snapshot). *Let $\mathcal{S}$ be the universe of snapshots. A snapshot $s \in \mathcal{S}$ is a description of a system's state. Such a description can be a text or an image (e.g., a screenshot).*

For this approach, events must have information related to snapshots, which we define in the following. Using this relationship, we can later add enabled activities.

Definition 3 (Snapshot Event Log). *A snapshot event log is a non-empty set of events $\mathcal{E}$ such that for any $e \in \mathcal{E}$: $\pi_{case}(e) \in \mathcal{C}$, $\pi_{act}(e) \in \mathcal{A}$, $\pi_{time}(e) \in \mathcal{T}$. In addition, for any $e \in \mathcal{E}$, $\pi_s(e) \in \mathcal{S}$, denotes the snapshot related to event e.*

Our goal is to convert snapshot event logs into translucent event logs. To do so, we need patterns.

Definition 4 (Pattern). *Let $\mathcal{P}$ be the universe of patterns. If a pattern $p \in \mathcal{P}$ appears in a snapshot $s \in \mathcal{S}$, this is denoted as $p \sqsubseteq s$.*

Since patterns can be of any form, it is necessary to convert their information into an event-log-friendly format. Therefore, the user has to label each pattern.

Definition 5 (Labeling). *A labeling function maps each pattern to an enabled activity: $\pi_{label} : \mathcal{P} \to \mathcal{A}$.*

Next, we define how we convert a snapshot event log into a translucent event log. For the conversion, we detect if patterns appear in snapshots, and if so, we add the corresponding labels as enabled activities.

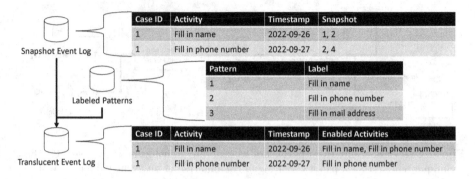

Fig. 3. Illustration about our approach of creating translucent event logs. A traditional event log is enriched with snapshots, i.e., each event has information about the system's state. In addition, there are labeled patterns. By matching all events' snapshots with patterns and the corresponding labels, we receive a translucent event log.

Definition 6 (Transform Snapshot Event Log to Translucent Event Log). *Let $\mathcal{E}$ be a snapshot event log and $\sqsubseteq$ and π_{label} defined as before. For any $e \in \mathcal{E}$, we set $\pi_{en} = \{\pi_{label}(p) | \exists p \in \mathcal{P} : p \sqsubseteq \pi_S(e)\}$*

As defined above, multiple activities can be enabled in an event. If we apply this function to each event, we receive a translucent event log as defined earlier. An application of this methodology in the field of RPM is shown in Sect. 5.1.

4.2   Alignment-Based Creation of Translucent Event Logs

In contrast to the formerly introduced creation of translucent event logs, the alignment-based creation takes a different angle. Instead of relying on patterns, pattern matching, and a snapshot event log, this technique needs a traditional event log and a process model. In this work, we focus on Petri nets as process model notation. An event log and a Petri net are used to compute alignments which we use in combination with a reachability graph to detect which activities are enabled besides the executed one. Important to note is that we add an artificial end-activity to each case, and as a result, to the process model.

As shown in Fig. 4, we compute an alignment by considering a Petri net and a process variant. Based on a Petri net with its initial marking, we can construct a reachability graph and, based on the graph, all paths which lead to the final marking. Given an alignment and the list of possible paths, the path which fits the order of executed non-τ-transitions and in which τ-transitions are executed latest is chosen. We can add the enabled activities by combining the chosen path and the reachability graph. To illustrate our approach, we refer to the Petri net shown in Fig. 5, the reachability graph depicted in Fig. 6, and the variant $\sigma = \langle c, b, e, end \rangle$.

There are two optimal alignments with the following moves on the model $\gamma_1^N(\sigma)$: $\langle t_1, t_2, t_4, t_5, t_7, t_8 \rangle$ and $\gamma_2^N(\sigma) = \langle t_1, t_4, t_2, t_5, t_7, t_8 \rangle$. As we observe in the Petri net shown in Fig. 5, $l(t_2) = l(t_5) = l(t_6) = \perp$. We can denote that the order

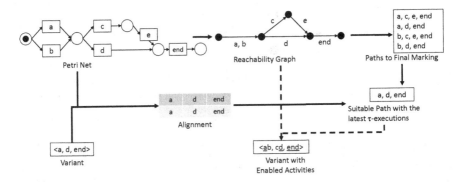

Fig. 4. Overview of creating translucent event logs using alignments. Starting from a Petri net and an event log, alignments are created for each variant. Moreover, using a Petri net and the corresponding initial marking, we create a reachability graph. Given this graph, we can generate all paths from the initial marking to the Petri net's final marking. Given a perfectly-fitting alignment and the list of paths, we can find the path where possible τ-transitions are executed as last. Given the selected path and the reachability graph, we can add enabled activities.

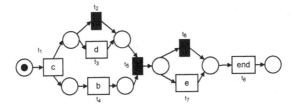

Fig. 5. Accepting labeled Petri net to illustrate creating translucent event logs.

of τ-executions differs. There are multiple approaches to deal with this situation, each leading to different results. We are interested in the alignment with the *latest* τ-executions. By doing so, we enforce the execution of non-τ-transitions that can lead to other enabled activities, and, therefore, to collect as much information about the process as possible. To decide which alignment has the latest execution of τ-transitions, we sum up the indices of τ-executions in each alignment. Then, the alignment with the greatest value is chosen. As a result, the sum of indices of τ-executions for $\gamma_1^N(\sigma)$ is 2+4=6 and for $\gamma_2^N(\sigma)$ it is 3+4=7. Therefore, we know that $\gamma_2^N(\sigma)$ is the alignment with the latest τ-executions. If non-τ-transitions can be swapped, it is up to the user which alignment to use for our technique. Next, we combine alignments and a reachability graph to get the information about enabled activities for each alignment step. To do so, we have to obtain the enabled activities per state. We use an alignment as a path through the reachability graph. At each state, we add from each outgoing arc the set of activities related to that arc. If $\perp$, a τ-execution, is an element of a set of an arc, we also consider the outgoing arcs of the target node. We proceed with this

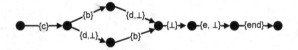

Fig. 6. Reachability graph based on Petri net shown in Fig. 5. Each node is a marking, and each arc is annotated with the set of activities leading from one marking to another.

procedure until no τ-executions are obtained anymore. Afterward, we remove the steps in the alignment that use τ-transitions. Given our example variant σ, the Petri net depicted in Fig. 5, and the reachability graph displayed in Fig. 6, we receive the following *translucent* variant: $\langle \underline{c}, \underline{bd}, \underline{eend}, \underline{end} \rangle$. In practice, not all optimal alignments are available. To overcome this, we need to compute all paths, bounded in their length by the longest alignment, to get all optimal alignments. Given an alignment, we collect all paths with the same order of non-τ-executions. Then, we search for the path with the latest τ-executions and continue as described before.

5   Proof of Concept

In this section, we provide a proof of concept. For our first technique related to pattern matching, we conduct a small case study using software created and maintained by a company. For our second technique, we discuss the approach and the general potential.

5.1   Task Mining with Screenshots

In the following, we give an overview of our implementation. Subsequently, we conduct an experiment to show the validity of our technique.

Overview. To annotate an event log used in RPM, we first have to create one. For creating user-interaction event logs, we use the software for task mining provided by Celonis[1]. The software enables us to record user interactions across different programs on a detailed level. Moreover, the software creates snapshots by taking user interface screenshots and linking them with the corresponding event. As a result, the application of Celonis generates snapshot event logs. To receive a translucent event log, we have to provide labeled patterns for the matching. In our case, patterns are snippets of the user interface. Figure 7 shows an overview of how to add information on enabled activities. As one can observe in Fig. 7, first, one has to record a task. After recording a task with the screen-shot functionality, which results in a snapshot event log, all possible enabled activities have to be defined using snippets of the user interface. To do so, one has to take pictures of possible activities and label them. These snippets are our

---

[1] https://www.celonis.com/.

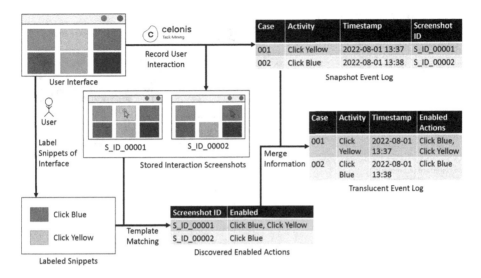

Fig. 7. Overview of adding enabled activities to user interaction logs. Starting from a user interface, snippets of the interface have to be labeled by a user. Using the tool offered by Celonis, user interactions are recorded, and screenshots are taken. We use these screenshots as snapshots, resulting in a snapshot event log. The labeled patterns are then compared with each taken snapshot. If a pattern appears in a snapshot, its label is added as enabled activity.

previously mentioned patterns. In our example, the corresponding activities are "Click Blue" and "Click Yellow". Given the previously taken snapshots during the recording and the labeled patterns, we detect if a pattern is contained in a snapshot. If we detect a pattern in a snapshot, we add the corresponding label to the enabled activities of the linked event. Given our example, we recognize that we can click blue and yellow in "S_ID_00001". In "S_ID_00002", we recognize that we can click blue but not yellow.

Case Study. We use the following example to show that our approach is applicable. Information is filled and pasted into a web form. This information contains a name, an email address, a subject, and a message. To record this process, we use the cross-program recording capability of the tool offered by Celonis. An overview of the different ingredients necessary for adding enabled activities is depicted in Fig. 8. After recording user interactions using the screenshot functionality, we receive an event log as shown in the first table in Figure 9. We can observe that user interface screenshots are linked to events, resulting in a snapshot event log. Based on our former explanations, we can transform the snapshot event log into a translucent event log. We use the stored screenshots as snapshots, the patterns shown in Fig. 8 and apply pattern matching by using template

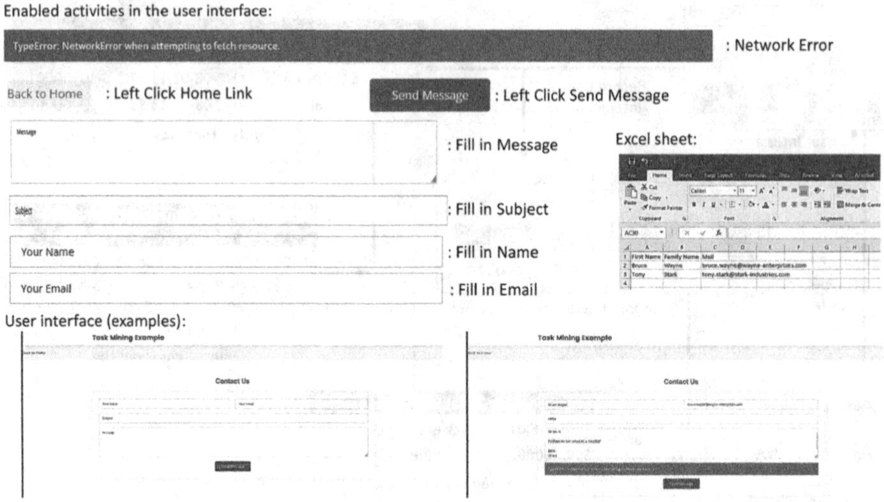

Enabled activities in the user interface:

Fig. 8. Overview of the required ingredients for our evaluation. We use small screenshots of the user interface to recognize enabled activities. Besides, we show two examples of the web form and the excel table that is a source of information.

matching provided in OpenCV[2]. The result of applying these techniques is the snapshot event log with enabled activities. However, to be a translucent event log, as defined earlier, we have to preprocess the data. Since the executed activity (*EventDescription*) has to be part of the enabled activities, we have to merge, respectively abstract, events. An overview of event abstraction is provided in [14]. The result of our applied event abstraction is the shown translucent event log.

An advantage of this technique is that we can observe how users interact with the form. We can discover lucent process models by using the discovery algorithm in [2].

5.2   Annotating Event Log

In this section, we discuss our second technique. As presented, we built our technique on existing work. Nevertheless, there are other techniques to receive information about enabled activities, for instance, a prefix-automaton. Moreover, annotating an event log from which a, perhaps, perfect process model has been generated might seem odd. However, there are several reasons why annotating a traditional event log can be beneficial.

First, translucent event logs become more available. As described, translucent event logs are rarely available. The lack of availability leads to a burden for developing new techniques. One reason is that benchmarks for different

---

[2] https://github.com/opencv/opencv-python.

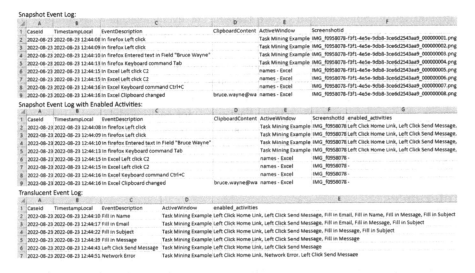

Fig. 9. Excepts of the recorded event log using the tool developed by Celonis. Applying template matching using the patterns shown in Fig. 8 leads to an intermediate log. Abstracting events results in the translucent event log.

algorithms cannot be created. Another reason is that the research area of translucent event logs might seem uninteresting due to the lack of available event logs.

Second, using the state-based discovery algorithm in [2], we can relate the different states of a system better to a model. Since enabled activities are used as states in an automaton, a Petri net can be discovered using region theory [6,7]. Depending on the circumstances, this Petri net can illustrate the system's behavior better than the original model. Nevertheless, the process model which is used for this approach influences the result.

As a result, creating translucent event logs based on an existing process model and an event log can still be beneficial for process mining.

6   Conclusion

In this work, we showed how translucent event logs could be created. Process mining can benefit from using this type of event log, and more concrete models can be discovered. We showed two techniques to create translucent event logs. The first technique, relying on labeled patterns, pattern matching, and snapshots, can be adopted in the area of RPM. However, preprocessing the data is still necessary, but this is outside this work's scope. Moreover, labeling each pattern can be an exhausting task. Nevertheless, this problem has the potential to be partially automated. For example, it might be possible to extract patterns from snapshots such that the user only has to label them. The second technique, using a traditional event log and a process model, can be used, for instance, to generate a ground truth. Since we can create translucent event logs, new techniques to improve process mining can be developed. However, multiple techniques can generate information on enabled activities given a traditional event log and a process model. Evaluating these techniques is a topic for future work. Nonetheless, the given process model influences the results of our shown technique and surely future techniques. Therefore, it seems helpful, given an event log, to generate multiple process models, generate enabled activities for each model, and later select the most suitable combination. We are sure that this process has the potential to be partly automated. We are confident that translucent event logs can help to tackle the challenges in RPM that are presented in [10].

References

1. van der Aalst, W.M.P.: Process Mining - Data Science in Action, 2nd edn. Springer, Heidelberg (2016). https://doi.org/10.1007/978-3-662-49851-4
2. van der Aalst, W.M.P.: Lucent process models and translucent event logs. Fundam. Informaticae **169**(1–2), 151–177 (2019). https://doi.org/10.3233/FI-2019-1842
3. van der Aalst, W.M.P.: Free-choice nets with home clusters are lucent. Fundam. Informaticae **181**(4), 273–302 (2021). https://doi.org/10.3233/FI-2021-2059
4. van der Aalst, W.M.P.: Reduction using induced subnets to systematically prove properties for free-choice nets. In: Buchs, D., Carmona, J. (eds.) PETRI NETS 2021, pp. 208–229. Springer, Cham (2021). https://doi.org/10.1007/978-3-030-76983-3_11
5. van der Aalst, W.M.P.: Using free-choice nets for process mining and business process management. In: Ganzha, M., Maciaszek, L., Paprzycki, M., Ślęzak, D. (eds.) FedCSIS 2021, pp. 9–15 (2021). https://doi.org/10.15439/2021F002
6. Badouel, E., Bernardinello, L., Darondeau, P.: Petri Net Synthesis. Texts in Theoretical Computer Science. An EATCS Series. Springer, Heidelberg (2015). https://doi.org/10.1007/978-3-662-47967-4
7. Cortadella, J., Kishinevsky, M., Lavagno, L., Yakovlev, A.: Deriving petri nets for finite transition systems. IEEE Trans. Comput. **47**(8), 859–882 (1998). https://doi.org/10.1109/12.707587
8. Dumas, M., La Rosa, M., Leno, V., Polyvyanyy, A., Maggi, F.M.: Robotic process mining. In: van der Aalst, W.M.P., Carmona, J. (eds) Process Mining Handbook, pp. 468–491. Springer, Cham (2022). https://doi.org/10.1007/978-3-031-08848-3_16
9. Leemans, S.J.J., Fahland, D., van der Aalst, W.M.P.: Discovering block-structured process models from event logs - a constructive approach. In: Colom, J.-M., Desel, J. (eds.) PETRI NETS 2013, pp. 311–329. Springer, Heidelberg (2013). https://doi.org/10.1007/978-3-642-38697-8_17
10. Leno, V., Polyvyanyy, A., Dumas, M., La Rosa, M., Maggi, F.M.: Robotic process mining: vision and challenges. Bus. Inf. Syst. Eng. **63**(3), 301–314 (2020). https://doi.org/10.1007/s12599-020-00641-4
11. Leno, V., Polyvyanyy, A., La Rosa, M., Dumas, M., Maggi, F.M.: Action logger: enabling process mining for robotic process automation. In: Proceedings of the Dissertation Award, Doctoral Consortium, and Demonstration Track at BPM 2019, pp. 124–128. CEUR-WS.org (2019)
12. Syed, R., et al.: Robotic process automation: Contemporary themes and challenges. Comput. Ind. **115**, 103162 (2020). https://doi.org/10.1016/j.compind.2019.103162

13. Zaman, R., Hassani, M., van Dongen, B.F.: Prefix imputation of orphan events in event stream processing. Front. Big Data **4**, 705243 (2021). https://doi.org/10.3389/fdata.2021.705243
14. van Zelst, S.J., Mannhardt, F., de Leoni, M., Koschmider, A.: Event abstraction in process mining: literature review and taxonomy. Granular Comput. **6**(3), 719–736 (2020). https://doi.org/10.1007/s41066-020-00226-2

7th International Workshop on Process Querying, Manipulation, and Intelligence (PQMI'22)

7th International Workshop on Process Querying, Manipulation, and Intelligence (PQMI 2022)

The aim of the Seventh International Workshop on Process Querying, Manipulation, and Intelligence (PQMI 2022) was to provide a high-quality forum for researchers and practitioners to exchange research findings and ideas on methods and practices in the corresponding areas. *Process Querying* combines concepts from Big Data and Process Modeling & Analysis with Business Process Analytics to study techniques for retrieving and manipulating models of processes, both observed in the real-world as per the recordings of IT systems, and envisioned as per their design in the form of conceptual representation. The ultimate aim is to systematically organize and extract process-related information for subsequent use. *Process Manipulation* studies inferences from real-world observations for augmenting, enhancing, and redesigning models of processes with the ultimate goal of improving real-world business processes. *Process Intelligence* looks into the application of representation models and approaches in Artificial Intelligence (AI), such as knowledge representation and reasoning, search, automated planning, natural language processing, explainable AI, autonomous agents, and multi-agent systems, among others, for solving problems in process mining, and vice versa using process mining techniques to tackle problems in AI.

Techniques, methods, and tools for process querying, manipulation, and intelligence have several applications. Examples of practical problems tackled by the themes of the workshop include business process compliance management, business process weakness detection, process variance management, process performance analysis, predictive process monitoring, process model translation, syntactical correctness checking, process model comparison, infrequent behavior detection, process instance migration, process reuse, and process standardization.

PQMI 2022 attracted eight high-quality submissions. Each paper was reviewed by at least three members of the Program Committee. The review process led to four accepted papers. The keynote by Timotheus Kampik and David Eickhoff entitled "Data-driven and Knowledge-based Process Querying across Processes and Organizations" opened the workshop. It gave an overview of ongoing and anticipated industry efforts that apply process querying, relating to traditional academic perspectives, as well as to industry challenges that appear to be flying under the radar of academic views. The paper by Gyunam Park and Wil van der Aalst introduced the Object-Centric Constraint Graphs (OCCGs) as a means to monitor object-centric process specifications, and present a technique to evaluate them on Object-Centric Event Logs (OCELs). The paper by Eva Klijn, Felix Mannhardt, and Dirk Fahland proposed new aggregation operations on event data for task analysis, expressed in the form of queries over Event Knowledge Graphs (EKG), alongside an implementation and evaluation thereof on a real-world event log. The paper by Diana Sola, Christian Warmuth, Bernhard Schäfer, Peyman Badakhshan, Jana-Rebecca Rehse and Timotheus Kampik presented a publicly accessible dataset with hundreds of thousands of process models extracted from academic.signavio.com, the

SAP Signavio web platform to create BPMN diagrams. Finally, the paper by Jing Xiong, Guohui Xiao, Tahir Emre Kalayci, Marco Montali, Zhenzhen Gu and Diego Calvanese described an approach to extract OCEL logs from relational databases leveraging Virtual Knowledge Graph (VKG) alongside its implementation in the OnProm system.

We hope the reader will enjoy reading of the PQMI papers in these proceedings to learn more about the latest advances in research in process querying, manipulation, and intelligence.

October 2022   Artem Polyvyanyy
Claudio Di Ciccio
Antonella Guzzo
Arthur ter Hofstede
Renuka Sindhgatta

Organization

Workshop Organizers

Artem Polyvyanyy — University of Melbourne, Australia
Claudio Di Ciccio — Sapienza University of Rome, Italy
Antonella Guzzo — Universitá della Calabria, Italy
Arthur ter Hofstede — Queensland University of Technology, Australia
Renuka Sindhgatta — IBM Research, India

Program Committee

Agnes Koschmider — Kiel University, Germany
Anna Kalenkova — University of Adelaide, Australia
Chiara Di Francescomarino — Fondazione Bruno Kessler-IRST, Italy
Fabrizio M. Maggi — Free University of Bozen-Bolzano, Italy
Hagen Völzer — University of St. Gallen, Switzerland
Han van der Aa — University of Mannheim, Germany
Hyerim Bae — Pusan National University, Korea
Jochen De Weerdt — Katholieke Universiteit Leuven, Belgium
Jorge Munoz-Gama — Pontificia Universidad Católica de Chile, Chile
Kanika Goel — Queensland University of Technology, Australia
María Teresa Gómez-López — University of Seville, Spain
Minseok Song — Pohang University of Science and Technology, Korea
Pablo David Villarreal — Universidad Tecnológica Nacional (UTN-FRSF), Argentina
Pnina Soffer — University of Haifa, Israel
Rong Liu — Stevens Institute of Technology, USA
Seppe Vanden Broucke — Katholieke Universiteit Leuven, Belgium

SAP Signavio Academic Models: A Large Process Model Dataset

Diana Sola[1,2] [iD], Christian Warmuth[1] [iD], Bernhard Schäfer[1,2] [iD],
Peyman Badakhshan[1] [iD], Jana-Rebecca Rehse[2] [iD],
and Timotheus Kampik[1(✉)] [iD]

[1] SAP Signavio, Berlin, Germany
{diana.sola,christian.warmuth,bernhard.schaefer,peyman.badakhshan,
timotheus.kampik}@sap.com
[2] University of Mannheim, Mannheim, Germany
rehse@uni-mannheim.de

Abstract. In this paper, we introduce the *SAP Signavio Academic Models* (SAP-SAM) dataset, a collection of hundreds of thousands of business models, mainly process models in BPMN notation. The model collection is a subset of the models that were created over the course of roughly a decade on academic.signavio.com, a free-of-charge software-as-a-service platform that researchers, teachers, and students can use to create business (process) models. We provide a preliminary analysis of the model collection, as well as recommendations on how to work with it. In addition, we discuss potential use cases and limitations of the model collection from academic and industry perspectives.

Keywords: Process models · Data set · Model collection

1 Introduction

Process models depict how organizations conduct their operations. They represent the basis for understanding, analyzing, redesigning, and automating processes along the business process management (BPM) lifecycle [9]. As such, many organizations posses large repositories of process models [11]. Having access to such repositories would be tremendously beneficial for developing and testing algorithms in the area of BPM, e.g., for process model querying [19] or reference model mining [20]. Also, the growing interest in applying machine learning in the BPM field, e.g., for process model matching [1], process model abstraction [27] or process modeling assistance [24], underlines the relevance for large model collections that can, for example, serve as training datasets.

However, researchers rarely have access to large collections of models from practice. Such models can contain sensitive information about the organization's internal operations. Legal aspects and the fear of losing competitive advantage thus discourage companies from publishing their business (process) models [25]. This inherent dilemma has so far largely prevented the publication of large-scale model collections for research, as they are common in related research fields [25].

© The Author(s) 2023
M. Montali et al. (Eds.): ICPM 2022 Workshops, LNBIP 468, pp. 453–465, 2023.
https://doi.org/10.1007/978-3-031-27815-0_33

In this paper, we introduce *SAP Signavio Academic Models* (SAP-SAM), a model collection that consists of hundreds of thousands of process and business models in different notations. We provide a basic overview of datasets related to SAP-SAM, as well as the origin and structure of it. Subsequently, we present selected properties and use cases of SAP-SAM. Finally, we discuss limitations of the dataset along with recommendations on how to work with it.

2   Related Datasets

Compared to SAP-SAM, existing process model collections are rather small. The hdBPMN [21] dataset, for example, contains 704 BPMN 2.0 models. This collection has the special feature that the models are handwritten and can be parsed as BPMN 2.0 XML. Another example is RePROSitory [5] (Repository of open PROcess models and logS) which is an open collection of business process models and logs, meaning users can contribute to the repository by uploading their own data. At the time of writing, RePROSitory also contains around 700 models. Some models included in SAP-SAM have already been published [28]. However, the previously published dataset contains only 29,810 models that were collected over a shorter period of time.

In the process mining community, the BPI challenge datasets, e.g., the BPI challenge 2020 [8], have become important benchmarks. Unlike SAP-SAM, these datasets consist of *event logs* from practice. Therefore, the applications of the BPI challenge datasets only partially overlap with those of SAP-SAM.

3   Origins and Structure of SAP-SAM

SAP-SAM contains 1,021,471 process and business models that were created using the software-as-a-service platform of the SAP Signavio Academic Initiative[1] (SAP-SAI), roughly from 2011 to 2021[2]. Most models are in Business Process Model and Notation (BPMN 2.0[3]). SAP-SAI allows academic researchers, teachers, and students to create, execute, and analyze process models, as well as related business models, e.g., of business decisions. The usage of SAP-SAI is restricted to non-commercial research and education. Upon registration, users consent that the models they create can be made available for research purposes, either *anonymized* or *non-anonymized*. SAP-SAM contains those models for which users have

---

[1] See: signavio.com/bpm-academic-initiative/ (accessed at 2022-07-25).

[2] The total number includes vendor-provided example models, which are automatically added to newly created workspaces (process repositories that users register). About 470,000 models in the dataset bear the name of an example model, but this can only be a rough estimate of the number of example models in the dataset.

[3] Technically, the latest version of BPMN is, at the time of writing, BPMN 2.0.2. However, little has changed between 2.0 and 2.0.2. We assume that the informal cross-vendor alignment efforts of the OMG BPMN Model Interchange Working Group are more substantial than formal progress between minor versions. In the following, we therefore use *BPMN 2.0* to refer to any version among 2.0 and 2.0.2.

consented to non-anonymized sharing. Still, anonymization scripts were run to post-process the models, in particular to remove email addresses, student registration numbers, and—to the extent possible—names.

The models in SAP-SAM were created between July 2011 and (incl.) September 2021 by a total of 72,996 users, based on a count of distinct user IDs that are associated with the creation or revision of a model. The models were extracted from the MySQL database of SAP-SAI and are in SAP Signavio's proprietary JSON-based data format. The BPMN models are conceptually BPMN-2.0-standard-compliant, i.e., individual models can be converted to BPMN 2.0 XML using the built-in functionality of SAP-SAI. Decision Model and Notation (DMN) models can be exported analogously. The dataset contains models in the following notations:

- Business Process Model and Notation (BPMN): BPMN is a standardized notation for modeling business processes [15]. SAP-SAM distinguishes between BPMN process models, collaboration models, and choreography models, and among BPMN process models between BPMN 1.1 and BPMN 2.0 models.
- Decision Model and Notation (DMN): DMN is a standardized notation for modeling business decisions, complementing BPMN [17].
- Case Management Model and Notation (CMMN): CMMN is an attempt to supplement BPMN and DMN with a notation that focuses on agility and autonomy [16].
- Event-driven Process Chain (EPC): EPC [22] is a process modeling notation that enjoyed substantial popularity before the advent of BPMN.
- Unified Modeling Language (UML): UML is a modeling language used to describe software (and other) systems. It is subdivided into class and use case diagrams.
- Value Chain: A value chain is an informal notation for sketching high-level end-to-end processes and process frameworks.
- ArchiMate: ArchiMate is a notation for the integrated modeling of information technology and business perspectives on large organizations [13].
- Organization Chart: Organization charts are tree-like models of organizational hierarchies.
- Fundamental Modeling Concepts (FMC) Block Diagram: FMC block diagrams support the modeling of software and IT system architectures.
- (Colored) Petri Net: Petri nets [18] are a popular mathematical modeling language for distributed systems and a crucial preliminary for many formal foundations of BPM. In SAP-SAM, colored Petri nets [12] are considered a separate notation.
- Journey Map: Journey maps model the customer's perspective on an organization's business processes.
- Yet Another Workflow Language (YAWL): YAWL is a language for modeling the control flow logic of workflows [26].
- jBPM: jBPM models allowed for the visualization of business process models that could be executed by the jBPM business process execution engine before the BPMN 2.0 XML serialization format existed. However, recent versions of jBPM rely on BPMN 2.0-based models.

- Process Documentation Template: Process documentation templates support the generation of comprehensive PDF-based process documentation reports. These templates are technically a model notation, although they may practically be considered a reporting tool instead.
- XForms: XForms is a (dated) standard for modeling form-based graphical user interfaces [2].
- Chen Notation: Chen notation diagrams [3] allow for the creation of entity-relationship models.

SAP-SAM is available at https://zenodo.org/record/7012043. Its license supports non-commercial use for research purposes, e.g., usage for the evaluation of academic research artifacts, such as algorithms and related software artifacts.

4   Properties of SAP-SAM

SAP-SAM comprises models in different modeling notations and languages, as well as of varying complexity. In this section, we provide an overview of selected properties of SAP-SAM. The source code that we used to examine the properties is available at https://github.com/signavio/sap-sam.

Modeling Notations. Figure 1 depicts the number of models in different notations in the dataset, as well as the according percentages (in brackets). We aggregate notations which are used for less than 100 models respectively into *Other*: Process Documentation Template (86 models), jBPM 4 (76 models), XForms (20 models), and Chen Notation (3 models). The primarily used modeling notation is BPMN 2.0, which confirms that it is the de-facto standard for modeling business processes [4]. Therefore, we will focus on BPMN 2.0 models as we examine further properties.

Languages. Since SAP-SAI can be used by academic researchers, teachers and students all over the world, the models in SAP-SAM are created using different languages. For example, SAP-SAM includes BPMN 2.0 models in 41 different languages. Figure 2 shows the ten most frequently used languages for BPMN 2.0 models. Note that the vendor-provided example models, which are added to newly created workspaces, exist in English, German, and French. When a SAP-SAI workspace is created, the example models added to it are in German or French if the language configured upon creation is German or French, respectively; otherwise, the example models are in English. This contributes to the fact that more than half of the BPMN 2.0 models (57.43 %) are in English.

Elements. Figure 3 illustrates the occurrence frequency of different element types in the BPMN 2.0 models of SAP-SAM. It can be recognized that the element types are not equally distributed, which confirms the findings of prior research [14]. The number of models that contain at least one instance of a particular element type is much higher for some types, e.g., sequence flow (98.88 %) or task (98.11 %), than for others, e.g., collapsed subprocess (25.23 %) or start message events (25.42 %). Note that Fig. 3 only includes element types that are

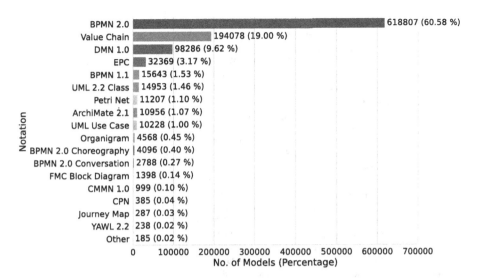

Fig. 1. Usage of different modeling notations.

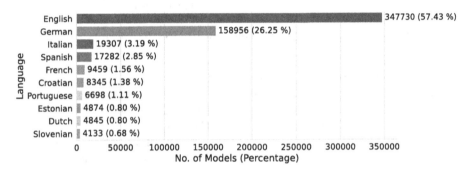

Fig. 2. Usage of different languages for BPMN 2.0 models.

used in at least 10 % of the BPMN 2.0 models. More than 30 element types are used by less than 1 % of the models. On average, a BPMN 2.0 model in SAP-SAM contains 11.3 different element types (median: 11) and 46.7 different elements, i.e., instances of element types (median: 40).

Table 1 shows the number of elements per model by type. For a compact representation, we aggregate similar element types by arranging them into groups. On average, connecting objects, which include associations and flows, make up the largest proportion of the elements in a model (mean: 23.1, median: 20).

Labels. All elements of a BPMN 2.0 model can be labeled by the modeler, which results in a total of 2,820,531 distinct labels for the 28,293,762 elements of all BPMN 2.0 models in SAP-SAM. Figure 4 depicts the distribution of label usage frequencies. We sorted the labels based on their absolute usage frequency in descending order and aggregated them in bins of size 10,000 to visualize the

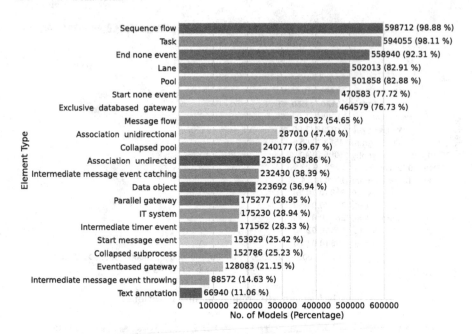

Fig. 3. Occurrence frequency of different BPMN 2.0 element types.

unevenness of the distribution. The first bin (leftmost bar in the chart) therefore contains the 10,000 most frequently used labels for the elements in the BPMN 2.0 models. Overall, 53.9 % of all elements in the BPMN 2.0 models are labeled with these first 10,000 labels. On the other hand, the long-tail distribution indicates that many of the labels are used for only one element of all BPMN 2.0 models. More precisely, 1,829,891 (64.9 %) of the labels are used only one time. The unevenness of the label usage distribution can again partly be explained by the vendor-provided examples in the dataset: The labels of the example processes appear very frequently in the dataset.

5   SAP Signavio Academic Models Applications

As pointed out above, large process model collections like SAP-SAM are a valuable and critical resource for BPM research. Process models from practice codify organizational knowledge about business processes and methodical knowledge about modeling practices. Both types of knowledge can be used by research, for example, for deriving recommendations for the design of future models. In addition, large process model collections are required for evaluating newly developed BPM algorithms and techniques regarding their applicability in practice.

To illustrate the potential value of SAP-SAM for the BPM community, the following list describes some application scenarios that we consider to be particularly relevant. It is neither prescriptive nor comprehensive; researchers can use SAP-SAM for many other purposes.

Table 1. Statistics of the number of elements per BPMN 2.0 model by type (grouped).

Element type groups	Mean	Std	Min	25%	50%	75%	Max
Activities	8.6	8.4	0	4	7	10	1543
Events	5.2	5.1	0	2	5	6	157
Gateways	3.7	4.4	0	2	3	4	303
Connecting objects	23.1	21.8	0	14	20	25	2066
Swimlanes	3.8	2.6	0	3	4	5	227
Data elements	1.3	3.4	0	0	0	2	266
Artifacts	0.9	4.0	0	0	0	1	529

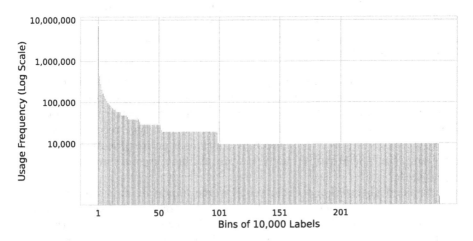

Fig. 4. Distribution of the label usage frequency in BPMN 2.0 models. Each bar represents a bin of 10,000 distinct labels.

Knowledge Generation. Process models depict business processes, codifying knowledge about the operations within organizations. This knowledge can be extracted and generalized to a broader context. Hence, SAP-SAM can be considered as a knowledge base to generate new insights into the contents and the practice of organizational modeling. Example applications include:

– Reference model mining [20]: Reference models provide a generic template for the design of new processes in a certain industry. They can be mined by merging commonalities between existing processes from different contexts into a new model that abstracts from their specific features. By applying this technique to subsets of similar models from SAP-SAM, we can mine new reference models for process landscapes or individual processes, including, e.g., the organizational perspective. Similarly, we could identify, analyze, and compare different variants of the same process.
– Identifying modeling patterns [10]: Process model patterns provide proven solutions to recurring problems in process modeling. They can help in

streamlining the modeling process and standardizing the use of modeling concepts. A dataset like SAP-SAM which contains process models from many different modelers, provides an empirical foundation both for finding new modeling patterns and for validating existing ones. This also extends to process model antipatterns, i.e., patterns that should be avoided, as well as modeling guidelines and conventions.

Modeling Assistance. The modeling knowledge that is codified in SAP-SAM can also be used for automated assistance functions in modeling tools. Such assistance functions support modelers in creating or updating process models, accelerating and facilitating the modeling process. However, many assistance functions are based on machine learning techniques and therefore require a large set of training data to generate useful results. With its large amounts of contained modeling structures and labels, SAP-SAM offers a substantial training set, for example, for the following applications:

- Process model auto-completion [23]. By providing recommendations on possible next modeling steps, process model auto-completion can speed up modeling and facilitate consistency of the terms and modeling patterns that are used by an organization. Besides structural next element type recommendations, text label suggestions or even recommendations of entire process segments are possible. SAP-SAM can be used to train machine learning models for these purposes.
- Automated abstraction techniques [27]: One important function of BPM is process model abstraction, i.e., the aggregation of model elements into less complex, higher-level structures to enable a better understanding of the overall process. Such an aggregation entails the identification and assignment of higher-level categories to groups of process elements. SAP-SAM can provide the necessary training data for an NLP-based automated abstraction.

Evaluation. Managing large repositories of process models is a key application of BPM [7]. Researchers have developed many different approaches to assist organizations with this task. To make these approaches as productive as possible, they need to be tested on datasets that are comparable to those within organizations. Since SAP-SAM goes well beyond the size of related datasets, it can be used for large-scale evaluations of existing process management approaches on data from practice. Examples for these approaches include process model querying [19], process model matching [1], and process model similarity [6].

6   Limitations and Recommendations for Usage

As explained in the previous section, SAP-SAM can be used by the academic community to test and evaluate a plethora of tools and algorithms that address a wide range of process querying and business process analytics use cases. However, in the context of any evaluation, the limitations of the dataset need to be taken into account. Considering the nature of SAP-SAM as a model collection that has been generated by academic researchers, teachers, and students, the following limitations must be considered:

- Many models in SAP-SAM exist multiple times, either as direct duplicates (copies) or as very similar versions. This includes vendor-provided example models or standard academic examples that are frequently used in academic teaching and research. The existence of these models can be used to evaluate variant identification and fuzzy matching approaches in process querying, but it negatively affects the diversity, i.e., the breadth of the dataset.
- Many models may be of low technical quality, in particular the models that are created by "process modeling beginners", i.e., early-stage students, for learning purposes. Although it can be interesting to analyze the mistakes or antipatterns in such models, flawed models can, for example, be problematic when using the dataset for generating modeling recommendations based on machine learning. Also, the mistakes that students make are most likely not representative of mistakes made by process modeling practitioners.
- Because many of the models have most likely been created for either teaching, learning, or demonstrating purposes, they presumably present a simplistic perspective on business processes. Even when assuming that all researchers, teachers, and students are skilled process modelers[4] and have a precise understanding of the underlying processes when modeling, the purpose of their models is typically fundamentally different from the purpose of industry process models. Whereas academic models often emphasize technical precision and correctness, industry models usually focus on a particular business goal, such as the facilitation of stakeholder alignment.

Let us note that this list may not be exhaustive; in particular, limitations that depend on a particular use case or evaluation scenario need to be identified by researchers who will use this dataset. Still, it is also worth highlighting that the rather "messy" nature of the model collection reflects the reality of industrial data science challenges, in which a sufficiently large amount of high-quality data (or models) is typically not straightforwardly available [11]; instead, substantial efforts need to be made to separate the wheat from the chaff, or to isolate use-cases in which the flaws in the data do not have an adverse effect on business value, or any other undesirable organizational or societal implications. However, most process models go beyond A-B-C toy examples from exercises and the overall SAP-SAM dataset is of sufficient relevance and quality for facilitating research, for example, in the directions that we have outlined in the previous section.

When using SAP-SAM for academic research purposes, it typically makes sense to filter it, i.e., to reduce it to a subset of models that satisfy desirable properties. Here, we provide some recommendations to help with this step.

---

[4] Considering the previous point, that means even when focusing on the subset of the model collection that only entails models carefully created by skilled advanced students, teachers, and researchers.

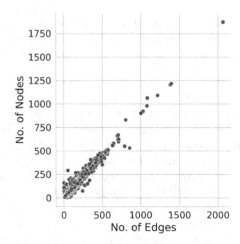

Fig. 5. Correlation of the number of nodes and edges in BPMN 2.0 models.

- It typically makes sense to filter out the vendor-provided example models that are created by the SAP-SAI system upon workspace creation.
- For many use cases, researchers may want to sort out process models that contain a very small or a very large number of elements. As can be expected for BPMN 2.0 models and is shown in Fig. 5, the number of nodes and the number of edges in a model are highly correlated. Hence, it is sufficient to filter according to the number of nodes. There is no need to additionally filter according to the number of edges.
- Similarly, researchers may want to sort out process models where the element labels have an average length of less than, for example, three characters to ensure that only models with useful labels are included.

Let us again highlight that example code that demonstrates how the dataset can be queried, as well as the code for the analysis in this paper is available at https://github.com/signavio/sap-sam.

7   Conclusion

In this paper, we have presented the SAP-SAM dataset of process and other business models. We are confident in our assumption that SAP-SAM is, by far, the largest publicly available collection of business process models. Hence, it can—despite the limitation that it entails "academic" models created by researchers, teachers, and students and not by process management professionals—serve as an excellent basis for developing and evaluating tools and algorithms for process model querying and analysis.

In the future, SAP-SAM can potentially be augmented by including the following additional data objects:

– Business objects/dictionary entries: In addition to models, SAP-SAI supports the creation of business objects, so-called *dictionary entries*. These objects represent, for example, organizational roles, documents, or IT systems and can be linked to models to then be re-used across a process landscape that entails many models. Dictionary entries facilitate process landscape maintenance, as well as reporting.

– Standard-conform XML serializations: The models in the SAP-SAM dataset are serialized using a non-standardized JSON format that *i)* supports a generalization of modeling notations and *ii)* is more convenient to use than XML-based serializations within the JavaScript-based front-ends of modern web applications. However, proprietary components exist that can—in the case of BPMN, DMN, and CMMN models—generate XML serializations which are compliant with the corresponding Object Management Group standards. Adding these XML serializations to the dataset can facilitate academic use, as many open-source and prototypical software tools support the open standards.

– PNG or SVG image representations: Similarly, to allow for a more straightforward visualization of models, PNG and SVG representations of the SAP-SAM models can be generated and included.

References

1. Antunes, G., Bakhshandelh, M., Borbinha, J., Cardoso, J., Dadashnia, S., et al.: The process model matching contest 2015. In: Enterprise Modelling and Information Systems Architectures, pp. 127–155. Köllen (2015)
2. Bruchez, E., Couthures, A., Pemberton, S., Van den Bleeken, N.: XForms 2.0. W3C Working Draft, World Wide Web Consortium (W3C) (2012). https://www.w3.org/TR/xforms20/
3. Chen, P.P.S.: The entity-relationship model-toward a unified view of data. ACM Trans. Database Syst. **1**(1), 9–36 (1976)
4. Chinosi, M., Trombetta, A.: BPMN: an introduction to the standard. Comput. Stan. Interfaces **34**(1), 124–134 (2012)
5. Corradini, F., Fornari, F., Polini, A., Re, B., Tiezzi, F.: Repository: a repository platform for sharing business process models. In: BPM (PhD/Demos), pp. 149–153 (2019)
6. Dijkman, R., Dumas, M., Van Dongen, B., Käärik, R., Mendling, J.: Similarity of business process models: metrics and evaluation. Inf. Syst. **36**(2), 498–516 (2011)
7. Dijkman, R., La Rosa, M., Reijers, H.: Managing large collections of business process models-current techniques and challenges. Comput. Ind. **63**(2), 91–97 (2012)
8. van Dongen, B.: Bpi challenge 2020: domestic declarations (2020). https://doi.org/10.4121/UUID:3F422315-ED9D-4882-891F-E180B5B4FEB5
9. Dumas, M., La Rosa, M., Mendling, J., Reijers, H.A.: Fundamentals of Business Process Management. Springer, Berlin (2013)
10. Fellmann, M., Koschmider, A., Laue, R., Schoknecht, A., Vetter, A.: Business process model patterns: state-of-the-art, research classification and taxonomy. Bus. Process Manag. J. **25**(5), 972–994 (2018)
11. Houy, C., Fettke, P., Loos, P., van der Aalst, W.M., Krogstie, J.: Business process management in the large. Bus. Inf. Syst. Eng. **3**(6), 385–388 (2011)

12. Jensen, K.: Coloured petri nets. In: Petri Nets: Central Models and their Properties, pp. 248–299. Springer, Heidelberg (1987)
13. Lankhorst, M.M., Proper, H.A., Jonkers, H.: The architecture of the archimate language. In: Halpin, T., et al. (eds.) BPMDS/EMMSAD -2009. LNBIP, vol. 29, pp. 367–380. Springer, Heidelberg (2009). https://doi.org/10.1007/978-3-642-01862-6_30
14. Muehlen, M., Recker, J.: How much language is enough? theoretical and practical use of the business process modeling notation. In: Seminal Contributions to Information Systems Engineering, pp. 429–443. Springer, Heidelberg (2013). https://doi.org/10.1007/978-3-642-36926-1_35
15. OMG: Business Process Model and Notation (BPMN), Version 2.0.2 (2013). http://www.omg.org/spec/BPMN/2.0.2
16. OMG: Case Management Model and Notation (CMMN), Version 1.1 (2016). http://www.omg.org/spec/CMMN/1.1
17. OMG: Decision Model and Notation (DMN), Version 1.3 (2021). http://www.omg.org/spec/DMN/1.3
18. Petri, C.A.: Kommunikation mit automaten. Westfäl. Inst. f. Instrumentelle Mathematik an der Univ, Bonn (1962)
19. Polyvyanyy, A.: Process querying: methods, techniques, and applications. In: Polyvyanyy, A. (ed.) Process Querying Methods, pp. 511–524. Springer, Cham (2022). https://doi.org/10.1007/978-3-030-92875-9_18
20. Rehse, J.R., Fettke, P., Loos, P.: A graph-theoretic method for the inductive development of reference process models. Softw. Syst. Model. 16(3), 833–873 (2017)
21. Schäfer, B., van der Aa, H., Leopold, H., Stuckenschmidt, H.: Sketch2bpmn: automatic recognition of hand-drawn BPMN models. In: La Rosa, M., Sadiq, S., Teniente, E. (eds.) Advanced Information Systems Engineering. Springer, Cham (2021). https://doi.org/10.1007/978-3-030-79382-1_21
22. Scheer, A.W., Thomas, O., Adam, O.: Process Modeling using Event-Driven Process Chains, Chapter 6, pp. 119–145. John Wiley & Sons Ltd., Hoboken (2005)
23. Sola, D., Aa, H.V.D., Meilicke, C., Stuckenschmidt, H.: Exploiting label semantics for rule-based activity recommendation in business process modeling. Inf. Syst. 108, 102049 (2022)
24. Sola, D., Meilicke, C., van der Aa, H., Stuckenschmidt, H.: On the use of knowledge graph completion methods for activity recommendation in business process modeling. In: Marrella, A., Weber, B. (eds.) BPM 2021. LNBIP, vol. 436, pp. 5–17. Springer, Cham (2022). https://doi.org/10.1007/978-3-030-94343-1_1
25. Thaler, T., Walter, J., Ardalani, P., Fettke, P., Loos, P.: The need for process model corpora. In: FMI 2014, p. 14 (2014)
26. van der Aalst, W., ter Hofstede, A.: Yawl: yet another workflow language. Inf. Syst. 30(4), 245–275 (2005)
27. Wang, N., Sun, S., OuYang, D.: Business process modeling abstraction based on semi-supervised clustering analysis. Bus. Inf. Syst. Eng. 60(6), 525–542 (2018)
28. Weske, M., Decker, G., Dumas, M., La Rosa, M., Mendling, J., Reijers, H.A.: Model collection of the business process management academic initiative (2020). https://doi.org/10.5281/zenodo.3758705

A Virtual Knowledge Graph Based Approach for Object-Centric Event Logs Extraction

Jing Xiong[1], Guohui Xiao[2,3,4] (✉), Tahir Emre Kalayci[5],
Marco Montali[1], Zhenzhen Gu[1], and Diego Calvanese[1,4,6]

[1] Free University of Bozen-Bolzano, Bolzano, Italy
[2] University of Bergen, Bergen, Norway
`guohui.xiao@uib.no`
[3] University of Oslo, Oslo, Norway
[4] Ontopic S.R.L, Bolzano, Italy
[5] Virtual Vehicle Research GmbH, Graz, Austria
[6] Umeå University, Umeå, Sweden

Abstract. Process mining is a family of techniques that support the analysis of operational processes based on event logs. Among the existing event log formats, the IEEE standard eXtensible Event Stream (XES) is the most widely adopted. In XES, each event must be related to a single case object, which may lead to convergence and divergence problems. To solve such issues, object-centric approaches become promising, where objects are the central notion and one event may refer to multiple objects. In particular, the *Object-Centric Event Logs* (OCEL) standard has been proposed recently. However, the crucial problem of extracting OCEL logs from external sources is still largely unexplored. In this paper, we try to fill this gap by leveraging the Virtual Knowledge Graph (VKG) approach to access data in relational databases. We have implemented this approach in the OnProm system, extending it to support both XES and OCEL standards. We have carried out an experiment with OnProm over the Dolibarr system. The evaluation results confirm that OnProm can effectively extract OCEL logs and the performance is scalable.

Keywords: Process mining · Object-Centric Event Logs · Virtual Knowledge Graphs · Ontology-based data access

1 Introduction

Process mining [1] is a family of techniques relating the fields of data science and process management to support the analysis of operational processes based on event logs. To perform process mining, normally the algorithms and tools expect that the event logs follow certain standards. However, in reality, most IT systems in companies and organizations do not directly produce such logs, and the relevant information is spread in legacy systems, e.g., relational databases. Event log extraction from legacy systems is a key enabler for process mining [6–8].

There have been several proposals for the representation of event logs, e.g., eXtensible Event Stream (XES) [16], JSON Support for XES (JXES) [15],

© The Author(s) 2023
M. Montali et al. (Eds.): ICPM 2022 Workshops, LNBIP 468, pp. 466–478, 2023.
https://doi.org/10.1007/978-3-031-27815-0_34

Open SQL Log Exchange (OpenSLEX) [14], and eXtensible Object-Centric (XOC) [12], where XES is the most adopted one, being the IEEE standard for interoperability in event logs [11]. In XES (and other similar proposals), each event is related to a single case object, which leads to problems with convergence and divergence [2], as later explained in Sect. 2.2. To solve these issues, object-centric approaches become promising, where objects are the central notion, and one event may refer to multiple objects. In particular, along this direction, the *Object-Centric Event Logs* (OCEL) standard [10] has been proposed recently.

To the best of our knowledge, the crucial problem of extracting OCEL logs from external sources is still largely unexplored. The only exception is [3], where OCEL logs are extracted by identifying the so-called master and relevant tables in the underlying database and building a *Graph of Relations (GoR)*. Though promising, this approach might be difficult to adopt when the underlying tables are complex and the GoR is hard to model because it does not separate the storage level (i.e., the database) from the concept level (i.e., domain knowledge about events).

In this work, we try to fill this gap by leveraging the OnProm framework [5,7] for extracting event logs from legacy information systems. OnProm v1 was already relying on the technology of Virtual Knowledge Graphs (VKG) [17] to expose databases as Knowledge Graphs that conform to a conceptual model, and to query this conceptual model and eventually generate logs by using ontology and mapping-based query processing. Using VKG, a SPARQL query q expressed over the virtual view is translated into a query $\mathcal{Q}$ that can be directly executed on a relational database $\mathcal{D}$, and the answer is simply the RDF graph following the standard SPARQL semantics. The workflow of OnProm v1 for extraction of event logs in XES format from relational databases consists of three steps: *conceptual modeling, event data annotations,* and *automatic event log extraction* [7]. OnProm came with a toolchain to process the conceptual model and to automatically extract XES event logs by relying on the VKG system Ontop [18].

We present here OnProm v2, which we have modularized so that it becomes easier to extend, and in which we have implemented OCEL-specific features to extract OCEL logs. We have carried out an experiment with OnProm over the Dolibarr Enterprise Resource Planning (ERP) & Customer Relationship Management (CRM) system. The evaluation results confirm that OnProm can effectively extract OCEL logs. The code of OnProm and the data for reproducing the experiment can be found on GitHub https://github.com/onprom/onprom.

2   Event Log Standards: XES and OCEL

A variety of event log standards have emerged in the literature. In this paper, we are mostly interested in the XES and OCEL standards.

2.1   XES Standard

The *eXtensible Event Stream* (XES) is an XML-based standard for event logs. It aims to provide an open format for event log data exchange between tools and applications. Since it first appeared in 2009, it has quickly become the de-facto standard in Process Mining and eventually became an official IEEE standard in 2016 [4]. The main elements of the XES standard are *Log*, *Trace*, *Event*, *Attribute*, *Extension*, and *Classifier*. We emphasize the following points:

– Log is the root component in XES.
– The Trace element is directly contained in the Log root element. Each trace belongs to a log, and each log may contain many traces.
– Each event belongs to a trace, and each trace usually contains many events.
– All information in an event log is stored in attributes. Both traces and events may contain an arbitrary number of attributes.

Example 1. Consider the order management process in an ERP system, and suppose there is an instance of order cancellation. Taking the order as a *case*, there is a trace containing *events* such as *create order*, *review order*, *cancel order*, and *close order*, as shown below.

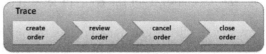

2.2 OCEL Standard

The purpose of the *Object-Centric Event Logs* (OCEL) standard is to provide a general standard to interchange event data with multiple case notions. Its goal is to exchange data between information systems and process mining analysis tools. It has been proposed recently as the mainstream format for storing object-centric event logs [10].

The main elements of the OCEL standard are *Log*, *Object*, *Event*, and *Element*. The main difference between XES and OCEL lies in the usage of *Case* in XES and *Object* in OCEL. Recall that XES requires a single case to describe events. In contrast, in OCEL the relationship between objects and events is many-to-many. This gives OCEL several advantages [10] compared with existing standards:

– It can handle application scenarios involving multiple cases, thus making up for the deficiencies of XES.
– Each event log contains a list of objects, and the properties of the objects are written only once in the log (and not replicated for each event).
– In comparison to tabular formats, the information is strongly typed.
– It supports lists and maps of elements, while most existing formats (such as XOC, tabular formats, and OpenSLEX) do not properly support them.

One main motivation for OCEL is to support multiple case notions. Using a traditional event log standard like XES may lead to problems of convergence (when an event is related to different cases and occurs repetitively) and divergence (when it is hard to separate events with a single case) [10]. We show these in the following example.

Example 2. Considering again an ERP system as in Example 1, when a valid order has been confirmed and payment has been completed, the goods are about to be delivered. Usually the items in the same order may come from different warehouses or suppliers, and may be packaged into different packages for delivery, as shown below.

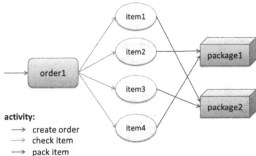

Suppose that we want to use XES to model this event log. If *item* is regarded as a case and *create order* is regarded as an activity, then *create order* will be repeated because there are multiple items (e.g., item1, item2, . . .), even if there is only one order *order1*. This is the *convergence* problem.

If *order* is regarded as a case and *pack item* and *check item* are regarded as activities, then in the same *order* case, there are multiple *pack item* events that should be executed after the *check item* events. However, we cannot distinguish different items in an *order*, and the order between the two activities may be disrupted. This is the *divergence* problem.

The OCEL standard is a good solution to these problems, since they can be easily solved by treating *order*, *item*, and *package* as objects, and then each event can be related to different objects. In this way, the properties of the objects are written only once in the event log and not replicated for each event.

3   The OnProm V2 Framework

We describe now the OnProm approach for event log extraction. OnProm v1, which supports only the XES standard, has been discussed extensively in [5, 7]. We describe here the revised version v2, which has a better modularized architecture and supports also OCEL. The architecture of OnProm v2 is shown in Fig. 1. We first briefly introduce the basic components of the framework.

To extract from a legacy *information system* $\mathcal{I}$, event logs that conform to an event log standard X, OnProm works as follows:

(A) *Creating a* VKG *specification.* The user designs a domain ontology $\mathcal{T}$ using the *UML Editor* of OnProm. Then they create a VKG mapping $\mathcal{M}$ (using, e.g., the Ontop plugin for Protégé [18]) to declare how the instances of classes and properties in $\mathcal{T}$ are populated from $\mathcal{I}$. This step is only concerned with modeling the domain of interest and is agnostic to the event log standard.

(B) *Annotating the domain ontology with the event ontology.* OnProm assumes that for the event log standard X, a specific event ontology $\mathcal{E}_X$ is available. The *Annotation Editor* of OnProm imports $\mathcal{E}_X$, and allows the user to create annotations $\mathcal{L}_X$ over the classes in $\mathcal{T}$ that are based on the classes of $\mathcal{E}_X$.

(C) *Extracting the event log.* OnProm assumes that for the standard X also a set of SPARQL queries for extracting the log information is defined. The *Log Extractor* of OnProm relies on a conceptual schema transformation approach [6] and query reformulation of Ontop, using $\mathcal{L}_X$, $\mathcal{T}$, $\mathcal{M}$, and

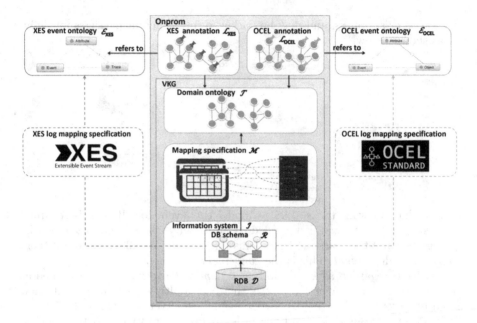

Fig. 1. OnProm event log extraction framework.

$\mathcal{R}$. It internally translates these SPARQL queries to SQL queries over $\mathcal{I}$, and evaluates the generated SQL queries to construct corresponding Java objects and serialize them into log files compliant with X.

In this work, we have first modularized the system, by separating the above steps into different software components, so as to make it more extensible. Then we have introduced OCEL-specific features in Steps (B) and (C). Hence, OnProm v2 is now able to extract OCEL logs from relational databases.

Below we detail these steps and provide a case study with the Dolibarr system. This example also serves as the base of the experiments in the next section. Dolibarr [9] is a popular open source ERP & CRM system. It uses a relational database as backend, and we consider a subset of the tables that are related to the *Sale Orders*. We model it as an information system $\mathcal{I} = \langle \mathcal{R}, \mathcal{D} \rangle$, where the schema $\mathcal{R}$ consists of 9 tables, related to product, customer, order, item, invoice, payment, shipment, etc., and the data $\mathcal{D}$ includes instances of the tables, a sample of which is shown in Table 1. Note that the table name is not immediately understandable (`llx_commande` is a table about orders).

Table 1. Table `llx_commande`.

rowid	fk_soc	ref	date_creation	date_valid	total_ttc
38	3	C07001-0010	2017-02-16 00:05:01	2021-02-16 00:05:01	200.00
40	10	C07001-0011	2017-02-16 00:05:10	2021-02-16 00:05:10	1210.00

3.1 Creating a VKG Specification

In this step, we define a domain ontology $\mathcal{T}$ and a mapping $\mathcal{M}$ for creating a VKG from $\mathcal{I} = \langle \mathcal{R}, \mathcal{D} \rangle$. This is to provide a more understandable knowledge graph view of the underlying data in terms of the domain.

The domain ontology $\mathcal{T}$ is a high-level abstraction of the business logic concerned with the domain of interest. The UML editor in OnProm uses UML class diagrams as a concrete language for ontology building and provides their logic-based formal encoding according to the OWL 2 QL ontology language [13]. In this case study, the domain ontology about *Sale Orders* is constructed using the UML editor as shown in Fig. 2.

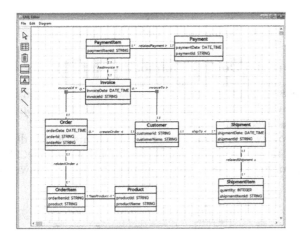

Fig. 2. Domain ontology in the UML editor.

In a VKG system, the domain ontology $\mathcal{T}$ is connected to the information system $\mathcal{I}$ through a declarative specification $\mathcal{M}$, called *mapping*. More specifically, $\mathcal{M}$ establishes a link between $\mathcal{I}$ and $\mathcal{T}$. The mapping $\mathcal{M}$ is a collection of mapping assertions, each of which consists of a SQL statement (called Source) over $\mathcal{I}$ and a triple template at the data concept schema level (called Target) over $\mathcal{T}$. For example, the following mapping assertion constructs instances of the Order class in $\mathcal{T}$, with their creation date, from a SQL query over the llx_commande table:

```
SELECT rowid, date_creation  FROM llx_commande                    (Source)
⤳ :Order/{rowid} a :Order; :createDate {date_creation}^^xsd:dateTime. (Target)
```

By instantiating rowid and date_creation with the values from the first row of llx_commande in Table 1, this mapping assertion would produce two triples: :Order/38 a :Order. :Order/38 :createDate "2017-02-16T00:05:01"8sd: dateTime.

The mapping can be edited using the Ontop plugin for Protégé. Figure 3 shows the mapping for the running example.

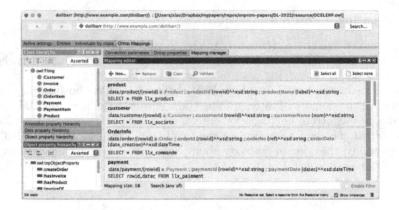

Fig. 3. Mapping in the Ontop plugin for Protégé.

3.2 Annotating the Domain Ontology with the Event Ontology

In this step, we establish the connection between the VKG and the event ontology. This is achieved by annotating the classes in the domain ontology using the elements from the event ontology.

An event ontology $\mathcal{E}$ is a conceptual event schema, which describes the key concepts and relationships in an event log standard. For the OCEL standard, we have created an ontology $\mathcal{E}_{\text{OCEL}}$, whose main elements are shown in Fig. 4.

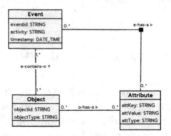

Fig. 4. OCEL event ontology.

In this ontology, the classes *Event* and *Object* are connected by the many-to-many relation *e-contains-o*. One event may contain multiple objects, and an object may be contained in multiple events. Events and objects can be related to attributes through the relations *e-has-a* and *o-has-a*, respectively. An attribute has a name (*attKey*), a type (*attType*), and a value (*attValue*).

Now, using the *Annotation Editor* in the OnProm tool chain, we can annotate the classes in $\mathcal{T}$ using the elements from $\mathcal{E}$ to produce an annotation $\mathcal{L}$. For OCEL, there are three kinds of annotations:

- The *event annotation* specifies which concepts in $\mathcal{T}$ are OCEL events. Each event represents an execution record of an underlying business process and contains mandatory (e.g., id, activity, timestamp, and relevant objects) and optional elements (e.g., event attributes). A screenshot of such example annotation is shown in Fig. 5(a), where we annotate the Order class with an *Event* and specify its properties label, activity, eventId, and timestamp.

- The *object annotation* specifies which concepts in $\mathcal{T}$ are OCEL objects. An OCEL object contains mandatory elements (e.g., id and type) and optional elements (e.g., price and weight). A screenshot of an example object annotation is shown in Fig. 5(b).
- The *attribute annotation* specifies the attributes attached to the events/objects. Both an event and an object may contain multiple attributes, and each attribute annotation consists of an *attKey*, an *attType*, and an *attValue*. A screenshot of an (event) attribute annotation using the *Annotation Editor* tool is shown in Fig. 5(c).

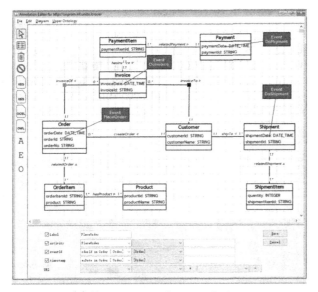

(a) Event annotation over Order.

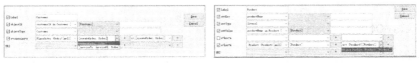

(b) Object annotation over Customer.   (c) Attribute annotation over Product.

Fig. 5. Annotation samples.

3.3 Extracting the Event Log

Once the annotation is concluded, OnProm will compute a new VKG specification $\mathcal{P}'$ with a new mapping $\mathcal{M}'$ and the event ontology $\mathcal{E}$, so that it exposes the information system $\mathcal{I}$ as an VKG using the vocabulary from the event standard.

For example, among others, OnProm produces a new mapping assertion in $\mathcal{M}'$ from the Dolibarr database to the *Event* classes in $\mathcal{E}_{\mathsf{OCEL}}$.

```
SELECT v1.'rowid', v1.'date_creation'                          (Source)
FROM 'llx_commande' v1 WHERE v1.'date_creation' IS NOT NULL
↝ :PlaceOrder/{rowid} a ocel:Event ;                          (Target)
   :timestamp {date_creation}^^xsd:dateTime .
```

Now all the information in an OCEL log can be obtained by issuing several predefined SPARQL queries over $\mathcal{P}'$. For example, the following query extracts all OCEL events and their attributes:

```
PREFIX ocel: <http://onprom.inf.unibz.it/ocel/>
SELECT DISTINCT * WHERE { ?event a ocel:Event .
   OPTIONAL { ?event ocel:e-has-a ?att. ?att a ocel:Attribute ;
      ocel:attType ?attType; ocel:attKey ?attKey; ocel:attValue ?attValue. }}
```

The following query extracts the relations between OCEL events and objects through the property *e-contains-o*:

```
SELECT DISTINCT * WHERE { ?event a ocel:Event ; ocel:e-contains-o ?object }
```

To evaluate these SPARQL queries, OnProm uses Ontop, which translates them to SQL queries over the database. In this way, extracting OCEL event logs boils down to evaluating some automatically generated (normally complex) SQL queries over the database directly. Finally, OnProm just needs to serialize the query results as logs in the XML or JSON format according to OCEL. Figure 6(a) shows a fragment in XML-OCEL and Fig. 6(b) shows its visualization.

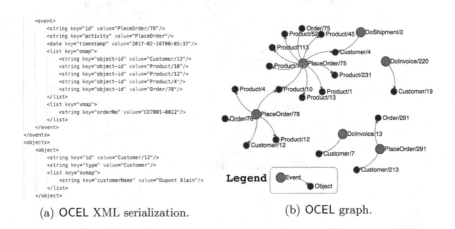

(a) OCEL XML serialization.   (b) OCEL graph.

Fig. 6. A fragment of the extracted OCEL log from the Dolibarr ERP system.

4   Experiments

We have conducted an evaluation of OnProm based on the scenario of Dolibarr. The experiments have been carried out using a machine with an Intel Core i7 2.0 GHz processor, 16 GB of RAM, Dolibarr v14, and MySQL v8. In order to test the scalability, we have generated 8 database instances of difference sizes from 2K to 1M. The size of a database is the number of rows.

Table 2. Extraction details of OCEL log elements.

Size	Attributes	Objects	Events	Relations	XML size (KB)
2 K	751	751	1000	1227	419
10 K	3750	3750	5000	6225	2094
50 K	18749	18749	24999	31222	10531
100 K	37448	37448	50000	62470	21093
250 K	93753	93789	125000	156218	52986
500 K	187502	187538	250000	312468	106112
750 K	281250	281286	374999	468712	159234
1 M	374999	374999	499997	624943	212682

Performance Evaluation. The running times are reported in Fig. 7. First, we notice that our approach scales well. The overall running time scales linearly with respect to the size of the database. In the biggest dataset of 1M rows, it takes less than 12 min to extract the event log. We also computed the division of the running time over the subtasks of log extraction. The upper left corner of Fig. 7 shows the proportion of the running time for each OCEL element. We observe that most of the time (98%) has been spent on the event, object, and attribute extraction, whose main tasks are to evaluate SPARQL queries and create corresponding Java objects in memory. The time for log serialization is almost negligible (2%). We note that since extracting these logs corresponds to evaluating the same SQL queries over databases of different sizes, it is actually not surprising to observe this linear behavior when the database tables are properly indexed.

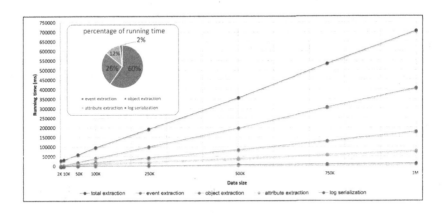

Fig. 7. Running times of the experiment.

We also report in Table 2 the number of OCEL elements extracted for each database size. At the size of 1M, OnProm extracts an OCEL event log with 374999 objects, 499997 events, 374999 attributes and 624943 relations, and it takes 207 MB to serialize the whole log in XML-OCEL.

Conformance Test. The OCEL standard comes also with a Python library and one of the main functionalities is the validation of JSON-OCEL and XML-OCEL. The library reports that the log obtained by our method is compliant with the OCEL standard.

5 Conclusions

In this work, we have presented how to extract OCEL logs using the revised version of the OnProm framework. OnProm uses an annotation-based interface for users to specify the relationship between a domain ontology and an event ontology. Then OnProm leverages the VKG system Ontop to expose the underlying sources as a Knowledge Graph using the vocabulary from the OCEL event ontology. Thus, extracting OCEL logs is reduced to evaluating a fixed set of SPARQL queries. Our experiments confirmed that the extraction is efficient and that the extracted logs are compliant with the standard. OnProm provides a flexible framework for users to choose XES or OCEL according to their needs. In the non-many-to-many business, the results are similar, but OCEL has higher extraction efficiency because it does not need to manage events in one case. In modeling many-to-many relations, OCEL has greater advantages because it is actually a graph structure.

There are several directions for future work. First of all, we would like to carry out a user-study to let more users try out our toolkit, and confirm that it is indeed easy-to-use. We are also interested in extracting logs from other sources beyond relational databases, e.g., from graph databases. Finally, the modularity of the approach makes it relatively straightforward to support other standards, and we will study this possibility.

Acknowledgements. This research has been supported by the Wallenberg AI, Autonomous Systems and Software Program (WASP) funded by the Knut and Alice Wallenberg Foundation, by the Italian PRIN project HOPE, by the EU H2020 project INODE (grant no. 863410), by the Free University of Bozen-Bolzano through the projects GeoVKG (CRC 2019) and SMART-APP (ID 2020), and by the Norwegian Research Council via the SIRIUS Centre for Research Based Innovation (grant no. 237898).

References

1. van der Aalst, W.M.P.: Process Mining - Data Science in Action, 2nd edn. Springer, Cham (2016)
2. Aalst, W.M.P.: Object-centric process mining: dealing with divergence and convergence in event data. In: Ölveczky, P.C., Salaün, G. (eds.) SEFM 2019. LNCS, vol. 11724, pp. 3–25. Springer, Cham (2019). https://doi.org/10.1007/978-3-030-30446-1_1
3. Berti, A., Park, G., Rafiei, M., van der Aalst, W.M.P.: An event data extraction approach from SAP ERP for process mining. CoRR Technical report (2021). arXiv:2110.03467, arXiv.org. e-Print archive

4. Calvanese, D., Kalayci, T.E., Montali, M., Santoso, A.: OBDA for log extraction in process mining. In: Ianni, G., et al. (eds.) Reasoning Web 2017. LNCS, vol. 10370, pp. 292–345. Springer, Cham (2017). https://doi.org/10.1007/978-3-319-61033-7_9

5. Calvanese, D., Kalayci, T.E., Montali, M., Santoso, A.: The onprom toolchain for extracting business process logs using ontology-based data access. In: Proceedings of the BPM Demo Track and BPM Dissertation Award (BPM-D&DA). CEUR Workshop Proceedings, vol. 1920. CEUR-WS.org (2017). http://ceur-ws.org/Vol-1920/BPM_2017_paper_207.pdf

6. Calvanese, D., Kalayci, T.E., Montali, M., Santoso, A., van der Aalst, W.: Conceptual schema transformation in ontology-based data access. In: Faron Zucker, C., Ghidini, C., Napoli, A., Toussaint, Y. (eds.) EKAW 2018. LNCS (LNAI), vol. 11313, pp. 50–67. Springer, Cham (2018). https://doi.org/10.1007/978-3-030-03667-6_4

7. Calvanese, D., Kalayci, T.E., Montali, M., Tinella, S.: Ontology-based data access for extracting event logs from legacy data: the onprom tool and methodology. In: Abramowicz, W. (ed.) BIS 2017. LNBIP, vol. 288, pp. 220–236. Springer, Cham (2017). https://doi.org/10.1007/978-3-319-59336-4_16

8. Calvanese, D., Montali, M., Syamsiyah, A., van der Aalst, W.M.P.: Ontology-driven extraction of event logs from relational databases. In: Reichert, M., Reijers, H.A. (eds.) BPM 2015. LNBIP, vol. 256, pp. 140–153. Springer, Cham (2016). https://doi.org/10.1007/978-3-319-42887-1_12

9. Dolibarr Open Source ERP CRM: Web suite for business. https://www.dolibarr.org/ (2021)

10. Ghahfarokhi, A.F., Park, G., Berti, A., van der Aalst, W.M.P.: OCEL: a standard for object-centric event logs. In: Bellatreche, L., et al. (eds.) ADBIS 2021. CCIS, vol. 1450, pp. 169–175. Springer, Cham (2021). https://doi.org/10.1007/978-3-030-85082-1_16

11. IEEE Computer Society: 1849–2016 - IEEE Standard for eXtensible Event Stream (XES) for Achieving Interoperability in Event Logs and Event Streams (2016). https://doi.org/10.1109/IEEESTD.2016.7740858

12. Li, G., de Murillas, E.G.L., de Carvalho, R.M., van der Aalst, W.M.P.: Extracting object-centric event logs to support process mining on databases. In: Mendling, J., Mouratidis, H. (eds.) CAiSE 2018. LNBIP, vol. 317, pp. 182–199. Springer, Cham (2018). https://doi.org/10.1007/978-3-319-92901-9_16

13. Motik, B., Cuenca Grau, B., Horrocks, I., Wu, Z., Fokoue, A., Lutz, C.: OWL 2 Web Ontology Language profiles, 2nd (edn). W3C Recommendation, World Wide Web Consortium (2012). http://www.w3.org/TR/owl2-profiles/

14. González López de Murillas, E., Reijers, H.A., van der Aalst, W.M.P.: Connecting databases with process mining: a meta model and toolset. Softw. Syst. Model. **18**(2), 1209–1247 (2018). https://doi.org/10.1007/s10270-018-0664-7

15. Shankara Narayana, M.B., Khalifa, H., van der Aalst, W.M.P.: JXES: JSON support for the XES event log standard. CoRR Technical report (2020). arXiv:2009.06363, arXiv.org. e-Print archive

16. Verbeek, H.M.W., Buijs, J.C.A.M., van Dongen, B.F., van der Aalst, W.M.P.: XES, XESame, and ProM 6. In: Soffer, P., Proper, E. (eds.) CAiSE Forum 2010. LNBIP, vol. 72, pp. 60–75. Springer, Heidelberg (2011). https://doi.org/10.1007/978-3-642-17722-4_5

17. Xiao, G., Ding, L., Cogrel, B., Calvanese, D.: Virtual knowledge graphs: an overview of systems and use cases. Data Intell. **1**(3), 201–223 (2019). https://doi.org/10.1162/dint_a_00011
18. Xiao, G., et al.: The virtual knowledge graph system Ontop. In: Pan, J.Z., et al. (eds.) ISWC 2020. LNCS, vol. 12507, pp. 259–277. Springer, Cham (2020). https://doi.org/10.1007/978-3-030-62466-8_17

Monitoring Constraints in Business Processes Using Object-Centric Constraint Graphs

Gyunam Park[✉] and Wil M. P. van der Aalst

Process and Data Science Group (PADS), RWTH Aachen University, Aachen, Germany
{gnpark,wvdaalst}@pads.rwth-aachen.de

Abstract. Constraint monitoring aims to monitor the violation of constraints in business processes, e.g., an invoice should be cleared within 48 h after the corresponding goods receipt, by analyzing event data. Existing techniques for constraint monitoring assume that a single case notion exists in a business process, e.g., a patient in a healthcare process, and each event is associated with the case notion. However, in reality, business processes are *object-centric*, i.e., multiple case notions (objects) exist, and an event may be associated with multiple objects. For instance, an Order-To-Cash (O2C) process involves *order*, *item*, *delivery*, etc., and they interact when executing an event, e.g., packing multiple items together for a delivery. The existing techniques produce misleading insights when applied to such object-centric business processes. In this work, we propose an approach to monitoring constraints in object-centric business processes. To this end, we introduce *Object-Centric Constraint Graphs* (OCCGs) to represent constraints that consider the interaction of objects. Next, we evaluate the constraints represented by OCCGs by analyzing Object-Centric Event Logs (OCELs) that store the interaction of different objects in events. We have implemented a web application to support the proposed approach and conducted two case studies using a real-life SAP ERP system.

Keywords: Constraint monitoring · Object-centric process mining · Compliance checking · Process monitoring

1 Introduction

It is indispensable for organizations to continuously monitor their operational problems and take proactive actions to mitigate risks and improve performance [2]. Constraint monitoring aims at detecting violations of *constraints* (i.e., operational problems) in business processes of an organization by analyzing event data recorded by information systems [8]. Once violations are detected, the organization can activate management actions to cover the respective violation [10].

A plethora of techniques has been suggested to implement constraint monitoring. For instance, a technique is proposed to detect events violating constraints, e.g., detecting an X-ray event with a long waiting time, using behavioral profiles and Complex Event Processing (CEP) [13]. Maggi et al. [9] propose a technique to detect process instances violating constraints, e.g., detecting a patient with multiple executions of X-rays, using Linear Temporal Logic (LTL).

© The Author(s) 2023
M. Montali et al. (Eds.): ICPM 2022 Workshops, LNBIP 468, pp. 479–492, 2023.
https://doi.org/10.1007/978-3-031-27815-0_35

The existing techniques assume that an event in event data is associated with a single object of a unique type (so-called case), e.g., a patient in a healthcare process. Thus, constraints are defined over the single case notion, e.g., each patient (i.e., case) should be registered before triage. However, in real-life business processes, an event may be associated with multiple objects of different types, i.e., real-life business processes are *object-centric* [1]. For instance, the omnipresent Purchase-To-Pay (P2P) process involves different object types, e.g., *purchase order*, *material*, *invoice*, *goods receipt*, etc., and an event may be associated with multiple objects of different types, e.g., clearing invoice is associated with a purchase order, an invoice, and a goods receipt to enable so-called *three-way matching*.

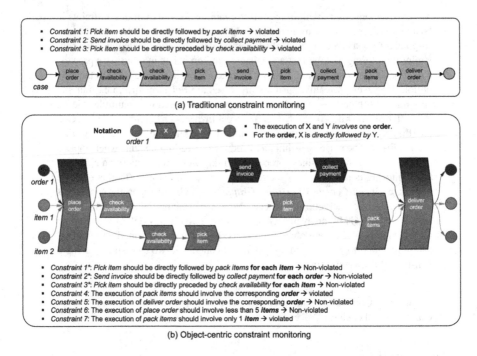

Fig. 1. Comparing (a) traditional and (b) object-centric constraint monitoring

Applying the existing techniques to such object-centric settings results in misleading insights. Figure 1(a) shows events of a "case" in an Order-To-Cash (O2C) process using *order* as the case notion. First, an order is placed, and the availability of two items of the order is checked, respectively. Next, one of the items is picked, and the invoice of the order is sent to the customer. Afterward, the other item is picked, and the payment of the invoice is collected. Finally, the items are packed and delivered to the customer. The three constraints shown in Fig. 1(a) are violated by the case. For instance, *Constraint 1* is violated since *pick item* is followed by *send invoice* in the case and *Constraint 3* is violated since *pick item* is preceded by *send invoice*.

However, in reality, the order and each item have different lifecycles as shown in Fig. 1(b). First, we place an order with two items. While the invoice is sent and the payment is collected for the order, we check the availability of each item and pick each of them. We finally deliver the order with two items after packing two items together. In this object-centric setting, constraints should be defined in relation to objects to provide accurate insights. For instance, *Constraint 1** extends *Constraint 1* with the corresponding object type (i.e., item). Contrary to *Constraint 1*, *Constraint 1** is not violated since *pick item* is directly followed by *pack item* for any items. Moreover, we can analyze more object-centric constraints by considering the interaction of different objects. First, we can analyze if an execution of an activity involves (un)necessary objects (cf. *Constraint 4* and *Constraint 5*). Also, we can analyze the cardinality of objects for executing an activity (cf. *Constraint 6* and *Constraint 7*).

In this work, we propose a technique for constraint monitoring in object-centric settings. To this end, we first introduce *object-centric behavioral metrics* that can be computed from Object-Centric Event Logs (OCELs), e.g., a metric to measure the degree to which *pick item* precedes *pack items* in the lifecycle of *items*. Next, we develop Object-Centric Constraint Graphs (OCCGs) to formally represent constraints using such metrics. Finally, *monitoring engine* evaluates the violation of the constraints represented by OCCGs by analyzing OCELs.

We have implemented a web application to support the approach. A demo video and a manual are available at https://github.com/gyunamister/ProPPa.git. Moreover, we have conducted case studies with a production process and a Purchase-To-Pay (P2P) process supported by an SAP ERP system.

The remainder is organized as follows. We discuss the related work in Sect. 2 and present the preliminaries, including OCELs in Sect. 3. In Sect. 4, we introduce object-centric behavioral metrics. Afterward, we present OCCGs to formally represent constraints and the monitoring engine to evaluate the violation of the constraints in Sect. 5. Next, Sect. 6 introduces the implementation of the proposed approach and case studies using real-life event data. Finally, Sect. 7 concludes the paper.

2 Related Work

Many approaches have been proposed to monitor the violation of constraints by analyzing event data. Weidlich et al. [13] propose a technique to abstract process models to behavioral profiles and produce event queries from the profile. Violated executions of events are monitored using Complex Event Processing (CEP) engines with the event queries. Awad et al. [5] define a set of generic patterns regarding the occurrence of tasks, their ordering, and resource assignments and generate anti-patterns from the generic patterns to monitor event executions. Maggi et al. [9] represent control-flow properties of a running process instance using Linear Temporal Logic (LTL) and evaluate their violations at runtime. Also, Petri-net-based constraints are aligned with event logs to evaluate whether the execution of business processes conforms to the constraints [12]. Indiono et al. [7] propose an approach to monitoring Instance-Spanning Constraints (ISCs) that span multiple instances of one or several processes based on Rete algorithm. However, the existing techniques may produce misleading insights in object-centric settings since it does not consider the interaction among objects of different types. Moreover, object-centric constraints, e.g., the cardinality of an object type for the execution of an activity, are not supported in the existing techniques.

Table 1. A fragment of an event log.

Event id	Activity	Timestamp	Order	Item
e_{93}	*place order (po)*	25-10-2022:09.35	$\{o_1\}$	$\{i_1, i_2, i_3\}$
e_{94}	*evaluate credit (ec)*	25-10-2022:13.35	$\{o_1\}$	$\emptyset$
e_{95}	*confirm order (co)*	25-10-2022:15.35	$\{o_1\}$	$\{i_1, i_2, i_3\}$

This paper is in line with the recent developments in object-centric process mining [1]. Object-centric process mining breaks the assumption of traditional process mining techniques that each event is associated with a single case notion (i.e., object), allowing one event to be associated with multiple objects. Moreover, a process discovery technique is proposed to discover Object-Centric Petri Nets (OCPNs) from OCELs [3]. Furthermore, Adams et al. [4] propose a conformance checking technique to determine the precision and fitness of the net, and Park et al. propose an approach to object-centric performance analysis [11]. Esser and Fahland [6] propose a graph database as a storage format for object-centric event data, enabling a user to use queries to calculate different statistics. This work extends the current development in the field of object-centric process mining by proposing a constraint monitoring technique in object-centric settings.

3   Preliminaries

Given a set X, the powerset $\mathscr{P}(X)$ denotes the set of all possible subsets. We denote a sequence with $\sigma = \langle x_1, \ldots, x_n \rangle$ and the set of all sequences over X with X^*. Given a sequence $\sigma \in X^*$, $x \in \sigma$ if and only if $\exists_{1 \leq i \leq |\sigma|} \sigma(i) = x$.

Definition 1 (Universes). $\mathbb{U}_{ei}$ *is the universe of event identifiers,* $\mathbb{U}_{oi}$ *is the universe of object identifiers,* $\mathbb{U}_{act}$ *is the universe of activity names,* $\mathbb{U}_{time}$ *is the universe of timestamps,* $\mathbb{U}_{ot}$ *is the universe of object types,* $\mathbb{U}_{attr}$ *is the universe of attributes,* $\mathbb{U}_{val}$ *is the universe of values, and* $\mathbb{U}_{map} = \mathbb{U}_{attr} \nrightarrow \mathbb{U}_{val}$ *is the universe of attribute-value mappings. For any* $f \in \mathbb{U}_{map}$ *and* $x \notin dom(f)$, $f(x) = \perp$.

Using the universes, we define an object-centric event log as follows.

Definition 2 (Object-Centric Event Log). *An object-centric event log is a tuple* $L = (E, O, \mu, R)$, *where* $E \subseteq \mathbb{U}_{event}$ *is a set of events,* $O \subseteq \mathbb{U}_{oi}$ *is a set of objects,* $\mu \in (E \rightarrow \mathbb{U}_{map}) \cup (O \rightarrow (\mathbb{U}_{time} \rightarrow \mathbb{U}_{map}))$ *is a mapping, and* $R \subseteq E \times O$ *is a relation, such that for any* $e \in E$, $\mu(e)(act) \in \mathbb{U}_{act}$ *and* $\mu(e)(time) \in \mathbb{U}_{time}$, *and for any* $o \in O$ *and* $t, t' \in \mathbb{U}_{time}$, $\mu(o)(t)(type) = \mu(o)(t')(type) \in \mathbb{U}_{ot}$. $\mathbb{U}_L$ *is the set of all possible object-centric event logs.*

For the sake of brevity, we denote $\mu(e)(x)$ as $\mu_x(e)$ and $\mu(o)(t)(x)$ as $\mu_x^t(o)$. Since the type of an object does not change over time, we denote $\mu_{type}^t(o)$ as $\mu_{type}(o)$. Table 1 describes a fraction of a simple event log $L_1 = (E_1, O_1, \mu_1, R_1)$ with $E_1 = \{e_{93}, e_{94}, e_{95}\}$, $O_1 = \{o_1, i_1, i_2, i_3\}$, $R_1 = \{(e_{93}, o_1), (e_{93}, i_1), \ldots\}$, $\mu_{act}(e_{93}) = po$, $\mu_{time}(e_{93}) = $ 25-10-2022:09.35, $\mu_{type}(o_1) = Order$, and $\mu_{type}(i_1) = Item$.
We define functions to query event logs as follows:

Definition 3 (Notations). *For an object-centric event log $L = (E,O,\mu,R)$, we introduce the following notations:*

- *$acts(L) = \{\mu_{act}(e) \mid e \in E\}$ is the set of activities,*
- *$events(L,a) = \{e \in E \mid \mu_{act}(e) = a\}$ is the set of the events associated to $a \in acts(L)$,*
- *$types(L) = \{\mu_{type}(o) \mid o \in O\}$ is the set of object types,*
- *$objects(L,ot) = \{o \in O \mid \mu_{type}(o) = ot\}$ is the set of the objects associated to $ot \in types(L)$,*
- *$events(L,o) = \{e \in E \mid (e,o) \in R\}$ is the set of the events containing $o \in O$,*
- *$objects(L,e) = \{o \in O \mid (e,o) \in R\}$ is the set of the objects involved in $e \in E$,*
- *$seq(o) = \langle e_1,e_2,\ldots,e_n\rangle$ such that $events(L,o) = \{e_1,e_2,\ldots,e_n\}$ and $\mu_{time}(e_i) \leq \mu_{time}(e_j)$ for any $1 \leq i < j \leq n$ is the sequence of all events where object $o \in O$ is involved in, and*
- *$trace(o) = \langle a_1,a_2,\ldots,a_n\rangle$ such that $seq(o) = \langle e_1,e_2,\ldots,e_n\rangle$ and $a_i = \mu_{act}(e_i)$ for any $1 \leq i \leq n$ is the trace of object $o \in O$.*

For instance, $acts(L_1) = \{po,ec,co\}$, $events(L_1,po) = \{e_{93}\}$, $types(L_1) = \{Order,Item\}$, $objects(L_1,Order) = \{o_1\}$, $events(L_1,o_1) = \{e_{93},e_{94},e_{95}\}$, $objects(L_1,e_{93}) = \{o_1,i_1,i_2,i_3\}$, $seq(o_1) = \langle e_{93},e_{94},e_{95}\rangle$, and $trace(o_1) = \langle po,ec,co\rangle$.

Using the notations, we characterize an event log as follows:

Definition 4 (Log Characteristics). *Let $L = (E,O,\mu,R)$ be an object-centric event log. For $ot \in types(L)$ and $a,b \in acts(L)$, we define the following characteristics of L:*

- *$\#_L(ot,X) = |\{o \in objects(L,ot) \mid \forall_{x \in X}\ x \in trace(o)\}|$ counts the objects of type ot whose trace contains $X \subseteq acts(L)$,*
- *$\#_L(ot,a,b) = |\{o \in objects(L,ot) \mid \exists_{1 \leq i < j \leq |trace(o)|}\ trace(o)(i) = a \land trace(o)(j) = b\}|$ counts the objects of type ot whose trace contains a followed by b,*
- *$\#_L^0(ot,a) = |\{e \in events(L,a) \mid |\{o \in objects(L,e) \mid \mu_{type}(o) = ot\}| = 0\}|$ counts the events relating no objects of type ot for the execution of a,*
- *$\#_L^1(ot,a) = |\{e \in events(L,a) \mid |\{o \in objects(L,e) \mid \mu_{type}(o) = ot\}| = 1\}|$ counts the events relating one object of type ot for the execution of a, and*
- *$\#_L^*(ot,a) = |\{e \in events(L,a) \mid |\{o \in objects(L,e) \mid \mu_{type}(o) = ot\}| > 1\}|$ counts the events relating more than one object of type ot for the execution of a.*

For instance, $\#_{L_1}(Order,\{po\}) = 1$, $\#_{L_1}(Item,\{po\}) = 3$, $\#_{L_1}(Item,\{po,ec\}) = 0$, $\#_{L_1}(Order,po,ec) = 1$, $\#_{L_1}^0(Order,ec) = 0$, $\#_{L_1}^0(Item,ec) = 1$, $\#_{L_1}^1(Order,po) = 1$, $\#_{L_1}^1(Item,po) = 0$, $\#_{L_1}^*(Order,po) = 0$, and $\#_{L_1}^*(Item,po) = 1$.

4   Object-Centric Behavioral Metrics

To introduce OCCGs, we first explain three types of object-centric behavioral metrics derived from an event log: *ordering relation*, *object involvement*, and *performance* metrics. Such metrics are used to define the semantics of OCCGs in Sec. 5.

An ordering relation metric refers to the strength of a causal/concurrent/choice relation between two activities in an OCEL w.r.t. an object type.

Definition 5 (Ordering Relation Metrics). *Let L be an object-centric event log. For* $ot \in types(L)$ *and* $a, b \in acts(L)$, *we define the following ordering relation metrics of L:*

$$- \ causal_L(ot,a,b) = \begin{cases} \frac{\#_L(ot,a,b)}{\#_L(ot,\{a,b\})}, if \ \#_L(ot,\{a,b\}) > 0 \\ 0, otherwise \end{cases}$$

$$- \ concur_L(ot,a,b) = \begin{cases} 1 - \frac{max(\#_L(ot,a,b),\#_L(ot,b,a)) - min(\#_L(ot,a,b),\#_L(ot,b,a))}{\#_L(ot,a,b) + \#_L(ot,b,a)}, \\ if \ \#_L(ot,a,b) + \#_L(ot,b,a) > 0 \\ 0, otherwise \end{cases}$$

$$- \ choice_L(ot,a,b) = \begin{cases} 1 - \frac{\#_L(ot,\{a,b\}) + \#_L(ot,\{a,b\})}{\#_L(ot,\{a\}) + \#_L(ot,\{b\})}, if \ \#_L(ot,\{a\}) + \#_L(ot,\{b\}) > 0 \\ 0, otherwise \end{cases}$$

$causal_L(ot,a,b)$, $concur_L(ot,a,b)$, and $choice_L(ot,a,b)$ all produce values between 0 (weak) and 1 (strong). For L_1 in Table 1, $causal_{L_1}(Order,po,co) = 1$, $concur_{L_1}(Order,po,co) = 0$, $choice_{L_1}(Order,po,co) = 0$, showing that po and co has a strong (not only directly, but also eventually) causal ordering relation.

Next, an object involvement metric quantitatively represents how the execution of an activity involves objects.

Definition 6 (Object Involvement Metrics). *Let L be an object-centric event log. For* $ot \in types(L)$ *and* $a \in acts(L)$, *we define three object involvement metrics of L in the following.*

- $absent_L(ot,a) = \frac{\#_L^0(ot,a)}{|events(L,a)|}$ *is the strength of ot's absence in a's execution.*
- $singular_L(ot,a) = \frac{\#_L^1(ot,a)}{|events(L,a)|}$ *is the strength of ot's singularity in a's execution.*
- $multiple_L(ot,a) = \frac{\#_L^*(ot,a)}{|events(L,a)|}$ *is the strength of ot's multiplicity in a's execution.*

All object involvement metrics produce values between 0 (weak) and 1 (strong). For L_1 in Table 1, $absent_{L_1}(Item,ec) = 1$, showing that items are not involved in the execution of ec. $singular_{L_1}(Order,po) = 1$ and $multiple_{L_1}(Item,po) = 1$, indicating that the execution of po involves only one order and multiple items.

Finally, a performance metric refers to a performance/frequency value related to the execution of an activity.

Definition 7 (Performance Metrics). *Let L be an object-centric event log. Let* $\mathbb{U}_{measure}$ *be the universe of performance/frequency measure names, e.g., the average waiting time. A performance metric of L,* $perf_L \in (acts(L) \times \mathbb{U}_{measure}) \nrightarrow \mathbb{R}$, *maps an activity and a performance/frequency measure to the value of the performance/frequency measure w.r.t. the activity.*

Note that we deliberately "underspecify" performance metrics, abstracting from the definition of individual performance metrics. Performance metrics may include the average number of objects per object type for the execution of an activity (e.g., the average number of *items* for placing an order), the average *sojourn time* for the execution of an activity (e.g., the average sojourn time for confirming an order), etc. For L_1 in Table 1, $perf_{L_1}(po, avg\text{-}num\text{-}items) = 3$, which denotes that the average number of *items* for po in L_1 is 3. Also, $perf_{L_1}(co, avg\text{-}sojourn\text{-}time) = 2$ h, which denotes that the average sojourn time for co in L_1 is 2 h.

5 Object-Centric Constraint Monitoring

In this section, we explain our proposed approach to object-centric constraint monitoring. To this end, we first introduce Object-Centric Constraint Graphs (OCCGs) to represent constraints. Next, we introduce a monitoring engine to evaluate the violation of constraints represented by OCCGs by analyzing OCELs.

5.1 Object-Centric Constraint Graphs (OCCGs)

An OCCG is a directed graph that consists of nodes and edges, as depicted in Fig. 2. Nodes consist of activities, object types, and *formulas*. A formula is a logical expression defined over performance measures of an activity using relational operators ($\leq, \geq, =$) as well as logical operators such as conjunction ($\wedge$), disjunction ($\vee$), and negation ($\neg$). Edges describe control-flow, object involvement, and performance edges.

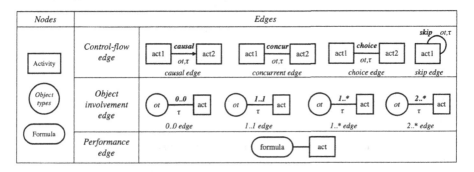

Fig. 2. Graphical notations of OCCGs. $act \in \mathbb{U}_{act}$, $ot \in \mathbb{U}_{ot}$, and $\tau \in [0, 1]$.

Definition 8 (Object-Centric Constraint Graph). *Let $F(X)$ be the set of all possible logical expressions with set X. Let $A \subseteq \mathbb{U}_{act}$, $OT \subseteq \mathbb{U}_{ot}$, and $\mathscr{F} \subseteq F(\mathbb{U}_{measure})$. Let $C = \{causal, concur, choice, skip\}$ be the set of control-flow labels and $I = \{0..0, 1..1, 1..*, 2..*\}$ the set of object involvement labels. An object-centric constraint graph is a graph $cg = (V, E_{flow}, E_{obj}, E_{perf}, l_c, l_i, l_\tau)$ where*

- *$V \subseteq A \cup OT \cup \mathscr{F}$ is a set of nodes,*
- *$E_{flow} \subseteq A \times OT \times A$ is a set of control-flow edges,*
- *$E_{obj} \subseteq OT \times A$ is a set of object involvement edges,*
- *$E_{perf} \subseteq \mathscr{F} \times A$ is a set of performance edges,*
- *$l_c \in E_{flow} \to C$ maps control-flow edges to control-flow labels such that, for any $(a, ot, b) \in E_{flow}$, if $l_c((a, ot, b)) = skip$, $a = b$,*
- *$l_i \in E_{obj} \to I$ maps object involvement edges to object involvement labels, and*
- *$l_\tau \in E_{flow} \cup E_{obj} \to [0, 1]$ maps control-flow and object involvement edges to thresholds.*

$\mathbb{U}_{cg}$ *denotes the set of all possible object-centric constraint graphs.*

Figure 3(a)-(k) introduces some example of OCCGs defined in an O2C process. For instance, Fig. 3(a) is formally represented as follows: $cg' = (V', E'_{flow}, \emptyset, \emptyset, l'_c, \emptyset, l'_\tau)$ where $V' = \{collect\ payment, send\ reminder\}$, $E'_{flow} = \{e_1 = (collect\ payment, Order, send\ reminder)\}$, $l'_c(e_1) = causal$, and $l'_\tau(e_1) = 0$.

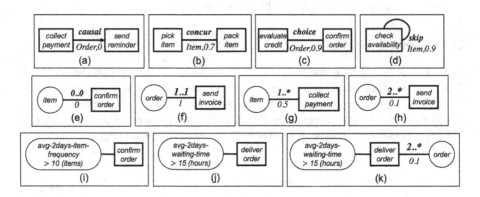

Fig. 3. Examples of object-centric constraint graphs.

We define the semantics of an OCCG with the notion of *violation*. An OCCG is *violated* in an OCEL if all constraints represented in its edges are satisfied.

Definition 9 (Semantics of object-centric constraint graphs). *Let L be an object-centric event log. An object-centric constraint graph* $cg = (V, E_{flow}, E_{obj}, E_{perf}, l_c, l_i, l_\tau)$ *is violated in L if*

1. *for any* $e = (a, ot, b) \in E_{flow}$ *s.t.* $ot \in types(L) \wedge a, b \in acts(L)$,
   - $causal_L(ot, a, b) > l_\tau(e)$ *if* $l_c(e) = causal$,
   - $concur_L(ot, a, b) > l_\tau(e)$ *if* $l_c(e) = concur$,
   - $choice_L(ot, a, b) > l_\tau(e)$ *if* $l_c(e) = choice$, *and*
   - $1 - \frac{\#_L(ot, \{a\})}{|objects(L, ot)|} > l_\tau(e)$ *if* $l_c(e) = skip$,
2. *for any* $e = (ot, a) \in E_{obj}$ *s.t.* $ot \in types(L) \wedge a \in acts(L)$,
   - $absent_L(ot, a) > l_\tau(e)$ *if* $l_i(e) = 0..0$,
   - $singular_L(ot, a) > l_\tau(e)$ *if* $l_i(e) = 1..1$,
   - $1 - absent_L(ot, a) > l_\tau(e)$ *if* $l_i(e) = 1..*$, *and*
   - $multiple_L(ot, a) > l_\tau(e)$ *if* $l_i(e) = 2..*$,
3. *for any* $(f, a) \in E_{perf}$ *s.t.* $a \in acts(L)$, *f evaluates to true w.r.t.* $perf_L$.

For instance, Fig. 3(a) is violated if *collect payment* is preceded by *send reminder* at all w.r.t. *Order*, Fig. 3(b) is violated if *pick item* and *pack item* are concurrently executed with the strength higher than 0.7 w.r.t. *Item*, Fig. 3(e) is violated if *confirm order* is executed without involving *Item* at all, Fig. 3(k) is violated if the average waiting time of the last two days for *deliver order* is longer than 15 h, and its execution involves multiple orders with the strength higher than 0.1, etc.

5.2 Monitoring Engine

A monitoring engine analyzes the violation of OCCGs by analyzing an OCEL.

Definition 10 (Monitoring Engine). *A monitoring engine monitor $\in \mathbb{U}_L \times \mathbb{U}_{cg} \rightarrow$ {true,false} is a function that maps an object-centric event log and an object-centric constraint graph to a Boolean value. For any $L \in \mathbb{U}_L$ and $cg \in \mathbb{U}_{cg}$, monitor$(L, cg) =$ true if cg is violated in L, and false, otherwise.*

We implement the monitoring engine by 1) computing the object-centric behavioral metrics of an event log and 2) evaluating the violation of OCCGs based on them. First, the derivation of ordering relation metrics and object involvement metrics is deterministic according to Definition 5 and Definition 6, respectively. However, the computation of performance metrics is non-trivial. In this work, we use the approach proposed in [11] to compute performance measures, such as *sojourn time, waiting time, service time, flow time, synchronization time, pooling time*, and *lagging time*, and frequency measures, such as *object count, object type count*, etc. Finally, using the object-centric behavioral metrics, we evaluate the violation of OCCGs according to Definition 9.

6 Implementation and Case Studies

This section presents the implementation of the approach presented in this paper and evaluates the feasibility of the approach by applying it to a production process and a P2P process of a real-life SAP ERP system.

6.1 Implementation

The approach presented in this work has been fully implemented as a web application[1] with a dedicated user interface. The following functions are supported:

- Importing OCELs in different formats, including OCEL JSON, OCEL XML, and CSV.
- Designing object-centric constraint graphs using graphical tools.
- Computing object-centric behavioral metrics of OCELs and evaluating the violation of object-centric constraint graphs based on the metrics.
- Visualizing monitoring results with detailed analysis results.

6.2 Case Study: Production Process

Using the implementation, we conduct a case study on a production process of a fictitious company supported by an SAP ERP system. The process involves four object types: *production order, reservation, purchase requisition*, and *purchase order*. Figure 4 shows a process model of the production process using Object-Centric Petri Nets (OCPNs) as a formalism. We refer readers to [3] for the details of OCPNs. We represent the following constraints using OCCGs:

---

[1] A demo video and sources: https://github.com/gyunamister/ProPPa.git.

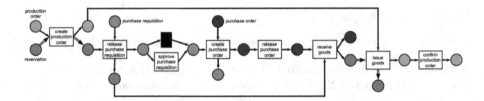

Fig. 4. Production process: First, a production order is created with a variable number of reservations (i.e., required materials). Next, a purchase requisition is released and approved. Afterward, a purchase order is created based on the purchase requisition. Once the order is released, the reservations are received and issued for production. Finally, the production order is confirmed.

- *Skipping Purchase Requisition Approval (PRA)*; A purchase requisition should not skip the approval step at all. Figure 5(a) represents the constraint.
- *No reservation for Purchase Requisition Approval (PRA)*; The execution of *approve purchase requisition* is supposed to include the corresponding reservation most of the time. Figure 5(b) represents the constraint.
- *Excessive reservations per Production Order (PO)*; The execution of *create production order* should not involve more than one reservation on average. Figure 5(c) represents the constraint.
- *Delayed Purchase Order Release (POR)*; The average sojourn time of *release purchase order* should be less than 15 days. Figure 5(d) represents the constraint.

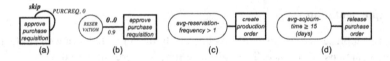

Fig. 5. OCCGs representing the constraints of the production process.

We monitor the process using three OCELs extracted from the SAP ERP system. Each event log contains events of different time windows; L_{prod}^{Jan22}, L_{prod}^{Feb22}, and L_{prod}^{Mar22} contain events of Jan., Feb., and Mar. 2022[2]. Table 2 shows the monitoring result. For instance, *no reservation for PRA* and *excessive reservations per PO* are violated for the three months. *Skipping PRA* only is violated in the last two months, while *delayed RPO* is violated only for Feb. 2022.

---

[2] Event logs are publicly available at https://github.com/gyunamister/ProPPa.git.

Table 2. Monitoring results of the production process. ✓ denotes the violation.

Constraints	Event log		
	L_{prod}^{Jan22}	L_{prod}^{Feb22}	L_{prod}^{Mar22}
Skipping PRA		✓	✓
No reservation for PRA	✓	✓	✓
Excessive reservations per PO	✓	✓	✓
Delayed POR		✓	

6.3 Case Study: Procure-to-Pay (P2P) Process

Next, we explain a case study on the P2P process. The process involves five object types: *purchase requisition*, *material*, *purchase order*, *goods receipt*, and *invoice*. Figure 6 shows a process model of the process.

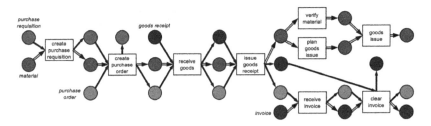

Fig. 6. P2P process: First, a purchase requisition is created with multiple materials. Next, a purchase order is created based on the purchase requisition and materials. Afterward, the materials are received and a goods receipt is issued. Then, the materials are verified and issued, and concurrently the invoice for the purchase order is received and cleared.

We represent the following constraints using OCCGs:

- *Concurrency between Verify Material (VM) and Plan Goods Issue (PGI)*; VM and PGI are usually not supposed to be concurrently executed. Figure 7(a) represents the constraint.
- *Clearance of multiple invoices*; The execution of *clear invoice* should not involve multiple invoices at all. Figure 7(b) represents the constraint.
- *Excessive materials per Purchase Order (PO)*; The execution of *create purchase order* should involve less than five materials on average. Figure 7(c) represents the constraint.
- *Delayed Purchase Order Creation (POC)*; The average sojourn time of *create purchase order* should be less than three days. Figure 7(d) represents the constraint.

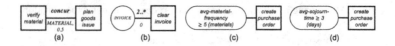

Fig. 7. OCCGs representing the constraints of the P2P process.

We monitor the process using three OCELs extracted from the SAP ERP system. Each event log contains events of different time windows; L^1_{p2p} starting from 01-Aug-2021 and ending at 14-Oct-2021, L^2_{p2p} starting from 15-Oct-2021 and ending at 18-Jan-2022, and L^3_{p2p} starting from 01-Feb-2022 and ending at 16-May-2022. Table 3 shows the monitoring result. *Concurrency between VM and PGI* and *clearance of multiple invoices* are only violated in the first two time windows, whereas *Excessive materials per PO* and *delayed POC* are only violated in the last time window.

Table 3. Monitoring results of the P2P process. ✓ denotes the violation.

Constraints	Event log		
	L^1_{p2p}	L^2_{p2p}	L^3_{p2p}
Concurrency between VM and PGI	✓	✓	
Clearance of multiple invoices	✓	✓	
Excessive materials per PO			✓
Delayed POC			✓

7 Conclusion

In this paper, we proposed an approach to process-level object-centric constraint monitoring. To this end, we first introduced object-centric behavioral metrics and defined OCCGs using the metrics. The proposed monitoring engine evaluates the constraints represented by OCCGs by analyzing OCELs. We have implemented the approach as a Web application and discussed two case studies.

This paper has several limitations. The suggested object-centric constraint graphs only represent the constraints selectively introduced in this work. More advanced constraints are not considered, e.g., ordering relations with the temporality (e.g., eventual or direct causality). Also, constraint graphs do not support timed constraints, e.g., no involvement of an object type during a specific period of time. In future work, we plan to extend the proposed approach to support more complete set of constraints, including more advanced constraints. Another interesting direction of future work is to apply the proposed approach to real-life business processes.

Acknowledgment. The authors would like to thank the Alexander von Humboldt (AvH) Stiftung for funding this research.

References

1. Aalst, W.M.P.: Object-centric process mining: dealing with divergence and convergence in event data. In: Ölveczky, P.C., Salaün, G. (eds.) SEFM 2019. LNCS, vol. 11724, pp. 3–25. Springer, Cham (2019). https://doi.org/10.1007/978-3-030-30446-1_1
2. van der Aalst, W.M.P.: Process Mining - Data Science in Action. Springer, Heidelbeerg (2016). https://doi.org/10.1007/978-3-662-49851-4
3. van der Aalst, W.M.P., Berti, A.: Discovering object-centric Petri nets. Fundam. Inform. **175**(1–4), 1–40 (2020)
4. Adams, J.N., van der Aalst, W.M.P.: Precision and fitness in object-centric process mining. In: Ciccio, C.D., Francescomarino, C.D., Soffer, P. (eds.) ICPM 2021, pp. 128–135. IEEE (2021)
5. Awad, A., et al.: Runtime detection of business process compliance violations: an approach based on anti patterns. In: Wainwright, R.L., et al. (eds.) 30th ACM SAC, pp. 1203–1210 (2015)
6. Esser, S., Fahland, D.: Multi-dimensional event data in graph databases. J. Data Semant. **10**(1–2), 109–141 (2021)
7. Indiono, C., Mangler, J., Fdhila, W., Rinderle-Ma, S.: Rule-based runtime monitoring of instance-spanning constraints in process-aware information systems. In: Debruyne, C., et al. (eds.) OTM 2016. LNCS, vol. 10033, pp. 381–399. Springer, Cham (2016). https://doi.org/10.1007/978-3-319-48472-3_22
8. Ly, L.T., Maggi, F.M., Montali, M., Rinderle-Ma, S., van der Aalst, W.M.P.: Compliance monitoring in business processes: functionalities, application, and tool-support. Inf. Syst. **54**, 209–234 (2015)
9. Maggi, F.M., Westergaard, M., Montali, M., van der Aalst, W.M.P.: Runtime verification of LTL-based declarative process models. In: Khurshid, S., Sen, K. (eds.) RV 2011. LNCS, vol. 7186, pp. 131–146. Springer, Heidelberg (2012). https://doi.org/10.1007/978-3-642-29860-8_11
10. Park, G., van der Aalst, W.M.P.: Action-oriented process mining: bridging the gap between insights and actions. Progr. Artif. Intell. 1–22 (2022). https://doi.org/10.1007/s13748-022-00281-7
11. Park, G., Adams, J.N., van der Aalst, W.M.P.: OPerA: Object-centric performance analysis. In: Ralyté, J., Chakravarthy, S., Mohania, M., Jeusfeld, M.A., Karlapalem, K. (eds.) ER 2022. LNCS, vol. 13607, pp. 281–292. Springer, Cham (2022). https://doi.org/10.1007/978-3-031-17995-2_20
12. Ramezani, E., Fahland, D., van der Aalst, W.M.P.: Where did i misbehave? Diagnostic information in compliance checking. In: Barros, A., Gal, A., Kindler, E. (eds.) BPM 2012. LNCS, vol. 7481, pp. 262–278. Springer, Heidelberg (2012). https://doi.org/10.1007/978-3-642-32885-5_21
13. Weidlich, M., Ziekow, H., Mendling, J., Günther, O., Weske, M., Desai, N.: Event-based monitoring of process execution violations. In: Rinderle-Ma, S., Toumani, F., Wolf, K. (eds.) BPM 2011. LNCS, vol. 6896, pp. 182–198. Springer, Heidelberg (2011). https://doi.org/10.1007/978-3-642-23059-2_16

Aggregating Event Knowledge Graphs for Task Analysis

Eva L. Klijn[✉][iD], Felix Mannhardt[iD], and Dirk Fahland[iD]

Eindhoven University of Technology, Eindhoven, The Netherlands
{e.l.klijn,f.mannhardt,d.fahland}@tue.nl

Abstract. Aggregation of event data is a key operation in process mining for revealing behavioral features of processes for analysis. It has primarily been studied over sequences of events in event logs. The data model of event knowledge graphs enables new analysis questions requiring new forms of aggregation. We focus on analyzing task executions in event knowledge graphs. We show that existing aggregation operations are inadequate and propose new aggregation operations, formulated as query operators over labeled property graphs. We show on the BPIC'17 dataset that the new aggregation operations allow gaining new insights into differences in task executions, actor behavior, and work division.

Keywords: Knowledge graph · Aggregation · Tasks

1 Introduction

Processes are executed by human actors and automated resources performing work on the cases of the process. For example, multiple employees of a bank jointly check a credit application, create (one or more) loan offers, contact the client for additional information, to finally decline or prepare a contract. Each case evolves by executing actions according to the process' control-flow [1]. Human actors (or resources) performing the actions often structure their work further by performing multiple actions on the same case before handing the case to the next actor, e.g., creating and sending two loan offers to the same client; such a larger unit of work is called *task* [13,19]. Routines research investigates thereby which patterns arise when actors jointly structure and divide work in a process into (recurring) tasks [10].

Task execution patterns can be identified from process event data when using graph-based data models. We can jointly model the synchronization of classical traces of all process cases and the traces of all actors working across all cases in an *event knowledge graph* [8]. Any sub-graph of this graph where an actor follows multiple events in a case corresponds to an execution of some task [13], as we recall in Sect. 2. Sub-graphs on real-life event logs can be identified through querying [14], e.g., 98% of the BPIC'17 [6] events are part of a larger task execution. But the structure of how task execution sub-graphs are related has not been described.

A key operation for describing structures in event data is *aggregation*. As the model of event knowledge graphs is novel, only limited aggregation operations have been proposed, but they either only aggregate events to actions [7], or task execution

© The Author(s) 2023
M. Montali et al. (Eds.): ICPM 2022 Workshops, LNBIP 468, pp. 493–505, 2023.
https://doi.org/10.1007/978-3-031-27815-0_36

sub-graphs to higher-level events [13]. We show in Sect. 3 that understanding tasks in a process requires (R1) to aggregate sets of similar higher-level events to suitable constructs while preserving their behavioral context, (R2) to aggregate events underlying higher-level events to study variations among actions, and (R3) that either aggregation requires parameters for filtering and for controlling the aggregation level.

We then propose in Sect. 4 two new parameterized aggregation operations, formalized as queries over event knowledge graphs, that address (R1–R3) and demonstrate in Sect. 5 their effectiveness for summarizing task executions of real-life event data in new kinds of global and local process models [4]. We compare our results to related work in Sect. 6 and conclude in Sect. 7.

2   Preliminaries

A process-aware system can record an action execution as an *event* in an event log. We require that each event records at least the *action* that occurred, the *time* of occurrence and at least two different entity identifiers of entities involved in the event: a data object or *case* in which the event occurred, and the *resource* (or actor) executing the action. An event can also record additional *attributes* describing the event further.

Event Knowledge Graphs. A classical event log orders all events by sequential traces according to a single entity identifier (also called case id). In contrast, an *event knowledge graph* (EKG) orders events wrt. multiple different entity identifiers [8]. EKGs are based on *labeled property graphs* (LPG), a graph-based data model supported by graph DB systems [3] that describes concepts as nodes and various relationships between them as edges. In an LPG $G = (X, Y, \Lambda, \#)$, each node $x \in X$ and each relationship $y \in Y$ with edge $\overrightarrow{y} = (x, x')$ from x to x' has a label $\ell \in \Lambda$, denoted $x \in \ell$ or $y \in \ell$ that describes the *concept* represented by x or y. $\#_{(a)(x)} = v$ and $\#_{(a)(y)} = v$ denotes that property a of x or y has value v; we use and $x.a = v$ and $y.a = v$ as short-hand.

In an EKG, each event and each entity (i.e., each data object or resource) is represented by a node with label *Event* and *Entity*, respectively. Each node $e \in Event$ defines *e.action* and *e.time*; each node $n \in Entity$ defines *n.type* and *n.id*. While EKGs allow to model arbitrarily many entity types, we subsequently restrict ourselves to EKGs with *two* entity types: *case* (any data object or a classical case identifier) and *resource* (the actors working in the process). Figure 1 shows an example graph: each square node is an *Event* node; each circle is an *Entity* node of the corresponding type (blue for *case*, red for *resource*). An EKG has relationship labels:

- *corr* (correlation): $y \in corr$, $\overrightarrow{y} = (e, n)$ iff event $e \in Event$ is correlated to entity $n \in Entity$; we write $(e, n) \in corr$ as short-hand.
- *df* (directly-follows): $y \in df$, $\overrightarrow{y} = (e, e')$ iff events e, e' are correlated to the same entity n $(e, n), (e', n) \in corr$, $e.time < e'.time$ and there is no other event $(e'', n) \in corr$ with $e.time < e''.time < e'.time$; we write $(e, e')^{n.type} \in df$ as short-hand, i.e., $(e, e')^c$ for entity type case and $(e, e')^r$ for resource.

In Fig. 1, *corr* relationships are shown as dashed edges, e.g., $e1, e2, e3, e4, e5$ are correlated to case $c3$ and $e3, e4, e9, e10$ are correlated to resource $a5$. *df*-relationships are

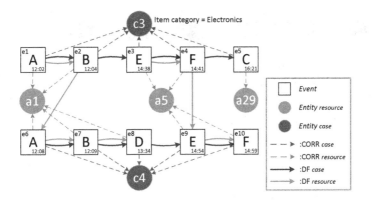

Fig. 1. Event knowledge graph.

shown as solid edges. The *df*-relationships between the events correlated to the same entity form a *df-path* for that entity; the graph in Fig. 1 has 2 df-paths for case entities, e.g., $\sigma_{c3} = \langle (e1, e2)^c, (e2, e3)^c, (e3, e4)^c, (e4, e5)^c \rangle$ and 3 df-paths for resource entities, e.g., $\sigma_{a5} = \langle (e3, e4)^r, (e4, e9)^r, (e9, e10)^r \rangle$. See [7] for details of how to create an EKG G from classical event data sources through graph DB queries.

Task Instance Sub-graphs. Where individual events record the execution of an atomic action, a resource often performs multiple subsequent actions in the same case. This is called a *task* [19]. A *task execution* materializes in an EKG as sub-graph, where a case and a resource df-path synchronize for several subsequent events [13]. While a variety of such task subgraphs can be characterized [13], we here recall the most simple one: a sub-graph of events $\{e_1, ..., e_k\}$ and adjacent df-edges that contains (1) exactly one (part of a) case df-path $\langle ... (e_1, e_2)^c, ..., (e_{k-1}, e_k)^c ... \rangle$ for a case c and (2) exactly one (part of an) actor df-path $\langle ... (e_1, e_2)^r, ..., (e_{k-1}, e_k)^r ... \rangle$ for an actor r, i.e., both paths synchronize over the same subsequent events. In Fig. 1, subgraphs of events that meet these criteria are $\{e_1, e_2\}$, $\{e_3, e_4\}$, $\{e_5\}$, $\{e_6, e_7, e_8\}$ and $\{e_9, e_{10}\}$. Each such subgraph ti describes one *task instance*. These sub-graphs $\{G_1, ..., G_k\} = TI(G)$ can be queried from G by (1) aggregating any two parallel df-edges $(e, e')^c$ and $(e, e')^r$ into a "joint" edge (e, e') with label *df-joint* and (2) then querying for maximal df-joint paths; see [13] for details.

3   Existing Aggregation Queries and Requirements

We first review existing aggregation operations on EKGs and present them systematically as three different types of aggregation queries. We then analyze their properties and shortcomings for summarizing task instances in (large) EKGs.

Node Aggregation. The first basic aggregation query $Agg_{nodes}(a, X', \ell, \ell')$ on an EKG $G = (X, Y, \Lambda, \#)$ proposed in [7] *aggregates nodes* $X' \subseteq X$ *by property* a *into concept* ℓ as follows: (1) query all values $V = \{x.a \mid x \in X'\}$, (2) for each value $v \in V$ add a new node $x_v \in \ell$ to G with label ℓ and set $x_v.id = v$, $x_v.type = a$, (3) for each $x \in X'$, add new relationship $y \in \ell'$ with label ℓ' from x to x_v, $\overrightarrow{y} = (x, x_v)$.

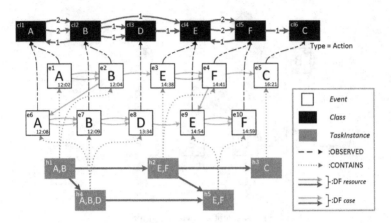

Fig. 2. Aggregation of the EKG of Fig. 1 by *action* into *Class* nodes (top), and by task instance sub-graphs into *TaskInstance* nodes (bottom).

For example, applying $Agg_{nodes}(action, Event, Class, observed)$ on the graph in Fig. 1 creates one new event *Class* node for each value of the *Event* nodes' *action* property, i.e., nodes $cl1, \ldots, cl6$ shown in Fig. 2, and links each event to the event class that was observed when the event occurred.

Event Sub-graph Aggregation. The query $Agg_{sub}(\mathcal{G}, \ell, \ell')$ proposed in [13] *aggregates given sub-graphs* $\mathcal{G} = \{G_1, \ldots, G_k\}$ *over Event nodes of G into high-level events with label ℓ as follows:* (1) the sub-graphs $\mathcal{G}$ have been obtained by a previous query, e.g., $\mathcal{G} = TI(G)$, see Sect. 2, (2) for each $G' \in \mathcal{G}$, create a new high-level event node $h_{G'} \in \ell$ with label ℓ and set $h_{G'}.time_{start} = \min\{e.time \mid e \in G'\}$ and $h_{G'}.time_{end} = \max\{e.time \mid e \in G'\}$, and (3) for each $e \in G'$ add new relationship $y \in \ell'$ with label ℓ' from $h_{G'}$ to e, $\overrightarrow{y} = (h_{G'}, e)$. Although $\ell \neq Event$, we interpret each new node $h_{G'}$ as a high-level event with duration as it has a start and an end timestamp.

For example, applying $Agg_{sub}(TI(G), TaskInstance, contains)$ on the graph in Fig. 1 materializes five task instance sub-graphs as *TaskInstance* high-level event nodes $h1, \ldots, h5$ shown in Fig. 2, and links each event to the *TaskInstance* in which it is contained.

Directly-Follows Aggregation. The query $Agg_{df}(t, \ell, \ell')$ proposed in [7] aggregates (or lifts) df-relationships between *Event* nodes for a particular entity type t to ℓ nodes along the ℓ' relationships as follows: (1) for any two nodes $x, x' \in \ell$ query the set $df_{x,x'}^t$ of all df-edges $(e, e')^t \in df$ where events $e, e' \in Event$ are related to x, x' via $y, y' \in \ell'$, $\overrightarrow{y} = (x, e)$, $\overrightarrow{y'} = (x', e')$, (2) if $df_{x,x'}^t \neq \emptyset$ create a new df-relationship $y^* \in df$, $\overrightarrow{y^*} = (x, x')$, $y^*.type = t$ and set $y^*.count = |df_{x,x'}^t|$. The variant $Agg_{df}^{\neq}(t, \ell, \ell')$ of the above query that requires $x \neq x'$ was proposed in [13].

For example, first aggregating events to *Class* nodes (as explained above), and then applying $Agg_{df}(t, Class, observed)$ for $t \in \{Case, Resource\}$ on the graph in Fig. 1 results in the df-edges between $cl1, \ldots, cl6$ shown in Fig. 2. For instance, $(cl2, cl1)^r$ originates from $(e2, e6)^r$ while $(cl1, cl2)^c$ originates from $(e1, e2)^c$

and $(e6, e7)^c$. Likewise, aggregating to *TaskInstance* nodes and then applying $Agg_{df}^{\neq}(t, TaskInstance, contains)$ for $t \in \{Case, Resource\}$ results in the df-edges between $h1, \ldots, h5$ shown in Fig. 2. For instance, $(h1, h4)^r$ originates from $(e2, e6)^r$.

Extensions. These basic aggregation queries can be extended for specific use cases. For instance, every task instance sub-graph is essentially a path $e_1, \ldots, e_k$ over event nodes. Aggregation into a *TaskInstance* node h_{ti} then allows to set property $h_{ti}.name = e_1.action, \ldots, e_k.action$ [13] describing the sequence of actions executed in the task, as shown in Fig 2. All these queries are implemented as Cypher queries over the graph DB system Neo4j [14].

Properties, Shortcomings, and Requirements. Agg_{nodes} together with Agg_{df} constructs directly-follows graphs where edges distinguish between multiple types of entities [8], i.e., nodes and edges are on the level of actions. Agg_{sub} together with $Agg_{df}^{\neq}$ constructs a "higher level" event graph, i.e., nodes and edges are on the level of *sets of events* but not on the level of actions.

Applying the aggregations in this way does not suffice to adequately summarize the process "as a whole" for analyzing task instances and tasks within a (larger) process. On one hand, task instances themselves are similar to events as they describe the specific execution of a task, i.e., multiple actions in a single case by a single resource. On the other hand, task instances are also not a hierarchical abstraction of the events wrt. actions: multiple different task instances overlap in their actions. The queries discussed so far do not take this nature of task instances into account.

In principle, the aim is to summarize the task instances (on the level of sets of *Event*s) as actual tasks (on the level of sets of actions or event *Class*es), and to lift the df-relationships accordingly.

A naive approach would be to aggregate *TaskInstance* nodes to *Task* nodes by their $h_{ti}.name$ property, i.e., $Agg_{nodes}(name, TaskInstance, Task, observed)$. However, as task instances are sequences of multiple actions, two different $h_{ti}.name$ values may be *different variants* of the same task. For example, $h1$ and $h4$ in Fig. 2 with $h1.name = A, B$ and $h4.name = A, B, D$ might be variants of the same task. Depending on the analysis, it may be desirable to (**R1**) aggregate *TaskInstance* nodes with similar (but not identical) *name* properties into the same *Task* node, which is not possible with the available queries.

If multiple task instances are considered as variants of the same task, it will be useful to summarize all the task instances on the level of actions to study the "contents" and "variability" of executions of a task. We seek to (**R2**) aggregate events and directly-follows relations that belong to similar *TaskInstance* nodes.

The presence of multiple types of DF-relationships (per entity type) increases the (visual) complexity of the aggregated graphs (see Fig. 2 (top)). Depending on the analysis, it may be desirable to (**R3**) control the aggregation through filtering and refinement to obtain more specific summaries in the form of smaller, simpler, or more precise aggregated graphs.

4   Queries for Summarizing Task Instances

To address requirements (R1-R3), we propose new queries for aggregating task instances in different ways, and discuss how to configure and combine aggregation queries with other queries to obtain specific graphs. In the following, let G be event knowledge graph $G = (X, Y, \Lambda, \#)$ after applying Agg_{sub} and $Agg_{df}^{\neq}$ as defined in Sect. 3, i.e., the graph as *Event* nodes and *TaskInstance* nodes connected by df-edges.

4.1   Aggregating Similar Task Instances

Addressing (R1) requires to (a) identify which task instances are *similar*, and (b) aggregating task instance nodes considered as similar.

The specific criteria when two *TaskInstance* nodes are similar depend on the concrete process, data, and analysis use case. For the scope of this work, we therefore assume an "oracle query" $O(h) = i$ that determines $O(h_{ti}) = O(h'_{ti})$ iff two task instances h_{ti} and h'_{ti} belong to the same task. $O(h)$ could, for instance, be implemented by agglomerative clustering wrt. the $h_{ti}.name$ values (with suitable parameters) [15].

Given such an oracle O, the query $Agg_{sim}(O, X')$ aggregates *TaskInstance* nodes $X' \subseteq TaskInstance$ wrt. oracle O to *Class* nodes as follows: (1) for each $h_{ti} \in X'$ set $h_{ti}.Task = O(h_{ti})$, (2) aggregate the *TaskInstance* nodes by property $h_{ti}.Task$ using $Agg_{nodes}(Task, TaskInstance, Class, observed)$ of Sect. 3.

For example, applying $Agg_{sim}(O, TaskInstance)$ on the graph in Fig. 2 creates the *Class* nodes $cl7, cl8, cl9$ of type *Task* shown in Fig. 3 (top). Further properties of a *Task* node t can be set based on the use case, e.g., setting $t.name$ as the set of (most frequent) $e.action$ of events *contained* in the h_{ti} nodes that *observed* t.

To also lift df-relationships from *TaskInstance* nodes to the *Class* nodes of type *Task* we have to generalize Agg_{df} to also consider high-level events such as *TaskInstance* and not just "regular" *Events*. The query $Agg_{df}(Z', t, \ell, \ell')$ aggregates df-relationships between nodes Z' for a particular entity type t to ℓ nodes along the ℓ' relationships as follows: (1) for any two nodes $x, x' \in \ell$ query the set $df_{x,x'}^t$ of all df-edges $(z, z')^t \in df$ where nodes $z, z' \in Z'$ are related to x, x' via $y, y' \in \ell'$, $\overrightarrow{y} = (z, x)$, $\overrightarrow{y'} = (z', x')$, (2) if $df_{x,x'}^t \neq \emptyset$ create a new df-relationship $y^* \in df$, $\overrightarrow{y} = (x, x')$, $y^*.type = t$ and set $y^*.count = |df_{x,x'}^t|$.

Applying $Agg_{df}(TaskInstance, t, Class, observed)$ for $t \in Case, Resource$ in our running example yields the df-edges between $cl7, cl8, cl9$ shown in Fig. 3 (top).

The sub-graph over the *Class* nodes of type *Task* and created in this way is a directly-follows graph on the level of tasks (instead of the DFG on the level of actions obtained in Sect. 3). We call this DFG an inter-task DFG to distinguish it from the DFG describing behavior *within* a task as we discuss next.

4.2   Aggregating Events Within Similar Task Instances

To address (R2) we need to aggregate only those events that are *contained* within task instances of the same task. Two previous aggregation operations already materialized this information. Each event e is connected to one task $t \in Class, t.type = Task$ via

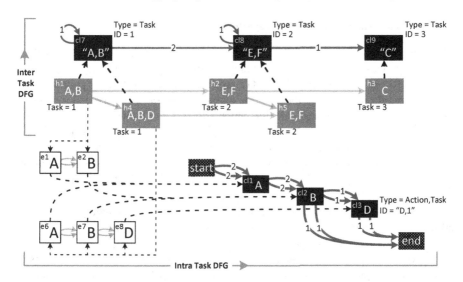

Fig. 3. Task instances aggregated into task classes for deriving inter-task dfGs (top). Subset of lower-level events aggregated into event classes for deriving intra-task dfGs (bottom).

$(h, e) \in contains$ and $(h, t) \in observed$ (created by Agg_{sub} of Sect. 3 and Agg_{sim} of Sect. 4.1, e.g., $(h1, e1)$ and $(h1, cl7)$ in Fig. 2).

Using these edges to task t as context, we adapt the node aggregation of Sect. 3 to be local to a task t. But as the same action may occur in different instances of different tasks, we have to distinguish to which task an action belongs. This requires to define an *event classifier* query $class(e)$ which returns for each event a value based on the properties of e or neighboring nodes. Agg_{node} of Sect. 3 used $class(e) = e.X$ for some property name X. To distinguish the task, we define event classifier $class_{task}(e) = (e.action, task(e))$ with $task(e) = i$ iff $(e, h_{ti}) \in contains, (h_{ti}, t) \in observed, t.ID = i$. Note that by basing $class_{task}(e)$ on the *Class* node, we become independent of the specific oracle O used to identify tasks.

The generalized aggregation query $Agg_{nodes}(class, X', \ell, \ell')$ on an EKG $G = (X, Y, \Lambda, \#)$ differs from $Agg_{nodes}(a, X', \ell, \ell')$ in the first step: (1) query all values $V = \{class(x) \mid x \in X'\}$, (2) for each value $v \in V$ add a new node $x_v \in \ell$ to G with label ℓ and set $x_v.id = v$, $x_v.type = class$, (3) for each $x \in X'$, add new relationship $y \in \ell'$ with label ℓ' from x to x_v, $\overrightarrow{y} = (x, x_v)$.

We then can aggregate the events per task $t \in Class, t.type = Task$ as follows. Query the events $E_t = \{e \in Event \mid \exists h(e, h) \in contains, (h, t) \in observed\}$ and aggregate by $Agg_{nodes}(class_{task}, E_t, Class, observes)$. Applying this query in our example for $cl7$ (Task with ID=1), we obtained the class nodes $cl1, cl2, cl3$ shown in Fig. 2 (bottom). The df-edges can be aggregated using Agg_{df} of Sect. 4.1.

In this way, Fig. 3 (bottom) shows how events $e1, e2, e6, e7, e8$ are aggregated to an "intra-task directly-follows graph" describing the local behavior within a task in one model. Analysts can use such an intra-task DFG to understand task contents and how homogeneous the task instances assigned to the same task are, e.g., to evaluate whether the chosen oracle O is of sufficient quality.

4.3   Parameterized, Specific Aggregation

The aggregations of Sect. 4.1 and 4.2 can result in a complex graph over two behavioral dimensions that is difficult to visualize and possibly not specific to answer an analysis question. To obtain more specific DFGs, we introduce the following parameters: (1) **node aggregation** by using more specific classifiers for *TaskInstance* nodes, (2) **filtering** by using different criteria to decide which *TaskInstance* nodes to keep and (3) **edge aggregation** by selecting which df-edges to aggregate. Each parameter is defined by the properties of the entire event knowledge graph, including the underlying events.

(1) We can refine the aggregation of *TaskInstance* nodes to *Class* nodes using a classifier over multiple properties. For example, the following classifier distinguishes tasks per actor: $class_{T \times R}(h) = (h.cluster, resource(h))$ with $resource(h) = a$ iff $(e, h) \in contains, e.resource = a$. The df-relationships are then aggregated per actor, allowing to compare different actors wrt. their behavior over tasks.

(2) To obtain a DFG for specific parts of the data, the *Agg* queries allow to limit the set of nodes to be aggregated to a subset $TI' \subseteq TaskInstance$. We can construct TI' by another query. For instance: (1) only $h_{ti} \in TaskInstance$ nodes correlated to an entity based on a specific property, e.g., in Fig. 2, related to resource entities where $n.ID = a5$, i.e., $h2$ and $h5$, or case entities where $n.item\_category =$ Electronics, i.e., $h1$, $h2$ and $h3$; or (2) based on temporal properties, e.g., only h_{ti} nodes in cases that end before 15:00, i.e., $(h_{ti}, e) \in contains, (e, n) \in corr, n.type = case$ and all events $(e', n) \in corr$ have $e'.time < 15 : 00$.

(3) We can limit the df-relationships to aggregate to a subset $df' \subseteq df$ determined by structural or temporal properties in the same way as in (2). Note that if df' is chosen independent of TI' there may be no aggregated df-edges between *Class* nodes.

Analysis typically requires to understand where behavior starts or ends. We summarize how often a *Class* node cl is a start node of the DFG (for entity type n) by querying the number of $h_{ti} \in TI'$ nodes with $(h_{ti}, cl) \in observed$ and no incoming df-edge $(h'_{ti}, h_{ti})^n \in df'$. For example, in Fig. 3, $cl7$ is start node once for r and twice for c. Correspondingly for end nodes. We visualize this as edges from/to artificial inserted start/end nodes.

5   Demonstration

We implemented the queries we proposed in Sect. 4 as naive, non-optimized Cypher queries invoked via parameterized Python scripts[1] on the graph database Neo4j. We applied the queries on the event knowledge graph [7] of the BPIC' 17 data [6] to evaluate and demonstrate the feasibility of the queries for obtaining new insight into the process on the level of tasks and task instances.

First, we materialized the task instance sub-graphs as *TaskInstance* nodes (see Sect. 2) which resulted in 171,200 task instances with 1,208 task variants (unique $h_{ti}.name$ values). Naively aggregating the *TaskInstance* nodes by $h_{ti}.name$ would lead to a graph too large to understand. We removed *TaskInstance* nodes describing variants occurring < 10 times (1%) and of length $= 1$ (6%). We then implemented a

---

[1] Available at: https://zenodo.org/record/6727896#.YrYcjXZBwuU.

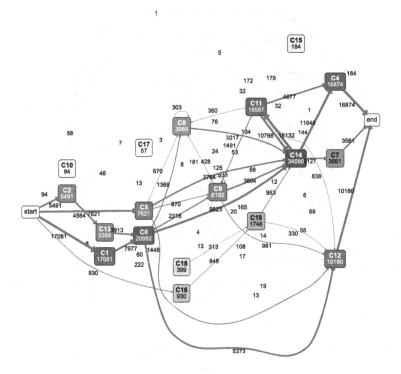

Fig. 4. Inter-task DFG over Task nodes obtained by aggregating case-df-edges wrt similar task instance sub-graphs.

simple oracle O for identifying tasks of similar task instances by agglomerative clustering as this method fits the bottom-up aggregation of instances into tasks. We used Euclidean distance between $h_{ti}.name$ as distance metric and chose the number of clusters by maximizing the silhouette index, see [15]. Applying $Agg_{sim}(O, TaskInstance)$ (Sect. 4.1) resulted in 20 *Class* nodes of type *Task*. Aggregating all case-df-edges results in the DFG shown in Fig. 4. For space limitations, we can explain only the contents of a few selected tasks. For example, C1,C2,C5 show the 3 most frequent ways actors group actions differently into tasks at the start of the process, with C1 containing actions *A_Create, A_Concept, W_Compl appl+Start*; C2 containing *A_Create, A_Submit, W_Handle Lds+Start* and while C5 contains more actions *A_Create, A_Concept, W_Compl appl+Start, A_Accept, O_Create, W_Call offers+Start, A_Complete*. Cases starting with C1 and C2 later go through C0 containing *A_Accept, O_Create, O_Sent, W_Compl appl+E, W_Call offers+S, A_Complete*, i.e., task C5 is done by a single actor combining tasks C1 and C0 done by two different actors.

We then evaluated whether aggregating events of task instances of the same task is effective to understand the contents of a task. We applied $Agg_{nodes}(class_{task}, E_t, Class, observes)$ of Sect. 4.2 for all tasks and obtained a corresponding intra-task DFG. Figure 5 shows the intra-task DFG of C14 (the most frequent task after C5 and

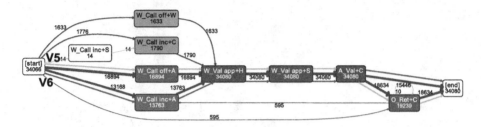

Fig. 5. Intra-task DFG of C14 with variants V5 and V6.

C0) highlighting two different variants of the task that differ in the actions executed. The intra-task DFGs of other tasks revealed also variability in the order of actions executed.

We then explored the more advanced capabilities of parameterizing aggregation with further queries explained in Sect. 4.3. We chose to compare how 2 different actors work and collaborate on a day-to-day basis in terms of tasks. For this, we constructed a composition of multiple actor DFGs interconnected by cases as follows: (1) classifier $class_{T \times R}(h)$ defined in Sect. 4.3, i.e., create class nodes task and actor, (2) TI' contains only *TaskInstance* nodes related to one of two specific resources, (3) include a resource df-edge $(h, h')^r \in df'$ only if $h.time_{end}$ and $h'.time_{start}$ occur on the same day, and include any case df-edge in df'.

Figure 6 shows an example of a specialized DFG; it summarizes for each actor the behavior executed over a day (no df-edges to a task on the next day) and the aggregated case DF-edges show how often an actor handed a case from one task to another actor with another task. U29 was working on 100 d while U113 worked on 43 d; U20 performs 4 tasks while U113 performs 3 tasks; both work on C4 and C8 but otherwise do disjoint work and hand work over between C11 and C14 and from C14 to C4.

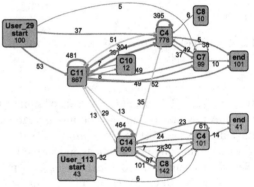

Fig. 6. Inter-task DFGs showing behavior of users 29 and 113 and handovers.

Our naive queries took 1.5 h to build the graph with similar tasks materialized as *Class* nodes and about 1 m for computing each of the DFGs, including filtering on an Intel i7 CPU @ 2.2 GHz machine with 32 GB RAM.

6 Related Work

We discuss how our findings relate to other works on aggregation and analyzing tasks and actor behavior in terms of sub-sequences or patterns in cases and/or actor behavior.

Kumar and Lui [16] analyze tasks by detecting frequent collaboration patterns in sequences of actor behavior; but the contents of work between hand-offs is disregarded and not the whole process can be summarized. Yang et al. [20] discover organizational models including grouping of resources and their relation to execution contexts; but an execution context consists of single activities disregarding work that may be aggregated into larger tasks. Hulzen et al. [11] cluster activity instance to activity instance archetypes related to actors; this technique corresponds to the oracle for identifying similar task executions used as input for aggregation in Sect. 4. Delcoucq et al. [5] aggregate frequent, gapped behavior of an actor over the entire trace into a local process model of a task; but the resulting models are not related to the case making it impossible to study the behavioral context in the case or to other actors as we allow. Jooken et al. [12] mine resource interactions as collaboration sessions of actors working on the same data objects within a specific time-window from multi-entity event table; the collaborations are then aggregated into a social network. This approach is an alternative to task instance querying [13] used in this paper, but their approach does not model task executions in the context of process executions allowing fewer types of aggregations compared to our approach. Leoni and Dündar [18] use waiting time between events as heuristic to group consecutive low-level events into "batch sessions" and cluster them using the most frequently executed activity in a cluster as label; our aggregation queries preserve the structure of task variants in the graph. Several task mining approaches [2, 17] aim to discover task executions by segmenting an event log of desktop interactions such that repetitive patterns or pre-identified routines are found similar to our previous work [15]. However, such tasks are limited to a single actor ignoring collaboration and do not investigate the process context. Finally, Genga et al. [9] used frequent sub-graph mining with SUBDUE to summarize graph-based event data; the approach enforces a hierarchical structure and cannot be configured to a desired abstraction level, e.g., task instances or specific subsets. In contrast, the query-based aggregation operations proposed in this paper offer the required flexibility.

7   Conclusion

We showed how to adapt and generalize existing aggregation queries on event knowledge graphs to preserve the intermediate abstraction level of *task instances* being multiple events executed by the one actor in the same case. These queries, implemented as Cypher queries on standard graph DB systems, allow us to generate three completely new types of event data summaries: global inter-task DFGs that summarize processes on the level of larger tasks (instead of atomic actions); local intra-task DFGs that summarize behavior within a task (similar to a local process model [4]); and inter-task DFGs modeling behavior and interactions of multiple actors.

Our demonstration on the BPIC'17 event data suggests that these data summaries are helpful in answering questions of how work is structured and divided among actors in different parts of the process. We believe that such analysis of event data can give new insights into actor behavior in the context of routines [10, 19] and organizational models [20]. Future work is to evaluate whether the aggregation operations are effective for analysts trying to *understand* tasks.

Our work has two limitations. We modeled behavior along the control-flow using a single entity identifier while many processes operate on multiple objects; task identification and queries have to be generalized in this regard. The aggregation queries share many elements, but are formalized independently as pattern matching and creation operations over LPGs. A necessary next step is to systematically inventorize query operators over event knowledge graphs and develop a formal query algebra that is natural to process concepts.

References

1. van der Aalst, W.M.P.: Process Mining: Data Science in Action. Springer (2016)
2. Agostinelli, S., Leotta, F., Marrella, A.: Interactive segmentation of user interface logs. In: ICSOC. LNCS, vol. 13121, pp. 65–80 (2021)
3. Bonifati, A., Fletcher, G.H.L., Voigt, H., Yakovets, N.: Querying Graphs. Morgan & Claypool Publishers, Synthesis Lectures on Data Management (2018)
4. Brunings, M., Fahland, D., van Dongen, B.: Defining meaningful local process models. In: TOPNOC XVI. LNCS, vol. 13220, pp. 24–48. Springer (2022)
5. Delcoucq, L., Lecron, F., Fortemps, P., van der Aalst, W.M.P.: Resource-centric process mining: clustering using local process models. In: SAC 2020. pp. 45–52. ACM (2020)
6. van Dongen, B.F.: BPI Challenge 2017. Dataset (2017), https://doi.org/10.4121/12705737.v2
7. Esser, S., Fahland, D.: Multi-dimensional event data in graph databases. J. Data Semant. **10**, 109–141 (2021)
8. Fahland, D.: Process Mining over Multiple Behavioral Dimensions with Event Knowledge Graphs. In: van der Aalst, W.M.P., Carmona, J. (eds.) Process Mining Handbook, LNBIP, vol. 448, pp. 274–319. Springer (2022)
9. Genga, L., Potena, D., Martino, O., Alizadeh, M., Diamantini, C., Zannone, N.: Subgraph mining for anomalous pattern discovery in event logs. In: NFMCP 2016. LNCS, vol. 10312, pp. 181–197. Springer (2016)
10. Goh, K., Pentland, B.: From actions to paths to patterning: Toward a dynamic theory of patterning in routines. Acad. Manage. J. 62, 1901–1929 (12 2019)
11. van Hulzen, G., Martin, N., Depaire, B.: Looking beyond activity labels: Mining context-aware resource profiles using activity instance archetypes. In: BPM (Forum). LNBIP, vol. 427, pp. 230–245 (2021)
12. Jooken, L., Jans, M., Depaire, B.: Mining valuable collaborations from event data using the recency-frequency-monetary principle. In: CAiSE 2022. LNCS, vol. 13295, pp. 339–354. Springer (2022)
13. Klijn, E.L., Mannhardt, F., Fahland, D.: Classifying and detecting task executions and routines in processes using event graphs. In: BPM Forum. LNBIP, vol. 427, pp. 212–229. Springer (2021)
14. Klijn, E.L., Mannhardt, F., Fahland, D.: Exploring task execution patterns in event graphs. In: ICPM Demo Track. pp. 49–50 (2021)
15. Klijn, E.L., Mannhardt, F., Fahland, D.: Analyzing Actor Behavior in Process Executions. Tech. rep., Zenodo, https://doi.org/10.5281/zenodo.6719505 (Jul 2022)
16. Kumar, A., Liu, S.: Analyzing a helpdesk process through the lens of actor handoff patterns. In: BPM (Forum). LNBIP, vol. 392, pp. 313–329. Springer (2020)
17. Leno, V., Augusto, A., Dumas, M., La Rosa, M., Maggi, F.M., Polyvyanyy, A.: Discovering data transfer routines from user interaction logs. Inf. Syst. **107**, 101916 (2022)
18. de Leoni, M., Dündar, S.: Event-log abstraction using batch session identification and clustering. In: SAC 2020. pp. 36–44. ACM (2020)
19. Pentland, B., Feldman, M., Becker, M., Liu, P.: Dynamics of organizational routines: A generative model. J. of Mngmt. Studies 49, 1484–1508 (12 2012)

20. Yang, J., Ouyang, C., van der Aalst, W.M.P., ter Hofstede, A.H.M., Yu, Y.: OrdinoR: A framework for discovering, evaluating, and analyzing organizational models using event logs. Decis. Support Syst. **158**, 113771 (2022)

1st International Workshop
on Education Meets Process Mining
(EduPM'22)

First International Workshop Education Meets Process Mining (EduPM'22)

Process Mining has proven to be a powerful interdisciplinary tool for addressing open challenges in several fields such as healthcare or finances, and Education is no exception. The recent Process Mining approaches proposed for learning analytics, curricular analytics, or MOOC analytics are just some examples. But the Education discipline is also contributing to Process Mining, providing best practices, lessons learned, and new artifacts for better teaching and assessing Process Mining.

The International Workshop Education meets Process Mining (EduPM) aims to provide a high-quality forum for research at the intersection of Education and Process Mining. This intersection goes in two directions: Firstly, Process Mining for Education (PM4Edu). How could process mining be used to address some of the challenges in the field of education? For example, Process Mining for learning analytics, curricular analytics, motivation trajectories, MOOCs and blended courses, self-regulated learning patterns, etc. Secondly, Education for Process Mining (Edu4PM). How could we improve the teaching of the Process Mining discipline? For example, novel learning strategies tailored for Process Mining, new instruments to automatically assess specific topics of Process Mining, systematic studies of how Process Mining is being taught on different educational programs or levels, or novel curricula around Process Mining, among others.

Two types of contributions were invited: regular papers and Show&Tell papers. Regular papers were required to have a research contribution, and were evaluated on the basis of their significance, originality, technical quality, and potential to generate relevant discussion. Show&Tell submissions were non-research contributions, where authors presented an interesting element or initiative for the EduPM community.

The first edition of EduPM received a total of 14 submissions, 12 of which were regular papers. Of the regular papers, all except one addressed the PM4Edu direction, while there was one Show&Tell submission in each of both directions. After thorough reviewing by the program committee members, six regular submissions were accepted for a full-paper presentation. Additionally, after careful consideration by the workshop chairs, one of the Show&Tell submissions was invited for a short presentation. A brief description of the accepted papers included in this proceeding is given below.

In the paper by Van Daele et al., the authors set out to investigate which specific steps are taken during exploratory data analysis and how they are structured. The motivation for which is that such understanding will possibly contribute to the development of structured procedures that will support training novice analysts and contribute to reducing the cognitive load of such analysis.

The paper by Hobeck et al. presents a case study-based process mining analysis of student traces in a data set of information system students at TU Berlin. The authors apply the PM^2 framework to identify the traces of students on their way to obtaining their Bachelor's degree.

The paper by Hildago et al. presents a methodology for domain-driven event abstraction from MOOCs data in order to be useful for process mining analysis. It shows how to leverage MOOC event data for understanding learning habits in working sessions, given that the high-level activities are defined correctly.

The paper by Wagner et al. describes an ongoing project that aims to discover, check, recommend, and predict the academic trajectories of students in higher education institutions from data stored in campus management systems. The novelty of the proposed approach lies in the combination of process mining with rule-based artificial intelligence.

The paper by Rohani et al. presents the discovery analysis of student learning strategies in a visual programming MOOC using process mining techniques. The authors use a combination of Markov models and expectation maximisation to identify four learning tactics and several learning strategies extracted from a large sample with 3k+ students.

Finally, the paper by Bala et al. presents the findings of a study that analyses student behavior in completing open-ended exams on digital platforms. To do so, the paper analyzed the trace data about student behavior with the use of process mining, descriptive statistics and correlation analysis. The paper specifically compares the assessment behavior between top and low performing students.

In addition to these papers, the workshop included a panel discussion on the best practices of process mining education, as well as the challenges that exist. Panel members were Francesca Zerbato (chair), Mieke Jans, Boudewijn van Dongen, Marcos Sepúlveda, and Wil van der Aalst. This discussion gave rise to much food for thought, including the lack of proper datasets for educational purposes, the need for more emphasis on the event log construction phase, as well as the possibility to organise process mining certifications in a similar vein as Lean Six Sigma belts.

Finally, two awards were presented: the Best Student Paper Award for the student Luciano Hidalgo et al. and his work "Domain-Driven Event Abstraction Framework for Learning Dynamics in MOOCs Sessions", and the Best Paper Award for the authors Richard Hobeck, Luise Pufahl and Ingo Weber and their work "Process Mining on Curriculum-based Study Data – A Case Study at a German University."

The organisers wish to thank the EduPM'22 Program Committee for their important work in reviewing the submissions, as well as all the authors who submitted papers and the workshop participants for making the first edition of this workshop a success. Furthermore, a word of thanks also goes to the organising committee of ICPM'22.

November 2022

Jorge Munoz-Gama
Francesca Zerbato
Gert Janssenswillen
Wil van der Aalst

Organization

Workshop Chairs

Jorge Munoz-Gama — Pontificia Universidad Católica de Chile, Chile

Francesca Zerbato — University of St. Gallen, Switzerland

Gert Janssenswillen — Hasselt University, Belgium

Wil van der Aalst — RWTH Aachen University, Germany

Program Committee

Wil van der Aalst — RWTH Aachen University, Germany

Mitchel Brunings — Eindhoven University of Technology, The Netherlands

Andrea Burattin — Technical University of Denmark, Denmark

Josep Carmona — Universitat Politècnica de Catalunya, Spain

Rebeca Cerezo — University of Oviedo, Spain

Jan Claes — Arteveldehogeschool, Belgium

Dragan Gasevic — Monash University, Australia

Jerome Geyer-Klingeberg — Celonis SE, Germany

Luciano Hidalgo — Pontificia Universidad Católica de Chile, Chile

Gert Janssenswillen — Hasselt University, Belgium

Manuel Lama Penin — University of Santiago de Compostela, Spain

Sander Leemans — RWTH Aachen University, Germany

Jorge Maldonado-Mahauad — Universidad de Cuenca, Ecuador

Felix Mannhardt — Eindhoven University of Technology, The Netherlands

Niels Martin — Hasselt University, Belgium

Jorge Munoz-Gama — Pontificia Universidad Católica de Chile, Chile

Peter Reimann — University of Sydney, Australia

Cristobal Romero — Universidad de Córdoba, Spain

Mar Pérez-Sanagustin — Institut de Recherce en Informatique Toulouse, France

Marcos Sepúlveda — Pontificia Universidad Católica de Chile, Chile

Pnina Soffer — University of Haifa, Israel

Ernest Teniente   Universitat Politècnica de Catalunya, Spain
Jochen De Weerdt   Katholieke Universiteit Leuven, Belgium
Francesca Zerbato   University of St. Gallen, Switzerland

A Combined Approach of Process Mining and Rule-Based AI for Study Planning and Monitoring in Higher Education

Miriam Wagner[1]([✉]), Hayyan Helal[2], Rene Roepke[3], Sven Judel[3],
Jens Doveren[3], Sergej Goerzen[3], Pouya Soudmand[1], Gerhard Lakemeyer[2],
Ulrik Schroeder[3], and Wil M. P. van der Aalst[1]

[1] Process and Data Science (PADS), RWTH Aachen University, Aachen, Germany
{wagner,pouya.soudmand,wvdaalst}@pads.rwth-aachen.de
[2] Knowledge-Based Systems Group, RWTH Aachen University, Aachen, Germany
{helal,gerhard}@kbsg.rwth-aachen.de
[3] Learning Technologies Research Group, RWTH Aachen University,
Aachen, Germany
{roepke,judel,doveren,goerzen}@cs.rwth-aachen.de,
schroeder@informatik.rwth-aachen.de

Abstract. This paper presents an approach of using methods of process mining and rule-based artificial intelligence to analyze and understand study paths of students based on campus management system data and study program models. Process mining techniques are used to characterize successful study paths, as well as to detect and visualize deviations from expected plans. These insights are combined with recommendations and requirements of the corresponding study programs extracted from examination regulations. Here, event calculus and answer set programming are used to provide models of the study programs which support planning and conformance checking while providing feedback on possible study plan violations. In its combination, process mining and rule-based artificial intelligence are used to support study planning and monitoring by deriving rules and recommendations for guiding students to more suitable study paths with higher success rates. Two applications will be implemented, one for students and one for study program designers.

Keywords: Educational Process Mining · Conformance checking · Rule-based AI · Study planning · Study monitoring

1 Introduction

In higher education, study programs usually come with an idealized, recommended study plan. However, given how students have different capacities to study due to circumstances like part-time jobs or child care, and how one deviation from the intended study plan can have ripple effects spanning several semesters, in reality, a large number of different study paths can be observed. Further, capacity limits like room sizes or the amount of supervision that lecturers can provide make the planning of study paths more complex. Even though

M. Montali et al. (Eds.): ICPM 2022 Workshops, LNBIP 468, pp. 513–525, 2023.
https://doi.org/10.1007/978-3-031-27815-0_37

individualized study paths are possible due to the flexibility in study programs and their curriculum, students may need assistance and guidance in planning their studies. Software systems that assist students and study program designers in planning might do so by analyzing the large amounts of data in higher education institutions [12]. Of particular interest in this context are event data extracted from *Campus Management Systems* (CMS) including course enrollments, exam registrations and grade entries. To this purpose the *AIStudyBuddy* project - a cooperation between RWTH Aachen University, Ruhr University Bochum and University of Wuppertal - is set up. For preliminary analyses, we received access to the CMS data of two Bachelor programs, Computer Science and Mechanical Engineering, at RWTH Aachen University. Within the project, it will be investigated how to preprocess the data of all partners to apply the preliminary as well as the further intended analyses.

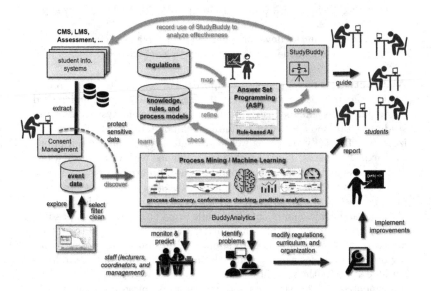

Fig. 1. Overview of the project, showing the two parts: *StudyBuddy* and *BuddyAnalytics* and their relationships to the different systems and techniques.

The aim of the project is to develop two applications: an intelligent planning tool for students and an analytics dashboard for study program designers (see Fig. 1). Both will be powered by a combination of rule-based *Artificial Intelligence* (AI) and *Process Mining* (PM) approaches. The implementation and evaluation of this combination's ability to efficiently generate rich feedback when checking the conformance to formal study plans is a key aspect of this project. This feedback will include PM results in the form of *recommendations*, which do not result from explicit regulations but rather historic study path data.

The planning tool for students, *StudyBuddy*, will use rule-based AI to check preliminary plans against an encoding of study program regulations. It will be able to provide immediate high-quality feedback regarding any potential conflicts in students' study plans. In addition to the rules explicitly codified in institutional regulations, the tool will have a notion of recommendations, which result from analyzing historical CMS data using PM approaches and finding characterizations of successful paths, e.g., finished in standard period of study.

The analytics dashboard, *BuddyAnalytics*, will enable study program designers to explore the PM results for the process of *Curriculum Analytics*. Process models of recommended study plans can be compared to study paths in the data to detect possible deviations or favorable routes. Various study path analyses could support monitoring and help study program designers as well as student counseling services to support successful study paths and intervene in misguided study planning by providing individualized plans.

The paper is structured as follows: Sect. 2 presents relevant related work in the fields of PM, rule-based AI and curriculum analytics. Section 3 introduces the aim of addressing individualized study planning for students and data-driven study monitoring for study program designers in a combined approach. The current state as well as challenges of the project are described in Sect. 4, while Sect. 5 presents objectives of future work. Section 6 concludes the paper.

2 Related Work

2.1 Process Mining in Education

Educational Process Mining (EPM) [4,27] is a sub-field of PM [28], using various, commonly known PM techniques in the educational context, e.g. higher education. While we focus on CMS data, most work in EPM has been done using *Learning Management Systems* (LMS) data with similar aims. In [20], two online exams have been analyzed using dotted chart analysis and process discovery with various miners. The applicability of standard methods provided in ProM in the context of LMS data is shown. In [5], course-related student data has been extracted to visualize the learning processes using an inductive miner to help preventing failing the course. "Uncover relationships between usage behavior and students' grades" is the aim of [13] by using *Directly-Follow Graph* (DFG). In [11], a case study is described in which the LMS data of one course is analyzed using among other things DFG. Also, in [18], data from an LMS is used and the creation of the event log is described in detail. Those event logs are used for the creation of DFG.

Analyses of LMS data show that the PM techniques can be used in the educational context but while concentrating on the behavior of students in one course, *Curriculum Mining* analyzes the different study paths a student can take [19] which is a substantial aspect in our work. Here, different approaches exist: [25,29] describe ways to use curriculum data to uncover the de-facto paths students take to, in the next step, recommend suitable follow-up courses. To our knowledge, this next step has not been done. [8] focuses on the study counselor perspective and uses, e.g., Fuzzy Miner and Inductive Visual Miner, to visualize the de-facto study paths and use those insights to improve the curriculum. In [23], the influence of failing a course on the study success is analyzed using mainly DFGs, while in [24], the analysis is done by modeling how students retake courses and the influence on study program dropouts.

Further, we will explore the application of conformance checking [10]. Therefore, similar approaches to ours are reviewed. An extended approach to conformance checking is multi-perspective conformance checking as in [17]. For our purpose, one reason to not extend this technique is that the Petri nets representing the study plan are hard to read when including all allowed behavior. For example, allowing a course to be in different semesters might lead to repositioning other courses as well. Furthermore, some rules that need to be represented are not connected to the model itself, e.g., credit point thresholds belonging to a semester and not to a course. Those could be modeled using invisible transitions, which makes the model more complicated and less intuitive.

2.2   Related Work on Rule-Based AI

The goal of rule-based AI is to model the examination regulations and the module catalog in a machine-readable language that allows for dealing with and planning events. For such scenarios, the combination of *Answer Set Programming* (ASP) and *Event Calculus* (EC) is applied. Both are based on a wider concept called *non-monotonic reasoning*, which differentiates from *monotonic reasoning* by the ability to retract already made implications based on further evidence [6].

Non-monotonic reasoning can model *defaults* as described in [22]. Defaults are assumed to hold, but do not necessarily have to. For instance, *Students typically take course X after they do course Y* will be modeled as a default, as it is a recommendation, not a requirement. As long as the student does not plan anything against it, it will be considered in their planning. Else, it will be ignored. A requirement on the other hand must be valid for all plans.

Looking for similar approaches, in [2], the problem of curriculum-based course timetabling was solved using ASP, however using a mechanism other than EC. While we consider recommendations to be defaults that must be typically followed, they should only ever result in a warning to the student, still giving the freedom to be deviated from. In [2], recommendations come in handy for planning, where the number of violations on them should be minimized. Furthermore, the timetabling problem focuses much more on the availability requirement for courses rather than also considering the results (e.g. success or failure, *Credit Points* (CPs) collected, ...) of these courses, which is the main focal point for us.

More generally, *Declarative Conformance Checking* [10] is a common application of rule-based AI to process models. In [9,16], declarative rules are used instead of classical conformance checking based on Petri nets. While [16] just covers the activities for constraints, [9] extended it with a data- and time-perspective. Furthermore, [1] has a wider model for requirements. It specifies three kinds of requirements, which refer to the relation in time between events, e.g. an event has a succession requirement if there is an event that must be done in the future after doing it. All three approaches use Linear Temporal Logic instead of ASP and EC, as it suitable for modeling the three mentioned requirements. For our purposes though, it makes the modeling of the contribution of an event to a specific result (e.g., CPs) harder, because our approach does not focus on the relation in time between events as much as the contributions of these events.

2.3 Curriculum Analytics and Planning

Having emerged as a sub-field of Learning Analytics, curriculum analytics aims to use educational data to drive evidence-based curriculum design and study program improvements [15]. Leveraging the data gathered in educational institutions, it can help identify student's needs and reduce dropout rates [12]. As such, different approaches and tools (e.g., [3,7,14,21]) have been developed to support the analysis of CMS or LMS data with the aim of helping instructors and program coordinators reflect on the curriculum and teaching practices. While various data and PM approaches have been used to analyze study paths provided through CMS event data [3,21], curriculum sequencing and study planning was explored using semantic web concepts applied on examination regulations, with the overall aim of supporting curriculum authoring, i.e., the design of personalized curricula fulfilling a set of constraints [1]. Other approaches include recommender systems [30] or genetic algorithms [26] to support students in course selection processes and fulfilling requirements of a study program. To the best of our knowledge, however, no joint approach of PM and rule-based AI has yet been explored in order to support study planning and monitoring for students and study program designers.

3   Approach

The aim of AIStudyBuddy is to support individualized study planning (for students) and monitoring (for study program designers). *Study planning* describes the students' activities of planning and scheduling modules, courses and exams throughout the complete course of a study program. The examination regulations provide recommendations and requirements to describe a study program and the conditions for students to successfully earn a degree. These may include a sample study plan recommending when to take which module or course and attempting to distribute CPs evenly over the standard period of study. Students choose from the module catalog, a list of mandatory and elective modules.

While most students may start with the same recommended plan in their first semesters, deviations due to various reasons can occur at any time, e.g., working part-time may result in a reduced course load and delaying courses to the next year, thus, changing the complete plan and its duration. Therefore, support for individualized planning as well as recommendations of suitable study paths are needed. Further, the diversity of study paths and deviations from recommended study plans raises questions of how different students move through a study program, if certain modules or courses cause delays in the study plan, or whether a study program may need revisions. Here, *study monitoring* can be provided by analyzing students' traces in various systems used in the university. In our project, we will initially focus on CMS data and might include LMS data later.

In order to support students and study program designers in their respective tasks, a modular infrastructure (see Fig. 1) with two primary applications for the target groups will be implemented. The application *StudyBuddy* presents a web interface to guide and engage students in study planning activities. As in many programs students do not necessarily have to follow a recommended plan and in later phases not even have recommendations. To help finding suitable courses historic data can be used to give hints which combinations have been successful. Furthermore, course-content is not always independent from other courses and a specific order might help to pass with higher chance. It offers an overview of a student's study program and allows for creation and validation of individual study plans. ASP and EC are used to model these regulations. Given a study plan, they can be used to generate feedback regarding violations and give recommendations. These recommendations are the result of mining historic data of previous study paths for those with high success rates.

For study program designers, the application *BuddyAnalytics* presents an interactive, web-based dashboard visualizing PM data analysis results. Different methods, i.e., process discovery and conformance checking, can help to understand how different student cohorts behave throughout the course of the study program and identify deviations from recommended study plans. Based on different indicators and questions by study program designers, student cohorts can be analyzed and insights into their paths can be gained. Study program designers can evaluate and compare different study paths and further develop new redesigned study plans in an evidence-based way.

4   Current State and Challenges

The main data source for this project is the CMS of a university, which contains information about the students, courses, exams and their combination. Later, the possibility to integrate LMS data will be explored. As the project aims to be independent from the systems and study programs at different universities, a general data model has been created (see Fig. 2). This model is the starting point for our project work and shows the general relation between courses and students as well as study programs. The diagram does not include all possible data fields as they differ depending on the available data of a university.

Students can have multiple study programs, e.g., first do a Bachelor in Computer Science followed by a Master. Each semester a student has a study status, e.g., *enrolled* or *semester on leave*. The same offered course is scheduled in different semesters, e.g., *Programming* is offered every winter semester, and in different study programs, e.g., *Introduction to Data Science* is mandatory for a Master in Data Science but elective for a Master in Computer Science. Students also have a status for scheduled courses during their study program, e.g., *course passed*.

Until now, we explored data on exam information (i.e., registrations and results). The analyzed data includes Bachelor and Master Computer Science

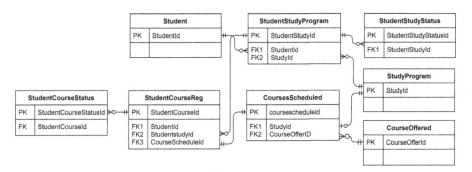

Fig. 2. A basic and generic data model for CMS data

students as well as Mechanical Engineering Bachelor of RWTH Aachen University. Some standard KPIs used in various departments of universities that give meaningful insights about students, study programs or cohorts are:

– Success rate of a course [in specific semesters] [for a cohort]
– Number of attempts a course is taken [on average] [for a cohort]
– Exams taken/passed in a [specific] semester [on average] [of a cohort]
– Average study duration [of a cohort]
– Percentage of dropouts [of a cohort] [in a predefined period]

A cohort can be defined based on the semester a group of students started, e.g., *cohort WS21* refers to all students that started in winter semester 2021/2022. It can also be defined by the amount of semesters students already studied or the examination regulations they belong to. Different cohort definitions are needed to answer various questions about the behavior of students. For more insights exceeding simple SQL queries used for descriptive statistics, the data is transferred into specific event logs, in which activities can be based just on courses and exams, or may even include additional information. First, we concentrated on events describing the final status of exams for students. A student can have multiple occurrences of a course, e.g. when they do not pass the exam in the first try or when they registered first, but in the end, they did not take it. As a timestamp, the semester or the exact exam date can be used. Also, some activities may have specific status dates, e.g., the date of the (de-)registration. Those event logs can be used to create de-facto models showing the actual behavior of a group of students. As model we use DFG, BPMN models, process trees and Petri nets, as shown in Fig. 3, because they are easy to read also for non-specialists in PM.

For useful insights, the multiple occurrence and the partial order of courses must be treated. The partial order is caused by using, e.g., the scheduled semester, instead of the arbitrarily set exam dates, based on among others room capacities. We tried out different solutions with the setting depending on the underlying questions that should be answered by the resulting model, e.g., when using a combination of exam attempt and course ID as the activity, the resulting de-facto model shows how courses are retried and visualizes better the real

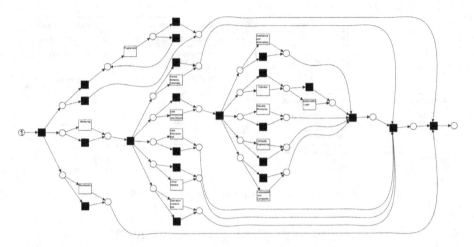

Fig. 3. Model created by ProM plugin "Mine Petri net with Inductive Miner" for data of students studying in examination regulation 2018 just using their mandatory courses

workload per semester. In Fig. 3, just the first occurrence of the course is used and all exams of a semester have the same date. Semester-blocks are visible, especially when the offered semester of a course is in mind, e.g., *Programming* and *Calculus* are offered in the winter semester. The examination regulation of 2018 states that it should be taken in the first semester. Compared to the (simplified) recommended plan (see Fig. 4) *Mentoring* occurs two semesters before *Calculus*, while they should be concurrent. *Data Communication and Security* is taken two semesters earlier than planned and before courses that should precede it, e.g., *Computability and Complexity*. Those models give a first impression of the actual study path but need interpretation.

As a simpler approach to the later proposed combination of ASP and classical PM conformance checking, we explored the possibility of creating de-jure models based on the recommended study plan. We used Petri nets since they can cover course concurrency and are still understandable by non-experts. The de-jure model in Fig. 4 shows the main recommended path. Note, the data was just available including the third semester and later courses are invisible. Using Petri nets and conformance checking this recommendation becomes a requirement.

The results of classical conformance checking are still useful to find typical deviation points, e.g., *Linear Algebra* tends to be taken in a different semester than proposed. Also, when filtering on the first exam attempts, the resulting insights are different from filtering on the successful passing of exams. Filtered on the first attempt, we can see how many students actually tried to follow the plan, while filtered on the passed exams indicates the success route. When we have a high percentage of students that try to follow the recommended study plan, but just a low percentage that succeeds, this may be a warning for study program designers that the rules may need to be adapted to improve the recommendation and thereby increase the study success of students.

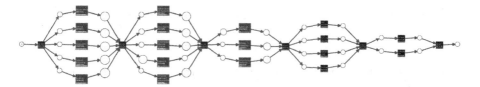

Fig. 4. Conformance checking result using ProM plugin "Replay a Log on Petri Net for Conformance Analysis" on data of students studying in examination regulation 2018 and a simplified Petri net model of the regulation

Our findings show that in later semesters, students deviate more from the recommended study plan, which can be explained by delays occurring earlier in their study. What is not modeled by the Petri net here is that for *Seminar* (semester 5), *Proseminar* (semester 2) is a prerequisite. Therefore, *Proseminar* has to be taken before *Seminar* and forms a *requirement*. Including those additional requirements and all already planned exceptions from the original plan, those models are fast becoming so called spaghetti models and lose a lot of their readability. Lastly, additional constraints, e.g., credit point constraints such as *at the end of the third semester, at least 60 CPs must have been earned*, are not taken into account using just the described approach.

For that matter, we used the combination of ASP and EC such that e.g. defaults can model recommendations. The first main issues concerning modeling study requirements in general and using EC was translating examination regulations given in natural languages into formal languages. We encountered the following problems and challenges:

– There are rules that are understood by any human and thus not written.
– There is a lot of human interference that allows for exceptions. Exceptions in study plans are not rare.
– There are older versions of the examination regulations, which certain students still follow.

The second problem we encountered with EC is that almost all events contribute to a single result (e.g. CPs), instead of a majority of events, each initiating new kinds of results. EC is designed for the latter, but in study plans the former holds. We thus adjusted the EC. One modification was to differentiate between events that happened and events that are planned. For planning in the future, one needs to follow the rules. For events in the past, a record is sufficient and there is no need for further requirement checking. This allows to add exceptions that are actually inconsistent with the examination regulations. It was also important to keep track of certain relevant numbers a student has at any point in time, in order to be able to do requirement checking. This was achieved through results, which events can contribute to. *Mathematics 1*, for example, adds 9 units to the result *credit points*, after the event of success at it. A requirement on CPs should consider the general number of CPs collected or just within a field or a time frame. For that matter we created the notion of a *result requirement*, which makes sure that the sum of results caused by a subset of events is less than, greater than, or equal to some value. With all of this in mind, we separated the required rules into three categories:

- *Invariant*: Rules about the requirements and the EC modified axiom system.
- *Variant by Admins*: Rules about modules and their availability.
- *Variant by Student*: Rules about the plan of the student.

After that, we were able to translate the examination regulations, module catalogs, and student event logs into rules. This enables us to perform model as well as conformance checking.

5   Future Steps

Until now, the data are limited to information about exams and is exclusively derived from the CMS. In a next step, course enrollments will be added to further analyze study behavior of students. This additional information will give more concrete insights about the students' intended study plan, since at many universities, course enrollments are not automatically coupled to exam registrations. While students might start to take a course in the intended semester, thus enroll in it, they might realize that the workload is too high or exam qualification requirements are not fulfilled and refrain from registering for the exam in the end. This may also be valuable information considering the instructors' workload as more course enrollments indicate more work during the course and may require larger lecture halls or additional support staff. As such, this workload needs to be balanced out when planning courses for upcoming semesters.

The information stored in the LMS contains valuable information to understand students' learning behavior, as shown in related work. When combined with activities in the CMS, a more complete view on students' behavior and more direct feedback about the success of the intended plan can be provided. This feedback can then be used in BuddyAnalytics to help study program designers in improving curricula and recommended study plans, as well as give more informed suggestions for individual study plans. Possibly, in StudyBuddy, students might be informed about their behavior deviating from a recommended plan and are presented with suggestions suitable to their individual circumstances.

On the theoretical side, the possibilities of a combination of AI and PM are further explored and implemented. The main focus will be to improve the conformance checking results. Also, PM conformance checking possibilities will be further explored. One planned aspect is the extraction of constraints from event logs directly. We expect to learn rules that are not intended but are beneficial, e.g., *Statistics* is a good preparation for *Introduction to Data Science* and when taken in order, the grade and success rate of the latter improves. Those rules could be added to the examination regulations rules as defaults.

6 Conclusion

The AIStudyBuddy project will combine different existing AI and PM frameworks and extend them with new features, making use of the already existing data at universities, to help students and study program designers make more informed decisions about study paths and curricula. The first results get positive feedback from students and study program designers. Currently, only a small fraction of available CMS data was used to produce these results, leaving a lot of potential for future steps. PM techniques already give valuable new insights to the study program designers and the combination of AI and PM for conformance checking in particular helps overcome restrictions due to the data and rule properties. Having requirements and recommendations, credit point boundaries, and long-term relations between courses should be included in the system to model examination regulations in a more accurate manner.

Acknowledgements. The authors gratefully acknowledge the funding by the Federal Ministry of Education and Research (BMBF) for the joint project AIStudyBuddy (grant no. 16DHBKI016).

References

1. Baldoni, M., Baroglio, C., Brunkhorst, I., Henze, N., Marengo, E., Patti, V.: Constraint modeling for curriculum planning and validation. Interact. Learn. Environ. **19**(1), 81–123 (2011)
2. Banbara, M., et al.: *teaspoon*: solving the curriculum-based course timetabling problems with answer set programming. Ann. Oper. Res. **275**(1), 3–37 (2018). https://doi.org/10.1007/s10479-018-2757-7
3. Bendatu, L.Y., Yahya, B.N.: Sequence matching analysis for curriculum development. J. Teknik Ind. **17**(1), 47–52 (2015)
4. Bogarín, A., Cerezo, R., Romero, C.: A survey on educational process mining. WIREs Data Min. Knowl. Discov. **8**(1), e1230 (2018)
5. Bogarín, A., Cerezo, R., Romero, C.: Discovering learning processes using inductive miner: a case study with learning management systems (LMSs). Psicothema (2018)
6. Brewka, G., Dix, J., Konolige, K.: Nonmonotonic Reasoning: An Overview, vol. 73. CSLI, Stanford (1997)
7. Brown, M., DeMonbrun, R.M., Teasley, S.: Taken together: conceptualizing students' concurrent course enrollment across the post-secondary curriculum using temporal analytics. Learn. Analytics **5**(3), 60–72 (2018)
8. Buck-Emden, R., Dahmann, F.D.: Analyse von Studienverläufen mit Process-Mining-Techniken. HMD Praxis der Wirtschaftsinformatik **55**(4) (2018)
9. Burattin, A., Maggi, F.M., Sperduti, A.: Conformance checking based on multi-perspective declarative process models. Expert Syst. Appl. **65**, 194–211 (2016)
10. Carmona, J., van Dongen, B., Solti, A., Weidlich, M.: Conformance Checking: Relating Processes and Models. Springer, Cham (2018)
11. Cenka, B.A.N., Santoso, H.B., Junus, K.: Analysing student behaviour in a learning management system using a process mining approach. Knowl. Manag. E-Learn. **14**(1), 62–80 (2022)

12. Daniel, B.: Big data and analytics in higher education: opportunities and challenges: the value of big data in higher education. Educ. Technol. **46**(5), 904–920 (2015)

13. Etinger, D.: Discovering and mapping LMS course usage patterns to learning outcomes. In: Ahram, T., Karwowski, W., Vergnano, A., Leali, F., Taiar, R. (eds.) IHSI 2020. AISC, vol. 1131, pp. 486–491. Springer, Cham (2020). https://doi.org/10.1007/978-3-030-39512-4_76

14. Heileman, G.L., Hickman, M., Slim, A., Abdallah, C.T.: Characterizing the complexity of curricular patterns in engineering programs. In: ASEE Annual Conference & Exposition (2017)

15. Hilliger, I., Aguirre, C., Miranda, C., Celis, S., Pérez-Sanagustín, M.: Lessons learned from designing a curriculum analytics tool for improving student learning and program quality. J. Comput. High. Educ. **34**, 1–25 (2022). https://doi.org/10.1007/s12528-022-09315-4

16. de Leoni, M., Maggi, F.M., van der Aalst, W.M.P.: Aligning event logs and declarative process models for conformance checking. In: Barros, A., Gal, A., Kindler, E. (eds.) BPM 2012. LNCS, vol. 7481, pp. 82–97. Springer, Heidelberg (2012). https://doi.org/10.1007/978-3-642-32885-5_6

17. Mannhardt, F., de Leoni, M., Reijers, H.A., van der Aalst, W.M.P.: Balanced multi-perspective checking of process conformance. Computing **98**(4) (2016). https://doi.org/10.1007/S00607-015-0441-1

18. Mathrani, A., Umer, R., Susnjak, T., Suriadi, S.: Data quality challenges in educational process mining: building process-oriented event logs from process-unaware online learning systems. Bus. Inf. Syst. **39**(4), 569–592 (2022)

19. Pechenizkiy, M., Trcka, N., de Bra, P., Toledo, P.A.: CurriM: curriculum mining. In: EDM (2012)

20. Pechenizkiy, M., Trcka, N., Vasilyeva, E., van der Aalst, W., de Bra, P.: Process mining online assessment data. In: International Working Group on Educational Data Mining (2009)

21. Priyambada, S.A., Mahendrawathi, E.R., Yahya, B.N.: Curriculum assessment of higher educational institution using aggregate profile clustering. Procedia Comput. Sci. **124**, 264–273 (2017)

22. Reiter, R.: A logic for default reasoning. Artif. Intell. **13**(1–2), 81–132 (1980)

23. Salazar-Fernandez, J.P., Munoz-Gama, J., Maldonado-Mahauad, J., Bustamante, D., Sepúlveda, M.: Backpack process model (BPPM): a process mining approach for curricular analytics. Appl. Sci. **11**(9), 4265 (2021)

24. Salazar-Fernandez, J.P., Sepúlveda, M., Munoz-Gama, J., Nussbaum, M.: Curricular analytics to characterize educational trajectories in high-failure rate courses that lead to late dropout. Appl. Sci. **11**(4), 1436 (2021)

25. Schulte, J., Fernandez de Mendonca, P., Martinez-Maldonado, R., Buckingham Shum, S.: Large scale predictive process mining and analytics of university degree course data. In: LAK'17: Proceedings of the Seventh International Learning Analytics & Knowledge Conference. Association for Computing Machinery (2017)

26. Srisamutr, A., Raruaysong, T., Mettanant, V.: A course planning application for undergraduate students using genetic algorithm. In: ICT-ISPC (2018)

27. Sypsas, A., Kalles, D.: Reviewing process mining applications and techniques in education. Artif. Intell. Appl. **13**(1), 83–102 (2022)

28. van der Aalst, W.M.P.: Process Mining: Data science in Action. Springer, Cham (2018)

29. Wang, R., Zaïane, O.R.: Discovering process in curriculum data to provide recommendation. In: EDM (2015)
30. Wong, C.: Sequence based course recommender for personalized curriculum planning. In: Penstein Rosé, C., et al. (eds.) AIED 2018. LNCS (LNAI), vol. 10948, pp. 531–534. Springer, Cham (2018). https://doi.org/10.1007/978-3-319-93846-2_100

Identifying the Steps in an Exploratory Data Analysis: A Process-Oriented Approach

Seppe Van Daele and Gert Janssenswillen[✉][iD]

Faculty of Business Economics, UHasselt - Hasselt University,
Agoralaan, 3590 Diepenbeek, Belgium
gert.janssenswillen@uhasselt.be

Abstract. Best practices in (teaching) data literacy, specifically Exploratory Data Analysis, remain an area of tacit knowledge until this day. However, with the increase in the amount of data and its importance in organisations, analysing data is becoming a much-needed skill in today's society. Within this paper, we describe an empirical experiment that was used to examine the steps taken during an exploratory data analysis, and the order in which these actions were taken. Twenty actions were identified. Participants followed a rather iterative process of working step by step towards the solution. In terms of the practices of novice and advanced data analysts, few relevant differences were yet discovered.

Keywords: Process mining · Deliberate practice · Learning analytics

1 Introduction

Data is sometimes called the new gold, but is much better compared to gold-rich soil. As with gold mining, several steps are needed to go through in order to get to the true value. With the amount and importance of data in nearly every industry [13–15], data analysis is a vital skill in the current job market, not limited to profiles such as data scientists or machine learning engineers, but equally important for marketing analysts, business controllers, as well as sport coaches, among others.

However, best practices in data literacy, and how to develop them, mainly remains an area of tacit knowledge until this day, specifically in the area of Exploratory Data Analysis (EDA). EDA is an important part in the data analysis process where interaction between the analyst and the data is high [3]. While there are guidelines on how the process of data analysis can best be carried out [15,18,21], these steps typically describe what needs to be done at a relatively high level, and do not precisely tell how best to perform them in an actionable manner. Which specific steps take place during an exploratory data analysis, and how they are structured in an analysis has not been investigated.

The goal of this paper is to refine the steps underlying exploratory data analysis beyond high-level categorisations such as transforming, visualising,

M. Montali et al. (Eds.): ICPM 2022 Workshops, LNBIP 468, pp. 526–538, 2023.
https://doi.org/10.1007/978-3-031-27815-0_38

and modelling. In addition, we analyse the order in which these actions are performed. The results of this paper form a first step towards better understanding the detailed steps in a data analysis, which can be used in future research to analyse difference between novices and experts in data analysis, and create better data analysis teaching methods focussed on removing these differences.

The next section will discuss related work, while Sect. 3 will discuss the methodology used. The identified steps are described in the subsequent section, while an analysis of the recorded data is provided in Sect. 5. Section 6 concludes the paper.

2 Related Work

A number of high-level tasks to be followed while performing a data analysis have already been defined in the literature [15,18], which can be synthesised as 1) the collection of data, 2) processing of data, 3) cleaning of data, 4) exploratory data analysis, 5) predictive data analysis, and 6) communicating the results. In [21] this process is elaborated in more detail, applied to the R language. Here the process starts with importing data and cleaning. The actual data analysis is subsequently composed of the cycle of transforming, visualising and modelling data, and is thus slightly more concrete than the theoretical exploratory and prescriptive data analysis. The concluding communication step is similar to [15,18].

That the different steps performed in a data analysis have received little attention, has also been recognised by [23], specifically focused on process analysis. In this paper, an empirical study has been done to understand how process analysts follow different patterns in analysing process data, and have different strategies to explore event data. Subsequent research has shown that such analysis can lead to the identification of challenges to improve best practices [24].

Breaking down a given action into smaller steps can reduce cognitive load when performing the action [20]. Cognitive load is the load that occurs when processing information. The more complex this information is, the higher the cognitive load is. Excessive cognitive load can overload working memory and thus slow down the learning process. Creating an instruction manual addresses The Isolated Elements Effect [4], when there is a reduction in cognitive load by isolating steps, and only then looking at the bigger picture [20]. In [5], this theory was applied using *The Structured Process Modeling Theory*, to reduce the cognitive load when creating a process model. Participants who followed structured steps, thus reducing their cognitive load, generally made fewer syntax errors and created better process models [5]. Similarly, in [10], participants were asked to build an event log, where the test group was provided with the event log building guide from [11]. The results showed that the event logs built by the test group outperformed those of the control group in several areas.

An additional benefit of identifying smaller steps is that these steps can be used in the creation of a *deliberate practice*—a training course that meets the following conditions [1,6] :

1. Tasks with a defined objective
2. Immediate feedback on the task created

3. Opportunity to repeat this task multiple times
4. Motivation to actually get better

Karl Ericsson [6] studied what the training of experts in different fields had in common [2], from which the concept of deliberate practice emerged. It was already successfully applied, for example, in [7] where a physics course, reworked to deliberate practise principles, resulted in higher attendance and better grades.

In addition to studying what kind of training experts use to acquire their expertise, it has also been studied why experts are better at a particular field than others. In [6], it is concluded that experts have more sophisticated mental representations that enable them to make better and/or faster decisions. Mental representations are internal models about certain information that become more refined with training [6]. Identifying actions taken in a data analysis can help in mapping mental representations of data analysis experts. This can be done by comparing the behaviour of experts with that of beginners. Knowing why an expert performs a certain action at a certain point can have a positive effect on the development of beginners' mental models. In fact, using mental representations of experts was considered in [19] as a crucial first step in designing new teaching methods.

3   Methodology

In order to analyse the different steps performed during an exploratory analysis, and typical flows between them, an experiment was conducted. The experiments and further data processing and analysis steps are described below.

Experiment. Cognitive Task Analysis (CTA) [22] was used as overall methodology for conducting the experiment described in this paper, with the aim to uncover (hidden) steps in a participant's process of exploratory data analysis. Participants were asked to make some simple analyses using supplied data and to make a screen recording of this process. The tasks concerned analysing the distribution of variables, the relationship between variables, as well as calculating certain statistics.

As certain steps can be taken for granted due to developed automatisms [8], the actual analysis was followed by an interview, in which the participants were asked to explain step by step what decisions and actions were taken. By having the interview take place after the data analysis, interference with the participants' usual way of working was avoided. For example, asking questions before or during the data analysis could have caused participants to hesitate, slow down, or even make different choices.

The general structure of the experiment was as follows:

1. **Participants:** The participants for this experiment were invited by mail from three groups with different levels of experience: undergraduate students, graduate students, and PhD students, from the degree Business and Information

systems engineering. These students received an introductory course on data analysis in their first bachelor year, where they work with the language R, which was subsequently chosen as the language to be used in the experiment. In the end, 11 students were convinced to participate in this experiment: two undergraduate students, four graduate students and 5 PhD students. The 11 participants each performed the complete analysis of three assignments, and thus results from 33 assignments were collected.

While having participants with different levels of experience is expected to result in a broader variety in terms of behaviour, the scale of the experiment and the use of student participants only will not allow a detailed analysis of the relationship between experience-level and analysis behaviour. Furthermore, disregarding the different level of students, the once accepting the invitation to participate might also be the more confident about their skills.

2. **Survey:** Before participants began the data analysis, they were asked to complete an introductory survey to gain insight into their own perceptions of their data analysis skill (in R).
3. **Assignment:** The exploratory analysis was done in the R programming language, and consisted of three independent tasks about data from a housing market: 2 involving data visualisation and 1 specific quantitative question. The analysis was recorded by the participants.
4. **Interview:** The recording of the assignment was used during the interview to find out what steps, according to the participants themselves, were taken. Participants were asked to actively tell what actions were taken and why.

Transcription. The transcription of the interviews was done manually. Because most participants actively narrated the actions taken, a question-answer structure was not chosen. If a question was still asked, it was placed in italics between two dashes when transcribed.

Coding and Categorization. To code the transcripts of the interviews, a combination of descriptive and process coding was used in the first iteration. Descriptive coding looks for nouns that capture the content of the sentence [16]. Process coding, in turn, attempts to capture actions by encoding primarily action-oriented words (verbs) [16]. These coding techniques were applied to the transcripts by highlighting the words and sentences that met them. A second iteration used open coding (also known as initial coding) where the marked codes from the first iteration were grouped with similarly marked codes [9,17]. These iterations were performed one after the other for the same transcription before starting the next transcription.

These resulting codes were the input for constructing the categories. In this process, the codes that had the same purpose were taken together and codes with a similar purpose were grouped together and given an overarching term. This coding step is called axial coding [9].

Event Log Construction. Based on the screen recording and the transcription, the actions found were transformed into an event log. In addition, if applicable, additional information was also stored to enrich the data such as the location where a certain action was performed (e.g. in the console, in a script, etc.), what exactly happened in the action (e.g. what was filtered on) and then an attribute how this happened (e.g. search for a variable using *CTRL+F*). Timestamps for the event log where based on the screen recordings.

Event Log Analysis. The frequency of activities, and typical activity flows were subsequently analysed. Next to the recorded behaviour, also the quality of the execution was assessed, by looking at both the duration of the analysis, as well as the correctness of the results. For each of these focus points, participants with differing levels of experiences where also compared.

For the analysis of the event log, the R package bupaR was used [12]. Because there were relatively few cases present in the event log, the analysis also consisted largely of qualitative analysis of the individual traces.

4   Identified Actions

Before analysing the executed actions and flows in relation to the different experiences, duration and correctness, this section describes the identified actions, which have been subdivided in the categories preparatory, analysis, debugging, and other actions.

Preparatory Actions. Actions are considered preparatory steps if they occurred mainly prior to the actual analysis itself. For the purpose of this experiment, actions were selected that had a higher relative frequency among the actions performed before the first question than during the analysis. An overview of preparatory actions is shown in Table 1.

Table 1. Preparatory actions

Action	Description
Check data	Check if the data met their expectations, if the data was tidy (each row is an observation and each column is a variable [21])
Explore data	Viewing the data itself, e.g., in the IDE or Excel, or by consulting the data description. Whereas data checking is really exploring the quality of the data, the act of data exploring looks at the content of the data
Load data	Checking what file type the data source had, whether column names were present, what the separator was if any, and in what directory the data file was present. This operation corresponds to importing data from [21]
Load library	In *R*, packages must be loaded before they can be used
Read assignment	Studying the assignment. This activity was performed both at the start of the assignment, as well as during the analysis

Analysis Actions. The steps covered within this category are actions that can be performed to accomplish a specific task, and are listed in Table 2. These are actions directly related to solving the data analysis task and not, for example, emergency actions that must be performed such as solving an error message.

Debugging Actions. Debugging is the third category of operations that was identified. Next to the actual debugging of the code, this category include the activities that (might) trigger debugging, which are *errors*, *warnings*, and *messages*.

Table 2. Analysis actions.

Action	Description
Evaluate results	Reflection on (intermediate) results. Is this the result I expect? Does it answer the question?
Execute code	Executing the written code
Manipulation data	This step covers the preparation of the data for a specific assignment. Eight types of data manipulation were identified. – Data grouping: looking at aggregate statistics – Data filtering: selecting rows in the data. – Data selection: selecting columns in the data. – Data joining – Data transformation: pivoting a dataset – Mutate data: add a column with calculated variables. – Change data type: changing the data type of a column. – Create object: e.g. to store intermediate results
Prepare plot	Determine the type of graph and data mapping
Search variable	Identifying a particular requested variable, by looking at the description file or the data itself
Show plot	Graph formatting
Summarize data	Calculating summary statistics such as frequency, centrality measures, and measures of variance

Executing the code 77 times out of 377 resulted in an error. Debugging is a (series of) action(s) taken after receiving an error or warning. Most of these errors were fairly trivial to resolve. In twenty percent of the loglines registered during debugging, however, additional information was consulted on, for example, the Internet.

Other Actions. The last category of actions includes adding structure, reasoning, reviewing the assignments, consulting information, and trial-and-error. Except for the review of the assignments, which was performed after completing all the assignments, these actions are fairly independent of the previous action

Table 3. Other actions

Action	Description
Add structure	Adding intermediate steps and comments and structuring code in chunks
Consult information	Four different sources were used: documentation of programming functions used, examples included in function documentations, returning to previous analyses, and consulting relevant programming course materials
Reasoning	Thinking about performing a task was undoubtedly performed by all participants, though only seven participants cited actively thinking at certain points during the analysis
Review solution	Before finishing, checking all the solutions whether they are correct and met the assignments
Trial-and-error	Experimenting, by just trying out some things or comparing the outcome of different types of joins

and thus were performed at any point in the analysis. An overview of these actions can be found in Table 3. Note that as trial-and-error is a method rather than a separate action, it was not coded separately in the event log, but can be identified in the log as a pattern.

5   Analysis

In the experiment, a total of 1674 activity instances were recorded. An overview of the identified actions together with summary statistics is provided in Table 4. It can be seen that the most often observed actions are *Execute code*, *Consult information*, *Prepare data* and *Evaluate results*. Twelve of the identified actions were performed by all 11 participants at some point. Looking at the summary statistics, we observe quite significant differences in the execution frequency of actions, such as the consultation of information (ranging from 4 to 63) and the execution of code (ranging from 16 to 48), indicating important individual differences. Table 5 shows for each participant the total processing time (minutes) together with the total number of actions, and the number of actions per category.

Flows. A first observation is that the log records direct repetitions of a certain number of actions. This is a natural consequence of the fact that information is stored in additional attributes. As such, when a participant is, for instance, consulting different sources of information directly after one another, this will not be regarded as a single "Consulting information" action, but as a sequence of smaller actions. Information of these repetitions is shown in Table 6. Because these length-one loops might clutter the analysis, it was decided to *collapse* them into single activity instances. After doing so, the number of activity instances was reduced from 1674 to 1572.

That the process of data analysis is flexible attests Fig. 1, which contains a directly-follows matrix of the log. While many different (and infrequent) flows can be observed, some interesting insights can be seen. Within the analysis actions, we can see 2 groups: actions related to manipulation of data, and actions

Table 4. Summary statistics of the identified actions.

Category	Action	#part	Total freq	Min. freq	Avg. freq	Max. freq
Preparatory	Check data	7	11	1	1.57	3
	Explore data	10	52	2	5.20	12
	Load data	10	35	2	3.50	6
	Load library	11	39	2	3.55	9
	Read assignment	11	84	4	7.64	14
Analysis	Evaluate results	11	182	5	16.55	33
	Execute code	11	377	16	34.27	48
	Manipulate data	11	195	6	17.73	34
	Prepare plot	11	70	2	6.36	14
	Search variable	11	81	4	7.36	10
	Show plot	8	40	1	5.00	12
	Summarize data	11	44	1	4.00	8
Debugging	Debug	11	48	1	4.36	12
	Error	11	77	2	7.00	14
	Message	1	2	2	2.00	2
	Warning	3	8	1	2.67	4
Other	Add structure	11	69	3	6.27	10
	Consult information	11	229	4	20.82	63
	Reasoning	7	17	1	2.43	4
	Review solution	9	14	1	1.56	3

Table 5. Statistics per participant

Participant	Proc. time	#actions	Preparatory	Analysis	Debugging	Other
1	26.20	139	19	75	26	19
2	32.87	159	16	110	12	21
3	42.98	172	15	117	19	21
4	52.63	172	31	88	6	47
5	39.67	151	21	87	8	35
6	43.15	155	19	93	14	29
7	38.08	155	14	109	10	22
8	36.17	104	11	54	8	31
9	17.52	97	23	55	5	14
10	38.75	170	28	112	12	18
11	71.52	200	24	89	15	72

Table 6. Direct repetitions of actions

Action	Number of repetitions	Action	Number of repetitions
Consult information	54.00	Load data	7.00
Prepare data	23.00	Load library	6.00
Search variable	19.00	Debug	2.00
Add structure	14.00	Check data	1.00
Execute code	13.00	Read assignment	1.00
Explore data	7.00	Review solution	1.00

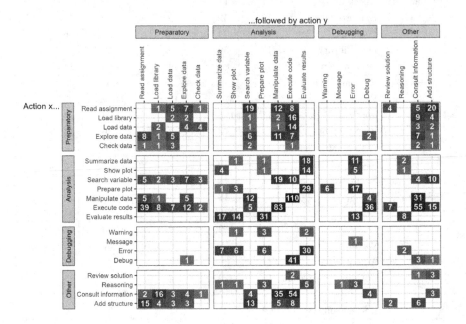

Fig. 1. Precedence flows between actions.

related to evaluation and visualising data. Furthermore, it can be seen that some analysis actions are often performed before or after preparatory actions, while most are not.

Duration. In Fig. 2, the total time spent on each of the 4 categories is shown per participant, divided in undergraduate, graduate and PhD participants. The dotted vertical lines in each group indicates the average time spent. While the limited size of the experiment does not warrant generalizable results with respect to different experience levels, it can be seen that Undergraduates spent the least time overall, while graduate spent the most time. In the latter group, we can however see a large amount of variation between participants. What is notable is that both graduate participants and PhDs spent a significantly larger amount of time on preparatory steps, compared to undergraduate students. On average, graduate students spent more time on other actions than the other groups. Predominantly, this appeared to be the consultation of information. This might be explained by the fact that for these students, data analysis (specifically the course in R) was further removed in the past compared to undergraduate students. On the other hand, PhDs might have more expertise about usage of R and data analysis readily available.

Correctness. After the experiment, the results where also scored for correctness. Table 7 shows the average scores in each group, on a scale from zero to 100%. While the differences are small, and still noting the limited scope of the experiment, a slight gap can be observed between undergraduates on the one hand, and PhDs and graduates on the other. The gap between the latter two is less apparent.

Table 7. Average scores per group.

Group	Avg score (out of 100)
Undergraduate	83.5
Graduate	91.5
PhD	93.5

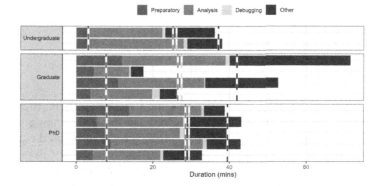

Fig. 2. Duration per category for each participant in each experience level.

Figure 3 shows a correlation matrix between the scores, the number of actions in each category, and the time spent on each category. Taking into account the small data underlying these correlations, it can be seen that no significant positive correlations with the score can be observed. However, the score is found to have a moderate negative correlation with both the amount and duration of debugging actions, as well as the duration of analysis actions. While the former seems logical, the latter is somewhat counter-intuitive. Given that no relation is found between with the number of analysis actions, the average duration of an analysis task seems to relevant. This might thus indicate that the score is negatively influenced when the analysis takes place slower, which might be a sign of inferior skills.

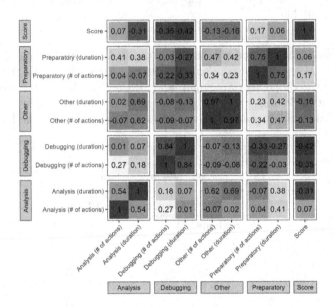

Fig. 3. Correlations between score, number of (distinct) actions in each category, and duration of each category.

6 Conclusion

The steps completed during an exploratory data analysis can be divided into four categories: the preparatory steps, the analysis steps, the debug step, and finally the actions that do not belong to a category but can be used throughout the analysis process. By further breaking down the exploratory data analysis into these steps, it becomes easier to proceed step by step and thus possibly obtain better analyses. The data analysis process performed by the participants appeared to be an iterative process that involved working step-by-step towards the solution.

The experiment described in this paper clearly is only a first step towards understanding the behaviour of data analysts. Only a small amount of people participated and the analysis requested was a relatively simple exercise. As a result, the list of operations found might not be exhaustive. Furthermore, the use of *R* and *RStudio* will have caused that some of the operations are specifically related to R. While R was chosen because all participants had a basic knowledge of *R* through an introductory course received in the first bachelor year, future research is needed to see whether these steps are also relevant with respect to other programming languages or tools. Moreover, this course may have already taught a certain methodology, which might not generalize to other data analyst. Additionally, the fact that the participants participated voluntarily, might mean they feel more comfortable performing a data analysis in R than their peers, especially among novices.

It is recommended that further research is conducted on both the operations, the order of these operations as well as the practices of experts and novices. By using more heterogeneous participants, a more difficult task and different programming languages, it is expected that additional operations can be identified as well as differences in practices between experts and beginners. These can be used to identify the mental representations of experts and, in turn, can be used to design new teaching methods [19]. In addition, an analysis at the sub-activity level could provide insights about frequencies and a lower-level order, such as in what order the sub-activities in the act of preparing data were usually performed.

References

1. Anders Ericsson, K.: Deliberate practice and acquisition of expert performance: a general overview. Acad. Emerg. Med. **15**(11), 988–994 (2008)
2. Anders Ericsson, K., Towne, T.J.: Expertise. Wiley Interdisc. Rev.: Cogn. Sci. **1**(3), 404–416 (2010)
3. Behrens, J.T.: Principles and procedures of exploratory data analysis. Psychol. Methods **2**(2), 131 (1997)
4. Blayney, P., Kalyuga, S., Sweller, J.: Interactions between the isolated-interactive elements effect and levels of learner expertise: experimental evidence from an accountancy class. Instr. Sci. **38**(3), 277–287 (2010)
5. Claes, J., Vanderfeesten, I., Gailly, F., Grefen, P., Poels, G.: The structured process modeling theory (SPMT) a cognitive view on why and how modelers benefit from structuring the process of process modeling. Inf. Syst. Front. **17**(6), 1401–1425 (2015). https://doi.org/10.1007/s10796-015-9585-y
6. Ericsson, A., Pool, R.: Peak: Secrets from the New Science of Expertise. Random House, New York (2016)
7. Ericsson, K.A., et al.: The influence of experience and deliberate practice on the development of superior expert performance. Cambridge Handb. Expertise Expert Perform. **38**(685–705), 2–2 (2006)
8. Hinds, P.J.: The curse of expertise: the effects of expertise and debiasing methods on prediction of novice performance. J. Exp. Psychol. Appl. **5**(2), 205 (1999)
9. Holton, J.A.: The coding process and its challenges. Sage Handb. Grounded Theory **3**, 265–289 (2007)
10. Jans, M., Soffer, P., Jouck, T.: Building a valuable event log for process mining: an experimental exploration of a guided process. Enterp. Inf. Syst. **13**(5), 601–630 (2019)
11. Jans, M.: From relational database to valuable event logs for process mining purposes: a procedure. Technical report, Hasselt University, Technical report (2017)
12. Janssenswillen, G., Depaire, B., Swennen, M., Jans, M., Vanhoof, K.: bupaR: enabling reproducible business process analysis. Knowl.-Based Syst. **163**, 927–930 (2019)

13. Kitchin, R.: The Data Revolution: Big Data, Open Data, Data Infrastructures and their Consequences. Sage, New York (2014)
14. Mayer-Schoenberger, V., Cukier, K.: The rise of big data: how it's changing the way we think about the world. Foreign Aff. **92**(3), 28–40 (2013)
15. O'Neil, C., Schutt, R.: Doing Data Science: Straight Talk from the Frontline. O'Reilly Media Inc, California (2013)
16. Saldaña, J.: Coding and analysis strategies. The Oxford handbook of qualitative research, pp. 581–605 (2014)
17. Saldaña, J.: The coding manual for qualitative researchers. The coding manual for qualitative researchers, pp. 1–440 (2021)
18. Saltz, J.S., Shamshurin, I.: Exploring the process of doing data science via an ethnographic study of a media advertising company. In: 2015 IEEE International Conference on Big Data (Big Data), pp. 2098–2105. IEEE (2015)
19. Spector, J.M., Ohrazda, C.: Automating instructional design: approaches and limitations. In: Handbook of Research on Educational Communications and Technology, pp. 681–695. Routledge (2013)
20. Sweller, J.: Cognitive load theory: Recent theoretical advances. (2010)
21. Wickham, H., Grolemund, G.: R for Data Science: Import, Tidy, Transform, Visualize, and Model Data. O'Reilly Media Inc, California (2016)
22. Yates, K.A., Clark, R.E.: Cognitive task analysis. International Handbook of Student Achievement. New York, Routledge (2012)
23. Zerbato, F., Soffer, P., Weber, B.: Initial insights into exploratory process mining practices. In: Polyvyanyy, A., Wynn, M.T., Van Looy, A., Reichert, M. (eds.) BPM 2021. LNBIP, vol. 427, pp. 145–161. Springer, Cham (2021). https://doi.org/10.1007/978-3-030-85440-9_9
24. Zimmermann, L., Zerbato, F., Weber, B.: Process mining challenges perceived by analysts: an interview study. In: Augusto, A., Gill, A., Bork, D., Nurcan, S., Reinhartz-Berger, I., Schmidt, R. (eds.) International Conference on Business Process Modeling, Development and Support, International Conference on Evaluation and Modeling Methods for Systems Analysis and Development, vol. 450, pp. 3–17. Springer, Cham (2022). https://doi.org/10.1007/978-3-031-07475-2_1

Discovering Students' Learning Strategies in a Visual Programming MOOC Through Process Mining Techniques

Narjes Rohani[1](✉), Kobi Gal[2](✉), Michael Gallagher[3](✉),
and Areti Manataki[4](✉)

[1] Usher Institute, University of Edinburgh, Scotland, UK
Narjes.Rohani@ed.ac.uk
[2] School of Informatics, University of Edinburgh, Scotland, UK
Kgal@inf.ed.ac.uk
[3] Moray House School of Education and Sport, University of Edinburgh, Scotland, UK
Michael.S.Gallagher@ed.ac.uk
[4] School of Computer Science, University of St Andrews, Scotland, UK
A.Manataki@st-andrews.ac.uk

Abstract. Understanding students' learning patterns is key for supporting their learning experience and improving course design. However, this is particularly challenging in courses with large cohorts, which might contain diverse students that exhibit a wide range of behaviours. In this study, we employed a previously developed method, which considers process flow, sequence, and frequency of learning actions, for detecting students' learning tactics and strategies. With the aim of demonstrating its applicability to a new learning context, we applied the method to a large-scale online visual programming course. Four low-level learning tactics were identified, ranging from project- and video-focused to explorative. Our results also indicate that some students employed all four tactics, some used course assessments to strategize about how to study, while others selected only two or three of all learning tactics. This research demonstrates the applicability and usefulness of process mining for discovering meaningful and distinguishable learning strategies in large courses with thousands of learners.

Keywords: Process mining · Massive open online courses · Educational data mining · Visual programming · Learning tactic · Learning strategy

1 Introduction

The increasing use of digital learning environments enables the collection of large amounts of data, which can be analysed through Educational Process Mining (EPM) to better understand educational processes [1,2]. A problem that has

© The Author(s) 2023
M. Montali et al. (Eds.): ICPM 2022 Workshops, LNBIP 468, pp. 539–551, 2023.
https://doi.org/10.1007/978-3-031-27815-0_39

recently attracted increasing research interest in the EPM community is around detecting students' learning tactics and strategies [19,20].

Identification of learning tactics and strategies can help customize course design, provide helpful feedback to students and assist them to adopt the best strategies for learning [20]. A learning tactic is defined as a series of actions that a student carries out to fulfil a specific task, such as passing an exam [7,13,17,21]; whereas, a learning strategy is "a coordinated set of learning tactics that are directed by a learning goal, and aimed at acquiring a new skill or gaining understanding" [17]. Identifying learning tactics and strategies is challenging, as they are invisible and latent [14]. It is even more challenging in courses with large cohorts, which may include more diverse student behaviour. Hence, appropriate analytical methods are needed, such as EPM. Most previous research that applied EPM methods to education are limited to traditional process mining methods, such as Alpha Miner, Heuristic Miner and Evolutionary Tree Miner [2,3]. On the other hand, Matcha *et al.* [19,20] proposed a novel EPM-based method for discovering students' learning tactics and strategies, which combines processes flow, frequency and distribution of learning actions, thus providing a more comprehensive view of student behaviour. However, the generalisability of this method needs to be further investigated, specifically in Massive Open Online Courses (MOOCs), which are less studied. To the best of our knowledge, only one MOOC [20] has been studied with the use of this method, and it involved a student cohort that is relatively small for a MOOC.

To take a step toward addressing this gap, we apply the EPM method by Matcha *et al.* [19] to study students' learning tactics and strategies in a large-scale visual programming MOOC with thousands of learners. The contributions of this paper are:

- We provide further evidence of the applicability of the method by Matcha *et al.* [19], by replicating their approach on large-scale data from a visual programming MOOC with thousands of students. To the best of our knowledge, this is the first time that this method is applied to such a large student cohort.
- We discover students' learning tactics and strategies in a visual programming MOOC. This is the first time that such learning patterns are investigated in a visual programming course.

2 Related Work

A growing number of studies have been conducted recently to analyse the educational behaviours of students, and detect their learning tactics and strategies using process mining and sequence mining [6,16,19]. Maldonado-Mahauad *et al.* [16] used the Process Mining PM^2 method [8] on three MOOCs in engineering, education, and management. They identified seven different learning tactics, such as only-video or only-assessment. Then, by applying hierarchical clustering, they discovered three learning strategies (i.e. comprehensive, targeting, and sampling) that involved different levels of self-regulated learning. In another study,

Jovanovic *et al.* [14] analysed trace data from an engineering course delivered in a flipped classroom. They discovered four learning tactics using sequence mining techniques and identified five learning strategies by applying hierarchical clustering to the tactics used by students. Fincham *et al.* [10] used the trace data from the same course and applied a different method. Instead of sequence mining, they used process mining based on Hidden Markov models, which resulted in the identification of eight learning tactics. Then, they clustered the students based on their used tactics and identified four learning strategies in two different periods. Matcha *et al.* [19] also studied the learning tactics and strategies in the same course. They employed a combination of First-order Markov models and the Expectation-Maximization algorithm for discovering learning tactics. This novel method is capable of considering not only the process flow of learning actions, but also their distribution and frequency. By applying hierarchical clustering, they also obtained three learning strategies.

In 2020, Matcha *et al.* applied the same methodology to two additional courses: a blended learning course in biology and a Python programming MOOC [20]. In the latter, they discovered four learning tactics (Diverse-Practice, Lecture-Oriented, Long-Practice, and Short-Practice) and three learning strategies (Inactive, Highly active at the beginning, and Highly active). By using the same methodology as in their previous work, they provided evidence of the generalisability of their method. However, further research is needed in order to draw solid conclusions about its i) generalisability to different learning contexts (e.g. different course designs) and ii) its scalability to large student cohorts and datasets. This is particularly important, as the MOOC analysed in [20] had only 368 students enrolled, which is a much smaller number than the average MOOC size of thousands of learners [4].

3 Materials and Methods

In this paper, we applied the EPM-based method in [19] on an introductory visual programming MOOC. We utilise course assessment and clickstream data from the *"Code Yourself! An Introduction to Programming" (CDY)* MOOC, which was delivered on Coursera [5] from January 2016 to December 2017.

CDY teaches the basics of programming using Scratch, which is one of the most popular visual programming languages [23]. It covers five topics (referred to as 'weeks' from now on) through 71 videos, 11 reading materials, 5 weekly discussion forums, 5 weekly quizzes/exams, and 2 peer-reviewed projects (on the third and fifth week). Notably, students can submit a quiz or project multiple times, and they receive the highest achieved score among all submissions.

The CDY dataset contains information about 46,018 enrolled students (45% male, 33% female, 22% unknown) and 55,485 learning sessions. A learning session is a series of clickstream actions that a student performs within one login into the platform. In this study, the sessions that have at least one of the following actions were considered for the analysis (i.e. 37,282 sessions in total):

1. **Video-start:** Starting to watch a video for the first time

2. **Video-play:** Playing a video lecture
3. **Video-end:** Watching a video until end
4. **Video-seek:** Skipping forward or backward throughout a video
5. **Video-pause:** Pausing a video lecture
6. **Video-revisit:** Watching a video for the second time or more
7. **Reading engagement:** Any activity related to the reading material such as visiting reading pages
8. **Discussion engagement:** Any activity related to the discussion forums
9. **Exam-visit:** Visiting exam-related pages without submitting answers
10. **Exam-failed:** Failing an exam (score lower than 50% of total score)
11. **Exam-passed:** Passing an exam
12. **Peer-reviewed project engagement:** Any activity related to the peer-reviewed projects, such as submitting or reviewing a submission

3.1 Pre-processing

Learning sessions were profiled for each student and analysed to identify their learning tactics. We considered two consecutive sessions with a time gap less than 30 min as one session. Due to the high variation between session lengths (i.e. between the number of actions in sessions), very long sessions (higher than the 95th quantile) and sessions with only one action were removed to obtain a more representative dataset. Since the course is a MOOC, there are numerous participants without the intention to take the quizzes and pass the course [15, 25]. Therefore, students without any attempt to submit an assessment were removed. A same approach for pre-processing was used in related work [6, 19]. The pre-processing steps resulted in 3,190 students (sample size 8 times larger than in [19]) and 34,091 sessions. The course completion rate among the 3,190 students considered in this study was 42%.

3.2 Detecting Learning Tactics and Strategies Through Process Mining and Clustering

To detect the learning tactics and strategies of CDY students, we followed the methodology in [19], the main steps of which are shown in Fig. 1. Learning tactics were detected with the use of process mining and clustering methods. In particular, First-order Markov Models, as implemented in the *pMineR* package [12], were employed to calculate the transition probability matrix of actions. The number of possible learning tactics (no. tactics=4) was estimated based on a process flow created by first-order Markov model, Elbow method, Hierarchical clustering dendrogram, and prior contextual knowledge. To identify the learning tactics, the Expectation-Maximisation algorithm [12] was applied to the obtained transition probability matrix. To shed light on the identified learning tactics, the *TraMineR package* [11] was used for analysing the distribution, duration and the order of employed learning actions. A student may apply a range of tactics throughout a course. Therefore, a learning strategy is defined as the goal-driven usage of a collection of learning tactics with the aim of obtaining knowledge or learning a new skill

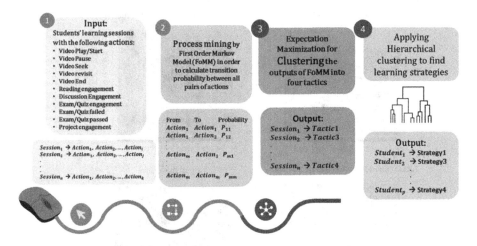

Fig. 1. Schema of the method: 1) Sessions with at least one coded action were selected. 2) First-order Markov Model was applied to create a process map and a transition matrix for all pairs of actions. 3) The transition matrix was used to cluster the sessions into four tactics using Expectation-Maximization method. 4) Hierarchical clustering was used to cluster students into four groups of strategies based on the frequency of their tactics.

[17]. To extract the various strategies adopted by students, and following methods established in related work [6,19], we calculated the number of occurrences of each tactic used by each student and we transformed it to the standard normal distribution. Finally, the strategies were identified by clustering the students using Agglomerative hierarchical clustering with Ward's linkage and Euclidean distance of the normalised vectors as the distance of students. The number of clusters (no. strategies = 4) was determined based on the dendrogram analysis, Elbow method, and contextual prior knowledge.

4   Results

Four learning tactics were discovered, which are characterised as follows.

Tactic1: Video-Oriented (17,819 sessions, 52.3% of all learning sessions) is the most commonly used learning tactic in CDY. It is characterized by relatively short sessions (median = 11 actions per session) that include mostly (over 99%) video-related learning actions. The high proportion of Video-end and Video-revisit actions indicate the high degree of interaction with videos (Fig. 2).

Tactic2: Long-Diverse and Video-Oriented (11,794 sessions, 35.12% of all learning sessions) are long sessions (median = 74 actions per session) composed of diverse actions, predominantly video-related. The majority of these sessions begin with a high peak in reading- and video-related actions, followed by a peak

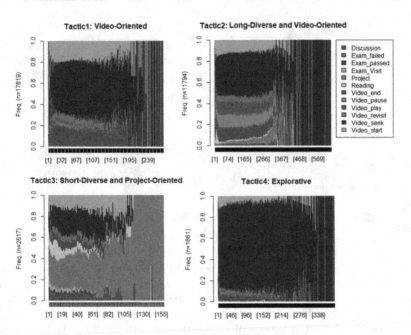

Fig. 2. Sequence distribution plot for the learning tactics. The X-axis presents the position of each learning action in the sessions and the Y-axis shows the relative frequency for each action in the corresponding position in the sessions. For example, the top right image for Tactic 2 shows that sessions in this cluster can contain over 500 actions. The relative frequency of reading-related actions decreases throughout these sessions, while the relative frequency of project-related actions increases.

in project engagement (Fig. 2). We can infer that students employed this tactic to first gain knowledge and then do the peer-reviewed projects.

Tactic3: Short-Diverse and Project-Oriented (2,617 sessions, 7.7% of all learning sessions) are the shortest (median = 8 actions per session) and most diverse sessions, shaped by a wide range of learning actions and dominated by project engagement (Fig. 2). The frequency of reading- and exam-related actions is much higher in this tactic than in other tactics. Figure 2 demonstrates that most of these sessions start with understanding theoretical concepts using video and reading actions, and continue with project actions. There is also a noticeable proportion of exam-related actions in these sessions, which indicates that students not only used video and reading materials to understand the concepts, but also they engaged in quizzes for self-assessment.

Tactic4: Explorative (1,861 sessions, 5.4% of all learning sessions) is the least frequent learning tactic. It involves relatively long sessions (median = 22 actions per session), largely dominated by video-seeking actions (Fig. 2). This indicates the exploratory behaviour of students, i.e. students may use this tactic to explore the videos or look for a specific concept.

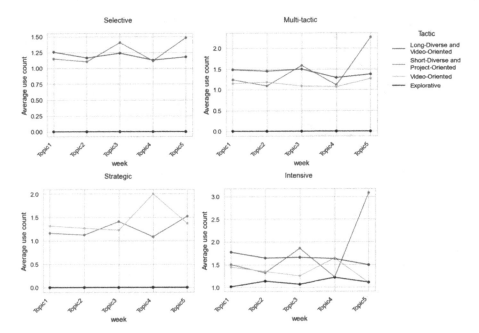

Fig. 3. Weekly changes in the applied learning tactics for the discovered learning strategies.

After finding the learning tactics, four learning strategies were identified following the methodology described in Sect. 3. It is worth noting that similarly to other MOOCs, the average number of sessions per student is low (avg: 2) and almost all students across all strategies have a relatively low level of engagement, especially with assessments [19]. The characteristics of the four learning strategies are as follows.

Strategy1, Selective: This strategy is followed by the majority of students (69.9% of students) and it is characterized mainly by using the *Long-Diverse and Video-Oriented*, and *Short-Diverse and Project-Oriented* learning tactics. In other words, this group of students are highly selective and use only two tactics. Based on the discussion in the learning tactics section, we can infer that students tend to use these two learning tactics to obtain knowledge, with the objective of answering questions in exams or doing peer-reviewed projects. Therefore, this group of students are characterized as *Selective* learners. Figure 4 indicates that the students using this strategy mainly start their learning process by a *Long-Diverse and Video-Oriented* tactic (p = 0.89). Afterwards, they tend to keep using this tactic (p = 0.7). The highest probable tactic to finish their learning process is also *Long-Diverse and Video-Oriented* (p = 0.24), and the most probable transition between the two tactics is the shift to a *Long-Diverse and Video-Oriented* tactic from a *Short-Diverse and Project-Oriented* tactic (p = 0.38).

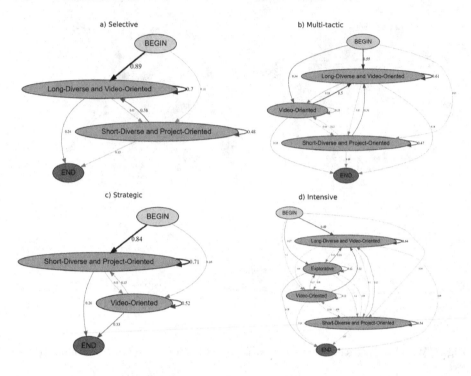

Fig. 4. Process models of the discovered learning strategies, which were created by *pMineR* package.

Strategy2, Multi-tactic: This strategy contains 13.5% of students who used multiple learning tactics each week (Fig. 3). In other words, all learning tactics except *Explorative* are employed in this strategy. Moreover, the frequency of *Long-Diverse and Video-Oriented*, and *Video-Oriented* tactics in this strategy remains almost the same during the course, while the frequency of *Short-Diverse and Project-Oriented* fluctuates throughout the different weeks. *Multi-tactic* students mainly tend to start their week with a *Long-Diverse and Video-Oriented* (p = 0.55) or *Video-Oriented* (p = 0.34) tactic; either way, they tend to continue the week with a *Long-Diverse and Video-Oriented*. The most probable shifts between used tactics are the transitions from any tactic to *Long-Diverse and Video-Oriented*, underlining this tactic as the predominantly used tactic by *Multi-tactic* learners (Fig. 4).

Strategy3, Strategic: This group contains 11.8% of all students, who mostly used the *Short-Diverse and Project-Oriented* and *Video-Oriented* learning tactics. *Short-Diverse and Project-Oriented* was mostly used at the time of submitting peer-reviewed projects, while the rest of the time these students primarily used *Video-Oriented* to learn the course materials (Fig. 3). On the other hand, the process flow of these students' sessions (Fig. 4) demonstrates that these students tend to start their learning process with a *Short-Diverse and*

Project-Oriented tactic (p = 0.84) and continue using this tactic until the end of the session (p = 0.71). The second most probable scenario is to start (p = 0.16) and continue (p = 0.52) to use only the *Video-Oriented* tactic with lower probability tactic. Alternatively, they might start the session with a *Short-Diverse and Project-Oriented* tactic and shift to *Video-Oriented* tactic. This strategy is named *Strategic* due to the high probability of using *Short-Diverse and Project-Oriented* tactic, which is a short tactic including a considerable number of project and exam-related actions along with the rest of the actions. Therefore, it can be inferred that the students strategically started their learning session with this tactic to achieve the required understanding for doing projects and exams.

Strategy4, Intensive: This is the smallest group of students (4% of all students) and they are very diligent, with relatively high engagement across all weeks (Fig. 3). These students used all learning tactics every week. Although the frequency of employed tactics varies across weeks, the least and most used tactics in this strategy are the *Explorative* and *Short-Diverse and Project-Oriented*, respectively. The *Video-Oriented* tactic was primarily used in the fourth week with two drops in the third and the fifth weeks, which is similar to the frequency trend of this tactic in the *Strategic* group. The average frequency of *Explorative* and *Long-Diverse and Video-Oriented* remains fairly steady throughout the course. Figure 4 shows the process flow of this strategy, which is not as straightforward as the process flow of the other strategies. The learning process in this strategy mainly starts with a *Long-Diverse and Video-Oriented* (p = 0.49) or an *Explorative* tactic (p = 0.27). Irrespective of the starting tactic, students tend to shift to *Long-Diverse and Video-Oriented* and continue using it with the highest probability. The process flow also highlights the diversity of tactics used in this strategy and the fact that there is no clear structure in terms of learning tactic transitions.

It is worth mentioning that we also investigated the association between learning strategies and academic performance, and found that the learning strategies in CDY do not correlate significantly with students' assessment scores. However, the discovered learning strategies in [20] were significantly associated with student performance. An explanation for this phenomenon can be the fact that the strategies discovered in [20] are indicative of students' engagement level, and students that engage more with a course tend to perform better. The strategies discovered in this study, however, are not indicative of engagement level and are rather characterised by different combinations of tactics.

5   Discussion

In this study, we applied an existing EPM-based method [19] to data from a large-scale course in visual programming, and detected novel learning tactics and strategies. Our main contribution is around evidence of the applicability of this method to a different learning context, namely a visual programming MOOC with thousands of learners. Only one other MOOC has been studied with the use of this method. Another important factor is student cohort size – our study involved 3,190 learners (after pre-processing), while the largest cohort analysed with this method in previous work was 1,135 students [20].

The learning tactics and strategies detected in our study are novel for programming and computing courses. In fact, it is the first time that such learning behaviours are investigated in a visual programming course. Most of the tactics detected include the high employment of video-related actions, which is reasonable given the high volume of video materials in the CDY course. This finding is in line with the fact that learning tactics can represent the different study approaches that are embedded in course designs and supplemented by course materials [9, 10, 18–20].

The four learning strategies discovered differ in terms of the learning tactics employed, whereas the engagement level does not vary much. However, the strategies found by Matcha et al. [20] were primarily focused on student engagement. In particular, most students in [20] used almost all learning tactics; therefore, clustering was based on the number of tactics used, which is an indicator of engagement. On the other hand, in CDY, clustering was based on the different combinations of tactics used. This demonstrates that the EPM method employed can effectively yield conceptually different strategies. Another advantage of this method is that it considers the process flow of learning tactics in order to group students, thus providing further insight into learning processes. Our findings indicate that the process flow of learning tactics in CDY is distinct in each group. For example, the process models of selective and strategic learners are composed of only two learning tactics; while multi-tactic and intensive students used multiple different learning tactics.

Moreover, the learning strategies extracted with the use of process mining are helpful resources for optimizing future course designs and understanding how the course design impacted the students' learning behaviour. The more insights we gain about the learning tactics and their relation to the course design, the better we can design future courses to achieve better student comprehension and fit with their learning preferences. As an example, the high rate of using the *Video-Oriented* tactic may be due to the high number of available videos in CDY. Therefore, the course design can be adjusted by supplementing more diverse resources, such as pre-lab reading, adding some programming lab notes, and making the exams or projects more interactive and attractive, so as to increase student engagement with assessments. Furthermore, informing students about their used learning strategies and other possible strategies that they can apply, can lead to better awareness and improvement of their learning approach. Also, teachers can consider students' learning strategies for providing personalized feedback [22]. For example, identifying a student that is erratic or that is only focusing on projects can help teachers provide personalized suggestions.

5.1 Limitations and Future Directions

The learning tactics and strategies that can be detected with the use of EPM methods are limited to the kind of data collected on the learning platform. For a programming course, it would have been interesting to also consider the programming process, for example when attempting assignments. This was not possible in the case of CDY, but it is worth addressing in future research. Another promising avenue for future research is to combine self-declared information and trace data [24] for analysing students' educational behaviour.

There is also a great opportunity to extend this work to investigate how student's demographic features, such as gender, academic degree, and age, impact the selection of learning tactics and strategies. This is particularly interesting to examine for courses with diverse student populations, such as MOOCs.

Similarly to related work, in this study we assume that learning strategies are static. However, it is plausible that students change their learning strategy throughout a course. Future studies should relax this assumption and consider changes in learning strategies over time.

Finally, we see great value in comparing learning strategies before and after the outbreak of the Covid-19 pandemic. An interesting methodological question is to what extend the method by Matcha *et al.* [19] enables such comparisons.

Acknowledgements. This work was supported by the Medical Research Council [grant number MR/N013166/1].

References

1. Baker, R.S.: Educational data mining: an advance for intelligent systems in education. IEEE Intell. Syst. **29**(3), 78–82 (2014)
2. Bogarín, A., Cerezo, R., Romero, C.: A survey on educational process mining. Wiley Interdisc. Rev.: Data Min. Knowl. Disc. **8**(1), e1230 (2018)
3. Cerezo, R., Bogarín, A., Esteban, M., Romero, C.: Process mining for self-regulated learning assessment in e-learning. J. Comput. High. Educ. **32**(1), 74–88 (2020)
4. Chen, Y.H., Chen, P.J.: MOOC study group: facilitation strategies, influential factors, and student perceived gains. Comput. Educ. **86**, 55–70 (2015)
5. Coursera: Code yourself! an introduction to programming. https://www.coursera.org/learn/intro-programming. Accessed 4 June 2022
6. Crosslin, M., Breuer, K., Milikić, N., Dellinger, J.T.: Understanding student learning pathways in traditional online history courses: utilizing process mining analysis on clickstream data. J. Res. Innovative Teach. Learn. (2021)
7. Derby, S.J.: Putting learning strategies to work. Educ. Leadersh. **46**(4), 4–10 (1989)
8. van Eck, M.L., Lu, X., Leemans, S.J.J., van der Aalst, W.M.P.: PM^2: a process mining project methodology. In: Zdravkovic, J., Kirikova, M., Johannesson, P. (eds.) CAiSE 2015. LNCS, vol. 9097, pp. 297–313. Springer, Cham (2015). https://doi.org/10.1007/978-3-319-19069-3_19
9. Fan, Y., Saint, J., Singh, S., Jovanovic, J., Gašević, D.: A learning analytic approach to unveiling self-regulatory processes in learning tactics. In: LAK21: 11th International Learning Analytics and Knowledge Conference, pp. 184–195 (2021)
10. Fincham, E., Gašević, D., Jovanović, J., Pardo, A.: From study tactics to learning strategies: an analytical method for extracting interpretable representations. IEEE Trans. Learn. Technol. **12**(1), 59–72 (2018)
11. Gabadinho, A., Ritschard, G., Mueller, N.S., Studer, M.: Analyzing and visualizing state sequences in R with TraMineR. J. Stat. Softw. **40**(4), 1–37 (2011)

12. Gatta, R., et al.: pMineR: an innovative R library for performing process mining in medicine. In: ten Teije, A., Popow, C., Holmes, J.H., Sacchi, L. (eds.) Artificial Intelligence in Medicine, pp. 351–355. Springer International Publishing, Cham (2017)

13. Hadwin, A.F., Nesbit, J.C., Jamieson-Noel, D., Code, J., Winne, P.H.: Examining trace data to explore self-regulated learning. Metacognition Learn. **2**(2), 107–124 (2007)

14. Jovanovic, J., Gasevic, D., Dawson, S., Pardo, A., Mirriahi, N., et al.: Learning analytics to unveil learning strategies in a flipped classroom. Internet High. Educ. **33**(4), 74–85 (2017)

15. Koller, D., Ng, A., Do, C., Chen, Z.: Retention and intention in massive open online courses: in depth. Educause Rev. **48**(3), 62–63 (2013)

16. Maldonado-Mahauad, J., Pérez-Sanagustín, M., Kizilcec, R.F., Morales, N., Munoz-Gama, J.: Mining theory-based patterns from big data: identifying self-regulated learning strategies in massive open online courses. Comput. Hum. Behav. **80**, 179–196 (2018)

17. Malmberg, J., Järvelä, S., Kirschner, P.A.: Elementary school students' strategic learning: does task-type matter? Metacognition Learn. **9**(2), 113–136 (2014)

18. Matcha, W., et al.: Detection of learning strategies: a comparison of process, sequence and network analytic approaches. In: Scheffel, M., Broisin, J., Pammer-Schindler, V., Ioannou, A., Schneider, J. (eds.) EC-TEL 2019. LNCS, vol. 11722, pp. 525–540. Springer, Cham (2019). https://doi.org/10.1007/978-3-030-29736-7_39

19. Matcha, W., Gašević, D., Uzir, N.A., Jovanović, J., Pardo, A.: Analytics of learning strategies: associations with academic performance and feedback. In: Proceedings of the 9th International Conference on Learning Analytics & Knowledge, pp. 461–470 (2019)

20. Matcha, W., et al.: Analytics of learning strategies: role of course design and delivery modality. J. Learn. Anal. **7**(2), 45–71 (2020)

21. Rachal, K.C., Daigle, S., Rachal, W.S.: Learning problems reported by college students: are they using learning strategies? J. Instr. Psychol. **34**(4), 191–202 (2007)

22. Reimann, P., Frerejean, J., Thompson, K.: Using process mining to identify models of group decision making in chat data (2009)

23. Resnick, M., et al.: Scratch: programming for all. Commun. ACM **52**(11), 60–67 (2009)

24. Ye, D., Pennisi, S.: Using trace data to enhance students' self-regulation: a learning analytics perspective. Internet High. Educ. **54**, 100855 (2022)

25. Zheng, S., Rosson, M.B., Shih, P.C., Carroll, J.M.: Understanding student motivation, behaviors and perceptions in MOOCS. In: Proceedings of the 18th ACM Conference on Computer Supported Cooperative Work & Social Computing, pp. 1882–1895 (2015)

Domain-Driven Event Abstraction Framework for Learning Dynamics in MOOCs Sessions

Luciano Hidalgo[(✉)] and Jorge Munoz-Gama

Department of Computer Science, Pontificia Universidad Católica de Chile,
Santiago, Chile
{lhidalgo1,jmun}@uc.cl

Abstract. In conjunction with the rapid expansion of Massive Open Online Courses (MOOCs), academic interest has grown in the analysis of MOOC student study sessions. Education researchers have increasingly regarded process mining as a promising tool with which to answer simple questions, including the order in which resources are completed. However, its application to more complex questions about learning dynamics remains a challenge. For example, do MOOC students genuinely study from a resource or merely skim content to understand what will come next? One common practice is to use the resources directly as activities, resulting in spaghetti process models that subsequently undergo filtering. However, this leads to over-simplified and difficult-to-interpret conclusions. Consequently, an event abstraction becomes necessary, whereby low-level events are combined with high-level activities. A wide range of event abstraction techniques has been presented in process mining literature, primarily in relation to data-driven bottom-up strategies, where patterns are discovered from the data and later mapped to education concepts. Accordingly, this paper proposes a domain-driven top-down framework that allows educators who are less familiar with data and process analytics to more easily search for a set of predefined high-level concepts from their own MOOC data. The framework outlined herein has been successfully tested in a Coursera MOOC, with the objective of understanding the in-session behavioral dynamics of learners who successfully complete their respective courses.

Keywords: Event abstraction · MOOC · Learning dynamics

1 Introduction

The use of technology in educational environments has increased the learning alternatives around the world. In this regard, Massive Open Online Courses (MOOCs) are one of the most popular alternatives, since they enable learners to operate through a completely online environment, across a variety of subjects,

This work is partially supported by ANID FONDECYT 1220202, IDeA I+D 2210048 and ANID-Subdirección de Capital Humano/Doctorado Nacional/2022-21220979.

M. Montali et al. (Eds.): ICPM 2022 Workshops, LNBIP 468, pp. 552–564, 2023.
https://doi.org/10.1007/978-3-031-27815-0_40

scaling seamlessly across hundreds or thousands of users [4]. These courses were originally conceived of as opportunities for personal capacity building and have now been integrated into the curricula of numerous educational institutions, in which the line between face-to-face and online learning has become increasingly blurred. This integration has led to an increase in the understanding of how users carry out their tasks and perform on these platforms, and this in itself has become both a topic of interest for all stakeholders and an open area of research [2,4]. In particular, there is a growing interest in understanding learner dynamics within a session, i.e., during an uninterrupted period of work [2,4].

Educational managers have considered process mining a promising tool with which to answer their research questions, given its ease of use for users who are not necessarily experts in data and process analytics [14]. A common approach in the literature consists of using fields directly from a database table as activities for process mining algorithms, e.g., the accessed MOOC resource [14]. The conclusions that can be drawn from this approach are limited. Given the number of possible activities and variants, the result may end up as a spaghetti process model. In such cases, a majority of authors opt to heavily filter the number of activities or arcs to achieve a readable albeit partial model and to limit the complexity of the questions that can be answered.

More complex questions necessarily require event abstractions, i.e., low-level events are combined in high-level patterns, creating logs that are better tailored to answering such questions and with less variability, thus improving interpretability. In the literature on process mining, there is a broad variety of event abstraction methods (for a literature review on the topic, readers should see [15]). Most event abstraction approaches are data-driven (bottom up), i.e., domain-agnostic and unsupervised methods to detect frequent patterns in data. In certain cases these frequent patterns are mapped according to the most fitting education concepts, e.g., self-regulated learning profiles. However, the application of these techniques, although possible, is difficult when there is a set of high-level activities that have already been defined and an attempt is made to determine such behaviors in the log in a domain-driven (top-down) manner. For example, in the case of learning dynamics, the same pattern of accessing a MOOC resource may reflect whether the learner is studying from a resource, or simply skimming over it to understand what will come next. Finally, defining an event abstraction can be a highly complex task for educational decision-makers who are not experts in process mining, since it requires a solid understanding of concepts such as case ID, activity ID and event ID. That is why it is necessary to define frameworks (or easy-to-follow recipes) in interdisciplinary scenarios, such as education, in order to apply process mining.

This paper proposes a domain-driven event abstraction framework specifically to analyze learning dynamics in MOOC sessions. The framework is simple enough to be replicated by educational managers and defines the following: 1) a minimal data model that can be adapted to most platforms (Coursera, FutureLearn, EdX); 2) the definition of a low-level event log, including the definition of case ID and session; and 3) the definition of seven high-level learning dynamics and their corresponding high-level log. In addition, this paper validates and illustrates the application of the framework by means of a case study: to determine the learning dynamics of the sessions of students who successfully complete the MOOC "Introduction to Programming in Python" on the Coursera platform. The remainder of the paper is structured as follows: Sect. 2 describes the most relevant research undertaken in the area; Sect. 3 presents the framework and its three core elements; Sect. 4 illustrates the application of the framework in the selected case study in order to validate the feasibility thereof; and Sect. 5 concludes the paper and outlines potential future work.

2   Related Work

Process Mining and MOOCs: Although MOOC systems generate a significant amount of data, their research using process mining techniques is just starting [14]. However, several authors have attempted to describe or explore student processes from this data. For example, [12] investigate the differences in the process between three different sets of students depending on whether they have completed all, some or none of the MOOC activities. On the other hand, by combining clustering techniques with process mining, [3] identify four sets of students, ranging from those who drop out at the very beginning of the course to those who successfully complete it. Their research shows how students who composed the cluster of individuals who successfully completed the course tended to watch videos in successive batches. In one of the most relevant works in this subject, [9] study the event logs of three MOOC Coursera courses and discovered six patterns of interaction among students. These patterns were also grouped into three clusters, identified as sampling learners, comprehensive learners and targeting learners, according to the behavior described. Furthermore, this work has incorporated the concept of "session" as a unit of analysis. [4] explore in greater depth the behavior of students in work sessions according to eight different possible interactions, segmenting them according to those who complete and those who do not complete the course. The aforementioned paper finds that students who complete the course are those who show more dedicated behavior and carry out a greater number of sessions.

Process Mining and Event Abstraction: Despite the utility of process mining techniques for understanding how organizations function, the systems that generate this data are not necessarily capable of handling the appropriate level of detail. Therefore, techniques that allow the abstraction of high-level activities from granular data are vital for the correct application of process mining techniques [15]. Currently, there are several strategies with which to address this problem. One family of techniques uses unsupervised machine learning by grouping events according to different dimensions, such as: the semantics of activity names [13], the physical proximity in which events occur [11], events that occur frequently together [10], and sub-sequences of activities that are repeated [5], among others. Additional authors have proposed less automated strategies, such as [7], who group elements according to the relationships between entities (ontologies) in order to abstract events using domain knowledge. This latter research was successfully applied in the medical domain. Similarly, [1] proposes a four-stage method based on the prior identification of process activities, a granular matching between activities and events according to their type, and certain context-sensitive rules. Indeed, this method proposes the grouping of different events into activities. Furthermore, in a combination of supervised and unsupervised methods, [8] propose a method for event abstraction in diffuse environments. As such, the aforementioned approach is based on the separation of events into sessions according to activity periods, prior to the generation of clusters of events, which are manually reviewed in a heat map in order to subsequently map them to high-level activities.

3   Domain-Driven Event Abstraction Framework

This section presents the domain-driven event abstraction framework to aid educational managers in building a high-level event log with which to analyze the learning dynamics of students during their MOOC work sessions. The framework is composed of three stages: 1) a minimal data model capable of being mapped to any MOOC system; 2) the definition of a low-level log from the minimal data model; and 3) the definition of a high-level log derived from the low-level log.

S1: Minimal Data Model. The first stage that defines the framework is the minimal data model. This is a data model with the minimum information necessary to build the low-level event log, which serves as a *lingua franca* among different MOOC systems, including Coursera, FutureLearn and edX, among others. Figure 1 shows the minimal data model, which is filled with information each time a user interacts with a MOOC resource. The model contemplates the identification of three main elements: the resource interacted with, the user who performs the interaction, and the time at which the interaction is made. Resources and users are identified with a unique identifier, present in all MOOC systems. In addition, the model determines that each resource adheres to an associated order within the MOOC. Utilizing this approach, it can be determined whether the user is interacting in a sequential or disorderly manner via the resources. The model also defines the type of resource in question. In this proposal, two generic types are defined: content resources (video-lectures, presentations, etc.) and assessments (quizzes, exams, etc.). However, the framework can be easily extended to include other types of resources, such as project or bibliographical resources. Finally, each interaction with a resource has an associated state (start or complete) in the event log. This makes it possible to identify whether the learning dynamics of students correspond to exploratory or in-depth work patterns. The majority of MOOC systems contain the necessary information to be able to determine status. In some cases, such as Coursera, state is explicitly recorded as two different interactions (one is "Started" and the other is "Completed") in its Course Progress table. In other systems, status can be determined from two timestamps ("Start" and "End") that are associated with the same interaction.

S2: Low-Level Log. The second stage of the framework describes how to build the low-level log, based on the information contained in the minimal data model,

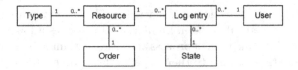

Fig. 1. Minimal data model suggested.

as defined in the previous stage. Each interaction with a MOOC resource recorded in the minimal data model represents an event in the low-level log. The transformation of the information in the minimal data model to the low-level log is straightforward, with the exception of two elements: the session and case ID.

This framework is designed to analyze the learning dynamics in student work sessions, i.e., an uninterrupted period of work. Therefore, it is necessary to define to which session each interaction with a resource pertains. Certain MOOC systems have their own built-in session definition and identification. However, in most MOOC systems this definition is not explicitly available, although it can be determined. For example, two consecutive interactions pertain to different sessions if, between their timestamps, a certain threshold of time has passed in which no interaction with the MOOC has been carried out. Different thresholds and the implications thereof have been reviewed in the literature [6]. Once the session has been determined, the framework defines the case ID of the low-level log as the pair (user ID, session ID), i.e., different sessions of the same student correspond to different cases in the log.

S3: High-level Log. The low-level event log obtained in stage two resembles the analysis input that a non-expert user in process mining would normally use directly in a tool such as Disco or ProM. However, the large amount of resources and variants that result from this type of log make it difficult to obtain process-driven answers. Therefore, stage three of the framework defines seven high-level activities (Fig. 2), with each one representing a different learning dynamic which reflects learner behavior, regardless of the resources consulted. In particular, this includes four dynamics associated with content consumption and three related to interaction with assessments.

– *Progressing*: this represents the learning dynamic of a student who consumes a resource and then continues, in the correct order, with the next resource in the course.
– *Exploring*: this represents the learning dynamic of a student who interacts in a superficial manner with new content, simply in order to know what to expect, for example, to determine the time needed to consume that content.
– *Echoing*: this represents the learning dynamic of a student who consumes a resource, and then continues on to the next resource in the correct order, but with resources that have already been previously completed. A good example is a learner who decides to review content prior to sitting an exam.
– *Fetching*: this represents the learning dynamic of a student who interacts with a previously completed resource, with or without completing it, and in no

particular order. A good example is a student who, after failing an assessment question, re-watches (partially or totally) a specific video in order to identify the answer.

- *Assessing*: this represents the learning dynamic of a student who interacts with and completes an assessment-type resource that has not been previously completed. In the case of a block of several Assessing dynamics in a row, regardless of their order, these are collapsed into a single dynamic.
- *Skimming*: this represents the learning dynamic of a student who initiates but does not complete interactions with assessments. For example, the student could be reviewing the questions before taking an assessment seriously or could be reviewing an assessment beforehand in order to understand where he/she went wrong.
- *Retaking*: this represents the learning dynamic of a student who initiates and completes assessments that have been previously completed. For example, a user who did not obtain a satisfactory score and who decides to retry in order to improve their previous result.

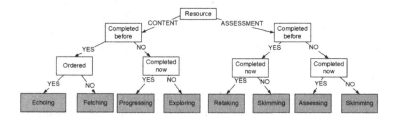

Fig. 2. Criteria to assign to each activity.

4   Case Study: Successful Student Sessions in Coursera

To illustrate the application of the framework and validate its applicability with real data, a case study was conducted using data from the "Introduction to Programming in Python" course on the Coursera platform. The objective of the case study was to examine the learning dynamics that took place in the sessions of students who successfully completed the course. Specifically, the following two questions are defined: *RQ1: What are the characteristics of the sessions that involve learning dynamics in which a resource is revisited?* and *RQ2: Are there differences in terms of learning dynamics between the first sessions and the final sessions carried out by students?* With that in mind, this section presents the following: first, the descriptive information of the course and the application of the three levels of the framework related to the case study; second, the results-based answers of the two research questions; and third, a brief discussion of the implications of these results.

Case Study and Framework: This study considers data generated from a Coursera course held during the period June 23, 2017 to April 14, 2018.

The course involved a total time commitment of 17 h and was organized into 6 modules, 1 for each week. In this analysis, consideration was taken of 58 possible resources with which to interact, 35 content resources (video lectures) and 23 assessment resources.

The first step in the application of the framework was to align the minimal data model available to Coursera with the minimal data model proposed herein. The Coursera data model contained more than 75 tables. The most relevant table for this study was the Course Progress table, which recorded the course ID, the resource interacted with, the user who performed the interaction, the status (start/complete) and the timestamp detailing when it occurs. However, as this table only contained IDs, it was necessary to supplement it with the course information tables (Course Item Types, Course Items, Course Lessons, Course Modules, Course Progress State Types) so as to establish the order of the resources within the course and obtain descriptive information.

The second step in the application of the framework was to build the low-level event log, including the concept of session ID. To do so, an activity was considered to occur in the same session as the previous activity if, between them, there was a lapse equal to or less than 60 min, which is the maximum limit for time-on-task, as established by [6]. Hence, the case ID for the low-level event log was established as the pair (user ID, session ID). Only users who began and completed the course during the observation period were used for this analysis. The criterion to determine whether a user completed the course was based on whether that learner completed either of the final two course assessments. This yielded 209 user cases for analysis and a total of 320,421 low-level events. Finally, Coursera recorded progress through each question within the assessment as each new event started, e.g., a student completing an assessment with 10 questions results in 11 events started and 1 completed. This duplication was subsequently condensed, resulting in a low-level event log of 39,650 events.

The final step in the application of the framework was the creation of the high-level event log from the definition of the seven high-level activities: *Progressing, Exploring, Echoing, Fetching, Assessing, Skimming and Retaking*. The resulting high-level log contained 18,029 events. This represented a 54.5% reduction of activities compared to the low-level log. As with the low-level log, the case ID for the high-level event log was established as the pair (user ID, session ID). From the 209 users, this generated 7,087 cases which were grouped into 1,237 distinct variants.

RQ1: This study detected differences between the various sessions that involved learning dynamics in which a resource was revisited, i.e., Echoing, Fetching, and Retaking. An exploratory analysis of the sessions showed that Fetching appeared in 13% of cases, and the interaction of this activity seems to be strongly related to assessment dynamics (i.e., Assessing, Skimming, Retaking); in 54.3% of cases in which this activity was detected, its occurrence was preceded by one of the activities related to assessment; and in 50.9% of cases, Fetching was followed by some form of assessment.

In this case, the Fetching of a content (totally or partially) suggests a specific search-related action, either in preparation for an assessment or in response to a certain element that appeared in an assessment and about which it is worth clarifying a particular doubt. However, when consideration is taken of the sessions that included an Assessing or Retaking activity besides Fetching, the proportion changed, with 25.6% performing the fetch prior to the assessment and 21.5% afterwards. Analysis of the content associated with Fetching showed that the most commonly fetched resources were *2.2.2 Input*, *3.1.1 If/Else*, *3.2.2 For*, *2.1.1. Data Types* (which can be understood as the first different elements for someone with no prior programming knowledge), and *6.1.4 List Functions* (following analysis, it could be seen that this particular content was poorly designed and suggestions were made to re-record the video using a new structure).

When comparing with cases in which Echoing appeared (as shown in Fig. 3), behavior was seen to have changed, since in the majority of cases this activity was directly related to Progressing, to the extent that in 35.9% of the cases with Echoing, the previous activity or the one that immediately succeeded it was Progressing. This indicates that the extensive repetition of content occurred in sessions in which the student was oriented towards studying content and that during these study sessions doubts arose, which therefore necessitates an in-depth review of previously seen content. This differs to the patterns generated with regards to Fetching, which appears more strongly related to assessment activities. Nonetheless, in this case a relationship also existed with the assessment activities. Yet, they differed in the sequence point in which they appeared, since a repetition of content occurred more frequently prior to the assessment, as opposed to the variants that included Fetching, whereby the content review occurred more frequently after the assessment was accessed.

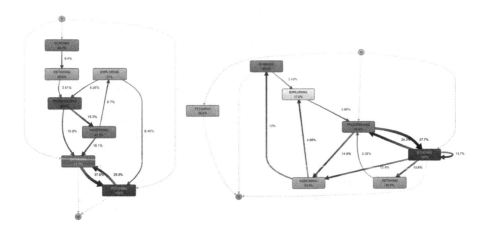

Fig. 3. Comparison between sessions fetching (left) and echoing (right) sessions.

Finally, when reviewing Retaking (Fig. 4) it can be assumed that the user entered the session directly with the intention of retaking assessments, since the most common variant (25.9% of cases) only repeated their assessments and then concluded the session. Similarly, the activity with which there was the strongest relationship in this case is Skimming, which indicates a dynamic whereby learners performed a self-evaluation and then reviewed the results, or looked at their previous results which they then attempted to improve. The transition from Retaking to Skimming occurred in 33.6% of cases in which repetition was present, while the reverse occurred in 32.1% of the cases. This implies that either (or both) of these interactions appeared in 43.0% of the cases with Retaking. By reviewing the most commonly repeated Retaking-related assessments, one assessment in particular was noted as having a significantly higher number of Retaking than the rest (597 occurrences out of an average of 285). In consultation with the course designers, this assessment, which measured the topics of variables and input/output, was found to have had a bug in one of the questions. The bug was subsequently corrected after the observation date had been recorded.

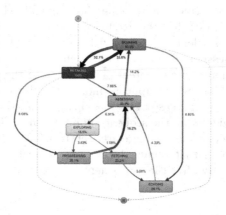

Fig. 4. Learning dynamics in sessions with retaking.

RQ2: The sessions of each student were divided into quintiles by considering the total number of sessions completed by each one. Thus, the sessions of the first and last quintile were compared. This made it possible to verify the existence of differences between behavior at the beginning and end of the course.

In the process model obtained from the analysis of the initial sessions (Fig. 5) it can be observed that the most common activities were associated with orderly and comprehensive learning (Progressing 63.9% and Echoing 29.7%). Furthermore, a relatively low commitment to assessment can also be seen at this point in the course, since although the Skimming activity appeared in 36.7% of cases, students were observed undertaking sessions without completing an assessment in 66.3% of cases. This idea is reinforced by the observation that in 5.78% of cases, the Progressing activity involved more than one piece of content being completed in the correct order. This suggests that students preferred not to interrupt their content study progression in order to carry out the interspersed assessments.

As the Progressing and Exploring activities refer to the very first time a piece of content was viewed, these activities were expected to be more frequent at the beginning of the course, showing a decreasing frequency towards the end of the course. However, it is noteworthy that the Echoing activity experienced a high frequency of 29.7% during the initial sessions.

Conversely, by grouping the sessions into quintiles it was possible to evince that sessions at the beginning of the course tended to experience the most changes in terms of learning dynamics. Indeed, despite comprising 19% of the sessions, 23% of all events in the high-level log were found to take place in these initial stages. By conducting the same exercise with each quintile in turn, it can be seen that the number of events grouped together in each one decreased, reaching a mere 15% of events in the final quintile.

It seems that with regards to the final sessions (Fig. 5) these were mainly carried out in relation to assessment activities, since all associated activities (Skimming, Assessing and Retaking) appeared more frequently than those associated with contents. For example, 39.9% of the former performed at least one Assessing or Retaking activity. However, it is striking to find that 40.4% of cases corresponded to students who only undertook Skimming and then finished the session, thus suggesting that a significant number of learners simply logged on to browse the questions without completing the broader assessment. Regarding the dynamics of the content activities, the Progressing activity tended to be the one that initiated the sessions in which it appeared, and was most frequently succeeded by assessment activities, particularly Assessing. This indicates changes from the beginning of the course, whereby the user tended to either continue to study or repeat content more frequently. In addition, from this perspective it should be noted that even at the end of the course the Progressing activity appeared more frequently than Echoing and with a higher average duration (23.5 min versus 9.6 min, on average). Similarly, the behavior of continuing to study by skipping an assessment drastically reduced its occurrence, accounting for merely 2 cases or 0.1% of these sessions.

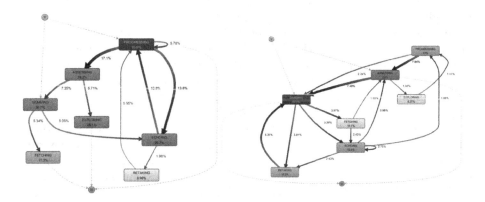

Fig. 5. Difference between initial sessions and ending sessions (30% paths).

Discussion: First, the results show that students varied their session behavior during the duration of the MOOC, given that at the beginning of the course they were more reluctant to assess themselves and preferred to review content rather that to measure the extent of their overall knowledge. The situation changed as they progressed through the course, as 25% of the total number of events recorded in the log ended up as completed assessments, either for the first time or by repeating an already-completed assessment. This indicates that student commitment to the course increased as they progress through it. By examining the detail of the cases, it was found that the most common variants were of a single activity and that the longest sequences commonly involved activities of the same type (e.g., Progressing and Echoing or Skimming and Retaking). This confirms the findings of [2] who suggest that successful students change the priority of the activities they complete between course sessions. On the other hand, the patterns observed are consistent with experiments that use other techniques or optics on MOOC data, such as machine learning or clustering.

One of the unexpected results in this research was the discovery that the sole, most common variant was the Skimming activity, which accounted for 26.7% of the high-level log. This could point to the need to refine the skimming activity, since the review of an unfinished assessment may be the result of several possible factors, including: that the difficulty of the content due to be assessed is being reviewed in preparation for a serious attempt to complete it; that mistakes made in previous attempts are being reviewed; and that the questions are being used as learning examples, among others.

5   Conclusions

This paper presents a domain-driven event abstraction framework that facilitates the construction of a high-level event log with which to analyze learning dynamics in MOOC sessions. Specifically, the framework is composed of three stages: 1) the minimal data model necessary; 2) the construction of a low-level event log; and 3) the definition of seven high-level activities that can be used to build the high-level event log: Progressing, Exploring, Echoing, Fetching, Assessing, Skimming, Retaking. The application of the framework in a real scenario was validated in a case study in which the learning dynamics of the sessions of students who successfully completed the course were analyzed. Specifically, analysis was undertaken of the behavior in the sessions in which a resource was reviewed and an error found in the course, in addition to the differences in behavior between the first and last sessions of the students.

This research should be considered as exploratory and preliminary in nature, with significant room for improvement in future work. First, the framework attempts to extrapolate the intentions of the students (e.g., progressing vs exploring) from the available data. Nevertheless, such extrapolations could be refined if the framework were complemented with certain additional instruments, for example, surveys and interviews, as has been carried out in other types of MOOC analysis, such as self-regulated learning [2]. Second, domain-driven event abstractions and data-driven event abstractions should not be considered as opposing techniques, but rather as two sides of the same coin that can complement one another. In this regard, rather than a purely domain-driven event abstraction, this investigation could be complemented by one of the data-driven event abstraction techniques outlined in [15], thus creating a hybrid method that combines the two approaches in an iterative manner. Third, it is crucial to test the framework in different courses and MOOCs to ensure its generality and usefulness.

References

1. Baier, T., Mendling, J., Weske, M.: Bridging abstraction layers in process mining. Inf. Syst. **46**, 123–139 (2014)
2. de Barba, P.G., Malekian, D., Oliveira, E.A., Bailey, J., Ryan, T., Kennedy, G.: The importance and meaning of session behaviour in a MOOC. Comput. Educ. **146**, 103772 (2020)
3. Van den Beemt, A., Buijs, J., Van der Aalst, W.: Analysing structured learning behaviour in massive open online courses (MOOCs): an approach based on process mining and clustering. Int. Rev. Res. Open Distrib. Learn. **19**(5) (2018)
4. Bernal, F., Maldonado-Mahauad, J., Villalba-Condori, K., Zúñiga-Prieto, M., Veintimilla-Reyes, J., Mejía, M.: Analyzing students' behavior in a MOOC course: a process-oriented approach. In: Stephanidis, C., et al. (eds.) HCII 2020. LNCS, vol. 12425, pp. 307–325. Springer, Cham (2020). https://doi.org/10.1007/978-3-030-60128-7_24
5. Günther, C.W., Rozinat, A., van der Aalst, W.M.P.: Activity mining by global trace segmentation. In: Rinderle-Ma, S., Sadiq, S., Leymann, F. (eds.) BPM 2009. LNBIP, vol. 43, pp. 128–139. Springer, Heidelberg (2010). https://doi.org/10.1007/978-3-642-12186-9_13
6. Kovanović, V., Gašević, D., Dawson, S., Joksimović, S., Baker, R.S., Hatala, M.: Penetrating the black box of time-on-task estimation. In: Proceedings of the Fifth International Conference on Learning Analytics and Knowledge, pp. 184–193 (2015)
7. Leonardi, G., Striani, M., Quaglini, S., Cavallini, A., Montani, S.: Towards semantic process mining through knowledge-based trace abstraction. In: Ceravolo, P., van Keulen, M., Stoffel, K. (eds.) SIMPDA 2017. LNBIP, vol. 340, pp. 45–64. Springer, Cham (2019). https://doi.org/10.1007/978-3-030-11638-5_3
8. de Leoni, M., Dündar, S.: Event-log abstraction using batch session identification and clustering. In: ACM Symposium on Applied Computing, pp. 36–44 (2020)
9. Maldonado-Mahauad, J., Pérez-Sanagustín, M., Kizilcec, R.F., Morales, N., Munoz-Gama, J.: Mining theory-based patterns from big data: identifying self-regulated learning strategies in massive open online courses. Comput. Hum. Behav. **80**, 179–196 (2018)
10. Mannhardt, F., Tax, N.: Unsupervised event abstraction using pattern abstraction and local process models. arXiv preprint arXiv:1704.03520 (2017)
11. Rehse, J.-R., Fettke, P.: Clustering business process activities for identifying reference model components. In: Daniel, F., Sheng, Q.Z., Motahari, H. (eds.) BPM 2018. LNBIP, vol. 342, pp. 5–17. Springer, Cham (2019). https://doi.org/10.1007/978-3-030-11641-5_1

12. Rizvi, S., Rienties, B., Rogaten, J., Kizilcec, R.F.: Investigating variation in learning processes in a FutureLearn MOOC. J. Comput. High. Educ. **32**(1), 162–181 (2020)
13. Sánchez-Charles, D., Carmona, J., Muntés-Mulero, V., Solé, M.: Reducing event variability in logs by clustering of word embeddings. In: Teniente, E., Weidlich, M. (eds.) BPM 2017. LNBIP, vol. 308, pp. 191–203. Springer, Cham (2018). https://doi.org/10.1007/978-3-319-74030-0_14
14. Wambsganss, T., et al.: The potential of technology-mediated learning processes: a taxonomy and research agenda for educational process mining. In: ICIS (2021)
15. van Zelst, S.J., Mannhardt, F., de Leoni, M., Koschmider, A.: Event abstraction in process mining: literature review and taxonomy. Granular Comput. **6**(3), 719–736 (2021)

Process Mining for Analyzing Open Questions Computer-Aided Examinations

Saimir Bala[✉][iD], Kate Revoredo[iD], and Jan Mendling[iD]

Humboldt University of Berlin, Berlin, Germany
{saimir.bala,kate.revoredo,jan.mendling}@hu-berlin.de

Abstract. Computer-based education relies on information systems to support teaching and learning processes. These systems store trace data about the interaction of the learners with their different functionalities. Process mining techniques have been used to evaluate these traces and provide insights to instructors on the behavior of students. However, an analysis of students behavior on solving open-questioned examinations combined with the marks they received is still missing. This analysis can support the instructors not only on improving the design of future edition of the course, but also on improving the structure of online and physical evaluations. In this paper, we use process mining techniques to evaluate the behavioral patterns of students solving computer-based open-ended exams and their correlation with the grades. Our results show patterns of behavior associated to the marks received. We discuss how these results may support the instructor on elaborating future open question examinations.

Keywords: Education · Process mining · Educational process mining · Exam process

1 Introduction

Educational process mining [1] analyzes data generated from educational systems using process mining techniques. These analyses may support the course instructors for example on understanding how students engage with self-assessment [2] or how the students behave while using the online educational systems [3]. Typically, these kind of analyses focus on online courses, such as the ones provided by Massive Open Online Course (MOOC) platforms like Coursera[1], Edx[2], etc. In these settings the courses are designed for being taught online. Consecutively also students assessments is performed online using closed-answer questions [3,4].

However, with the advent of the COVID-19 pandemic, a new reality emerged: courses that were designed to be held in presence had to switch to online mode

---

[1] https://www.coursera.org.
[2] https://www.edx.org.

This work was supported by the Einstein Foundation Berlin [grant number EPP-2019-524, 2022].

M. Montali et al. (Eds.): ICPM 2022 Workshops, LNBIP 468, pp. 565–576, 2023.
https://doi.org/10.1007/978-3-031-27815-0_41

due to the various lockdowns. Oftentimes this transfer from physical mode to online mode had to be performed with short notice, leaving the instructors little or not time to design the course anew. As a result, many courses "switched" to online by simply mimicking their in-presence version. Thus, previously planned on-paper exams, were simply replaced by online documents to be downloaded by the students, performed within a remotely-controlled environment (i.e., monitoring students via webcam, microphone, screenshots) and uploaded again to the system [5]. These kind of exams are referred to as *open questions computer-aided examinations*.

In order to make it possible for the teacher or other authorities to check for students misconduct during the exam at a later stage, the monitoring data are usually persisted in event logs as *trace data* [6]. In this way, such setting opens up to a unique opportunity to use process mining to gain further insights on the *exam-taking process*. Specifically, mining techniques can be used to support the instructors on understanding how the students behave when solving the exam, for example to understand which question was more or less demanding. Also, confronting the behavior for solving the exam with the marks the students received may provide other insights to the instructors. For example, if certain behavior leads to better performance, if the most demanding question was also the one with lower marks meaning that the students did not acquire the knowledge.

In this paper, we use a multi-method approach based on process mining [7] to analyze the trace data generated from the interaction of students with an online system while doing an exam with open questions. We used data from two master course exams. We enriched the trace data with the marks the students received for each of the questions. The results show that there is a pattern on solving the exam when considering the topmost performers students. Also, there is a relation between the time spent by the students on solving the question with the marks they received for the question. With this research we contribute to the area for educational process mining by showing how process mining can be used also to support courses designed as physical.

The rest of the paper is structured as follows. Section 2 discusses the related work. Section 3 presents our method for evaluating students behavior on solving an online exam. Section 4 describes our scenario of application including the setting, results and some discussions. Section 5 concludes our work and provide some future directions.

2   Related Work

Educational data has been exploited by process mining techniques for various analyses [8] and in several ways. In [3] the data is grouped considering the grades and the behavior of the students while using an online educational tool. Process mining techniques are then applied to the different groups showing that the models discovered are more comprehensible and with higher fitness than the models learned using the whole data. In [9] data from a Massive Open Online Course (MOOC) was used to analyze the behavior of the students during the learning phase confronted with the final marks they achieve in the course.

Our literature review did not find many works related to ours, i.e., that focus on using process mining for analyzing the behavior of the students considering an *online assessment*. In the remaining of this section we outline the contributions of works who take online assessment into account.

In [2] process mining is used to evaluate how students engage with self-assessment and formative assessment and how these two types of assessments are related. In [4] process mining is used to evaluate the navigation behavior of students when answering to a close-ended online test. Also, a navigation reference model is used for conformance checking. The results of the paper show that the navigation behavior impacts on the performance of the students. In [10] a system to automatically evaluate the performance of students was proposed. Process discovery is used to learn the process used by the students when doing an online test that requires the use of a special software, e.g., ERP system. The process discovered represent how the student behaved to achieve the given business scenario. Based on the learned model students' performance is automatically evaluated. In [11] different techniques of process mining were used to evaluated assessment data from online multiple choice tests. Data from two exams were considered where in a first study the questions must be answered in a strict order and immediately after the students could receive feedback and learn the correct answer. In the second study, the student could choose the order for answering the questions and they could revisit earlier questions and their answer. In [12] process mining was used to examine self-regulated learning (SRL) of students. By analyzing data recorded during think-aloud sessions, differences were found in the frequency and order of the regulatory activities. In [13] a framework called Trace-SRL was proposed to analyze SRL processes, using stochastic process mining under the theoretical lens of SRL. Findings include the discovery of different learner-strategy types along with specific patterns.

While related, none of the above-mentioned works focuses on evaluating *computer-aided examinations with open-ended questions*. In the following section, we describe how this format of examination can be evaluated. Also, we compare the behavior of the students when answering the test with the marks they received for the questions.

3   Method

Computer-aided examinations with open-ended questions belong to the context of computer-aided teaching and learning, In this environment there are two main actors, the instructor and the student. The instructor is responsible for *designing* the course, *teaching* and *grading* the students. The students are responsible for *learning* the content taught to them and perform an *examination* that assesses how well they acquired the content taught in the course. During the course design phase the instructor designs the classes to be taught and also how the examination will be. In this environment, the examination is performed using an online system that is able to store the interactions of the students with the system during the examination. Also, the grading of the examination is made available digitally.

Our method aims at improving the instructors knowledge about the exam-process. To this end, its input is constituted by the generated trace data and the grades of the students. Next, it encodes them onto an enriched event log. Process mining techniques and statistical methods are used to analyze this enriched event log, presenting the discovered knowledge to the instructor. Based on this knowledge the instructor may change the design of future editions of the course, which may include more teaching time on concepts that were shown to be not clear to the students or changing the order of the concepts being evaluated (i.e., questions) in the examination. Figure 1 depicts a sketch of our method. The shaded steps are the steps of the computer-aided teaching and learning process on which this research focuses.

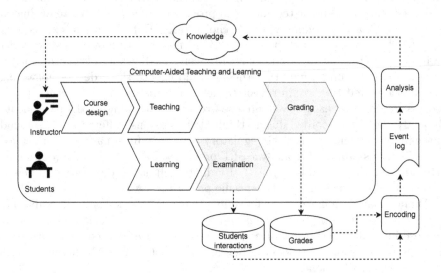

Fig. 1. Exploiting process mining to analyze exams in order to gather knowledge for improving computer-aided teaching & learning processes.

The encoding of the event log is done in two steps. The first step creates a standard event log in the XES [14] format with case ID, activity and timestamp. And the second enriches the created event log with attributes that correspond to the grades received in the questions and in the overall exam. Also, attributes that store the duration of working on each question are included in the event log.

For generating the event log the method requires that the online system being used stores data that allow one to identify when the student was working in each of the questions. Given that the goal is to analyze the student behavior on performing an online exam, the student matriculation number defines a case in the event log and the student interactions with the system define the activities.

We focus on collecting insights on how the students answered the questions of the exam, therefore we created four activity templates: *Look Question X*, *Work on Question X*, *Save Draft of Question X* and *Submit Question X*, where X is a placeholder for the question number. The first activity starts when the student opens question X and finishes when the student either closes question X, starts working on question X or save or submit question X. The second activity starts when the student starts writing on the environment and finishes when the student closes the question or presses the save or submit button in the system. The third activity happens when the student pushes the button to save a draft of the question. The fourth activity happens when the student pushes the button to submit the question. Saving a draft or submitting a question do not have a meaningful duration. The duration that we are interested on is the duration of the *Work on Question X* activity, which represents the overall time that the student took to answer the question. The structure of the final traces in the event log is $Trace_i = \langle Student_i, Activity, Time, Grade_{Q_1}, ..., Grade_{Q_n}, Duration_{Q_1}, ..., Duration_{Q_n}\rangle$.

For the analysis phase process mining techniques [7] are used. Process discovery is used to explore the sequence behavior of solving the exam searching for possible patterns. Process data such as duration of the activities, activities most frequently executed wee collected for the analysis. The choice of the process data collected is of the instructor depending on the investigation he or she wants to do.

4 Application

As an application scenario, we applied our method on a case of open question examinations, henceforth called *Exam1* and *Exam2*. These examinations stemmed from two master courses of an Austrian university. The two courses were designed for in-presence teaching and examinations. However, due to a COVID-19 wave the classes and the exams were moved to online.

For what concerns the exams, all the setup was kept the same as to a written exam taken physically. All the questions were made available online in the Teaching and Learning information system in the same way that they were available in the paper format. The students could visit the questions in the order they wanted and as many times as they wanted. It was possible to save a draft of the answers until the submission of the final answers. Each exam had to be performed in 90 min, however the students were given 10 min more than planned for the physical exam to compensate any possible infrastructure issue, summing up a maximum of 100 min for doing the exam.

In the following, we describe the details of applying our method to analyze the behavior of the students when answering the questions of *Exam1* and *Exam2* and how this behavior is related to the grades they achieved. Section 4.1 describes the event logs generated from the data logged by the Moodle system and the grades achieved by the students. Section 4.2 presents the results found. And, Sect. 4.3 discusses our findings.

4.1   Setting

Exam1 had 8 questions and *Exam2* had 4 questions. Thus, the event log for each of the exams were composed by 32 and 16 distinct activities, respectively. The teaching and learning system stored every interaction event along with a timestamp. This timestamp was used to set when each activity started. The students matriculation identifiers defined the cases in the event log. For *Exam1* 61 students completed the exam and for *Exam2* 27 students. Thus, the event logs had 61 and 27 cases, respectively.

The event log was enriched with the grade received for each of the questions and also the final grade on the exam. Both exams have a maximum of 100 points. For *Exam1* the points were split equally, i.e., each of the questions had a maximum of 12.5 points. For *Exam2*, three questions (1,2 and 4) had maximum of 20 each and one question (3) had a maximum of 40 points. The event logs where then filtered by the achieved final grade generating two event logs for each exam. One event log was composed by the traces of the students that achieved more than 80 (inclusive) in the exam, i.e., the topmost performers (TP) of the exam. The other event log was composed by the traces of the students that achieved less than 50 (inclusive), i.e., the lowermost performers (LP) of the exam. Table 1 provides details on the event logs generated. For analyzing the data we used the Disco[3] tool for process mining and R[4] software for correlation analysis and plot generation. The analyses were guided by the following questions:

Table 1. Event logs description

Event log	Cases	Events	Activities	Median case duration	Mean case duration	Min. activity frequency	Median act. freq.	Mean act. freq.	Max act. frequency	Act. frequency std. dev.
Exam1	61	7173	32	88.9 min	86.7 min	2	178	224.16	769	199.15
Exam1$_{TP}$	24	2708	31	89.4 min	87.6 min	1	76	87.35	349	84.85
Exam1$_{LP}$	7	820	29	87.8 min	82.5 min	1	27	28.28	85	23.26
Exam2	27	2892	16	99.3 min	91 min	2	115	180.75	707	203.53
Exam2$_{TP}$	7	698	15	84.1 min	84.4 min	1	27	46.53	163	50.58
Exam2$_{LP}$	10	1144	16	103.8 min	97.2 min	1	52	71.5	274	75.2

Q1: What are patterns in the behavior of exam solving?
Q2: How does the grade correlate with the time spent to solve a question?

4.2   Results

The number of variants is the same as the number of cases, amounting to 61 variants for *Exam1* and 27 variants for *Exam2*, which shows that every student used a different strategy to solve the exam.

Figure 2 and Fig. 3 depict the process models learned from the event logs generated for *Exam1* and *Exam2*, respectively. The processes on the left (a)

---

[3] https://fluxicon.com/disco.
[4] https://www.r-project.org.

were learned from $Exam1_{TP}$ and $Exam2_{TP}$ event logs, while the processes on the right (b) were learned from $Exam1_{LP}$ and $Exam2_{LP}$ event logs.

The activities most executed in all cases are the *Work on Question X*, given that these activities are executed when the students are working on the answers for question X. By analyzing the difference in the color of these activities it is possible to notice which question the students took more time for answering. There are self cycle in some of these activities, which means that the teaching and learning information system automatically saved the draft of the answer. This happens when the student is continually changing the content of the question, so periodically the system auto saves the content. Cycles are observed in all processes, meaning that the students did not work in one question and submitted it. They chose to save the draft of the answers and they returned to the question either to change its content or to validate before submitting it. Also, the control flow analysis of the processes show that in general the topmost performer students solved the exam following the order presented while the lowermost performer students solved the exam in a more chaotic way.

Figure 4 depicts the distribution of points for each question. For *Exam1* the majority of the students achieved the maximum points for questions 2, 6 and 8, given the median close to 12.5. Question 7 has a diversity of points, which indicate that it was the most controversial question in this exam. It is potentially a question about concepts not well understood by the students and thus a concept more deeply discussed with the students in future editions of the course. *Exam2* seems a more hard exam given that the majority of the students did not score the maximum points of the questions. Question 3 is the question with more variation on the points received by the students. It seems the hardest question in this exam, which it is expected given that it is the only question with maximum of 40 points. Some of the outliers presented in *Exam1* correspond to students in the lowermost performers students. The rest correspond to students that achieve between 50 and 80 points.

Figure 5 depicts the distribution of the time spent to solve each of the questions. The duration considers only the time spent on working on a particular question. It is expressed in seconds. For *Exam1* the question that was done faster by the students were Question 6, while the question that demanded more time was question 5. When confronting this result with the one presented in Fig. 4 it seems that Question 6 was the easiest, given that it was the fasted to be executed and the majority of the students score the maximum points. Also, it may indicate a concept well understood by the students. When confronting the data for Question 5, it was the second question with more spread points and given that it was the question with higher duration, it may indicate that it was a hard question or the concepts discussed in it were not well understood by the students. In *Exam2*, Question 2 was the question that demanded less time from the students. It was also the question where the students achieved highest points and there was a less variation on the points achieved. This result indicate to the instructor that either the question was easy or the concept discussed in it was well understood by the students. Question 3 had a duration higher than

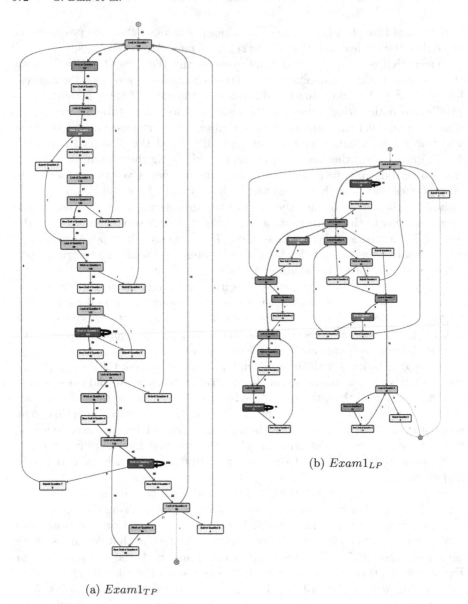

(a) $Exam1_{TP}$

(b) $Exam1_{LP}$

Fig. 2. Exam solving processes for the *Exam1* exam. Left (a): top performers (students who achieved more than 80 points). Right (b): lowermost performers (students who achieved less than 50 points)

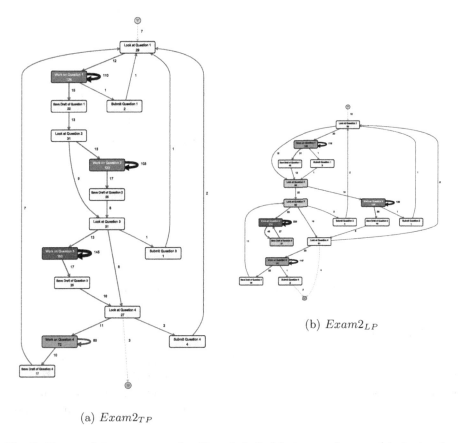

(b) $Exam2_{LP}$

(a) $Exam2_{TP}$

Fig. 3. Exam solving processes for *Exam2*. Left (a): top performers (students who achieved more than 80 points). Right (b): lowermost performers (students who achieved less than 50 points)

the other, but this was an expected result given that it was the biggest question. As the maximum points of this question is double the points of each of the other questions, it was also expected to be normal a duration of double the duration of each of the other questions. However, considering the medians this situation was not observed. Given the variation on points achieved it seems that the content of this question was not fully understood by some of the students.

A correlation analysis between the duration and the points for each question using Pearson correlation showed that only Question 2 in *Exam2* presents a correlation between these two attributes considering 95% confidence level. Correlation 0.418 and p-value 0.0299. In *Exam1* questions 1, 2, 3, 5 and 6 showed a correlation between the two attributes. The correlations and p-values were (0.461, 0.000185), (0.289, 0.0241), (0.399, 0.00144), (0.492, 0.0000572) and (0.347, 0.00617) respectively.

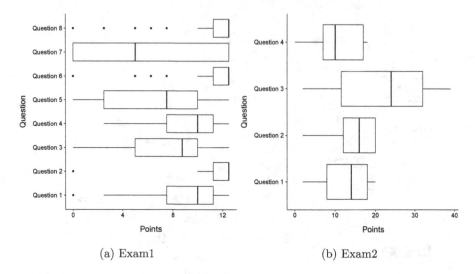

(a) Exam1 (b) Exam2

Fig. 4. Questions versus points achieved on them

4.3   Discussion

From the results observed it is not possible to state that there is not a common behavior on solving the exams ($Q1$). Each student created their own strategy for solving the exam. However, when evaluating groups of students based on their performance, it was possible to observe a pattern in the behavior of the topmost

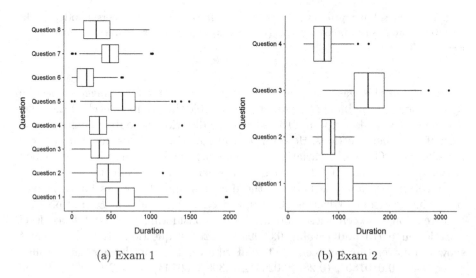

(a) Exam 1 (b) Exam 2

Fig. 5. Questions versus time (in seconds) spent on solving them

performers students. This group solved the questions in the same order in which they were presented in the exam.

When evaluating the correlation between the time spent for answering the questions and the points received for each of the questions only Question 2 in *Exam2* showed a correlation. This result conforms with the previous analysis that showed that the highest points were achieved in Question 2 and this question was the one with lower duration. It means that the students were confident when answering this question. It seems that its content was well assimilated by the students.

5 Conclusion

Process mining has been used in the education area to support the analysis of the behavior of students in online educational environments. In this paper, we used process mining to analyze the behavior of students when solving an exam with open ended questions. Trace data generated from the online teaching and learning environment was used to generate a event log. This event log was enriched with attributes that encoded the points received in each question and the time spent by the students to solve the questions.

We applied our approach in two exams performed by students from two master courses of an Austrian university. The results raised interesting questions for the instructor to investigate further, which may support them on the design of future editions of the courses. Especially, when designing further editions of the course, our method can help at better content and granularity of the questions.

Future work shall increment the depth and scope of the analysis of the educational data at hand. More specifically, we want to improve our analysis in two ways. First, we want to improve the encoding and consider more cases for the analysis, such as for example differentiating between students that receive zero points in a question because they answered it wrongly from those that did not answer the question. Second, we want to apply other kind of process mining techniques, such as conformance checking, in order to quantify how much deviation is associated to a good or a bad grade.

References

1. Trcka, N., Pechenizkiy, M., van der Aalst, W.: Process mining from educational data. In: Handbook of Educational Data Mining, pp. 123–142 (2010)
2. Domínguez, C., Izquierdo, F.J.G., Elizondo, A.J., Pérez, B., Rubio, Á.L., Zapata, M.A.: Using process mining to analyze time distribution of self-assessment and formative assessment exercises on an online learning tool. IEEE Trans. Learn. Technol. **14**(5), 709–722 (2021)
3. Bogarín, A., Romero, C., Cerezo, R., Sánchez-Santillán, M.: Clustering for improving educational process mining. In: LAK, pp. 11–15. ACM (2014)
4. Aisa, V., Kurniati, A.P., Firdaus, A.W.Y.: Evaluation of the online assessment test using process mining (case study: intensive English center). In: ICoICT, pp. 472–477 (2015)

5. Ali, L., Dmour, N.A.: The shift to online assessment due to COVID-19: an empirical study of university students, behaviour and performance, in the region of UAE. Int. J. Educ. Technol. High. Educ. **11**, 220–228 (2021)

6. Berente, N., Seidel, S., Safadi, H.: Research commentary - data-driven computationally intensive theory development. Inf. Syst. Res. **30**(1), 50–64 (2019)

7. van der Aalst, W.M.P.: Process Mining - Data Science in Action, 2nd edn. Springer, Heidelberg (2016). https://doi.org/10.1007/978-3-662-49851-4

8. Bogarín, A., Cerezo, R., Romero, C.: A survey on educational process mining. WIREs Data Mining Knowl. Discov. **8**(1), e1230 (2018)

9. Mukala, P., Buijs, J.C.A.M., Leemans, M., van der Aalst, W.M.P.: Learning analytics on coursera event data: a process mining approach. In: SIMPDA, ser. CEUR Workshop Proceedings, vol. 1527, pp. 18–32. CEUR-WS.org (2015)

10. Baykasoglu, A., Özbel, B.K., Dudakli, N., Subulan, K., Senol, M.E.: Process mining based approach to performance evaluation in computer-aided examinations. Comput. Appl. Eng. Educ. **26**(5), 1841–1861 (2018)

11. Pechenizkiy, M., Trcka, N., Vasilyeva, E., Van der Aalst, W., De Bra, P.: Process mining online assessment data. ERIC (2009)

12. Bannert, M., Reimann, P., Sonnenberg, C.: Process mining techniques for analysing patterns and strategies in students' self-regulated learning. Metacogn. Learn. **9**(2), 161–185 (2014)

13. Saint, J., Whitelock-Wainwright, A., Gasevic, D., Pardo, A.: Trace-SRL: a framework for analysis of microlevel processes of self-regulated learning from trace data. IEEE Trans. Learn. Technol. **13**(4), 861–877 (2020)

14. Verbeek, H.M.W., Buijs, J.C.A.M., van Dongen, B.F., van der Aalst, W.M.P.: XES, XESame, and ProM 6. In: Soffer, P., Proper, E. (eds.) CAiSE Forum 2010. LNBIP, vol. 72, pp. 60–75. Springer, Heidelberg (2011). https://doi.org/10.1007/978-3-642-17722-4_5

Process Mining on Curriculum-Based Study Data: A Case Study at a German University

Richard Hobeck[✉], Luise Pufahl[✉], and Ingo Weber[✉]

Software and Business Engineering, Technische Universitaet Berlin,
Berlin, Germany
{richard.hobeck,luise.pufahl,ingo.weber}@tu-berlin.de

Abstract. On their trajectory through educational university systems, students leave a trace of event data. The analysis of that event data with a process lens poses a set of domain-specific challenges that is addressed in the field of Educational Process Mining (EPM). Despite the vast potential for understanding the progress of students and improving the quality of study programs through process mining, a case study based on an established process mining methodology is still missing. In this paper, we address this gap by applying the state-of-the-art process mining project methodology (PM^2) in an EPM case study with a focus on student trajectory analysis at a German university. We found that process mining can create actionable items to improve the quality of university education. We also point out domain-specific challenges, like handling reoccurring exams (retaken after failing) for future research in EPM. Finally, we observe insights of some value in our case.

Keywords: Educational Process Mining · Curriculum mining · Case study

1 Introduction

Students are the lifeblood of universities and their main reason for existence. Universities' role in society is unquestionably large, with more than 40% of the population in Europe[1] and 24% in the U.S.[2] attaining at least a Bachelor degree. We aim to recruit young academic talents from the best graduating students to sustain excellent work across sectors. But talent is not spread equally: the international competition among universities for top students is largely driven

---

[1] https://www.statista.com/statistics/1093466/eu-28-adults-with-tertiary-education-attainment/, 2020 data, accessed 2022-08-22.

[2] Estimated population: 328.24M; Bachelor, Master, and Doctoral degrees: 80.33M; both for 2019. Sources: https://www.statista.com/statistics/183489/population-of-the-us-by-ethnicity-since-2000/ and https://www2.census.gov/programs-surveys/demo/tables/educational-attainment/2019/cps-detailed-tables/table-1-1.xlsx, accessed 2022-08-22.

© The Author(s) 2023
M. Montali et al. (Eds.): ICPM 2022 Workshops, LNBIP 468, pp. 577–589, 2023.
https://doi.org/10.1007/978-3-031-27815-0_42

by university rankings, in which the quality of teaching is a pivotal factor. On the other end of the spectrum, unfortunately large shares of students leave colleges and universities without a degree – for the U.S., this was the case for at least 20 million inhabitants in 2019[3]. In summary, universities can be expected to have a high level of motivation to increase student success.

Once students enroll in a program, they complete courses to receive their degrees – with varying levels of freedom, depending on the respective university system. On their trajectory through the university system, those students leave a trace of data. Some universities analyze that data with basic statistics, others employ more elaborate data mining techniques [4]. Insights from such analyses inform refinement of curricula and course offerings, to improve the quality of teaching and (global) competitiveness, and to lower drop-out rates [13].

As a set of process-focused data science techniques, process mining is widely used in various business environments [1]. A core value proposition of process mining is an increased understanding of the actual execution of processes and leveraging that knowledge for process improvements. Those benefits are not limited to an industrial or business context and can also be applied in other domains, such as education [16]. The process perspective on education interprets learning and teaching as an ordered number of activities (such as taking an exam) that are being executed over time (like each semester) [5]. The term *Educational Process Mining (EPM)* [9,15] covers the analysis of execution data with process mining techniques in the education domain. As the limited number of case studies and publications on process mining on student trajectory data [5] shows, the potential of process mining for improving university teaching has rarely been unlocked.

In this paper, we add a case study to the EPM field that has been conducted at a German university. In contrast to former case studies, our initiative is guided by the Process Mining Project Management methodology [7] (PM^2). Our main contributions are two-fold: (i) we document our lessons learned and motivate potential refinements to cater for the application of PM^2 to student data; and (ii) through the case study, we obtain insights which, in some instances and for some contexts, indicate a rather clear value of educational process mining.

In the remainder, we elaborate on preliminary work in the field (Sect. 2), present our research methodology (Sect. 3) and execute the methodology based on a case study at a German university (Sect. 4). Section 5 sums up our lessons learned, before Sect. 6 concludes.

2   Related Work

Data analysis in education is widely applied and has drawn research attention in the past decades under the umbrella term Educational Data Mining (EDM) [2,13]. The process perspective on courses taken by students is covered in the subfield Educational Process Mining (EPM) [9,15,16], which by itself spans

---

[3] See source in footnote 2, "Some college, no degree", and https://www.statista.com/statistics/235406/undergraduate-enrollment-in-us-universities/ for current enrollment numbers; accessed 2022-08-22.

a spectrum of application areas. In our paper, however, the focus lies on curriculum mining – a term covering course-based analysis of student trajectories in educational institutions [5]. In its original meaning, curriculum mining described the pattern-based discovery of a curriculum from observed study data and its subsequent usage for process mining [11,16]. From this origin, authors picked up on the term curriculum mining and extended it, adding comparisons between individual curricula of successful and less successful students, while "success" was measured in course or program grading [18]. Due to the extension of the term curriculum mining, earlier case studies may be subsumed under the term in retrospect such as [17]. [10, Ch.8] explored student's paths with a focus on the impact of failure on their trajectories. [18] furthermore proposed a process-based recommender system for students to provide guidance when choosing courses, which they published in 2018 [19]. Other initiatives aimed at creating specific techniques for curriculum mining. [3] contributed an approach for conformance checking multiple events with the same timestamps (e.g., courses taken in the same semester). However, they excluded student's option to retake courses (e.g., after failing them) in their method, leaving room for improvement. Notably, some recent attempts to apply EPM on student curricula lagged behind expectations due to domain-specific challenges [14] that in part remained unsolved as yet. One of the related case studies [6] (in German) presents a method for a curriculum mining initiative, although that method focuses on gaining insights from three specific techniques: bubble-chart-analysis, fuzzy mining and inductive mining; disregarding established process mining methodologies such as PM^2 [7].

3   Research Method and Case

We employ a case study-based method to explore how student trajectories can be analyzed in a process mining project. A case study, as a qualitative research method, analyzes a phenomenon in its natural setting to gain insights into emerging topics [12, Ch.5]. With this work, we address the research question: *Does curriculum-based EPM with PM^2 provide benefits for the study program analysis and improvement?* In the process, we explore the arising challenges.

The case we selected deals with the study progress of Bachelor of Science students in Information Systems Management (B.Sc. ISM) at Technische Universität Berlin (TUB). B.Sc. ISM is the third-largest study program of the department for Electrical Engineering and Computer Science comprising 985 students (winter term 2021/22). The department provides a study plan which recommends taking certain courses in certain semesters. We chose this case study, due to our high influence on the study process (one of the authors of this paper serves as program director[4]) and our domain expertise as we teach in the program. In that respect, our team encompassed all roles for a process mining project. Next, the case and study design are described.

---

[4] https://www.eecs.tu-berlin.de/menue/studium_und_lehre/studiengaenge/wirtschaft sinformatik_information_systems_management/beratung_und_service/studiengangsb eauftragter/, accessed 22-08-2022.

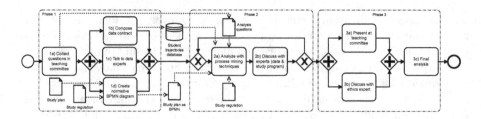

Fig. 1. BPMN diagram representing the case study design.

Case. TUB has around 34.000 enrolled students (winter term 2021/22) and 335 professors. The program B.Sc. ISM has existed since 2013. Currently, 717 B.Sc. ISM students are studying based on the study regulation from 2015, and 268 B.Sc. ISM students are studying based on the study regulation from 2021. To increase the data quality for the case study, we focus on trajectories of the 696 students that started their program with or after the effective date of the 2015 study regulation (01-10-2017). (Bi-)Yearly study program meetings are a central element of the teaching quality management at TUB. In such meetings, the study program director, lecturers, and students discuss development and improvement options for the program based on experiences, teaching evaluations, and a high-level analysis of student trajectory data (e.g., cohort analysis of students in the program, dropout rates, etc.). The controlling department of TUB collects student trajectory data of all study programs. Process mining for a more detailed analysis of student trajectory data was applied for the first time at TUB in this case study.

Case Study Design. The BPMN diagram in Fig. 1 provides an overview of our main case study that consisted of (1) a *preparation phase*, (2) a *process mining analysis*, and (3) a *finalization phase*. We prepared the case study in two teaching committee meetings, in which we gathered questions (1a) for a (process-centered) analysis of student trajectory data. Next, we composed a data contract (1b) between the controlling department and our research group to define the appropriation for the data usage, required data attributes, data storage means with respect to data security, and privacy protection mechanisms. This step was supported by the privacy protection department of the TUB. As an output, we received a defined subset of the student trajectory database for doing the process mining analysis. In parallel, we talked to the system experts (1c) from the controlling department regularly to understand the different data tables and attributes of the database and their quality issues. Finally, we also reviewed study program regulations as well as the study plan, and (1d) created a normative BPMN process diagram based on the study plan. After these preparation steps, we started with the analysis (2a). The first step was the creation of an event log from the database tables that suited a process representation of a student curriculum and qualified for answering the analysis questions. After mining and analysis of the event log, the results were discussed with the data and study program experts (2b). In the final phase, the resulting analysis was presented at the meeting of the teaching committee (3a). Feedback and further questions were collected. In parallel, the results and further ideas for analysis were presented to an ethics expert (3b) to discuss how and in which way the results should be used. Based on these insights, we finalized our analysis of the student trajectories (3c), which is presented in the following section.

4   Applying PM² for Educational Process Mining

The PM² [7] is the defacto standard process mining methodology and consists of six main phases: (1) project planning, (2) extraction and (3) data processing of the event log, (4) mining and analysis, (5) evaluation and (6) process improvement & support. In the following, we describe them for our EPM case.

4.1   Planning

The process under scrutiny was the trajectory of students through the university course system. The goal of the project was 1) to learn about student's paths through the university system, and 2) to find deviations from recommended path (the study plan) through the university system provided by the department.

Selecting Business Processes. As described in Sect. 3, the program B.Sc. ISM was well known to the members of the project team. Also, the project had lively support of the program director, which provided a lever on changeability of the process. Additionally, availability of the necessary data in the university's information systems was given, following the signing of the data contract.

Identifying Research Questions. To avoid confusion with the research question in this paper, we refer to research questions of the project as "project question (PQ)". The mentioned study plan recommends a certain order of courses to Bachelor students. The teaching committee did not yet have information about:

PQ1 Do B.Sc. ISM students follow the study plan?
PQ2 Are students that follow the study plan successful in their studies?
PQ3 Which behavioral patterns can be observed in the data?

Composing the Project Team. The project team comprised four people with the following roles: the study program manager (process owner), three lecturers in the study program (business experts), a member of the controlling team with experience of data warehousing at TUB (system expert) and three process analysts. Additionally, we frequently sought feedback from TUB's data protection unit about the use of the data. We also incorporated ethical advice for result exploitation.

4.2   Extraction

For data extraction, we had different sources of input. On the one hand, the university operates partially self-deployed information systems building on off-the-shelf student lifecycle management systems holding all available data

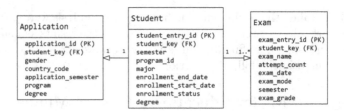

Fig. 2. Data scheme showing a subset of available data attributes. Note that the tables were not normalized (PK ... Primary key; FK ... Foreign key).

about students' study progress. On the other hand, several documents officially issued by the university contained descriptions of the process students go through at TUB.

Determining the Scope. With respect to the project questions, two levels of granularity were required: 1) exams taken by the students on specific days during a semester, and 2) the semester the students were enrolled in, including the status of the semester (actively studying, sabbatical, exmatriculated, etc.). The relevant time-frame for B.Sc. ISM students of the most recent long-running version of the program was from September 2017 to January 2021. We were provided with a data schema covering student-related data attributes. An abbreviated version is depicted in Fig. 2. Note that student's study data are considered *personal data* according to the European Union's General Data Protection Regulation and thus have to be handled with additional care (GDPR Art. 4). To sustain the ability to assign courses to individual students, we created pseudonyms for student ID numbers to which courses were assigned. Additionally, the data was delivered using an encrypted and secure data transfer mechanism.

Extracting Event Data. The data was delivered as a multi-table SQL dump. The tables, as we received them, were not normalized. As notion of an instance, we selected the student with the pseudonym of the matriculation number (student_key) and selected some case-specific attributes from the student table. The main two extracted event types are the (re-)enrollment of a student for a semester and their exams taken for which we also consider event-specific attributes (e.g., timestamp, name of the exam, (non-)compulsory exam). Fundamentally, we joined the tables Student and Exam based on the attribute student_key to generate the event log. Note that we did not make use of the data in the table Application. Including the following additional preparatory steps to transform the data, the SQL commands for the event log generation amounted to 150 lines of code: 1) filtering for time frame the program B.Sc. ISM; 2) unifying event labels; 3) flagging compulsory and elective courses; 4) flagging events by their type; 5) initial filters, e.g. for the study program and its version; 6) creating and re-labeling semester re-enrollment events; and 7) adjust the timestamps for discovery of parallelism.

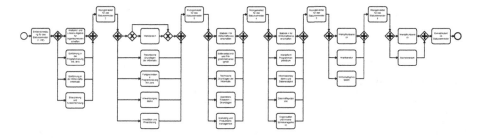

Fig. 3. Normative BPMN diagram capturing the study plan for B.Sc. ISM.

Transferring Process Knowledge. We transferred knowledge from written document-bound information issued by TUB that described the study process such as the *General Study and Examination Regulations of TUB* (university-wide). For the project, we created a normative BPMN diagram shown in Fig. 3 representing the study plan. We had to take a few aspects into consideration during modeling. First, how can we model the structure of semesters? To this end, the first activity in the process corresponds to initial enrollment (i.e., the registration for the first semester). This is followed by the activities for the first four modules in parallel (between a parallel split and a parallel join). Subsequently comes the activity to re-enroll for the second semester. In the parallel construct that follows, the top branch of the process has an optional activity, labeled "Wahlbereich", i.e., free electives, while the other modules are compulsory. The rest of the process follows the same logic.

4.3   Data Processing

Creating Views. To create meaningful views on the event data for the purposes of our project (analyzing course sequences taken by students) we chose student ID (pseudonyms) as a case notion. That way, for each student their exams as well as their status for a semester were aligned as a series of events.

Aggregating Events. One major challenge of the event log are the two levels of granularity in the events: exams taken and semesters studied, while multiple exams can be taken in one semester. Since the study plans suggested an order of taking exams, there was a de facto part-of relation between the exams and the semesters. We thus aggregated the exams to the semester level for parts of the analysis.

Enriching Logs. For this project, answering the project questions did not require enriching the log with additional information.

Filtering Logs. The applied filters concerned various attributes. Most frequently, we filtered for particular cohorts of students (e.g., only students that enrolled in a specific semester) or particular courses (e.g., to learn about the order in which

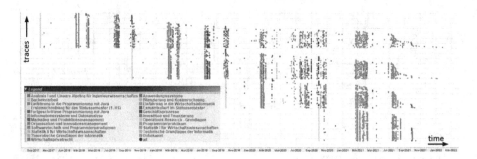

Fig. 4. High-level view on the event data in a dotted chart.

two exams were taken). Lastly, in April 2021, TUB was the target of an IT hack that led to multiple services being interrupted, including the exam database. Hence, most exams taken since could not be tracked as complete entries and were available to us as "unknown", which caused a data quality issue for this case study. The "unknown" events were filtered out in almost all analyses, except for investigating the count of exams over the observed time period.

4.4   Mining and Analysis

Mining and Analysis started with applying process discovery techniques to answer PQ2 and PQ3. PQ1 was approached with conformance checking.

Process Discovery. To gain an overview of the data and its time distribution, we generated a dotted chart[5] from the filtered data, which is shown in Fig. 4. The different cohorts of students starting in the five years appear clearly separated, with the yellow dots for matriculation forming basically solid lines in October of the respective years. Most students attend classes for the first semester before sitting their first exam, but interestingly some students do not; these might have transferred from a different university or program, or might have prior knowledge that allows them to sit an exam. The dots corresponding to some exams form almost solid lines, like the ones shown in blue, green, and pink after the first semester – e.g., in February–April 2018 – indicating that the corresponding cohorts take these exams in unison.

Very noticeable is also the decline of participation in exams over the years (e.g., following the first cohort at the top of Fig. 4): while almost all students sit some exam after the first and second semester, the number of exam events is subject to a sharp decline from the second to the third semester and slowly drops further. To understand this decline, it is worth noting that German universities often have a low bar for matriculation into a study program – first-semester

---

[5] A number of events highlighted in green appears in the observed traces as of spring 2021 across cohorts. These are the "unknown" events that resulted from the TUB's IT being compromised. Exams that are "unknown" were filtered out in all analysis (as described above), but included in the dotted chart for illustration purposes.

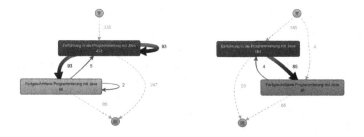

Fig. 5. Order of programming courses (left: all attempts; right: passed attempts).

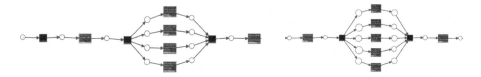

Fig. 6. Conformance in semester 1   **Fig. 7.** Conformance in semester 3

students are then admitted without a test to measure their qualification for a particular program. Other students might have started a program without a solid understanding about its content, and decide that they prefer a different one. For these or similar reasons, it is rather common that about one third to half of the students drop out of a study program without a degree. One concrete question in our case was, whether students attempted (or passed) the advanced programming course ("Fortgeschrittene Programmierung mit Java") before the introductory programming course ("Einführung in die Programmierung mit Java"). To examine this, we filtered the DFG of individual exam attempts to only show these two exams – depicted in Fig. 5 in terms of all attempts (left) and passed attempts (right). Clearly the answer is "no": 93 (85) times the introductory course is attempted (passed) before the advanced one, and only 5 (4) times the opposite is true. This is one of the more concrete questions that we have collected for the B.Sc. ISM program.

Conformance Checking. For evaluating the question: "To which degree do students follow the study plans of their programs?" conformance checking can be applied. As the variance in non-compulsory modules is high, we projected the process model (see Fig. 3) and the log to only re-enrollments and compulsory exams. We focused only on the first cohort of students that matriculated in September 2017 and had a chance to finish their studies (participate in all courses) to avoid result distortions from non-finalized cases of early semester students. With the help of ProM[6] 6.9, we converted the normative BPMN diagram into a Petri net and then, used it for the alignment-based conformance checking. The resulting Petri net's layout is very long, hence we only show results for the first and the third semester, in Figs. 6 and 7, respectively. Clearly observable

---

[6] https://www.promtools.org/doku.php, accessed 2022-08-22.

is that the percentage of adherence (shown by the green bar at the bottom of a transition in the net) to recommended modules (i) varies somewhat within a semester, and (ii) decreases considerably from the first to the third semester. This trend continues further after the third semester, though at varying speeds as observed from the dotted chart above. In addition, we obtain statistics for the entire log: The average trace fitness was approx. 29% – for the compulsory modules. This indicates that students make ample use of the freedom provided by the study regulation at TUB.

4.5   Evaluation

For the diagnosis as well as the verification, we conferred with the teaching committee yet again. Most of the results of the study confirmed speculations, in particular the decreasing conformance of student trajectories with the study plan. Given the novelty of the study results for the committee, the meeting was largely used to define further research questions, e.g.: How can the findings be incorporated in study plans? Can process mining techniques be used to predict drop-outs? What are ethical ways to communicate potential prediction findings to students?

4.6   Process Improvement and Support

The implementation of this phase is still in progress. For process improvements, we identified two areas to take action: 1) the study plan that could be adapted following the findings, 2) communicating results of the project to students and providing them an outside perspective on how they advanced in their studies. In both scenarios, ethical considerations ought to play a crucial role: e.g., nudging students away from using their freedom of choice in courses is disputable. Supporting operations, i.e., including process mining in the stable set of analysis tools to inform the university directors and teaching committees, was at the heart of the case study and is ongoing in collaboration with the controlling department.

5   Lessons Learned

In this section, we report on our lessons learned from the case study in the different phases of the PM^2 methodology.

Planning. Our *research questions* such as "Do B.Sc. ISM students follow the study plan?" were defined based on the related work (in particular [11] and [10, Ch.8]) and the discussion in the study program meeting. More specific questions can be added for each study program. Besides, data on students' studies are considered as *personal data* that need to be handled with special care according to the GDPR. We worked with the TUB data privacy department for consultancy in this regard and recommend allocating time for these matters. *Defining student* *success* over the course of the whole degree is a non-obvious question. We could distinguish levels of success by the GPA, like [19], or overall grade, but might run the risk of overly simplifying.

Extraction. We showed a first approach to define a *normative process* diagram in BPMN representing the study plan for a program and the challenges thereby.

Data Processing. Due to experiences with *existing regulations and new requirements*, study regulations are regularly changing (also see [11,14]). This leads to different student cohorts that should be analyzed independently (also see [17]). It is challenging to define consistent student cohorts for different event log views. In this study, we filtered for time-frame in which the regulation was valid. Additionally, timestamps of events of student trajectories are usually on different levels of granularity, discussed as one of the *timestamp imperfections* of event logs by [8]. Whereas the information about the re-registration for a semester and its status is on a semester level, exams are captured finer-grained on a day-level. Also, German universities offer a very high degree of flexibility in (compulsory) *electives*. Based on our observations, for most analyses it makes sense to aggregate such courses.

Mining and Analysis. In this phase we encountered several challenges. To many of them the obvious solution would have been to apply strong event filters to reduce noise in the log and simplify the analysis, coming at the cost of reducing the expressiveness of the log. These challenges include handling *exam repetitions* after failing (also see [3,14]), *semesters abroad* students spend trying to recognize modules as equivalent to offerings at their home university, *lateral program entry* by students switching programs at various points (also see [14]), and *handling non-finalized cases* which poses a particular challenge in conformance checking.

Evaluation. Students of TUB have access to a wide variety of (compulsory) electives in their B.Sc. studies. This results in many *snow flakes*, i.e., unique traces. As above, aggregation might be necessary to be able to obtain insights from this data, since the raw data might be too fragmented.

Process Improvement and Support. *Communicating* individual data analysis results back to students may cause unease, or be stressful to students. Additionally, purely data-based results do not include alternative cause of action yet. Opt-in options or coupling the communication with consultation offers should be considered. Lastly, the results of the case study analysis may nudge students to follow very specific succession of courses, which is opposing the *Humboldtian ideal*[7] of freedom of study for students – one of the basic principles of the German university system. Hence, there is an area of conflict between educational ideals and efficiency goals of EPM projects that need to be debated.

---

[7] https://en.wikipedia.org/wiki/Humboldtian_model_of_higher_education, accessed 2022-08-22.

6 Conclusion

In this paper, we study how to apply process mining to curriculum-based study data. Our case encompasses a major Bachelor program at TU Berlin, a leading university in Germany. Section 4 describes our approach using the PM² methodology. We were able to answer concrete questions about student behavior and adherence to the study plan; as such, with regards to our research question we observe an indication that indeed curriculum-based EPM can provide insights of some value – e.g., checking if contents of succeeding lectures are coordinated in a way that lets students advance, or potential to translate student trajectories into curriculum recommendations which we expect to reduce study time and eventually (personal and social) costs. In Sect. 5 we reflected on specific challenges encountered during our study. If similar challenges appear in coming curricular EPM case studies, we suspect future domain-specific alterations of PM² might be justified considering its objective to "overcome common challenges" [7]. Given the research method, case study, we inherit typical threats to validity of such research [12, p.125], specifically threats of limited replicability and generalizability. Also, the analysis team was also responsible for data preparation, which might have introduced bias.

Acknowledgments. We are very thankful for the input of Patrick Russ, data analyst at TUB's controlling department.

References

1. Van der Aalst, W.M.: Process Mining: Data Science in Action. Springer, Heidelberg (2016)
2. Baker, R.S., Inventado, P.S.: Educational data mining and learning analytics. In: Larusson, J.A., White, B. (eds.) Learning Analytics, pp. 61–75. Springer, New York (2014). https://doi.org/10.1007/978-1-4614-3305-7_4
3. Bendatu, L.Y., Yahya, B.N.: Sequence matching analysis for curriculum development. Jurnal Teknik Industri **17**(1), 47–52 (2015)
4. Berland, M., Baker, R.S., Blikstein, P.: Educational data mining and learning analytics: applications to constructionist research. Technol. Knowl. Learn. **19**(1), 205–220 (2014)
5. Bogarín, A., Cerezo, R., Romero, C.: A survey on educational process mining. WIREs Data Min. Knowl. Discov. **8**(1), e1230 (2018)
6. Buck-Emden, R., Dahmann, F.D.: Zur Auswertung von Studienverläufen mit Process-Mining-Techniken. Technical report, Hochschule Bonn-Rhein-Sieg (2017)
7. van Eck, M.L., Lu, X., Leemans, S.J.J., van der Aalst, W.M.P.: PM²: a process mining project methodology. In: Zdravkovic, J., Kirikova, M., Johannesson, P. (eds.) CAiSE 2015. LNCS, vol. 9097, pp. 297–313. Springer, Cham (2015). https://doi.org/10.1007/978-3-319-19069-3_19
8. Fischer, D.A., Goel, K., Andrews, R., van Dun, C.G.J., Wynn, M.T., Röglinger, M.: Enhancing event log quality: detecting and quantifying timestamp imperfections. In: Fahland, D., Ghidini, C., Becker, J., Dumas, M. (eds.) BPM 2020. LNCS, vol. 12168, pp. 309–326. Springer, Cham (2020). https://doi.org/10.1007/978-3-030-58666-9_18

9. Ghazal, M.A., Ibrahim, O., Salama, M.A.: Educational process mining: a systematic literature review. In: EECS Conference, pp. 198–203 (2017)
10. Janssenswillen, G.: Unearthing the Real Process Behind the Event Data. LNBIP, vol. 412. Springer, Cham (2021). https://doi.org/10.1007/978-3-030-70733-0
11. Pechenizkiy, M., Trcka, N., De Bra, P., Toledo, P.: CurriM: curriculum mining. In: International Conference on Educational Data Mining, EDM, pp. 216–217 (2012)
12. Recker, J.: Scientific Research in Information Systems: A Beginner's Guide. PI, Springer, Cham (2021). https://doi.org/10.1007/978-3-030-85436-2
13. Romero, C., Ventura, S.: Educational data mining and learning analytics: an updated survey. Wiley Interd. Rev.: Data Min. Knowl. Disc. 10(3), e1355 (2020)
14. Schulte, J., Fernandez de Mendonca, P., Martinez-Maldonado, R., Buckingham Shum, S.: Large scale predictive process mining and analytics of university degree course data. In: International Learning Analytics & Knowledge Conference, pp. 538–539 (2017)
15. Sypsas, A., Kalles, D.: Reviewing process mining applications and techniques in education. Int. J. Artif. Intell. Appl. 13, 83–102 (2022)
16. Trcka, N., Pechenizkiy, M.: From local patterns to global models: towards domain driven educational process mining. In: International Conference on Intelligent Systems Design and Applications, pp. 1114–1119. IEEE (2009)
17. Trcka, N., Pechenizkiy, M., van der Aalst, W.: Process mining from educational data. Handb. Educ. Data Min. 123–142 (2010)
18. Wang, R., Zaïane, O.R.: Discovering process in curriculum data to provide recommendation. In: EDM, pp. 580–581 (2015)
19. Wang, R., Zaïane, O.R.: Sequence-based approaches to course recommender systems. In: Hartmann, S., Ma, H., Hameurlain, A., Pernul, G., Wagner, R.R. (eds.) DEXA 2018. LNCS, vol. 11029, pp. 35–50. Springer, Cham (2018). https://doi.org/10.1007/978-3-319-98809-2_3

Author Index

Printed in the United States
by Baker & Taylor Publisher Services